Pharmacotherapy for Depression and Treatment-Resistant Depression

Pharmacotherapy for Depression and Treatment-Resistant Depression

George I. Papakostas
Maurizio Fava
Massachusetts General Hospital and Harvard Medical School, USA

World Scientific

NEW JERSEY • LONDON • SINGAPORE • BEIJING • SHANGHAI • HONG KONG • TAIPEI • CHENNAI

Published by

World Scientific Publishing Co. Pte. Ltd.

5 Toh Tuck Link, Singapore 596224

USA office: 27 Warren Street, Suite 401-402, Hackensack, NJ 07601

UK office: 57 Shelton Street, Covent Garden, London WC2H 9HE

British Library Cataloguing-in-Publication Data
A catalogue record for this book is available from the British Library.

PHARMACOTHERAPY FOR DEPRESSION AND TREATMENT-RESISTANT DEPRESSION

ISBN-13 978-981-4287-58-6
ISBN-10 981-4287-58-X

Typeset by Stallion Press
Email: enquiries@stallionpress.com

Printed in Singapore by World Scientific Printers.

I dedicate this book to my children Yanni and Ellie.

George

I am extremely grateful to my wife Stefania
and our son Giovanni
for their incredible support of my work.

Maurizio

About the Authors

George I. Papakostas

George I. Papakostas is Associate Professor of Psychiatry at Harvard Medical School and Director of Treatment-Resistant Depression Studies in the Department of Psychiatry at Massachusetts General Hospital in Boston, Massachusetts, USA. The focus of Dr. Papakostas' research includes the pharmacotherapy of major depressive disorder including treatment-resistant depression, the study of the "placebo" effect and its relevance to clinical trial design in major depressive disorder, and the study of clinical and biologic predictors, moderators, and mediators of treatment outcome in major depressive disorder. Dr. Papakostas has received numerous national and international research awards from sources including the American College of Neuropsychopharmacology, the Collegium Internationale Neuropsychopharmacologium, the New Clinical Drug Evaluation Unit of the National Institute of Mental Health, the American Psychiatric Association, the World Federation of Societies of Biological Psychiatry, the American Academy of Clinical Psychiatrists, the International College of Psychosomatic Medicine, and the American Foundation for Suicide Prevention. He is the author or co-author of over 150 clinical and scientific publications and book chapters, his publications appearing in prominent journals, including the *American Journal of Psychiatry*, *Biological Psychiatry*, the *Journal of Clinical Psychiatry*, and the *Journal of Clinical Psychopharmacology*. He is also on the editorial board of the journal *Psychiatry Research*, and a field editor for psychopharmacology for the *World Journal of Biological Psychiatry*. Dr. Papakostas is often invited throughout the United States and abroad to lecture on a wide range of topics pertaining to the treatment of depression. To date, he has delivered more than 100 lectures at national or international meetings in more than 30 countries.

Dr. Papakostas attended Medical School at the New York University School of Medicine. He completed his residency in adult psychiatry at Massachusetts General Hospital and McLean Hospital, and a fellowship in Clinical Neuropsychopharmacology at Massachusetts General Hospital that was funded by the American College of Neuropsychopharmacology.

Maurizio Fava

Dr. Fava obtained his medical degree from the University of Padova School of Medicine, USA, and completed a residency training in endocrinology at the same university. After completing a residency training in psychiatry at the Massachusetts General Hospital (MGH), he has been Director of the MGH Depression Clinical and Research Program since 1990 at the same hospital. Under Dr. Fava's direction, the MGH Depression Clinical and Research Program has become one of the most highly regarded depression programs in the country. Dr. Fava has authored or co-authored more than 400 original articles published in medical journals with international circulation. He has also edited five books, and published more than 50 chapters and 500 abstracts. Dr. Fava is also a well-known national and international speaker, and has also been the recipient of many honors and awards. He is currently Executive Vice Chair for the MGH Department of Psychiatry, Executive Director, MGH Clinical Trials Network and Institute, and Director of the MGH Depression Clinical and Research Program, and Professor of Psychiatry at Harvard Medical School.

Preface

Major depressive disorder (MDD) is a highly prevalent and, often, chronic illness, which has been shown to result in considerable patient suffering and distress, as well as significant disability, morbidity and mortality. Despite more than half a century of intensive research, contemporary therapies for MDD demonstrate, at best, modest overall efficacy, most often resulting in either a complete lack of or insufficient symptom improvement. In addition, the tolerability profile of all contemporary pharmacotherapies for MDD, although greatly improved since their first appearance in the mid-1950s, can often contribute to poor treatment adherence, as well as patient discomfort and disability. Furthermore, many patients who experience robust antidepressant effects may still suffer a relapse or recurrence of MDD shortly after the full eradication of symptoms, and despite full compliance with their treatment. As a result, patients with depression often describe feelings as if they are caught in a vicious cycle, with only brief periods of complete symptom recovery that are not sufficient in duration to allow for a return to the pre-morbid level of functioning.

When depression strikes, clinicians, patients, their families and their loved ones are on the front line. Supporting them are those working vigorously to enhance our ability to effectively treat depression: those working in academic clinical care and research centers, government sources including the National Institutes of Health, the pharmaceutical industry, as well as private donors and fundraisers. This book is intended as a review on the state of our knowledge regarding pharmacologic treatments for depression. It is divided into four parts. The first three parts focus on

"Life-Cycle" of Depression
Step-wise Contributing Factors

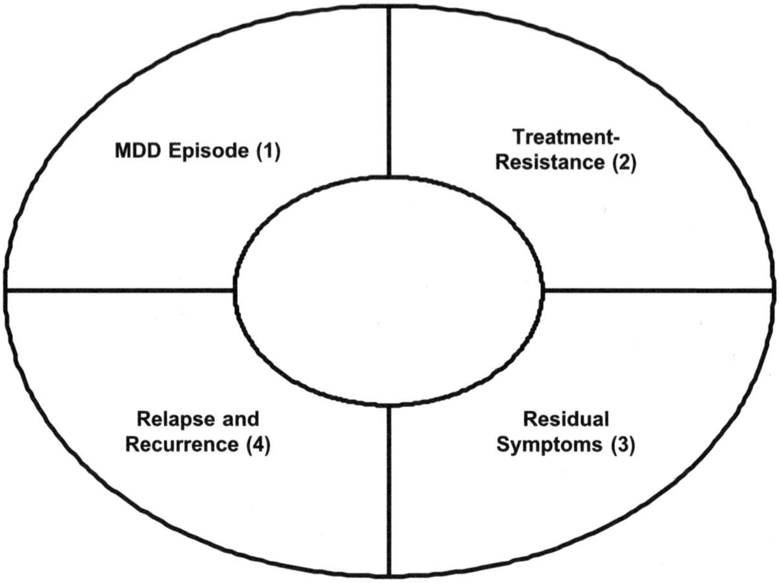

1: Relative high prevalence of MDD in the general population.
2: Limited efficacy of first-line treatments for MDD contributing to TRD.
3: Modest efficacy of subsequent treatment strategies for MDD contributing to residual symptomatology.
4: History of treatment-resistance, presence of residual symptoms, and partial or non-adherence to treatment (poor tolerability) contributing to depressive relapse or recurrence.

contemporary pharmacologic treatment strategies for MDD, as well as non-pharmacologic strategies for treatment-resistant MDD. These include a description of first-line pharmacotherapy strategies (Part I), next-step treatment strategies (Part II), and pharmacologic strategies to help maintain treatment gains (Part III). The final part of the book (Part IV) focuses on describing emerging leads that may help improve our ability to treat MDD (novel treatments and biological markers in depression).

When writing this book, it was our intention to combine a comprehensive and detail-oriented approach, so that this work may have broader appeal to all those who have an interest in the field, including clinicians, researchers, those who fund research, and those who provide direction and leadership. Thus, it was our hope that this work could, simultaneously, provide the readers with either an overview of our current state of understanding of the treatment of MDD, or with more selective knowledge that would enhance their understanding of a specific topic or topic area. Ultimately, such knowledge may lead to novel hypotheses and insights that, in turn, could help improve the standard of care for depression.

G. I. Papakostas and M. Fava

Contents

About the Authors vii

Preface ix

1. Major Depressive Disorder and Treatment-Resistant Depression 1

1.1 Major Depressive Disorder 1
1.1.1 Definition 1
1.1.2 Prevalence and disease burden 2
1.2 Treatment-Resistant Depression (TRD) 4
1.2.1 Definition and staging 4
1.2.2 Prevalence 10
1.2.3 "Pseudo-resistance" 12
1.3 Demographic and Clinical Risk Factors for Resistant Depression 15
1.3.1 Studies focusing on SSRI therapy 16
1.3.2 Studies focusing on therapy with older antidepressants 20
1.3.3 Studies focusing on therapy with newer antidepressants 22
Summary and Conclusion of Chapter 1 25

Part I: First-Line Pharmacotherapy Strategies 27

2. Monoaminergic-Based Strategies: "Single-Acting" Agents 29
   - 2.1 Monoamine Precursors for Depression 29
   - 2.2 Selective Serotonin Reuptake Inhibitors (SSRIs) 31
     - 2.2.1 Neuropharmacology 31
     - 2.2.2 Efficacy (general) 32
     - 2.2.3 Efficacy in patients with medical conditions 37
       - 2.2.3.1 Diabetes mellitus 37
       - 2.2.3.2 Coronary artery disease and myocardial infarction 38
       - 2.2.3.3 Pulmonary and sleep disorders 39
       - 2.2.3.4 Cerebrovascular illness and stroke 39
       - 2.2.3.5 Movement disorders 40
       - 2.2.3.6 Epilepsy 41
       - 2.2.3.7 Dementia 42
       - 2.2.3.8 Renal insufficiency 42
       - 2.2.3.9 Hepatitis, cirrhosis, and interferon therapy 43
       - 2.2.3.10 Human immunodeficiency virus 43
       - 2.2.3.11 Malignancy 44
       - 2.2.3.12 Transplant recipients 45
     - 2.2.4 Side effect profile 45
       - 2.2.4.1 General 45
       - 2.2.4.2 Central nervous system 46
       - 2.2.4.3 Cardiovascular 51
       - 2.2.4.4 Hematologic 52
       - 2.2.4.5 Endocrine 54
       - 2.2.4.6 Metabolic 57
       - 2.2.4.7 Immunologic 61
       - 2.2.4.8 Dermatologic 61
       - 2.2.4.9 Risk of malignancy 62

2.2.4.10 Risk of teratogenicity 62
2.2.4.11 Risk of transmission during breastfeeding 65
2.2.4.12 Discontinuation syndrome 65
2.2.5 Dosing 66
2.2.5.1 Initial and optimal dose 66
2.2.5.2 Serotonin transporter occupancy as a function of dose 67
2.2.5.3 Plasma levels and clinical efficacy 68
2.2.5.4 Cytochrome enzyme genotype and plasma levels 69
2.2.5.5 P-glycoprotein interactions . . . 70
2.2.6 Drug interactions 70
2.3 Serotonin Receptor Antagonists and Agonists . . 70
2.3.1 Trazodone and nefazodone 70
2.3.1.1 Neuropharmacology 70
2.3.1.2 Efficacy 71
2.3.1.3 Side effect profile 73
2.3.1.4 Dosing 76
2.3.2 Other 5HT-2 active agents 76
2.3.2.1 Ritanserin 76
2.3.2.2 Fenfluramine and dexfenfluramine 76
2.3.2.3 Agomelatine 77
2.3.3 5HT-1 active agents 78
2.3.3.1 Agonists 78
2.3.3.2 Antagonists 80
2.3.4 Agents acting on 5HT-3 and 5HT-4 80
2.4 Serotonin Reuptake Enhancers 81
2.5 α-2 Adrenergic Receptor Agonists and Antagonists 82
2.6 Norepinephrine Reuptake Inhibitors (NRIs) . . . 82
2.6.1 Reboxetine 82
2.6.2 Atomoxetine 85
2.6.3 Viloxazine 85

2.7 Selective β Adrenergic Receptor Agonists 85
2.8 Dopamine-Selective Agents 86
2.8.1 Receptor agonists 86
2.8.2 Reuptake inhibitors 87
2.8.3 Receptor antagonists 89

3. Monoaminergic-Based Strategies: "Dual-Acting" Agents 91

3.1 Tricyclic Antidepressants (TCAs) 91
3.1.1 Neuropharmacology 91
3.1.2 Classification 92
3.1.3 Efficacy 92
3.1.4 Side effect profile 95
3.1.5 Dosing 100
3.2 Serotonin-Norepinephrine Reuptake Inhibitors (SNRIs) 102
3.2.1 Venlafaxine 102
3.2.1.1 Neuropharmacology 102
3.2.1.2 Efficacy 102
3.2.1.3 Side effect profile 106
3.2.1.4 Dosing 109
3.2.2 Desvenlafaxine 110
3.2.3 Duloxetine 111
3.2.3.1 Efficacy 111
3.2.3.2 Side effect profile 113
3.2.3.3 Dosing 114
3.2.4 Milnacipran 115
3.3 5HT-2 and α-2 Adrenergic Receptor Antagonists 116
3.3.1 Mirtazapine 116
3.3.1.1 Neuropharmacology 116
3.3.1.2 Efficacy 117
3.3.1.3 Side effect profile 119
3.3.1.4 Dosing 121
3.3.2 Mianserin 121

3.4 Norepinephrine-Dopamine Reuptake Inhibitors 122
3.4.1 Bupropion 122
3.4.1.1 Neuropharmacology 122
3.4.1.2 Efficacy 123
3.4.1.3 Side effect profile 127
3.4.1.4 Dosing 131
3.4.2 Nomifensine 132

4. Monoaminergic-Based Strategies: "Triple-Acting" Agents 133

4.1 Monoamine Oxidase Inhibitors (MAOIs) 133
4.1.1 Neuropharmacology 133
4.1.2 Efficacy 134
4.1.3 Side effect profile 137
4.1.3.1 Dietary restrictions and drug interactions 141
4.1.4 Dosing 141
4.2 Serotonin-Norepinephrine-Dopamine Reuptake Inhibitors 142
4.3 Catechol-O-Methyltransferase (COMT) Inhibitors 143

5. Polypharmacy from the Onset of Treatment 144

5.1 Adjunctive Treatment with Monoaminergic Agents 144
5.1.1 Tryptophan 144
5.1.2 Pindolol 145
5.1.3 Typical antipsychotic agents 148
5.1.4 5HT2 and α-2 adrenergic receptor antagonists 149
5.1.5 Other antidepressants 152
5.1.6 Atypical antipsychotic agents 154
5.1.7 Dopaminergic agents 156
5.1.8 Other monoaminergic agents 156

5.2 Adjunctive Treatment with Neuroendocrine Agents 157
5.2.1 Thyroid hormones 157
5.2.2 Estrogen 159
5.2.3 Other neuroendocrine agents 159
5.3 Other Agents 161
5.3.1 Lithium 161
5.3.2 GABA-ergic agents 162
5.3.3 Folates and s-adenosylmethionine (SAMe) 165
5.3.4 Anticonvulsants 167
5.3.5 Miscellaneous other agents 168

Summary and Conclusion of Part I 174

Part II: Next-Step Treatment Strategies **177**

6. Polypharmacy Strategies for Treatment-Resistant Depression 179

6.1 Adjunctive Treatment with Monoaminergic Agents 179
6.1.1 Pindolol 179
6.1.2 5HT2 and α-2 adrenergic-receptor antagonists 181
6.1.3 Tricyclic antidepressants 184
6.1.4 Selective 5HT1A agonists 184
6.1.5 Other antidepressants 185
6.1.6 Atypical antipsychotic agents 188
6.1.7 Dopaminergic agents 193
6.1.8 Other monoaminergic agents 194
6.2 Adjunctive Treatment with Neuroendocrine Agents 195
6.2.1 Thyroid hormones 195
6.2.2 Androgens 198
6.2.3 Estrogens 199

6.2.4 Steroids and steroid synthesis inhibitors 199
6.2.5 Melatonin 200
6.3 Other Agents 200
6.3.1 Lithium 200
6.3.2 ω-3 fatty acids 205
6.3.3 Modafinil 206
6.3.4 Glutamatergic agents 208
6.3.5 Anticonvulsants 209
6.3.6 Inositol 211
6.3.7 Folates, s-adenosyl methionine (SAMe) and B-vitamins 211
6.3.8 Cholinergic agents 213
6.3.9 Miscellaneous other agents 214

7. Monotherapy Strategies for Resistant Depression 215

7.1 Increasing the Dose of Antidepressants 215
7.2 Switching Antidepressants Due to Lack of Efficacy 219
7.2.1 Switching from a TCA to an SSRI or MAOI and *vice versa* 219
7.2.2 Switching to a TCA or an MAOI following the failure of multiple antidepressants 222
7.2.3 Switching from one SSRI to another, or to a non-SSRI antidepressant 223
7.2.4 Other switch strategies 227

8. Non-pharmacologic Approaches for Resistant Depression 229

8.1 Device-Based Therapies 229
8.1.1 Electroconvulsive therapy 229
8.1.2 Vagus nerve stimulation 231
8.1.3 Transcranial magnetic stimulation 233
8.1.4 Deep brain stimulation 235

8.1.5 Transcranial direct current stimulation (tDCS) 235
8.1.6 Bright light therapy 235
8.1.7 Acupuncture 236
8.2 Psychotherapy 236
8.3 Exercise 239
8.4 Yoga and Meditation 240

Summary and Conclusion of Part II 241

Part III: Maintaining Treatment Gains **245**

9. Pharmacotherapy of Relapse/Recurrence Prevention and Treatment 247

9.1 Antidepressant Continuation and Maintenance Therapy Studies 247
9.1.1 Tricyclic antidepressants (TCAs) 247
9.1.2 Monoamine oxidase inhibitors (MAOIs) 247
9.1.3 Selective serotonin reuptake inhibitors (SSRIs) 251
9.1.4 Newer antidepressants 251
9.1.5 Summary of continuation and maintenance trials 251
9.2 Special Topics in the Pharmacotherapy of Relapse Prevention 258
9.2.1 Long-term efficacy differences among antidepressants 258
9.2.2 Optimal duration of long-term therapy 260
9.2.3 Long-term dosing and risk of relapse 262
9.2.4 Continuing adjunctive agents during long-term therapy 263
9.2.5 Instituting antidepressants among non-medicated remitters 266

9.2.6 Timing of symptom improvement and risk of relapse 267
9.2.7 Treatment-resistance and risk of relapse . 268
9.3 Treatment of Depressive Relapse/Recurrence . . 270

10. Pharmacologic Strategies to Enhance Antidepressant Tolerability 272

10.1 Adjunctive Therapy 272
10.1.1 Sexual dysfunction 272
10.1.2 Fatigue and hypersomnia 275
10.1.3 Insomnia, anxiety, and "activation" 277
10.1.4 Akathisia and bruxism 280
10.1.5 Gastrointestinal symptoms 280
10.1.6 Weight gain 281
10.1.7 Anticholinergic and other side effects . . . 282
10.1.8 Cognitive side effects 283
10.2 Switching Antidepressants Due to Intolerance 283

Summary and Conclusion of Part III 285

Part IV: Future Directions in Treatment Development 289

11. Agents Operating on Non-monoaminergic Neurotransmitter Systems 291

11.1 GABA-ergic Treatments 291
11.1.1 Benzodiazepines 291
11.1.1.1 Clinical evidence 291
11.1.1.2 Treatment limitations 300
11.1.1.3 Neuropharmacology of GABA-A receptors 301
11.1.1.4 Conclusion 302
11.1.2 Barbiturates 303
11.1.3 Other GABA-ergic agents 303

11.2 Glycine and Glutamate-Based Treatments 306
11.2.1 Neuropharmacology 306
11.2.2 NMDA-active agents 307
11.2.3 Other glutamatergic agents 309
11.2.4 Glycinergic agents 311
11.3 Agents with Combined GABA-ergic and Glutamatergic Activity 311
11.3.1 Anticonvulsants 311
11.4 Other Anticonvulsants 314
11.5 Neurokinin-Receptor Antagonists 316
11.5.1 Neuropharmacology 316
11.5.2 Clinical evidence 316
11.6 Nicotinic Receptor–Based Treatments 319
11.6.1 Neuropharmacology 319
11.6.2 Nicotinic-receptor agonists 319
11.6.3 Cholinesterase inhibitors 321
11.6.4 Nicotinic-receptor antagonists 322
11.7 Cannabinoids and Endocannabinoids 322
11.8 Opioidergic Therapies 324
11.8.1 Opioid-receptor antagonists 324
11.8.2 Opioid-receptor agonists 324
11.8.3 Mixed agonists/antagonists 325
11.9 Other Neurotransmitter Systems 326

12. Neuroendocrine-Based Agents 328
12.1 Hypothalamic-Pituitary-Gonadal Axis (HPG) 328
12.1.1 Estrogen 328
12.1.2 Progesterone 332
12.1.3 Androgens 333
12.1.4 Dehydroepiandrosterone (DHEA) 337
12.1.5 Other gonadotropic agents 338
12.2 Hypothalamic-Pituitary-Adrenal Axis (HPA) 338
12.2.1 Corticosteroids 338
12.2.2 Steroid synthesis inhibitors 339

12.2.3 Steroid- and CRF-receptor antagonists 340
12.3 Hypothalamic-Pituitary-Thyroid Axis (HPT) 342
12.4 Melatonin and Melatonergic Agents 343
12.5 Other Hormones 345

13. Metabolic-Based and Other Agents 348

13.1 Metabolic-Based Agents 348
13.1.1 Elements of the "one carbon cycle" 348
13.1.1.1 S-adenosylmethionine (SAMe) 348
13.1.1.2 Folates and other B-vitamins . . 353
13.1.2 Agents acting on neuronal "second messenger" systems 353
13.1.2.1 Anatomy of the "second messenger" system 353
13.1.2.2 Phosphodiesterase inhibitors 354
13.1.2.3 Inositol 355
13.1.2.4 Other agents 355
13.1.3 Essential fatty acids 356
13.1.3.1 Overview 356
13.1.3.2 Clinical studies 357
13.1.4 Carnitine 360
13.1.5 Minerals, trace elements, and vitamins (non-B vitamins) 362
13.2 Agents with Unknown Mechanism of Action 363
13.2.1 Herbal remedies 363
13.2.1.1 *Hypericum perforatum* 363
13.2.1.2 Ginseng 368
13.2.1.3 Kava kava 368
13.2.1.4 Valerian root and *Ginkgo bilboa* . 369
13.2.2 Modafinil 369
13.2.3 Pivagabine 370

14. Biological Predictors, Moderators, and Mediators of Efficacy 371

14.1 Definition and Significance of Mediators of Outcome 371

14.2 Genetic Markers 373

14.2.1 Studies involving SSRI therapy 376

14.2.1.1 Genes coding for TPH and 5HTT 376

14.2.1.2 Genes coding for 5HT-receptors 377

14.2.1.3 Genes coding for NET or NE-receptors 377

14.2.1.4 Genes coding for MAO and COMT 378

14.2.1.5 Genes coding for other proteins 378

14.2.2 Studies involving therapy with other antidepressants 380

14.2.3 Studies comparing antidepressants 382

14.3 Neurophysiology 385

14.3.1 Brain functioning and metabolism 385

14.3.1.1 Positron emission tomography 385

14.3.1.2 Functional magnetic resonance imaging 386

14.3.1.3 Magnetic resonance spectroscopy 387

14.3.2 Electroencephalography 388

14.3.2.1 Traditional electroencephalography 388

14.3.2.2 Quantitative electroencephalography 389

14.3.2.3 Loudness Dependence of Auditory Evoked Potentials (LDAEP) . . . 391

14.3.3 Brain functional asymmetry (dichotic listening) 392
14.4 Molecular Biology 393
14.4.1 Receptor and transporter kinetics 393
14.4.2 Intracellular signal transduction 394
14.4.3 Inflammatory markers 396

Summary and Conclusion of Part IV 399

Appendix A 401

Appendix B 403

Appendix C 405

Appendix D 407

Bibliography 409

Chapter 1 409
Chapter 2 422
Chapter 3 493
Chapter 4 535
Chapter 5 544
Chapter 6 560
Chapter 7 587
Chapter 8 594
Chapter 9 601
Chapter 10 610
Chapter 11 625
Chapter 12 650
Chapter 13 662
Chapter 14 676

Index 695

Chapter 1

Major Depressive Disorder and Treatment-Resistant Depression

1.1 Major Depressive Disorder

1.1.1 *Definition*

The Diagnostic and Statistical Manual of Mental Disorders (DSM) — 4th Edition (DSM-IV; APA 1994) — defines major depressive disorder (MDD) as the presence of depressed mood (can be irritable mood in children/adolescents) and/or reduced interest/pleasure (core symptoms), accompanied by at least four accompanying symptoms (three if both core symptoms are present), lasting for at least two weeks. The accompanying symptoms include sleep disturbance (insomnia or hypersomnia), a disturbance in appetite or weight (increased or decreased), loss of energy (fatigue), diminished ability to think or concentrate or indecisiveness, psychomotor disturbance (either agitation or retardation), feelings of worthlessness or excessive guilt, and recurrent thoughts of death or suicide. In addition, according to the DSM classification, the sum of these symptoms must result in significant psychosocial impairment in order to differentiate depressive disorders from physiological mood variability. Chronic depression is defined as the persistence of this syndrome for at least two years. Minor depression (MiD) is defined as the presence of depressed mood and/or lack of interest or pleasure associated with fewer of the previously mentioned accompanying symptoms (not exceeding three or not exceeding two if both core symptoms are present) (APA, 1994). Dysthymic disorder (DD) is defined as the persistence of this syndrome for at least two years (without an intervening two-month period during which these symptoms are absent). It is also worth noting that patients who suffer from depressive disorders (MDD, DD, MiD) can also present with a combination of psychological (e.g., anxiety, irritability, hostility), behavioral (e.g., aggressiveness, self-mutilation, crying spells, anger attacks, social withdrawal), and physical (e.g., headaches, limb and back pain, shortness of breath, palpitations, panic attacks, paresthesias, constipation, upper and lower GI upset) symptoms presently not recognized by the DSM.

1.1.2 *Prevalence and disease burden*

MDD is highly prevalent in the general population. The results of a large epidemiological study (the national comorbidity survey) report the current (past six months) prevalence of MDD in the general population at, nearly, 5% (Blazer *et al.*, 1994). More recently, Lepine *et al.* (1997) report the six-month prevalence of major depression in Western Europe as, approximately, 17%. Depression also appears to be more common among women than men (Weissman *et al.*, 1984), younger than older adults (Blazer *et al.*, 1994), urban-dwellers than rural-dwellers (Blazer *et al.*, 1985), patients with a history of sexual abuse (Breslau *et al.*, 1997), substance abuse (Grant, 1995), insomnia (Foley *et al.*, 2004), a chronic medical illness (Patten, 1999), alcohol abuse (Grant & Harford, 1995), an anxiety disorder (Kessler *et al.*, 1996), or a family history of depression or other comorbid axis-I disorders (Kendler *et al.*, 1997).

MDD is characterized by a significant burden of subjective suffering, increased morbidity, and impaired social and work functioning (Papakostas *et al.*, 2004a). During the mid-1990s, unipolar depression was estimated to be the leading cause of disability in developed countries (Wells *et al.*, 1996), and the fourth leading cause of disability worldwide (Murray & Lopez, 1997a). At the time, projections estimated that MDD would rise to be the second leading cause of disability worldwide by the year 2020 (Murray & Lopez, 1997b).

MDD has also been shown to account for a 23-fold increase in social disability, even after controlling for physical disease (Ormel *et al.*, 1999), as well as an almost five-fold increase in short-term work-disability (Broadhead *et al.*, 1990). This may account for the fact that individuals with a history of a depressive episode are also at increased risk for chronic financial stress (Maciejewski *et al.*, 2000). Patients with MDD have also been found to score lower than those with a number of medical conditions on physical functioning, role functioning and emotional functioning (Stewart *et al.*, 1989), and to have long-lasting decrements in psychosocial functioning that are equal to or greater than those of patients with chronic medical illness such as diabetes and osteoarthritis (Hayes *et al.*, 1995). In a study of 11,242 outpatients from three health-care provision systems, for example, Wells *et al.* (1989) reported worse physical, social, and role functioning in MDD patients than patients with no chronic conditions. Similarly, a large study of 25,916 primary care patients from 14 countries revealed that patients with MDD were more likely to report disability than those without, controlling for the severity of physical disease (Ormel *et al.*, 1994). In fact, in a Western European study, the degree of disability was directly related to the severity of depression in patients with MDD (Lepine *et al.*, 1997). The presence of less severe depressive disorders such as sub-syndromal depression and MiD have also been shown to have a negative impact on psychosocial functioning (Judd *et al.*, 1996).

Perhaps the most disabling aspect of depression is its adverse impact on psychosocial functioning and quality of life. For example, women with MDD were reported to have more impairment in familial, marital and occupational roles than non-depressed women in one study (Weissman *et al.*, 1978). Similarly, a separate study comparing social functioning in outpatients with MDD, bipolar depression and dysthymia revealed significant and profound disturbances in most areas of functioning in all three groups, with disturbances being most apparent with regards to occupational and leisure activities (De Lisio *et al.*, 1986). In parallel, in a community sample of nearly 5,000 patients, Fredman *et al.* (1988) reported poorer intimate relationships and less satisfying social interactions in patients with MDD compared to individuals without MDD. In addition, results stemming from the National Institutes of Mental Health (NIMH) Epidemiological Catchment Area Program (Eaton *et al.*, 1981) revealed that subjects with major depression or sub-syndromal depression had higher levels of household strain, social irritability, financial strain, limitations in occupational functioning, poor health status (Judd *et al.*, 1996), and days lost from work (Johnson *et al.*, 1992) than subjects without any depressive disorder or symptoms. Finally, data stemming from the National Comorbidity Survey (Kessler *et al.*, 1994) revealed that patients with depression (defined as either MDD, bipolar depression or dysthymia) were less likely to complete high school or college (Kessler *et al.*, 1995), more likely to experience teenage pregnancy (Kessler *et al.*, 1997), and more likely to experience divorce (Kessler *et al.*, 1998) than non-depressed subjects, while patients with MDD were less likely to be satisfied with their marriage (Whisman, 1999), and more likely to report poorer quality of interpersonal relationships (Zlotnick *et al.*, 2000) than subjects without MDD.

MDD is also characterized by an increase in mortality (Zheng *et al.*, 1997; Bruce *et al.*, 1994; Pennix *et al.*, 1999). For example, a study of 4,000 patients reveals that in depression, the standardized mortality rate is double for all causes of death and 26-fold for death from suicide (Newman *et al.*, 1991). Overall, the lifetime risk for suicide in depressed patients has been estimated at 2.2% (Bostwick *et al.*, 2000). Other complications of MDD include the presence and/or worsening of aggressive behavior, as well as an increased risk of alcohol and/or substance-use disorders (Marzuk *et al.*, 1992; Nunes *et al.*, 1996).

1.2 Treatment-Resistant Depression (TRD)

1.2.1 *Definition and staging*

Treatment-resistant depression (TRD) typically refers to an inadequate symptom improvement following one antidepressant trial of adequate dose and duration among patients suffering from MDD.

The definition of adequate dose varies widely from agent to agent, with values deriving from double-blind, placebo-controlled trials or dose-comparator studies (see Table 1.1 as well as Chaps. 2–4 for more details).

Adequate duration is often defined as a minimum of six weeks (Fava, 2003), stemming from the observation that fewer than 7% of patients who show little improvement following six weeks of treatment with fluoxetine eventually respond (50% decrease in symptom severity) following an additional two weeks of treatment (Nierenberg *et al.*, 1995) (see Fig. 1.1), while only 12% of patients who show little or no improvement following six weeks of treatment experience at least a partial response following an additional two weeks of treatment (Nierenberg *et al.*, 2000).

Although similar analyses of clinical trials of longer duration (12 weeks) have provided evidence arguing that six weeks may be too short a duration in order to declare an antidepressant trial ineffective (Quitkin *et al.*, 2003), it is also important to keep in mind that spontaneous remission rates can be substantial over time (Posternak & Zimmerman, 2000; Posternak & Miller, 2001), and may be responsible for the majority of symptom improvement seen following eight weeks of antidepressant therapy. Nevertheless, it is important to point out that the adequacy of duration issue is complicated by the fact that the original analyses by Nierenberg *et al.* (1995) were based on data derived from a fixed-dose trial of fluoxetine 20 mg/day, and that delayed dose escalations are likely to affect how long clinicians need to wait before they assume that the duration of the trial is adequate.

Definitions of "adequate symptom improvement" have varied throughout the course of the past few decades, ranging from the more traditional view in which treatment-resistance is defined as strict non-response, to the broadest definition, i.e., failure to achieve remission of the depressive episode (Nierenberg & DeCecco, 2001) (Table 1.2). Nowadays, most experts would agree that inadequate symptom improvement represents the failure to achieve remission of a depressive episode for several reasons (Fava, 2003). First of all, as first pointed out by Nierenberg and Amsterdam (1990), patients

Table 1.1 Minimally effective and optimal (daily) doses of common antidepressants.[a]

Agent	Minimally Effective Dose	Optimal Dose
Monoamine Oxidase Inhibitors		
Phenelzine (Nardil)	45 mg	90 mg
Tranylcypromine (Parnate)	30 mg	60 mg
Isocarboxazid (Marplan)	30 mg	60 mg
Selegiline Patch (Emsam)	6 mg	??[b]
Tricyclic Antidepressants	150 mg[c]	250 mg[d]
Selective Serotonin Reuptake Inhibitors		
Fluoxetine (Prozac)	20 mg	40 mg
Sertraline (Zoloft)	50 mg	100 mg
Paroxetine (Paxil)	20 mg	40 mg
Paroxetine CR (Paxil CR)	25 mg	50 mg
Citalopram (Celexa)	20 mg	40 mg
Escitalopram (Lexapro)	10 mg	20 mg
Fluvoxamine (Luvox)	50 mg	100 mg
Serotonin-Norepinephrine Reuptake Inhibitors		
Venlafaxine (Effexor) (IR or XR)	75 mg	150 mg
Duloxetine (Cymbalta)	60 mg	90 mg
Milnacipran (Ixel)	100 mg	200 mg
Desvenlafaxine (Pristiq)	50 mg	100 mg
Other Agents		
Bupropion (Wellbutrin) (IR, SR, or XL)	150 mg	300 mg
Mirtazapine (Remeron)	15 mg	30 mg
Reboxetine (Edronax)	8 mg	10 mg
Agomelatine	25 mg	50 mg
Serzone (Nefazodone)	300 mg	600 mg
Trazodone (Desyrel)	300 mg	600 mg

[a]Fava, M. (2003). Diagnosis and definition of treatment-resistant depression. *Biological Psychiatry*, 53(8), 649–659.
[b]??: Insufficient information at this time.
[c]Except nortriptyline (75 mg), Protriptyline (30 mg).
[d]Except nortriptyline (125 mg), Protriptyline (60 mg).

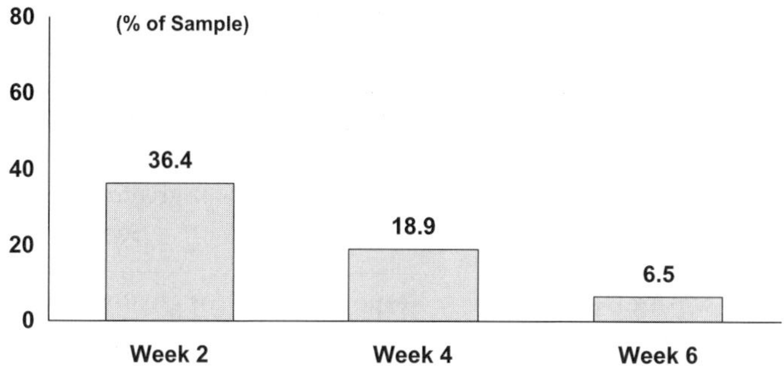

Fig. 1.1 Proportion of MDD patients with minimal symptom improvement* who eventually experience clinical response** following eight weeks of treatment with fluoxetine (SSRI). *Defined as less than 20% reduction in symptom severity. **Defined as a greater than 50% reduction in symptom severity during the course of eight weeks. [Data extracted from: Nierenberg, A.A., McLean, N.E., Alpert, J.E., Worthington, J.J., Rosenbaum, J.F., & Fava, M. (1995). Early nonresponse to fluoxetine as a predictor of poor eight-week outcome. *American Journal of Psychiatry*, 152, 1500–1503.]

presenting with moderate to severe depression may still be quite symptomatic despite a 25–50% improvement in depressive symptoms. In addition, residual symptoms have been associated with poorer psychosocial functioning (Papakostas *et al.*, 2004b), as well as increased relapse rates (Paykel *et al.*, 1995). Finally, incomplete response (defined as a 25% or greater improvement in depressive symptoms failing to achieve remission) appears to be more than twice as common as strict non-response in naturalistic treatment settings (28.7% versus 12.9%, respectively; Petersen *et al.*, 2005). Therefore, defining TRD as strict non-response following adequate treatment rather than failure to achieve remission would actually exclude the majority of patients who have not been successfully treated.

In recent years, an increasing amount of attention has also been paid to developing methods to stage the degree of resistance in patients with MDD. Based on models widely used in the field of oncology, Thase and Rush (1997) proposed a five-stage model that yields a categorical assignment of the degree of resistance. According to this model, failure of one trial of one major class of antidepressants

Table 1.2 Definitions of efficacy for common clinician-administered scales used in depression trials.[a]

Scale	Outcome	Definition
Hamilton Depression Rating Scale (17-item)[b]	Response Remission	50% or greater score reduction Score < 8
Montgomery-Asperg Depression Rating Scale[c]	Response Remission	50% or greater score reduction Score < 11
Quick Inventory of Depressive Symptomatology[d]	Response Remission	50% or greater score reduction Score < 6
Clinical Global Impression — Severity[e]	Response Remission	N/A Score = 1
Clinical Global Impression — Improvement[e]	Response Remission	Score < 3 N/A

[a]Nierenberg, A.A., & DeCecco, L.M. (2001). Definitions of antidepressant treatment response, remission, nonresponse, partial response, and other relevant outcomes: A focus on treatment-resistant depression. *Journal of Clinical Psychiatry*, 62 Suppl 16, 5–9.
[b]Hamilton, M. (1960). A rating scale for depression. *Journal of Neurology, Neurosurgery and Psychiatry*, 23, 56–62.
[c]Montgomery, S.A., & Asberg, A. (1979). A new depression scale designed to be sensitive to change. *British Journal of Psychiatry*, 134, 382–389.
[d]Trivedi, M.H., Rush, A.J., Ibrahim, H.M., Carmody, T.J., Biggs, M.M., Suppes, T., Crismon, M.L., Shores-Wilson, K., Toprac, M.G., Dennehy, E.B., Witte, B., & Kashner, T.M. (2004). The Inventory of Depressive Symptomatology, Clinician Rating (IDS-C) and Self-Report (IDS-SR), and the Quick Inventory of Depressive Symptomatology, Clinician Rating (QIDS-C) and Self-Report (QIDS-SR) in public sector patients with mood disorders: A psychometric evaluation. *Psychological Medicine*, 34(1), 73–82.
[e]Guy, W. (Ed). (1976). *ECDEU Assessment Manual for Psychopharmacology*, revised. Rockville, MD: National Institute of Mental Health.

constitutes stage I antidepressant-resistance, failing an additional antidepressant trial from a *different* class constitutes stage II resistance, failing an additional TCA trial stage III resistance, and failing an additional MAOI trial stage IV resistance. Finally, failing a trial of electro-convulsive therapy (ECT) has been defined as stage V treatment-resistance according to this model (Table 1.3).

Several methodological issues have been raised with respect to this staging model, including: (1) that the degree of intensity of each trial in terms of dosing and duration is not accounted for, (2) that the model assumes that non-response to two agents of different class is more difficult to treat than non-response to two agents of the same class, and (3) that the role of augmentation or combination strategies is not considered. An additional limiting factor is the implicit hierarchy of treatments, with the MAOIs considered superior to the TCAs.

More recently, the Massachusetts General Hospital (MGH) staging method was proposed (Fava, 2003). According to this model, non-response to each adequate trial increases the overall degree of resistance by one point, while optimization of dose and duration, augmentation, or combination increase the degree of resistance by 0.5 points. Finally, ECT was proposed to increase the degree of resistance by three points according to this model (Table 1.4).

Recently, empirical testing of these two models with the use of outcome data derived from outpatients receiving treatment for MDD in one of two hospital-based, academically-affiliated depression specialty clinics revealed that, although highly correlated, the MGH staging model demonstrated significantly greater ability to

Table 1.3 The Thase–Rush staging model for TRD.

Stage 1	Failure of at least one adequate trial of one major class of antidepressants
Stage 2	Failure of an additional antidepressant from a distinct class
Stage 3	Failure of an additional trial involving a tricyclic antidepressant
Stage 4	Failure of an additional trial involving a monoamine-oxidase inhibitor
Stage 5	Failure of an additional trial of electroconvulsive therapy

Thase, M.E., & Rush, A.J. (1997). When at first you don't succeed: Sequential strategies for antidepressant nonresponders. *Journal of Clinical Psychiatry*, 58, Suppl 13, 23–29.

Table 1.4 The Massachusetts General Hospital staging model for TRD.

1 Point	Non-response following an adequate trial of antidepressants
0.5 Points	Non-response following dose-optimization
	Non-response following an adequate augmentation or combination trial
3 Points	Non-response following a trial of electroconvulsive therapy

Fava, M. (2003). Diagnosis and definition of treatment-resistant depression. *Biological Psychiatry*, 53(8), 649–659.

predict remission status than the Thase–Rush model (Petersen *et al.*, 2005).

1.2.2 *Prevalence*

Prevalence estimates for TRD are available from several sources, including large clinical trials (Trivedi *et al.*, 2006), large meta-analyses (Papakostas & Fava, 2009), or naturalistic studies (Corey-Lisle *et al.*, 2004; Petersen *et al.*, 2005; Rush *et al.*, 2004). For example, in the first level of the Sequenced Treatment Alternatives to Relieve Depression (STAR*D) trial, only about 30% of patients were in remission following up to 12 weeks of therapy with the SSRI citalopram (Trivedi *et al.*, 2006). In addition, 15.8% of patients developed an intolerable adverse event, 38.6% developed moderate to severe impairment due to an adverse event, 8.6% discontinued treatment due to adverse events, and 2% developed a serious adverse event — findings that underscore efficacy and tolerability limitations of treatment with a typical first-line agent (Fig. 1.2).

Papakostas and Fava (2009) reviewed 182 randomized, double-blind, placebo-controlled trials involving the use of antidepressants for MDD. Approximately 53.4% of patients responded following treatment with an antidepressant, compared to 36.6% of patients who responded following the administration of a placebo pill (see Fig. 1.3).

Corey-Lisle *et al.* (2004) reported that approximately 22% of patients who received treatment for depression by their primary-care physicians remitted following six months of treatment,

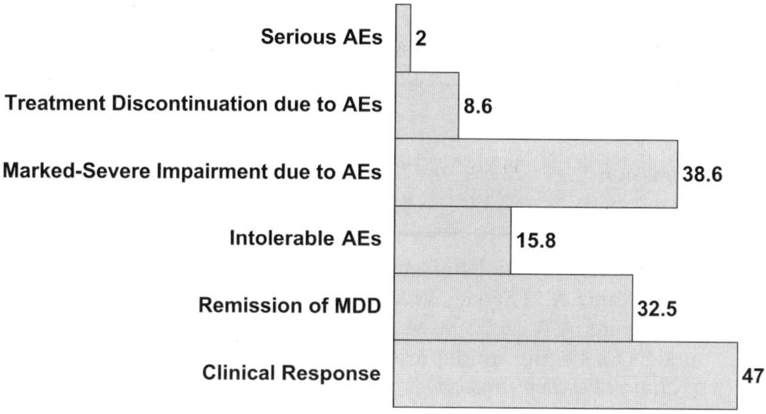

Fig. 1.2 STAR*D level 1: efficacy, tolerability and safety of citalopram (SSRI) monotherapy in MDD (% of sample) (n = 2,876). AEs: Adverse events. [Data extracted from: Trivedi, M.H., Rush, A.J., Wisniewski, S.R., *et al.* & STAR*D Study Team (2006). Evaluation of outcomes with citalopram for depression using measurement-based care in STAR*D: Implications for clinical practice. *American Journal of Psychiatry*, 163, 28–40.]

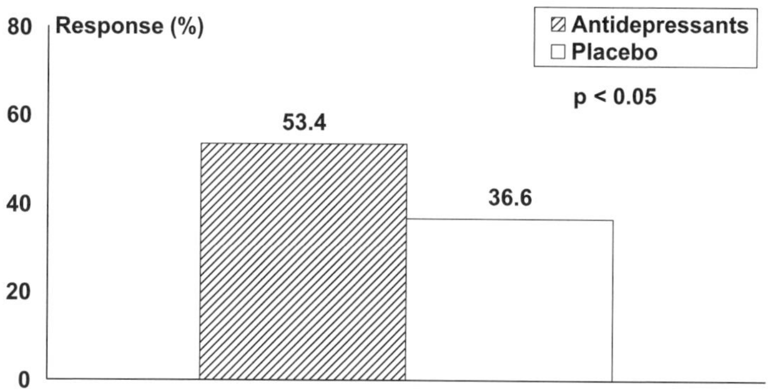

Fig. 1.3 Relative efficacy of antidepressants versus placebo: meta-analysis of 182 RCTs (n = 36,385). RCT: Randomized, Controlled Trial. [Data extracted from: Papakostas, G.I., & Fava, M. (2009). Does the probability of receiving placebo influence clinical trial outcome? A meta-regression of double-blind, randomized clinical trials in MDD. *European Neuropsychopharmacology*, 19(1), 34–40.]

Table 1.5 Outcome of MDD following each sequential treatment administered in a depression specialty clinic (n = 115).

Treatment	1st	2nd	3rd	"Endpoint"
Remission	22.6%	23.5%	20.5%	50.4%
No response	57.3%	41.1%	29.4%	12.9%

Data extracted from: Petersen, T., Papakostas, G.I., Posternak, M.A., Kant, A., Guyker, W.M., Iosifescu, D.V., Yeung, A.S., Nierenberg, A.A., & Fava, M. (2005). Empirical testing of two models for staging antidepressant treatment resistance. *Journal of Clinical Psychopharmacology*, 25, 336–341.

32% were partial responders, while 45% were non-responders. Similarly, Rush *et al.* (2004) reported an 11% remission rate and 26.3% response rate among depressed outpatients following 12 months of treatment of depression in one of several public-sector community clinics. Petersen *et al.* (2005) reported a 50.4% remission rate among outpatients with MDD enrolled in one of two hospital-based, academically affiliated depression specialty clinics (Massachusetts General Hospital, an affiliate of Harvard Medical School and Rhode Island Hospital, an affiliate of Brown University) following an average of 25.8 weeks of treatment (Table 1.5).

Finally, it is also worth noting that while partial or non-response are common, residual symptoms among remitters are also highly prevalent (Fava *et al.*, 2006; Nierenberg *et al.*, 1999), and associated with poorer psychosocial functioning (Papakostas *et al.*, 2004b) as well as increased relapse rates (Paykel *et al.*, 1995) (see Figs. 1.4 and 1.5).

1.2.3 *"Pseudo-resistance"*

In contrast to "true" treatment resistance, "pseudo-resistance" can arise during any of several clinical scenarios including:

1. Declaration of a depressive episode as "resistant" in light of a treatment of either inadequate dose or duration.

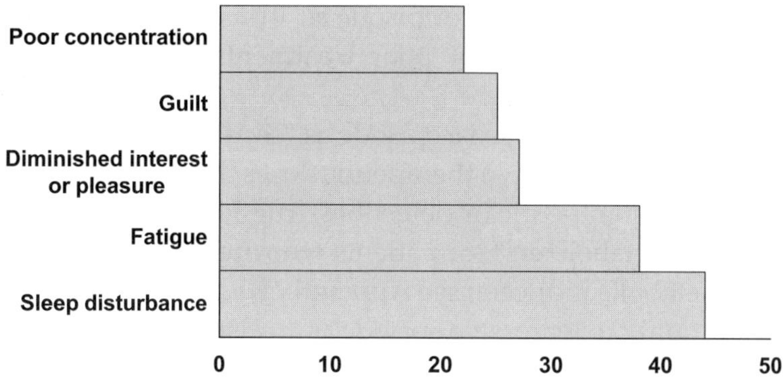

Fig. 1.4 Common residual MDD (DSM) symptoms among fluoxetine (SSRI)-remitters (% of sample) ($n = 108$). DSM: Diagnostic and Statistical Manual of Mental Disorders. [Data extracted from: Nierenberg, A.A., Keefe, B.R., Leslie, V.C., Alpert, J.E., Pava, J.A., Worthington, J.J. 3rd., Rosenbaum, J.F., & Fava, M. (1999). Residual symptoms in depressed patients who respond acutely to fluoxetine. *Journal of Clinical Psychiatry*, 60, 221–225.]

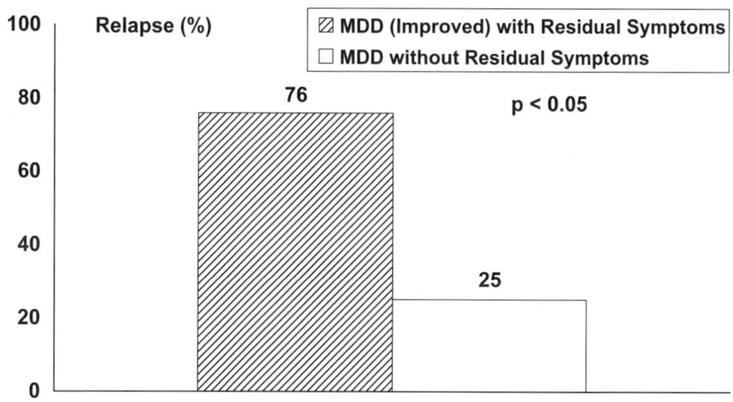

Fig. 1.5 MDD relapse rates following 15 months of continued treatment: Comparison of antidepressant responders/remitters with or without residual symptoms — observational study ($n = 57$). [Data extracted from: Paykel, E.S., Ramana, R., Cooper, Z., Hayhurst, H., Kerr, J., & Barocka, A. (1995). Residual symptoms after partial remission: An important outcome in depression. *Psychological Medicine*, 25, 1171–1180.]

2. Declaration of a depressive episode as "resistant" following adequate therapy in light of poor treatment adherence or nonadherence.
3. Declaration of a depressive episode as "resistant" following therapy prescribed at known therapeutic doses that, nevertheless, fail to result in therapeutic or detectible drug levels (i.e., in the case of "rapid metabolizers", or patients who are also being administered metabolic inducers; see Appendix I).
4. Declaration of a depressive episode as "resistant" following inappropriate treatment in light of misdiagnosis (for example, when a bipolar depressive episode has been diagnosed as a unipolar one, or when unipolar psychotic depression has been diagnosed as unipolar non-psychotic depression).
5. Misclassification of a depressive relapse during the long-term treatment with a previously effective agent as a depressive episode resistant to treatment with that agent.

Therefore, the following steps can often be helpful in the face of TRD:

1. Ensuring the adequacy of dose and duration of antidepressant treatment.
2. Ensuring adequate treatment adherence.
3. Diagnostic clarification: ruling out bipolar disorder, psychotic MDD, or misclassification of a depressive relapse as treatment resistance.
4. Antidepressant levels may be checked, particularly among patients on optimal or higher levels of antidepressants that are not experiencing side effects. Although, with the exception of TCAs, antidepressant levels cannot be used to guide treatment, the absence of detectible antidepressant levels may suggest the need for genotyping (when available, particularly for "rapid metabolizers") or a comprehensive examination of the drug regimen to exclude the possibility of drug interactions (presence of metabolic inducers).

1.3 Demographic and Clinical Risk Factors for Resistant Depression

Several factors have been examined as potential predictors of outcome (efficacy) in MDD. Efficacy outcomes commonly include either the resolution of depressive symptoms during treatment (the magnitude of reduction in depressive symptoms), the rapidity of response (the time-course of symptom reduction), the attainment of a treatment response, or the attainment of episode remission (see Table 1.2).

A predictor of outcome (efficacy) can involve factors (demographic, clinical, or biological), the presence or magnitude of which at baseline (immediately before treatment is initiated) influences the likelihood of a particular outcome occurring following treatment. *"Differential predictors"* or *"moderators"* of efficacy outcome are a special sub-category of outcome predictors. Moderators of outcome involve factors (demographic, clinical, or biological), the presence or magnitude of which at baseline (immediately before treatment is initiated) influences the *relative* likelihood of a particular outcome occurring following treatment with one agent versus another. Thus, moderators of response can help predict differential efficacy between two or more treatments (for example, MDD patients who also present with a given moderator are more likely to respond to treatment X than treatment Y, than patients who do not) (see Chap. 14, Fig. 1).

Identifying reliable, robust and feasible (from a clinical practice perspective) predictors of outcome (efficacy) can be useful for several reasons:

1. They can help stratify patients according to their risk for treatment-resistance, thereby leading to the development of tailored approaches to help optimize the overall efficacy of treatment.
2. Upon further research, they may prove to be moderators of efficacy outcome.

Identifying reliable, robust and feasible moderators of outcome can, in turn, be useful for several reasons (in addition to risk stratification):

1. They can lead to the development of tailored treatment approaches (algorithms) for a given subgroup of MDD patients (depressive subtype).
2. They can help further our understanding of the underlying pathophysiology (ies) of the various forms of depression, and mechanism(s) that constitute recovery from depression.

Unfortunately, only a handful of moderators of efficacy outcome have been suggested by the literature. These factors are, at best, preliminary although highly promising, and will be discussed within the context of each pertaining antidepressant agent (for further details, see Chaps. 2–4). Biological predictors represent a select subgroup of predictors in terms of their relevance and potential, and will be discussed separately (see Chap. 14).

1.3.1 *Studies focusing on SSRI therapy*

To date, the overwhelming number of published studies focusing on identifying predictors of response during the acute-phase of treatment of MDD involve the SSRIs. In general, the presence and/or extent of factors associated with personality or temperament, including the presence of a DSM-defined personality disorder (Fava *et al.*, 1994a and 1997a; Hirschfeld *et al.*, 1998; Russell *et al.*, 2001), neuroticism (Petersen *et al.*, 2002), hypochondriacal concerns (Demopulos *et al.*, 1996), dysfunctional attitudes (Fava *et al.*, 1994b), or temperamental style (Newman *et al.*, 2000) do not appear to predict response to the SSRIs. However, a high degree of perceived stress combined with dysfunctional attitudes was found to predict poorer response to the SSRI fluoxetine in a more recent study (Pedrelli *et al.*, 2008).

In contrast, the presence and or degree of general (Iosifescu *et al.*, 2003) as well as specific medical comorbidity including hypercholesterolemia (Sonawalla *et al.*, 2002), greater body weight (Papakostas *et al.*, 2004c), risk factors for vascular disease (Iosifescu *et al.*, 2005; Papakostas *et al.*, 2005b), hypofolatemia (Fava *et al.*,

1997b; Papakostas *et al.*, 2005a and b), and MRI white-matter hyperintensities (Iosifescu *et al.*, 2006; Papakostas *et al.*, 2005b; Alexopoulos *et al.*, 2008) consistently appear to predict poorer outcome during the acute-phase of treatment of MDD with the SSRIs, although other factors such as the presence of mild hypothyroidism (Fava *et al.*, 1995; Iosifescu *et al.*, 2001) and anemia (Mischoulon *et al.*, 2000) do not.

The presence and severity of several symptoms of depression have also been linked to poorer prognosis, including hopelessness (Papakostas *et al.*, 2007a), cognitive symptoms of depression including executive dysfunction (Alexopoulos *et al.*, 2005), physical symptoms of depression (somatic symptoms including pain, fatigue, physical symptoms of anxiety and gastrointestinal symptoms) (Burns *et al.*, 1995; Denninger *et al.*, 2006; Papakostas *et al.*, 2004d and 2008), and psychomotor retardation (Burns *et al.*, 1995; Caligiuri *et al.*, 2003; Taylor *et al.*, 2006). In fact, a greater resolution of somatic symptoms (Farabaugh *et al.*, 2005; Denninger *et al.*, 2006) including pain (Arnold *et al.*, 2008) was found to correlate with a greater probability of achieving remission of MDD during the course of treatment. Early improvement in overall depressive symptom burden has also been found to predict better outcome during the acute phase of treatment of MDD with fluoxetine (Farabaugh *et al.*, in press; Nierenberg *et al.*, 1995 and 2000; Papakostas *et al.*, 2007b and c).

Several other illness features including greater chronicity (Fava *et al.*, 1997a; Gilmer *et al.*, 2008; Hirschfeld *et al.*, 1998), early versus late onset of illness among elderly depressed patients (Kozel *et al.*, 2008), atypical depression (Fava *et al.*, 1997a), depression with anger attacks (Fava *et al.*, 1997a), depression with comorbid ADHD (Alpert *et al.*, 1996), or the presence of insomnia (Fava *et al.*, 2002; Hirschfeld *et al.*, 1998; Simon *et al.*, 1998) do not appear to confer a worse prognosis. For melancholic depression, the results of one study suggest a trend towards statistical significance for better outcome among SSRI-treated patients with melancholic MDD than those without (Heiligenstein *et al.*, 1994). However, subsequent analyses of three different datasets did not demonstrate an independent, predictive role for melancholic depression status (presence versus absence) on SSRI response in MDD (Burns *et al.*, 1995; Fava *et al.*, 1997a; McGrath *et al.*, 2008). Evidence on the potential moderating effects of a melancholic MDD subtype on the relative likelihood of responding to an SSRI versus a TCA is presented in Chap. 3, while evidence on the potential moderating effects of depression severity on the relative likelihood of responding to venlafaxine or escitalopram versus an older SSRI (fluoxetine, sertraline, paroxetine, citalopram) is presented in Chaps. 2 and 3.

The presence of an anxious MDD subtype (defined using the "syndromal" approach as MDD presenting with at least one comorbid DSM anxiety disorder) was found to result in poorer outcome during the acute-phase of treatment of MDD with fluoxetine (Fava *et al.*, 1997a), and citalopram (Howland *et al.*, 2009; Trivedi *et al.*, 2006), but not sertraline (Hirschfeld *et al.*, 1998). Until recently, however, several relatively small studies (Feiger *et al.*, 2003; Lenze *et al.*, 2002; Russell *et al.*, 2001; Sir *et al.*, 2005; Tollefson *et al.*, 1994) defining anxious MDD using the "dimensional" approach (most commonly defined as a score of seven or more on the anxiety-somatization sub-scale (HDRS-AS — Cleary & Guy, 1977) of the Hamilton Depression Rating Scale (HDRS — Hamilton, 1960), had not demonstrated lower remission rates among patients with anxious MDD than those without. Other studies (Rush *et al.*, 2001a and b; Simon *et al.*, 1998) that employed a scale different than the HDRS-AS to define anxious MDD (dimensional approach) had, also, not demonstrated lower remission rates among patients with anxious MDD than those without. However, recently, evidence stemming from Levels 1 and 2 of STAR*D does suggest significantly lower remission rates following the treatment of MDD with either first-line (citalopram) or second-line treatment strategies (switching to antidepressants versus augmentation or combination strategies — see Chaps. 6 and 7 for further details) (Fava *et al.*, 2008; Trivedi *et al.*, 2006). Evidence on the potential moderating effects of the presence of the anxious MDD subtype on the relative likelihood of responding to an SSRI versus the norepinephrine-dopamine reuptake inhibitor (NDRI) bupropion is presented in Chap. 3.

Several demographic and psychosocial factors also appear to predict poorer response to the SSRIs, including unemployment

(Frank *et al.*, 2002; Trivedi *et al.*, 2006), not living with a partner or spouse (Hirschfeld *et al.*, 1998; Trivedi *et al.*, 2005), and a lower educational status (Hirschfeld *et al.*, 1998; Trivedi *et al.*, 2006), although not all studies support these findings (Papakostas *et al.*, 2004b). A STAR*D-based report suggested lower remission rates for African-American patients with MDD than patients of other races (Lesser *et al.*, 2007; Trivedi *et al.*, 2006). A separate STAR*D report also found poorer remission rates among single mothers than mothers in two-parent households (Talati *et al.*, 2007). However, a subsequent report did not find language preference (Spanish versus English) among Hispanic outpatients to predict citalopram response (Lesser *et al.*, 2008). A separate analysis of STAR*D data does not suggest family history of depression to predict poorer acute-phase treatment outcome with citalopram monotherapy (Husain *et al.*, 2009). The degree of alcohol consumption, even in the absence of a frank alcohol-use disorder, but not the degree of caffeine or tobacco consumption also appears to a worse prognosis during the acute-phase of treatment of MDD with the SSRIs (Worthington *et al.*, 1996). A STAR*D-based report identified gender status to influence the relative likelihood of achieving remission during citalopram monotherapy in MDD, favoring women over men (Young *et al.*, 2009). Evidence on the potential moderating effects of age and gender on the relative likelihood of responding to an SSRI versus a TCA or SNRI in MDD is presented in Chap. 3.

Most studies described above that examine the potential role of several factors as possible predictors of outcome following the acute-phase of treatment of MDD with an SSRI share two major limitations: (1) they involve a relatively small sample size, resulting in limited statistical power to detect an effect of a factor on treatment outcome, and (2) they present results of analyses conducted in either univariate or bivariate fashion (i.e., simply controlling for overall depression severity at baseline). More recently, Trivedi *et al.* (2006) conducted multivariate analyses from STAR*D data, examining potential predictors of response to open-label citalopram (up to 60 mg, up to 14 weeks of treatment) in MDD, utilizing a dataset of unprecedented statistical power ($n = 2{,}876$). Variables examined as potential predictors of outcome included the following: race, gender, age, marital status, employment status, education, insurance status, family history of depression, history of suicide attempt, treatment setting (primary case versus specialty setting), age of onset of MDD, duration of current MDD episode, whether the episode was a first or recurrent, the presence of anxious depression, the presence and number of comorbid axis-I disorders (generalized anxiety disorder, obsessive-compulsive disorder, panic disorder, social phobia, post-traumatic stress disorder, agoraphobia, alcohol-use disorders, drug-use disorders, the presence of a somatoform disorder, hypochondriasis, or bulimia nervosa), the presence and extent of general medical comorbidity, overall depression symptom severity, quality of life and psychosocial functioning. Participants who were Caucasian, female, employed, or had higher levels of education or income had higher chances of success. Longer depressive episodes, more concurrent psychiatric (especially anxiety disorders and/or drug abuse) and general medical disorders, and lower baseline psychosocial functioning and quality of life were associated with poorer chances of success.

1.3.2 *Studies focusing on therapy with older antidepressants*

In general, results of these studies parallel those focusing on the use of SSRIs in MDD. While the results of two studies suggest that the presence of a comorbid personality disorder confers an increased risk of poor outcome during the treatment of MDD with the TCAs (Patience *et al.*, 1995; Reich *et al.*, 1990), the majority of studies do not support this relationship (Friedman *et al.*, 1995; Hirschfeld *et al.*, 1998; Joffe & Regan, 1989; Joyce *et al.*, 1994; Kocsis *et al.*, 1989; Mynors-Wallis & Gath, 1997; Papakostas *et al.*, 2003a; Shea *et al.*, 1990; Zuckerman *et al.*, 1980). However, two independent studies do report poorer outcome among MDD patients with than without a comorbid cluster C personality disorder during TCA treatment (Papakostas *et al.*, 2003a; Peselow *et al.*, 1992).

Neuroticism does not appear to predict TCA response in MDD (Kocsis *et al.*, 1989; Zuckerman *et al.*, 1980; Joyce *et al.*, 1994; Mynors-Wallis & Gath, 1997). The interactions of certain elements of temperament (novelty seeking, harm avoidance, and reward dependence) were found to help predict response to TCAs in one (Joyce *et al.*, 1994), but not a subsequent study (Sato *et al.*, 1999).

Some studies suggest the presence of certain demographic and psychosocial factors including the extent and quality of education (Hirschfeld *et al.*, 1998), better work functioning (Papakostas *et al.*, 2003b), living with a spouse or partner (Hirschfeld *et al.*, 1998), and the absence of marital disputes (Rounsaville *et al.*, 1979) to predict better outcome during TCA treatment of MDD, although others do not suggest a predictive role for employment (Friedman *et al.*, 1995; Hirschfeld *et al.*, 1998), marriage status (Friedman *et al.*, 1995; Kocsis *et al.*, 1989; Mynors-Wallis & Gath, 1997), or the quality of interpersonal relationships (Papakostas *et al.*, 2003b). Evidence on the potential moderating effects of age and gender on the relative likelihood of responding to TCA versus an SSRI in MDD is presented in Chap. 3.

Symptom chronicity was found to result in poor outcome during treatment of MDD with the TCAs in one (Mynors-Wallis & Gath, 1997), but not a second study (Hirschfeld *et al.*, 1998). Age of onset of depression does not appear to be predictive of TCA treatment outcome (Friedman *et al.*, 1995; Kocsis *et al.*, 1989; Valleo *et al.*, 1991). In addition, specific symptoms including insomnia (Hirschfeld *et al.*, 1998; Simon *et al.*, 1998), and suicidal ideation (Papakostas *et al.*, 2003c) do not appear to predict response to TCA treatment. However, the presence of somatic symptoms of depression (Papakostas *et al.*, 2003d), elevated cholesterol levels (Papakostas *et al.*, 2003e), but not the presence and/or extent of medical comorbidity (Papakostas *et al.*, 2003f) have been linked to lower chances of responding to the TCA nortriptyline in MDD.

Although earlier studies had suggested that patients with anxious MDD might respond more poorly to treatment with the TCAs and/or MAOIs (Flint & Rifat, 1997; Grunhaus *et al.*, 1986 and 1988), a number of studies did not find a significant relationship between the presence of an anxious MDD subtype and poorer outcome following treatment with an MAOI (Angst *et al.*, 1993; Delini-Stula *et al.*, 1995; Liebowitz *et al.*, 1988; Quitkin *et al.*, 1988 and 1990; Robinson *et al.*, 1985), or TCA (Angst *et al.*, 1993; Delini-Stula *et al.*, 1995; Friedman *et al.*, 1995; Hirschfeld *et al.*, 1998; Lenze *et al.*, 2002; Liebowitz *et al.*, 1988; Quitkin *et al.*, 1988 and 1990; Robinson *et al.*, 1985; Russell *et al.*, 2001; Simon *et al.*, 1998; Tollefson *et al.*, 1994). Evidence on the potential moderating effects of the presence of a melancholic subtype on the relative likelihood of responding to TCA versus an SSRI in MDD is presented in Chap. 3. Similarly, evidence on the potential moderating effects of the presence of an atypical MDD subtype on the relative likelihood of responding to an MAOI versus a TCA in MDD is presented in Chap. 4.

The literature focusing on other predictors of efficacy outcome during the treatment of MDD with the MAOIs is quite limited. Specifically, the presence and severity of psychomotor retardation has been found to confer a poorer chances of symptom improvement (Caligiuri *et al.*, 2003), while the extent of social support or the age of onset do not appear to be related to the likelihood of symptom improvement (Vallejo *et al.*, 1991).

1.3.3 *Studies focusing on therapy with newer antidepressants*

Relatively fewer studies specifically focus on identifying predictors of acute-phase treatment outcome (efficacy) during the treatment of MDD with newer agents. Nelson and Cloninger (1995) reported the interaction of several temperamental factors including reward dependence and harm avoidance to predict response to the serotonin-2–receptor antagonist nefazodone in MDD ($n = 18$). This was confirmed shortly thereafter using a larger database ($n = 1,119$) (Nelson & Cloninger, 1997). However, the predictive power of neuroticism in the latter study accounted for a trivial 1.1% of the total variance in outcome, raising questions regarding the clinical relevance of this finding. In a study comparing nefazodone, cognitive-behavioral analysis system of psychotherapy (CBASP), and their combination for MDD, treatment preference was found to predict treatment outcome (i.e., patients who were randomized to a treatment modality they preferred were more likely to experience remission of symptoms than patients who were not) (Kocsis *et al.*, 2009). In that same study, however, the presence of a comorbid axis-II disorder was not found to predict treatment outcome (Maddux *et al.*, 2009). Finally, the presence of a melancholic subtype did not appear to predict nefazodone response in one study (Marcus & Mendels, 1996).

The presence of a greater degree of psychomotor retardation at baseline was found to predict poorer response to bupropion (Caligiuri *et al.*, 2003). However, Rush *et al.* (2001a, 2001b, 2005) did not find the presence of pre-treatment anxiety or insomnia to confer a better or poorer prognosis during treatment with the NDRI bupropion. As discussed above, further evidence on the potential moderating effects of the presence of anxious MDD subtype on the relative likelihood of responding to an SSRI versus bupropion is presented in Chap. 3.

Sir *et al.* (2005) and Davidson *et al.* (2002) did not find that the presence of an anxious subtype of MDD or anxious symptoms in MDD influenced the likelihood of responding to venlafaxine in MDD, although Silvestone and Salinas (2001) found a slower onset of antidepressant effects among venlafaxine-treated patients with MDD and comorbid generalized anxiety disorder (GAD) than those without comorbid GAD. Similarly, patients with anxious depression, as defined by elevated scores on the HDRS-AS scale, were significantly less likely to remit following venlafaxine treatment in Level 2 of STAR*D than those without anxious MDD (Fava *et al.*, 2008). Howland *et al.* (2008) reported greater pain scores at baseline as well as greater HDRS-AS scores at baseline to predict poorer response to the SNRI duloxetine in MDD. Although in a separate analysis of the same database, Fava *et al.* (2007) reported no difference in acute treatment outcome for patients with versus without anxious depression (defined using a cut-off on the HDRS-AS subscale) during duloxetine treatment. Kornstein *et al.* (2006) found that neither age nor gender influenced efficacy outcome following treatment with the SNRI duloxetine, while Mallinckrodt *et al.* (2005) did not find the presence of a melancholic subtype to influence efficacy outcome following treatment with duloxetine. As discussed above, evidence on the potential moderating effects of age and gender on the relative likelihood of responding to an SSRI venlafaxine in MDD is presented in Chap. 3. Further evidence on the potential moderating effects of depression severity on the relative likelihood of responding to duloxetine versus an SSRI is also presented in Chap. 3.

Finally, Rush *et al.* (2008) examined multiple clinical and sociodemographic features as potential predictors of efficacy outcome for patients from STAR*D who had failed to respond to treatment with escitalopram, who were then switched to treatment with venlafaxine, bupropion, or sertraline. The presence of anxious depression (defined either as syndromal or dimensional), severe depression, melancholic depression, medical comorbidity, as well as lack symptom improvement during phase 1 of STAR*D were found to predict lower chances of remission. The presence of atypical depression was not found to be predictive. Similarly, African American patients, unemployed patients, as well as single patients were less likely to remit, while the age of onset of depression or the presence of a family history were not found to be predictive of symptom improvement. None of these factors were found to serve as moderators of differential symptom improvement during treatment with any of these three agents.

Summary and Conclusion of Chapter 1: Treatment Approaches for Patients at Risk of Treatment-Resistance

A number of potential risk factors for treatment-resistance have been identified to date, mostly from studies focusing on the acute phase of treatment of MDD with the SSRIs. These include greater illness chronicity, the presence of a greater number of concurrent psychiatric (especially anxiety disorders and or drug abuse) or general medical disorders, and the presence of poorer psychosocial functioning and quality of life. In light of (1) the paucity of studies examining predictors of efficacy outcome among newer antidepressants, (2) the multitude of studies suggesting that the overall efficacy of modern antidepressants is equivalent, and (3) the modest advantage in efficacy of antidepressants versus placebo (which suggests that the majority of symptom improvement in traditional clinical trials following the treatment of MDD with conventional antidepressants is due to non-specific therapeutic effects rather than specific drug effects), at the present time it is probably safe to assume that predictors of efficacy outcome identified from studies focusing on treatment with the SSRI can be generalized to other antidepressants as well (with few exceptions, i.e., moderators of response described in subsequent chapters). The presence of one or more of these factors should alert clinicians to alter their treatment approach in order to help optimize the chances of patients recovering from depression. Such measures may include:

1. Maintaining optimism and offering hope. In light of the considerable placebo-response seen in MDD, this may enhance the overall efficacy of treatment.
2. Identifying and then minimizing potential risk factors for resistance. This may include a standard medical work-up to identify any underlying physical illness, or a thorough psychiatric evaluation to examine for the presence of comorbid conditions including the presence of an anxiety disorder, or an alcohol/drug use disorder (or even the presence of moderate to heavy alcohol

consumption even in the absence of an alcohol-use disorder). Treatment approaches can then be employed to specifically target these comorbid conditions.

3. Educating patients about the likelihood of success of treatment and, in the possible case of non-response, about next-step treatment options available. This would help dispel any misconceptions patients often have regarding the nature of non-response to treatment in MDD. In turn, minimizing catastrophic-type thinking (i.e., "if this treatment doesn't work, I will never get better") may enhance overall treatment efficacy (Papakostas *et al.*, 2007) and adherence.
4. Educating patients regarding the time course of symptom improvement during treatment with antidepressants. Specifically, in most cases, several weeks of treatment are required before any benefits are manifested. This, in turn, may reduce the likelihood of patients discontinuing treatment early-on due to inefficacy as well as reassure patients early-on and minimize catastrophic-type thinking (thereby potentially improving outcome).
5. Educating patients regarding common and uncommon side effects of treatment, as well as strategies that may alleviate such side effects. In turn, this may reduce the likelihood of treatment non-adherence.
6. Choosing treatments that may result in better outcome than standard treatment (i.e., antidepressant monotherapy or the use of psychotherapy alone). This may include a combination of two drugs from the onset of treatment (see Chap. 5 for further details), or a combination of pharmacotherapy and psychotherapy from the onset of treatment (Pampallona *et al.*, 2004; Thase *et al.*, 1997).
7. Instituting more frequent follow-up periods in order to address side effects and non-response in a timelier manner.
8. Requiring shorter time-periods before declaring a treatment ineffective and moving to a subsequent treatment (particularly in light of strict non-response).

Part I

First-Line Pharmacotherapy Strategies

Introduction to Part I: The Discovery of the First Antidepressants

A number of key observations in the 1950s and 60s linking the monoamines (serotonin, norepinephrine and dopamine) to mood, perception and cognition were pivotal in the formulation of the monoamine hypothesis of depression, published the same year (1965) by Schildkraut in the *American Journal of Psychiatry* (Schildkraut, 1965) and by Bunney and Davis in the *Archives of General Psychiatry* (Bunney & Davis, 1965). The antihypertensive reserpine, which was noted to precipitate depression in some cases (Muller *et al.*, 1955), was also found to decrease urine serotonin (5HT) levels (Shore *et al.*, 1955), an effect reversed by administration of the dopamine and norepinephrine precursor DOPA (Degkewitz *et al.*, 1960).

These initial observations were followed by the serendipitous discovery of the precursors of two of the major contemporary antidepressant families, the monoamine oxidase inhibitors (MAOIs) and the tricyclic antidepressants (TCAs). Specifically, the administration of iproniazid, an antimycobacterial agent, was first noted to possess antidepressant effects in depressed patients suffering from tuberculosis (Crane, 1956). Shortly there after, iproniazid was found to inhibit the monoamine oxidase enzyme, involved in the catabolism of serotonin, norepinephrine and dopamine. In parallel, imipramine was initially developed as an antihistamine, but Kuhn *et al.* (1958)

discovered that of some 500 patients with various psychiatric disorders treated, only those with endogenous depression with mental and motor retardation showed a remarkable improvement after about one to six weeks of daily imipramine therapy. The same compound was subsequently found to inhibit the reuptake of serotonin and norepinephrine (Gershon *et al.*, 1962; Glowinski & Axelrod, 1964). Thus, it was the discovery of the antidepressant effects of iproniazid and imipramine that led to the development of the MAOIs and TCAs, but also such discovery was instrumental in the formulation of the monoamine theory of depression in 1965. In turn, guided by this theory, the subsequent development of compounds selective for the reuptake of either serotonin or norepinephrine or both was designed, rather than accidental. As a result, over the last few decades, these focused efforts have resulted in the creation of a wide variety of monoamine-based antidepressants with a variety of, even opposing (selective serotonin reuptake inhibitors — SSRIs and tianeptine, for example), mechanisms of action.

In this first part of the book, we discuss the use of various pharmacologic strategies used as first-line treatment for MDD. The first three chapters of this section focus on the use of monoaminergic agents as treatments for MDD. Drugs are grouped according to the number of monoaminergic systems involved with respect to their immediate mechanism of action (single-acting agents are described in Chap. 2, dual-acting agents are described in Chap. 3, and triple-acting agents are described in Chap. 4), and their indications, efficacy, safety, and tolerability are discussed in detail. The final chapter in Part I will focus on reviewing studies which examine whether it is possible to optimize treatment outcome by initiating therapy with two agents rather than one, termed co-initiation therapy or co-therapy. Co-initiation therapy strategies will be described as belonging to one of three families: (1) monoamine-based, (2) neuroendocrine-based, and (3) miscellaneous agents. The review will focus on co-therapy studies that do not exclusively involve treatment-resistant populations, since the use of polypharmacy strategies for treatment-resistant depression represents a distinct clinical challenge, and is described in Part II of this book.

Chapter 2

Monoaminergic-Based Strategies: "Single-Acting" Agents

2.1 Monoamine Precursors for Depression

Tryptophan and 5-hydroxytryptophan (5HTP) are precursors of serotonin, and have been studied for decades as a treatment for depression (Fugh-Bergman & Cott, 1999), although it has been suggested that tryptophan itself may be insufficient to boost Central Nervous System (CNS) serotonin levels (van Praag, 1981; van Praag *et al.*, 1986). 5HTP has the advantage of bypassing the conversion of tryptophan into 5HTP by the enzyme tryptophan hydroxylase, which is the rate-limiting step in serotonin synthesis. Numerous mostly small uncontrolled studies but also some double-blind studies have shown positive effects for tryptophan and 5HTP in the treatment of depression (Birdsall, 1998; Fugh-Berman & Cott, 1999; Meyers, 2000). However, the results of a meta-analysis of studies on the use of tryptophan and 5HTP in depression reveal that, while tryptophan and 5HTP appear to be more effective than placebo, the present evidence is inconclusive, due to the large number of underpowered studies or studies with methodological limitations (Shaw *et al.*, 2002a and b). In fact, of 108 studies reviewed in that meta-analysis, only two were found suitable for inclusion.

Tryptophan is no longer available in the United States due the emergence of eosinophilia-myalgia syndrome (EMS) associated with its use, characterized by eosinophilia, fever, abdominal pain, dyspnea, skin rash, and elevated serum concentrations of aminotransferase and aldolase (Hertzman *et al.*, 1990). Cases of EMS with

5HTP have also been reported (Michelson *et al.*, 1994). The role of a β-carbolene derivative in the development of EMS, found to contaminate the tryptophan and 5HTP preparations of some of those affected, has been postulated (Fugh-Berman & Cott, 1999; Michelson *et al.*, 1994; Williamson *et al.*, 1997, 1998a, b, c, and d). There are also reports of serotonin syndrome when tryptophan was combined with SSRIs (Steiner & Fontaine, 1986), as well as reports of fatalities when tryptophan was combined with MAOIs (Brennan *et al.*, 1988; Staufenberg & Tantam, 1989).

Tyrosine is the precursor of norepinephrine, and L-phenylalanine is the direct precursor of tyrosine. In a double-blind study, DL-phenylalanine (150–200 mg/day) or imipramine were administered to 40 depressed patients (20 in each group) for one month. No statistically significant difference in the resolution of depressive symptoms was found between the two groups, leading to the conclusion that DL-phenylalanine (DLPA) might have antidepressant properties (Beckmann *et al.*, 1979). A subsequent open trial of oral phenylalanine (Sabelli *et al.*, 1986) also reported a significant decrease in depressive symptoms during the treatment of depression. Two small case studies suggested L-tyrosine might have potential as an antidepressant as well (Gelenberg *et al.*, 1980; Goldberg, 1980). However, a four-week, double-blind clinical trial involving 65 outpatients with major depression randomized to receive L-tyrosine (100 mg/kg per day), imipramine, or placebo did not demonstrate an antidepressant effect for L-tyrosine (Gelenberg *et al.*, 1990). The development of phenylalanine-derivative compounds as antidepressants has been underway for some time (Amsterdam *et al.*, 2002). However, trials involving the use of such agents for depression have yet to be published.

Levodopa (L-Dopa, Sinemet) is the immediate precursor of dopamine, and is approved by the U.S. Food and Drug Administration (FDA) for the treatment of Parkinson's disease. A single controlled trial did not reveal levidopa/carbidopa (Sinemet) to be more effective than placebo in the treatment of seasonal affective disorder (Oren *et al.*, 1994). No other studies involving the use of Levodopa for depression have been published.

2.2 Selective Serotonin Reuptake Inhibitors (SSRIs)

2.2.1 *Neuropharmacology*

The immediate mechanism of action of the SSRIs is to inhibit the neuronal reuptake of serotonin by blocking the serotonin transporter (Bolden-Watson *et al.*, 1993; Owens *et al.*, 2001). In addition to this, some SSRIs appear to have effects at other monoamine receptors, with sertraline demonstrating mild dopaminergic reuptake inhibition and paroxetine demonstrating mild noradrenergic reuptake inhibition (Bolden-Watson *et al.*, 1993; Owens *et al.*, 2001). In addition, fluoxetine, particularly its R stereo-isomer, has been found to possess mild 5HT2A and 5HT2C antagonist activity, which may explain the increase in norepinephrine and dopamine in the prefrontal cortex of animals treated with fluoxetine (Koch *et al.*, 2002), as well as mild noradrenergic reuptake inhibition (Koch *et al.*, 2002; Owens *et al.*, 2001).

The SSRIs have minimal or no affinity for cholinergic receptors, with the exception of paroxetine which is a weak cholinergic receptor antagonist (Koch *et al.*, 2002; Owens *et al.*, 2001). The effects of the SSRIs on various histaminergic and α-adrenergic receptors are negligible (Koch *et al.*, 2002; Owens *et al.*, 2001). For these reasons, treatment with the SSRIs is associated with greater improvements in memory and cognitive performance than the TCAs (Keegan *et al.*, 1991; Levkovitz *et al.*, 2002). This, in turn, may explain the greater improvement in psychosocial and work functioning in patients with major depressive disorder (MDD) treated with SSRIs than TCAs (Finkel *et al.*, 1999; Lydiard *et al.*, 1997). Treatment with the SSRIs also appears to be associated with lower rates of gait disturbance than the TCAs (Lemke & Wendorff, 2000), an important consideration in the medically ill and the elderly.

Various non-monoaminergic effects have also been described for these agents. Paroxetine, for instance, also appears to inhibit the enzyme nitric oxide synthase (NOS), resulting in a decrease in nitric oxide and an increase in the metabolic end products of nitric oxide in humans (Finkel *et al.*, 1996; Lara *et al.*, 2003a). Fluoxetine has also been found to depress glutamate exocytosis in the rat cerebrocortical nerve terminals (synaptosomes) via inhibition of P/Q-type Ca^{2+} channels (Wang *et al.*, 2003). Fluoxetine (Fryer & Lukas, 1999; Maggi *et al.*, 1998), sertraline, and paroxetine also appear to act as non-competitive antagonists of nicotinic acetyl cholinergic receptors (Fryer and Lukas, 1999). In addition, fluoxetine (Choi *et al.*, 1999; Choi *et al.*, 2001; Hajdu *et al.*, 2003; Terstappen *et al.*, 2003; Thomas *et al.*, 2002; Yeung *et al.*, 1999), norfluoxetine (Choi *et al.*, 2001), and fluvoxamine (Milnes *et al.*, 2003) have also been reported to inhibit potassium channels, while fluoxetine also appears to be a weak inhibitor of sodium channels in some laboratory studies as well (Pancrazio *et al.*, 1998). Finally, fluvoxamine also appears to possess affinity for the σ-1 receptors (Ishikawa *et al.*, 2007).

2.2.2 *Efficacy (general)*

Zimeldine (Normud, Zelmid) and Indalpine (Upstene) were the first marketed SSRIs. However, zimeldine has been banned worldwide in 1983 due to serious, sometimes fatal cases of central and/or peripheral neuropathy known as Guillain–Barre syndrome (Bengtsson *et al.*, 1994; Fagius *et al.*, 1985; Naranjo *et al.*, 1990; Xiang *et al.*, 1997). Similarly, Indalpene was withdrawn due to reports of neutropenia (Grosbois *et al.*, 1985). To date, six SSRIs are available in the U.S. [fluoxetine (Prozac), paroxetine (Paxil and Paxil CR), sertraline (Zoloft), fluvoxamine (Luvox), citalopram (Celexa), and escitalopram (Lexapro)]. All but one (fluvoxamine) have been approved by the FDA for the treatment of MDD.

Abundant evidence in support of the SSRIs for the treatment of MDD in adults comes by way of more than 60 double-blind, placebo-controlled trials, more than any other antidepressant class (Papakostas & Fava, 2006b). The overall efficacy of the SSRIs in the treatment of adults with MDD is equivalent to the efficacy of the older TCAs (Anderson, 2001), and the MAOIs moclobemide (Papakostas & Fava, 2006a) and phenelzine (Pande *et al.*, 1996), while five of the SSRIs (fluoxetine, sertraline, paroxetine, citalopram, fluvoxamine) appear to be relatively equally effective in the treatment of MDD. In addition, the SSRIs appear to be as effective as the TCAs in the treatment of anxious MDD (Hoehn-Saric *et al.*, 2000; Marchesi *et al.*, 1998; Moon *et al.*, 1994; Simon *et al.*, 1998; Tollefson *et al.*, 1994a; Versiani *et al.*, 1999), or MDD presenting with prominent agitation (Tollefson *et al.*, 1994b), or insomnia (Simon *et al.*, 1998). There is some evidence to suggest that the SSRI escitalopram may be more effective than the remaining five SSRIs when treating MDD, particularly for patients with severe depression (Kennedy *et al.*, 2009) (Figs. 2.1 and 2.2).

The SSRIs also appear to be effective in the treatment of a number of MDD symptoms in addition to depressed mood, including suicidal ideation (Beasley *et al.*, 1991a and 2007; Montgomery *et al.*, 1995; Pedersen, 2005 and 2006), anxiety (Bandelow *et al.*, 2007; Fava *et al.*, 1998), anger/hostility (Fava *et al.*, 1993), fatigue (Judge *et al.*, 2000; Papakostas *et al.*, 2006a), and insomnia (Fava *et al.*, 2002; Lader *et al.*, 2005), but not hypersomnia (Papakostas *et al.*, 2006a). Overall, to date, the SSRIs enjoy the broadest spectrum of efficacy in the treatment of depressive disorders as well as in the treatment of psychiatric disorders often encountered in patients with MDD (see

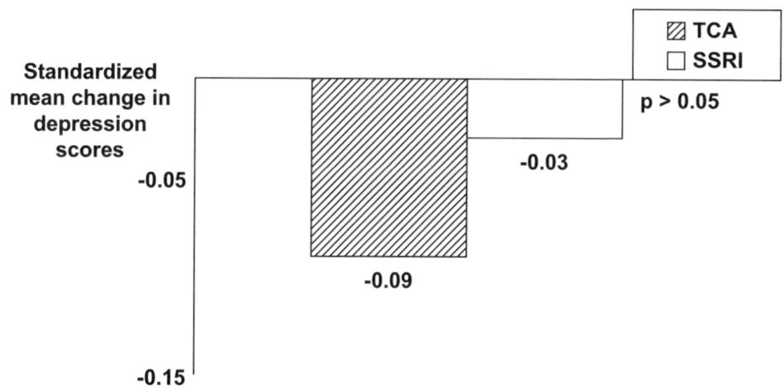

Fig. 2.1 Comparative efficacy of TCAs versus SSRIs in Depression: Meta analysis of 102 RCTs ($n = 10{,}706$) RCT: Randomized, Controlled Trial. [Data extracted from: Anderson, I.M. (2000). Selective serotonin reuptake inhibitors versus tricyclic antidepressants: A meta-analysis of efficacy and tolerability. *Journal of Affective Disorders*, 58, 19–36.]

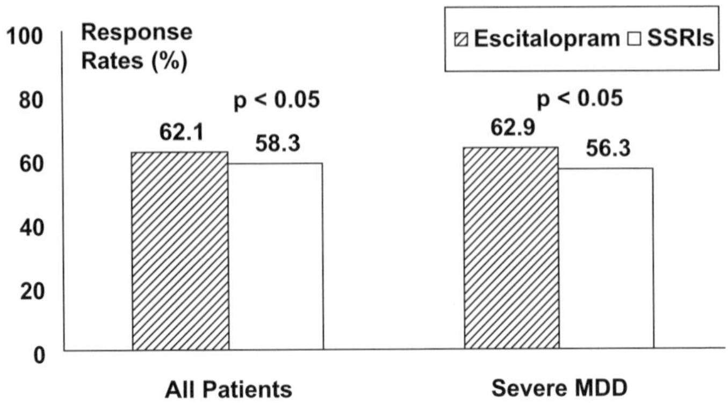

Fig. 2.2 Escitalopram versus the other SSRIs in MDD: Pooled analysis of 12 RCTs. [Data extracted from: Kennedy, S.H., Andersen, H.F., & Thase, M.E. (2009). Escitalopram in the treatment of major depressive disorder: A meta-analysis. *Current Medical and Research Opinion*, 25(1), 161–175.]

Appendices 2, 3 and 4 for a summary). Due to the ample evidence supporting their efficacy in a variety of populations and depressive disorders, as well as their favorable safety and tolerability profile, the SSRIs are used as first-line treatment in the overwhelming majority of cases, with more than 90% of clinicians in one survey indicating SSRIs as their first-line treatment preference (Petersen *et al.*, 2002).

Specifically, the efficacy of the SSRIs in the treatment of MDD in children/adolescents (Emslie *et al.*, 1997, 2002 and 2009; Wagner *et al.*, 2003 and 2004), and the elderly (Rapaport *et al.*, 2003 and 2009; Schneider *et al.*, 2003; Tollefson *et al.*, 1995) has been demonstrated in several double-blind, placebo-controlled trials. The efficacy of the SSRIs has also been established in other depressive disorders including dysthymic disorder (Hellerstein *et al.*, 1993; Ravindran *et al.*, 2000; Thase *et al.*, 1996; Vanelle *et al.*, 1997), minor depressive disorder (Judd *et al.*, 2004), and seasonal affective disorder (Lam *et al.*, 1995).

The efficacy of the SSRI antidepressants specifically, as well as all antidepressants in general, whether used as monotherapy or adjunctive therapy for the treatment of major depressive episodes in patients with bipolar disorder remains questionable.

Specifically, although the results of one (Cohn *et al.*, 1989), but not a second small, randomized, double-blind, placebo-controlled study (Amsterdam & Shults, 2005) supports the use of the SSRI fluoxetine as monotherapy for the treatment of major depressive episodes in patients with bipolar disorder, the results of larger, placebo-controlled trials do not support the use of the SSRIs either as monotherapy (McElroy *et al.*, 2008) or as an adjunct to mood-stabilizer treatment for bipolar depression (Nemeroff *et al.*, 2001; Sachs *et al.*, 2007). Similarly, although the results of a recent placebo-controlled study support the use of fluoxetine as an adjunct to the atypical antipsychotic olanzapine for bipolar depression (Tohen *et al.*, 2003), this finding has yet to be replicated. Randomized, double-blind, placebo-controlled studies focusing on the use of escitalopram (clinicaltrials.gov, NCT00464191), and citalopram (clinicaltrials.gov, NCT00562861) as an adjunct to mood-stabilizer therapy for the treatment of major depressive episodes in patients with bipolar disorder are pending.

The results of one randomized, placebo-controlled trial also support the use of fluoxetine as an adjunct to the atypical antipsychotic agent olanzapine for the treatment of MDD with psychotic symptoms (Rothschild *et al.*, 2004). This was recently replicated in a study examining the use of the SSRI sertraline as an adjunct to olanzapine for MDD with psychotic features (Meyers *et al.*, 2009).

Double-blind, randomized, placebo-controlled trials also support the use of fluoxetine and sertraline for the treatment of patients with MDD and comorbid alcohol use disorders (Cornelius *et al.*, 1997; Roy, 1998). However, the SSRIs do not appear to be more effective than placebo in the treatment of comorbid MDD and substance use disorders (Dean *et al.*, 2002; Petrakis *et al.*, 1998; Schmit *et al.*, 2001). There are also data from placebo-controlled trials supporting the use of the SSRIs for the treatment (fluoxetine — Appleby *et al.*, 1997) or prevention (sertraline — Wisner *et al.*, 2004) of post-partum depression, although a second placebo-controlled trial of SSRIs (paroxetine) for the treatment of post-partum MDD demonstrated greater antidepressant effects for paroxetine than placebo on

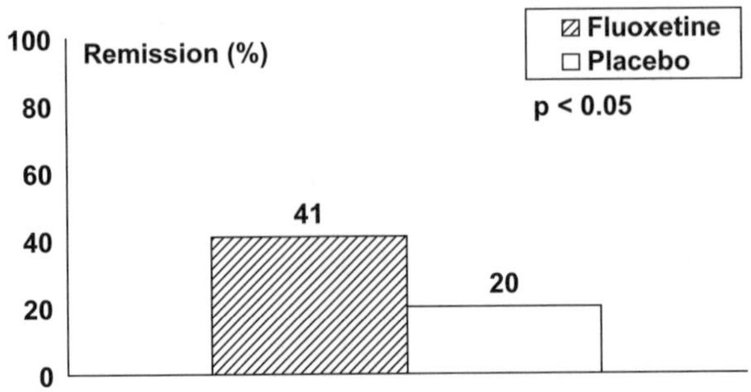

Fig. 2.3 Fluoxetine (SSRI) for the treatment of MDD in children and adolescents: A randomized, double-blind study ($n = 219$). [Data extracted from: Emslie, G.J., Heiligenstein, J.H., Wagner, K.D., *et al.* (2002). Fluoxetine for acute treatment of depression in children and adolescents: A placebo-controlled, randomized clinical trial. *Journal of the American Academy of Child and Adolescent Psychiatry*, 41, 1205–1215.]

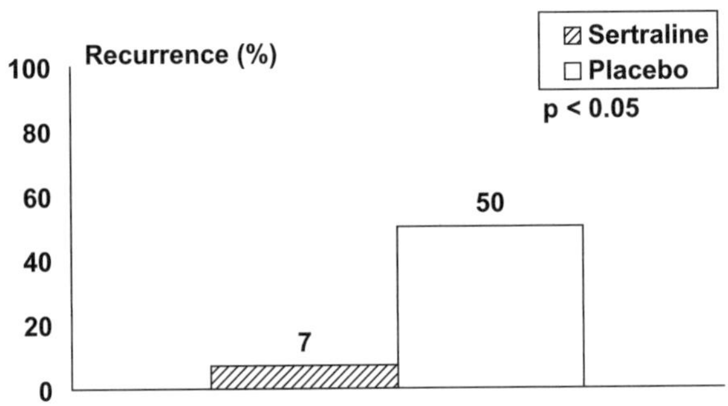

Fig. 2.4 Prevention of postpartum depression: A randomized, double-blind trial ($n = 22$). [Data extracted from: Wisner, K.L., Perel, J.M., Peindl, K.S., *et al.* (2004). Prevention of postpartum depression: A pilot randomized clinical trial. *American Journal of Psychiatry*, 161, 1290–1292.]

secondary but not primary efficacy measures (Yonkers *et al.*, 2008) (Figs. 2.3–2.5).

Finally, there is evidence from randomized, double-blind, placebo-controlled trial(s) to support the use of the SSRIs in psychiatric disorders often found comorbid in patients with MDD including generalized anxiety disorder (GAD) (Rickels *et al.*, 2006), panic disorder and agoraphobia (Bakker *et al.*, 2000), obsessive compulsive

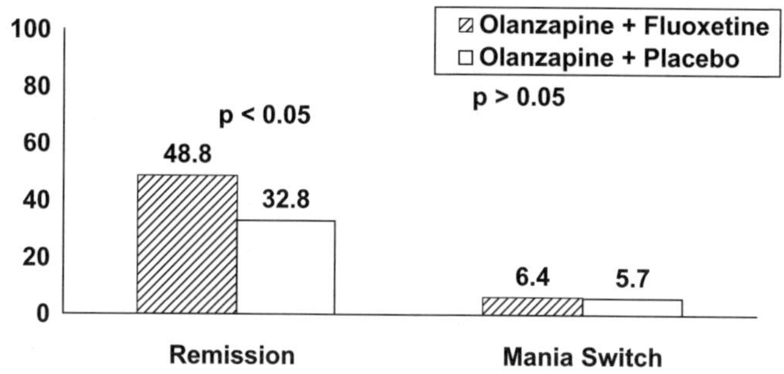

Fig. 2.5 Olanzapine plus fluoxetine (SSRI) in bipolar I depression: A randomized, double-blind study (n = 456). [Data extracted from: Tohen, M., Vieta, E., Calabrese, J., *et al.* (2003). Efficacy of olanzapine and olanzapine-fluoxetine combination in the treatment of bipolar I depression. *Archives of General Psychiatry*, 60, 1079–1088.]

disorder (OCD) (Pigott & Seay, 1999), social anxiety disorder (SAD) (Blanco *et al.*, 2003), post-traumatic stress disorder (PTSD) (Stein *et al.*, 2000), fibromyalgia (Arnold *et al.*, 2002; Patkar *et al.*, 2007), anorexia nervosa (Kaye *et al.*, 2001), bulimia nervosa (Fluoxetine Bulimia Nervosa Collaborative Study Group, 1992), and binge eating disorder (Arnold *et al.*, 2002) but not attention deficit (hyperactivity) disorder [AD(H)D].

2.2.3 *Efficacy in patients with medical conditions*

The safety, tolerability, and efficacy of the SSRIs for the treatment of MDD in patients with comorbid medical disorders has been extensively studied.

2.2.3.1 *Diabetes mellitus*

There have been several uncontrolled studies focusing on the use of fluoxetine for the treatment of depression in diabetic patients (Goodnick, 2001). The majority of these studies suggest that the use of SSRIs in diabetic patients represents a relatively safe treatment approach, although there have been case reports of hypo- (Deeg & Lipkin, 1996; Pollak *et al.*, 2001) or hyper-glycemia (Oswald *et al.*,

2003; Petty, 1996; Sansone & Sansone, 2003) during SSRI treatment. At least four randomized, double-blind, placebo-controlled trials focusing on the prevention or treatment of MDD in diabetic patients have been published to date. Specifically, there is evidence to support the use of sertraline for the prevention of depression recurrence for patients with diabetes (Lustman *et al.*, 2006), as well as for fluoxetine (Lustman *et al.*, 2000), but not escitalopram (Pollock *et al.*, 2006), or paroxetine (Paile-Hyvairinen *et al.*, 2007) for the treatment of depression in patients with diabetes.

2.2.3.2 *Coronary artery disease and myocardial infarction*

The results of a large ($n = 369$) randomized clinical trial of sertraline versus placebo for the treatment of MDD in patients hospitalized for an acute myocardial infarction (MI) or unstable angina revealed sertraline to be safe and effective, without significant adverse effects on left ventricular ejection fraction, ventricular premature complex (VPC) runs, or QTc interval length (Glassman *et al.*, 2002). The treatment of MDD with sertraline for patients hospitalized for an acute MI or unstable angina has also been shown to be more effective than placebo in restoring psychosocial functioning (Swenson *et al.*, 2003). Sertraline has also been found to accelerate the rate of autonomic recovery in post-MI depressed patients (McFarlane *et al.*, 2001). More recently, the results of a double-blind, placebo-controlled trial also support the safety and efficacy of citalopram for patients with MDD and comorbid coronary artery disease (Lesperance *et al.*, 2007). However, a double-blind, placebo-controlled trial failed to demonstrate the efficacy of fluoxetine for depression in the post-MI setting (Strik *et al.*, 2000). Finally, there is also a case report of SSRIs being useful for the treatment of recurrent syncope due to carotid sinus hypersensitivity resistant to dual chamber cardiac pacing (Grubb *et al.*, 1994).

Some SSRIs have also been shown to reduce markers of cardiovascular system activation or inflammation, including cytokine (TNF-α)-induced endothelial adhesion molecule (VCAM-1 and ICAM-1) expression, endothelial adhesiveness to monocytes (U937) and the circulating levels of vascular adhesion molecules (VCAM-1 and ICAM 1) *in vitro* (Lekakis *et al.*, in press). Escitalopram, similar to other SSRIs (Hayes, 2004), also appears to exhibit antiplatelet activity in humans, which may render it an attractive treatment option for depression in the post-MI setting (Atar *et al.*, 2006 and 2007), while treatment with sertraline in depressed post-acute coronary syndrome patients also appears to be associated with reductions in markers of platelet/endothelial activation (β-thromboglobulin and P-selectin) (Serebruany *et al.*, 2003).

2.2.3.3 *Pulmonary and sleep disorders*

The use of SSRIs in patients with MDD and chronic obstructive pulmonary disease (COPD) has not been systematically assessed. However, administration of SSRIs in patients with obstructive sleep apnea has been shown to result in various beneficial effects in a number of patients including an increase in the minimum night-time percentage of oxygen saturation (Kopelman *et al.*, 1992), a decrease in the apnea/hypopnea ratio during non-random eye movement (REM) sleep (Kopelman *et al.*, 1992; Kraiczi *et al.*, 1999), a decrease in the number of apneas and hypopneas during non-REM sleep (Hanzel *et al.*, 1991), and an increase in peak genioglossus muscle activity during non-REM sleep (Berry *et al.*, 1999). Due to their REM-suppressing effects (Winokur *et al.*, 2001), the SSRIs may also relieve symptoms of cataplexy in patients with narcolepsy (Frey & Darbonne, 1994; Schachter & Parkes, 1980; Thirumali & Shubin, 2000). More recently, a double-blind, placebo-controlled trial failed to demonstrate the efficacy of citalopram for the treatment of MDD in patients with asthma, although citalopram-treated patients required fewer corticosteroid treatments during the trial (Brown *et al.*, 2005). Finally, the results of an epidemiological study suggest that SSRI treatment may decrease mortality among patients with primary pulmonary hypertension and depression/anxiety (Shah *et al.*, 2009).

2.2.3.4 *Cerebrovascular illness and stroke*

A number of placebo-controlled trials focus on the use of the SSRIs for the *treatment* of post-stroke depression. Fluoxetine, for example, has been found to be safe and more effective than placebo in the treatment of post-stroke depression in some (Fruehwald *et al.*, 2003; Wiart *et al.*, 2000), but not other trials (Choi-Kwon *et al.*, 2006; Robinson *et al.*, 2000). Sertraline was not found to be more effective than placebo when treating minor or mild depression in post-stroke depression in one study (Murray *et al.*, 2005). However citalopram was found to be effective when treating post-stroke depression in a separate study (Andersen *et al.*, 1994). The results of a double-blind, randomized, placebo-controlled trial do not support the use of paroxetine for the treatment of post-stroke depression (GSK study PAR625).

There are also studies focusing on the use of SSRIs to *prevent* rather than treat post-stroke depression. Fluoxetine, more so than placebo, was also found to increase the survival of both depressed and non-depressed stroke patients after a six-month follow-up (Jorge *et al.*, 2003). Non-depressed patients randomized to sertraline (Rasmussen *et al.*, 2003), escitalopram (Robinson *et al.*, 2008), or fluoxetine (Narushima *et al.*, 2002) were also less likely to develop depression after a stroke than those randomized to placebo, although the results of a subsequent study by Almeida *et al.* (2006) involving the use of sertraline for the prevention of post-stroke depression were not consistent with that of the earlier trial by Rasmussen *et al.* (no statistically significant treatment effect).

2.2.3.5 *Movement disorders*

Non-placebo-controlled studies also support the use of the SSRI sertraline in the treatment of depression (Mohr *et al.*, 2001a), and fatigue (Mohr *et al.*, 2003) in patients with multiple sclerosis (MS). Sertraline also appears to concomitantly reduce interferon-γ production by peripheral blood mononuclear cells in MS patients (Mohr *et al.*, 2001b). There is also preliminary evidence to suggest that fluoxetine may reduce or slow the formation of new enhancing lesions in non-depressed patients with MS (Mostert *et al.*, 2008). However, a randomized, double-blind, placebo-controlled trial of the SSRI paroxetine for the treatment of MDD in patients with multiple sclerosis did not demonstrate greater antidepressant effects for paroxetine than placebo (Ehde *et al.*, 2008). There is also anecdotal evidence supporting the use of citalopram for the treatment of MDD in patients with tuberous sclerosis (Muzykewicz *et al.*, 2007), or in patients with MDD following a traumatic brain injury (Rapoport *et al.*, 2008).

Although some patients with Parkinson's disease may experience a worsening of motor symptoms during SSRI administration, these effects do not appear to be consistent (Ceravolo *et al.*, 2000; Dell'Agnello *et al.*, 2001; Devos *et al.*, 2008; Tesei *et al.*, 2000). In fact, a small open trial also suggests treatment with citalopram to improve bradykinesia in many patients with Parkinson's disease (Rampello *et al.*, 2002). However, the efficacy of the SSRIs in the treatment of MDD in Parkinson's disease is unclear. Specifically, a number of open-label trials had suggested that the SSRIs may alleviate MDD in some patients with Parkinson's disease (Ceravolo *et al.*, 2000; Dell'Agnello *et al.*, 2001; Devos *et al.*, 2008; Hauser & Zesiewicz, 1997; Marino *et al.*, 2008; Tesei *et al.*, 2000). However, the results of double-blind, placebo-controlled trials do not support the use of citalopram (Wermuth *et al.*, 1998), or paroxetine controlled release formulation (CR) (Menza *et al.*, 2009) for the treatment of depression in patients with Parkinson's disease. Finally, a more recent, subsequent randomized, double-blind, placebo- and desipramine-controlled trial did demonstrate greater antidepressant effects following treatment of MDD in patients with Parkinson's disease with the SSRI citalopram or the noradrenergic TCA desipramine, although desipramine treatment led to a more rapid improvement of depressive symptoms than citalopram treatment (Devos *et al.*, 2008).

2.2.3.6 *Epilepsy*

Open trials of citalopram support its use in patients with MDD and comorbid epilepsy (Hovorka *et al.*, 2000; Kuhn *et al.*, 2003). The SSRIs also appear to have some anticonvulsant effects *in vitro* (Leander,

1992; Pasini *et al.*, 1992; Prendiville & Gale, 1993), and in clinical trial populations (Alper *et al.*, 2007), while there is anecdotal evidence for an anticonvulsant role for the SSRIs in epilepsy (Favale *et al.*, 1995 and 2003), perhaps related to GABA-ergic effects of some SSRIs (Bhagwagar *et al.*, 2004; Członkowska *et al.*, 2003; Sanacora *et al.*, 2002).

2.2.3.7 *Dementia*

Several placebo-controlled studies have also examined the role of the SSRIs for the treatment of depression in patients with dementia. Specifically, double-blind, placebo-controlled trials support the efficacy of sertraline (Lyketsos *et al.*, 2003), but not fluoxetine (Petracca *et al.*, 2001) in the treatment of MDD in patients with Alzheimer's dementia. However, sertraline was not found to be more effective in relieving depression than placebo among nursing home–bound patients with late-stage Alzheimer's dementia (Magai *et al.*, 2000). Finally, Nyth *et al.* (1992) reported a greater resolution of depressive symptoms among citalopram- than placebo-treated patients with depression and dementia.

2.2.3.8 *Renal insufficiency*

Treatment of depression in hemodialysis patients with fluoxetine appears safe, yielding fluoxetine and norfluoxetine blood levels comparable to those of patients with normal renal function (Blumenfield *et al.*, 1997; Levy *et al.*, 1996), and more effective than placebo (Blumenfield *et al.*, 1997). In fact, the SSRIs fluoxetine and sertraline may also be beneficial with regards to alleviating postural hypotension in hemodialysis patients, present in up to 50% of patients with end-stage renal disease (Brewster *et al.*, 2003; Chin *et al.*, 1996; Dheenan *et al.*, 1998; Parazella, 2001). There is also an open-label study describing the use of fluvoxamine for depression in patients on hemodialysis (Kamo *et al.*, 2004), as well as an open-label study focusing on the use of citalopram for the treatment of depression in this patient population (Kalender *et al.*, 2007).

2.2.3.9 *Hepatitis, cirrhosis, and interferon therapy*

Several open-label trials support the use of citalopram and escitalopram for patients with MDD and hepatitis C (Gleason *et al.*, 2002, 2004, and 2005). The use of citalopram for the treatment of depression in patients with hepatitis C also appears not to worsen aspartate aminotransferase, alanine aminotransferase, or γ-glutamyltransferase levels (Gleason *et al.*, 2002) and, in the absence of severe hepatic impairment, does not result in toxic citalopram levels (Gleason *et al.*, 2004). However, the results of a literature review suggest caution when combining SSRIs with non-steroidal anti-inflammatory drugs (NSAIDs) in patients who are at risk of bleeding (i.e., cirrhosis) (Weinrieb *et al.*, 2003). The SSRIs appear to be useful and safe for the treatment of interferon-α (INF-α) related depressive disorder (Farah, 2002; Hauser *et al.*, 2002; Kraus *et al.*, 2002 and 2008; Levenson & Fallon, 1993; Schramm *et al.*, 2000), and for the prevention of INF-α related depressive disorders (Capuron *et al.*, 2002; Hauser *et al.*, 2000; Musselman *et al.*, 2001), perhaps by attenuating the behavioral consequences of interferon-α mediated tryptophan depletion (Capuron *et al.*, 2003). On the other hand, nitric oxide has also been implicated in INF-α related depression (Suzuki *et al.*, 2003). However, not all placebo-controlled studies examining the role of the SSRIs in preventing interferon-α-induced depression have been positive (Raison *et al.*, 2007).

2.2.3.10 *Human immunodeficiency virus*

The SSRIs appear to be safe in the treatment of depression in patients tested positive for human immunodeficiency virus (HIV+) (Cazzullo *et al.*, 1998; Currier *et al.*, 2004; Ferrando *et al.*, 1999 and 1997; Grassi *et al.*, 1997; Judd *et al.*, 1995; Rabkin *et al.*, 1999), with no significant reductions in CD4 cell count (Ferrando *et al.*, 1999), and more effective than placebo in the treatment of depression in HIV+ patients (Elliott *et al.*, 1998; Rabkin *et al.*, 1999; Zisook *et al.*, 1998). There is potential, however, for drug interactions between antiretroviral agents and the SSRIs that must be taken into consideration when treating MDD in HIV+ patients (Desilva *et al.*, 2001; Eralp Bellibas, 1999; Ouellet *et al.*, 1998).

2.2.3.11 *Malignancy*

There are reports of using the SSRIs for the treatment of depression in advanced cancer (Fisch *et al.*, 2003; Holland *et al.*, 1998; Torta *et al.*, 2007), breast cancer (Pezzella *et al.*, 2001), hematological malignancy (Pae *et al.*, 2004), and for the treatment of hot flashes in women with breast cancer (Weitzner *et al.*, 2002). The results of a placebo-controlled study of paroxetine in cancer patients on chemotherapy also reported a significantly greater reduction in depressive symptoms but not fatigue in the paroxetine group (Morrow *et al.*, 2003). In addition, in a separate study, paroxetine appeared to be more effective in reducing depressive symptoms but not fatigue among women with breast cancer undergoing chemotherapy (Roscoe *et al.*, 2005). A double-blind, placebo-controlled trial failed to demonstrate the efficacy of fluoxetine for the treatment of depression among women with breast cancer (Musselman *et al.*, 2006). However, a more recent randomized, double-blind, placebo-controlled trial of fluoxetine for the treatment of depression in women with end-stage breast cancer undergoing adjuvant therapy revealed a greater reduction in depressive symptoms, as well as a greater probability of completion of adjuvant therapy and better quality of life among fluoxetine- than placebo-treated patients (Navari *et al.*, 2008). In parallel, the results of a randomized, double-blind, placebo-controlled trial of citalopram for the prevention of MDD during the treatment of head and neck cancer demonstrated lower rates of emergence of MDD following administration of citalopram than placebo (Lydiatt *et al.*, 2008). There is also an open-label trial of sertraline for depression in patients treated with gonadotropin-releasing hormone agonists (Warnock *et al.*, 1998). The use of SSRIs in conjunction with tamoxifen does not appear to alter the protective effects of tamoxifen with regards to the prevention of breast-cancer recurrence (Lash *et al.*, 2008).

2.2.3.12 *Transplant recipients*

There is limited data on the use of the SSRIs in transplant recipients. A single chart review involving 13 depressed organ transplant recipients treated with fluoxetine revealed no serious adverse events, and no significant alterations in cyclosporine levels or graft function in fluoxetine-treated patients (Strouse *et al.*, 1996). There is also a case report of depression after cardiac transplant treated with paroxetine and psychotherapy (Miller, 2002).

2.2.4 *Side effect profile*

2.2.4.1 *General*

Nausea and upper gastro-intestinal (GI) upset are the most common side effects associated with SSRI treatment (Hu *et al.*, 2004; Papakostas, 2007). Although SSRI-emergent nausea appears to be well tolerated by most patients (Papakostas *et al.*, 2003), for patients complaining of GI side effects with paroxetine, the continued release formulation (Paxil-CR), reported to have a lower incidence of nausea early on during the course of treatment, may be used in place of the standard formulation (Golden *et al.*, 2002). The daily dose range for continued release of paroxetine is 25–62.5 mg, with the starting daily dose often being 12.5 mg.

Other common side effects include sexual dysfunction, headaches, insomnia/activation or sedation, fatigue, and jitteriness (Hu *et al.*, 2004; Masand & Gupta, 1999; Papakostas, 2007). The early recognition and management of SSRI-associated adverse events is critical, since these side effects have been reported as a common cause of discontinuing or switching treatment (Bull *et al.*, 2002).

SSRIs-induced sexual dysfunction is quite common, and can present with a variety of symptoms, including decreased libido; arousal dysfunction (i.e., inhibited sexual excitement, diminished genital sensation, erectile dysfunction, and failure to achieve or maintain vaginal lubrication), and orgasm disorders (i.e., delayed orgasm, partial or complete anorgasmia) (Clayton *et al.*, 2002; Montejo *et al.*, 2001; Papakostas, 2007) (Fig. 2.6). Although these

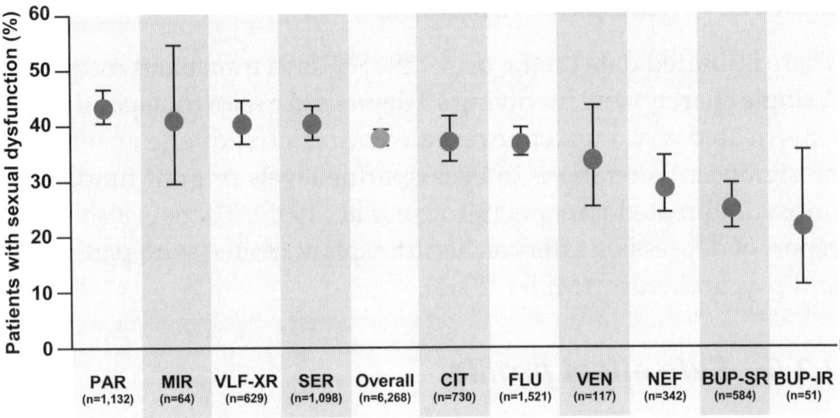

Fig. 2.6 Prevalence of sexual-dysfunction with antidepressants. *Notes*: PAR: paroxetine; MIR: mirtazapine; VLF-XR: venlafaxine xr; SER: sertraline; CIT: citalopram; VEN: venlafaxine; NEF: nefazodone; BUP-SR: bupropion SR; BUP-IR: bupropion. Error bars represent 95% confidence intervals. [Clayton, A.H., Pradko, J.F., Croft, H.A., Montano, C.B., Leadbetter, R.A., Bolden-Watson, C., Bass, K.I., Donahue, R.M., Jamerson, B.D., & Metz, A. Prevalence of sexual dysfunction among newer antidepressants. *Journal of Clinical Psychiatry*, 63, 357–366, 2002. Copyright 2002, Physicians Postgraduate Press. Reprinted by permission.]

side effects tend to improve rapidly after temporary ("drug holiday") discontinuation of the SSRIs, particularly those SSRIs with shorter half-life (Rothschild, 1995), such drug holidays carry a risk of withdrawal effects and depressive relapse. Adjunctive treatments to help alleviate sexual dysfunction and other SSRI- or antidepressant-induced side effects are described in Chap. 10. Details regarding adverse events reported with SSRI use are listed in the following paragraphs.

2.2.4.2 *Central nervous system*

Adverse events that rarely occur represent a significant challenge for researchers and clinicians alike. In order to study rare adverse events, large sample sizes and/or long follow-up periods are required. The emergence and/or worsening of suicidal ideation during antidepressant treatment represent one such example.

Specifically, during the early 1990s, a number of case reports were published (Fava & Rosenbaum, 1991; Masand *et al.*, 1991a; Papp & Gorman, 1900; Teicher *et al.*, 1990) regarding the potential for the SSRIs to worsen suicidal ideation or contribute to the emergence of suicidal ideation during the treatment of adults with MDD. These concerns were quickly followed by a number of pooled analyses (Beasley *et al.*, 1991a; Letizia *et al.*, 1996; Montgomery *et al.*, 1995), which suggested that SSRIs were no more likely to worsen suicidal ideation or result in suicide attempts than placebo treatment.

Recently, concerns resurfaced regarding the potential for antidepressants to contribute to the emergence and/or worsening of suicidal ideation during the treatment of children, adolescents, and young adults with MDD. This time, concerns were voiced by drug regulatory authorities in the U.S. and U.K., and were followed by several large, pooled analyses. These analyses suggest a small increase in the proportion of children and adolescents with MDD who experience treatment-emergent suicidal ideation during the first few weeks of treatment with the SSRIs (Apter *et al.*, 2006; Bridge *et al.*, 2007; Moscholder & Willy, 2006; Whittington *et al.*, 2004). An increase risk in suicide during antidepressant treatment, however, was not demonstrated (Bridge *et al.*, 2007). These findings underscore the need for good clinical practice, which includes the education of patients and families regarding antidepressant side effects (including the possible emergence of suicidal thoughts and behaviors), close monitoring of patients (especially early-on during treatment), and the need for rapid clinical intervention should suicidality emerge or worsen during treatment. A general consensus remains that the risks associated with withholding antidepressant treatment from patients, including pediatric patients, with serious depression vastly outweigh the risks associated with these drugs.

Pooled analyses of randomized, controlled trials of the SSRIs in adults (Beasley *et al.*, 2007; Hammad *et al.*, 2006; Khan *et al.*, 2003; Pedersen, 2005 and 2006; ctr.gsk.co.uk/Summary/bupropion/IV_suicide_observational.pdf) found no relationship between an emergence of suicidal ideation, a worsening of suicidal ideation or an increase in completed suicides during the treatment of MDD compared to placebo, although a recent study by Thase *et al.* (2006) demonstrated a numerically but not statistically higher rate of suicidal behavior among young adults (18–24 years old) treated with paroxetine than placebo for MDD. This finding was recently replicated for all antidepressants by the FDA (Stone *et al.*, in press). Risk factors for the emergence/worsening of suicidal ideation among adults with MDD during treatment with antidepressants include a history of alcohol use disorders, greater symptom severity, and the presence of melancholic features (Zisook *et al.*, 2009).

Although studies suggest that treatment with the TCAs may result in higher rates of abnormal mood elevations (mania and hypomania) during the treatment of bipolar depression than the SSRIs paroxetine (Nemeroff *et al.*, 2001), and fluoxetine (Cohn *et al.*, 1989), there is a paucity of studies comparing this adverse event among the remaining SSRI agents. Specifically, Post *et al.* (2006) reported lower rates of switching to mania or hypomania among patients with bipolar depression treated with bupropion or sertraline compared to venlafaxine (Fig. 2.7). Similarly, Vieta *et al.* (2002) found

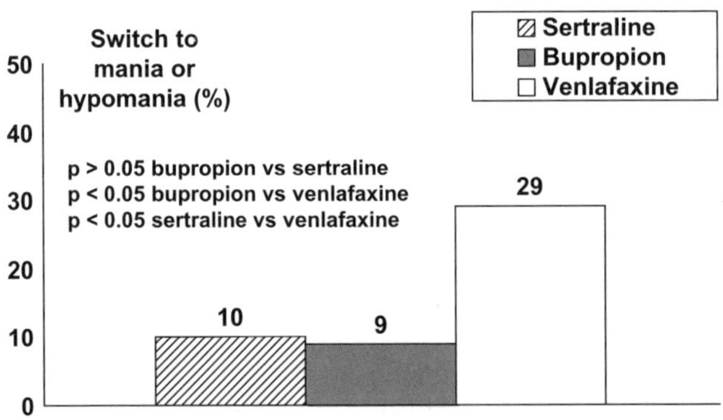

Fig. 2.7 Abnormal mood switch in bipolar depression: A randomized, double-blind comparison of adjunctive venlafaxine (SNRI), bupropion (NDRI) and Sertraline (SSRI) ($n = 174$). [Data extracted from: Post, R.M., Altshuler, L.L., Leverich, G.S., *et al.* (2006). Mood switch in bipolar depression: Comparison of adjunctive venlafaxine, bupropion and sertraline. *British Journal of Psychiatry*, 189, 124–131.]

lower rates of switching to mania or hypomania among paroxetine- than venlafaxine-treated patients with bipolar depression. More recently, the results of two large placebo-controlled studies focusing on the use of antidepressants either as monotherapy (McElroy *et al.*, 2008) or adjunctive therapy (Sachs *et al.*, 2008) for the treatment of a major depressive episode among patients with bipolar disorder have raised skepticism regarding whether the magnitude of the risk of abnormal mood elevations following the treatment of major depressive episodes among patients with bipolar disorder with newer antidepressants, including the SSRIs, is somewhat exaggerated. Specifically, rates of abnormal mood elevations in those two studies were comparable for SSRI- and placebo-treated patients in both studies.

There have been case reports of SSRI-related seizures, mostly occurring following overdoses of SSRIs (Braitberg & Curry, 1995; Caracci & Decina, 1991; Engebretsen *et al.*, 2003; Fisher *et al.*, 2002; Goldstein *et al.*, 1996; Graudins *et al.*, 1997; Gross *et al.*, 1998; Hargrave *et al.*, 1992; Kim *et al.*, 2000; Neely *et al.*, 1998; Oke *et al.*, 2001; Prasheer, 1993; Raju *et al.*, 2000; Riddle *et al.*, 1989; Saraf & Schrader, 1999; Spivey & Wait, 1993; Trabert *et al.*, 1995; Ware & Stewart, 1989; Waring *et al.*, 2008), although it was noted in one review that a significant proportion of antidepressant-related seizures occurs in individuals with an identifiable predisposition, such as previous seizures, sedative or alcohol withdrawal, and multiple concomitant medications (Rosenstein *et al.*, 1993). The co-administration of agents that inhibit CYP2D6 enzymatic activity, but not CYP2D6 or CYP2C19 genotype, has been identified as a risk factor for antidepressant-related seizures (Spigset *et al.*, 1997).

In one prospective, 12-month study of 100 patients with partial or generalized epilepsy treated with sertraline for either depression or OCD, six patients experienced an increase in seizure frequency that was thought to be probably or definitely associated with sertraline treatment (Kanner *et al.*, 2000). In a comprehensive literature review, the SSRIs fluoxetine and fluvoxamine were reported to carry the lowest seizure risk of all antidepressants examined (Pisani *et al.*, 2002). Interestingly, there is some animal model evidence suggesting that SSRIs such as fluoxetine may have anticonvulsant properties; for example, dietary fluoxetine supplementation appears to abolish handling-induced seizure susceptibility in El mice via a neural remodeling mechanism independent of energy balance (Richman *et al.*, 2007). The SSRI citalopram has not been found to alter seizure threshold during electroconvulsive therapy (ECT) in a double-blind, placebo-controlled study (Papakostas *et al.*, 2000).

Some patients treated with SSRIs may also experience cognitive side effects such as mental slowing and worsened attention (Fava *et al.*, 2006; Wadsworth *et al.*, 2005), psychological side effects such as apathy and emotional blunting (Bertschy & Vandel, 1993; Ellison & Stanziani, 1993; Garland & Baerg, 2001; Hoehn-Saric *et al.*, 1990 and 1991; Opbroek *et al.*, 2002), and motor side effects such as bruxism, akathisia, and extrapyramidal symptoms (Adler & Angrist, 1995; Altshuler *et al.*, 1994; Bauer *et al.*, 1996; Bertschy & Vandel, 1993; Bhakta & Andrade, in press; Black, 1992; Boffa & Lofchy, 2000; Bostwick & Jaffee, 1999; Chelben *et al.*, 2001; Chong, 1995; Chong & Tan, 1996; Dave, 1994; Dominguez-Moran *et al.*, 2001; Fleischhacker, 1991; Freidman, 1989; George & Trimble, 1993; Gerber & Lynd, 1998; Gill *et al.*, 1997; Glowinski *et al.*, 1989; Hansen, 2003; Klee & Kronig, 1993; Lambert *et al.*, 1998; Lee & Nam, 2000; Lipinski *et al.*, 1989; Lobbezoo *et al.*, 2001; Maany & Dhopesh, 1990; Mander *et al.*, 1994; Olivera, 1996; Olivera, 1997; Opler, 1994; Page *et al.*, 2008; Reccoppa *et al.*, 1990; Romanelli *et al.*, 1996; Settle, 1993; Shihabuddin & Rapport, 1994; Spigset, 1999; Stanislav & Childs, 1999; Perucca *et al.*, 1997; Walker, 2002; Wise, 2001). There are also case reports of the SSRIs worsening motor symptoms in patients with Parkinson's Disease (Leo *et al.*, 1995; Leo, 1996; Steur, 1993), as well as increased requirements of levodopa in Parkinson's patients following initiation of an SSRI for depression (van de Vijver *et al.*, 2002).

Finally, there have been several hundred reports of cerebrovascular disease in the setting of SSRI use (Ramasubbu, 1999). However, two case-control studies failed to show an association between SSRI use and intracranial hemorrhage, and one of these failed to show an association between SSRI use and ischemic stroke (Ramasubbu, 1999).

2.2.4.3 *Cardiovascular*

Although there are sporadic case reports of SSRI-associated arrhythmias, electrocardiographic (ECG) changes (Aström-Lilja *et al.*, 2008; Catalano *et al.*, 2001; Graudins *et al.*, 1997; Isbister *et al.*, 2001; Kanjanauthai *et al.*, 2008; Riddle *et al.*, 1989; Scharko & Schumacher, 2008; Tarabar *et al.*, 2008), or tachycardia (Neely, 1998), a large number of studies support the relative safety of the SSRIs with respect to cardiovascular effects. In fact, of all antidepressants, the SSRIs appear to possess the lowest toxicity in overdose (Henry *et al.*, 1995; White *et al.*, 2008).

Fluoxetine does not appear to alter QT variability, or heart period variability (Pohl *et al.*, 2003) in healthy volunteers, or to affect cardiac conduction in post-MI patients (Strik *et al.*, 2000), or left ventricular ejection fraction (LVEF) in elderly depressed patients (Strik *et al.*, 1998). For example, Roose *et al.* (1998a) studied fluoxetine in 27 MDD patients with cardiac disease and reported that fluoxetine induced a statistically significant 6% decrease in heart rate, a 2% increase in supine systolic pressure, and a 7% increase in ejection fraction. There was no effect on cardiac conduction, ventricular arrhythmia, or orthostatic blood pressure. Fluvoxamine also does not appear to alter LVEF in elderly depressed patients (Strik *et al.*, 1998) or to alter ECG intervals (Hewer *et al.*, 1995).

Similarly, treatment with sertraline does not appear to result in significant changes in heart rate, blood pressure, cardiac conduction, LVEF, or ventricular ectopic activity in post-MI MDD patients (Glassman *et al.*, 2002; Shapiro *et al.*, 1999). The use of sertraline also appears free of cardiovascular adverse events in children and adolescents (Wilens *et al.*, 1999). Paroxetine also does not appear to significantly alter blood pressure, conduction intervals, heart rate or rhythm, or indexes of heart rate variability in MDD patients with ischemic heart disease (Roose *et al.*, 1998b). No significant changes in heart rate, PR, and QTc intervals or in T-wave height were found after treatment with paroxetine in MDD (Edwards *et al.*, 1989). Citalopram also does not appear to alter PQ, QRS, or QTc intervals (Rasmussen *et al.*, 1999). Finally, the results of one study suggest the use of the

SSRIs combined with β-blockers in patients with depression and end-stage heart failure to reduce cardiovascular mortality compared to the use of β-blockers without antidepressants (Tousoulis *et al.*, 2008).

2.2.4.4 *Hematologic*

SSRIs have been associated with abnormal bleeding (e.g., bruising, epistaxis) in patients who have unremarkable routine hematologic laboratory results except for abnormal bleeding time or platelet counts (Calhoun & Calhoun, 1996; Fountoulakis *et al.*, 2007; Humphries *et al.*, 1990; Lake *et al.*, 2000; Pai & Kelly, 1996). Paroxetine has been reported to decrease platelet serotonin storage and platelet function (lowered expression of the platelet activation marker CD63 in response to two different concentrations of thrombin receptor-activating peptide) (Hergovich *et al.*, 2000) without altering plasma concentrations of prothrombin fragment, von Willebrand factor antigen, or circulating P-selectin in humans.

There are also reports of an increased risk of upper gastrointestinal (Dalton *et al.*, 2003; De Abajo & Garcia-Rodriguez, 2008; van Walraven *et al.*, 2001), or postoperative (Movig *et al.*, 2003), but not central nervous system bleeding with the SSRIs (Bak *et al.*, 2002; De Abajo *et al.*, 2000; Kharofa *et al.*, 2007), although not all studies suggest an increased risk of upper GI bleeding with the SSRIs (Layton *et al.*, 2001). However, systematic study of this issue has failed to reveal abnormalities in platelet aggregation, hematopoiesis, or coagulation profile in SSRI-treated patients (Alderman *et al.*, 1996). For instance, treatment with fluoxetine was not found to alter international normalized ratio, partial thromboplastin time, factors II, V, VII, VIII: C, IX, X, XI, XII, fibrinogen, thrombin time, bleeding time, euglobulin lysis time, protein kinase C, antithrombin, platelet counts, D dimer, lupus inhibitor, and platelet sensitivity studies to the following agonists: adenosine diphosphate, epinephrine, collagen, and arachidonic acid in MDD patients (Berk *et al.*, 1995). Sertraline also did not appear to alter bleeding time in MDD patients who were post-MI (Shapiro *et al.*, 1999), while

20 mg daily of paroxetine did not appear to increase bleeding time in MDD patients, although, in the latter study, patients with a specific serotonin transporter promoter polymorphism who underwent a dose escalation of paroxetine to 40 mg did demonstrate a statistically significant prolongation of bleeding time (Abdelmalik *et al.*, 2008). More recent studies have shown that the combined use of SSRIs and non-steroidal anti-inflammatory agents (NSAIDs) may potentiate the risk of GI adverse events than the use of SSRIs alone, or the combination of NSAIDs and non-SSRI antidepressants (De Abajo & Garcia-Rodriguez, 2008; de Jong *et al.*, 2003), although this finding could not be replicated in a subsequent study (Vidal *et al.*, 2008).

The results of one study suggest an increased risk of non-GI but not of GI bleeding when the SSRIs are combined with coumarin (Schalekamp *et al.*, 2008). There is also a case report of severe bleeding associated with use of low-molecular-weight heparin and SSRIs (de Maistre *et al.*, 2002), as well as drug interactions between SSRIs and warfarin (Claire *et al.*, 1991; Dent & Orrock, 1997; Limke *et al.*, 2002; Woolfrey *et al.*, 1993; Yap & Low, 1999), although interactions between SSRIs and warfarin do not consistently occur (Ford *et al.*, 1997). Potential interactions between SSRIs and warfarin may be mediated through the CYTP450 system (Duncan *et al.*, 1998; Sayal *et al.*, 2000), or protein binding (Apseloff *et al.*, 1997). Citalopram does not appear to alter the pharmacokinetics and pharmacodynamics of racemic warfarin (Priskorn *et al.*, 1997).

There are no reports of thrombosis or embolism during SSRI treatment. The results of one retrospective analysis report low rates of abnormal bleeding (1 case in 303) among patients with hepatitis C who were also administered an SSRI (the patient in this case also suffered from hemophilia) (Martin *et al.*, 2007). However, it has also been suggested that the concomitant use of NSAIDS with SSRIs may increase the risk of bleeding in this population (Weinrieb *et al.*, 2003). Clearly, the role of the SSRIs in potentiating the adverse GI effects of NSAIDs or increasing the risk of bleeding among coumarin-, warfarin-, or heparin-treated patients needs further exploration.

There have only been sporadic case reports of SSRI-related agranulocytosis (Trescoli-Serrano & Smith, 1997), aplastic anemia (Bosch & Vera, 1998), or leukopenia (Vilinsky & Lubin, 1997). However, treatment of depression with a number of agents, including SSRIs, did not appear to alter the number of red blood cells, hemoglobin and hematocrit concentrations, or reticulocyte count in one study (Maes *et al.*, 1996).

2.2.4.5 *Endocrine*

The endocrine effects of the SSRIs are less well characterized. There are numerous case reports of hyponatremia or syndrome of inappropriate anti-diuretic hormone secretion (SIADH) during treatment with the SSRIs (Agrawal *et al.*, 2007; Arinzon *et al.*, 2002; Ayonrinde *et al.*, 1995; Baliga & McHardy, 1993; Ball, 1993; Barclay & Lee, 2002; Bouman *et al.*, 1998; Bourgeois *et al.*, 2002; Burke & Franker, 1996a and b; Druckenbrod & Mulsant, 1994; Fisher *et al.*, 2002; Flores *et al.*, 2004; Girault *et al.*, 1997; Hull *et al.*, 2002; Iraqi & Baickle, 2004; Kazal *et al.*, 1993; Levsky & Schwartz, 1998; Liu *et al.*, 1996; Lowenthal, 1999; Marik *et al.*, 1990; Odeh *et al.*, 2001; Ota *et al.*, 2008; Portilla-Botelho *et al.*, 2008; Schattner & Skurnik, 1996; Siah *et al.*, 2007). Initially, the results of a small ($n = 8$), four-week study involving daily fluvoxamine administration in healthy subjects did not reveal any changes in serum sodium levels during administration, although a small increase in serum sodium levels (mean increase 1.9 mmol/L) was noted following the discontinuation of fluvoxamine (Spigset & Mjorndal, 1997). However, a subsequent, large chart review did suggest an increased risk of hyponatremia in SSRI- or venlafaxine-treated elderly patients (Kirby *et al.*, 2002). In fact, in a more recent, prospective study, 12% of elderly MDD patients were reported to develop hyponatremia during a 12-week trial with paroxetine (Fabian *et al.*, 2004).

The mechanism of SSRI-associated hyponatremia is unclear. The results of one study did not reveal any significant changes in afternoon basal arginine vasopressin (AVP) levels in fluoxetine-treated patients (Inder *et al.*, 2001), although an earlier study had shown a significant decrease in CSF AVP levels in fluoxetine-treated patients (De Bellis *et al.*, 1993). A separate study also did not show any difference in AVP release, plasma osmolality, or urine osmolality following a hyper or hypo-osmotic fluid challenge between fluoxetine- and placebo-administered subjects (Faull *et al.*, 1991). Similarly, administration of paroxetine also did not appear to interfere with free water excretion following hyposmotic fluid challenge in humans (Marar *et al.*, 2000). Finally, administration of citalopram versus placebo for seven days to healthy volunteers did not result in significant differences in renin levels between the two treatment groups (Jezova & Duncko, 2002).

Results from studies focusing on the effect of SSRIs on prolactin secretion in humans appear to be quite inconsistent. There are reports of hyperprolactinemia (Meltzer *et al.*, 1979; Peterson, 2001), and galactorrhea (Arya & Taylor, 1995; Peterson, 2001) during treatment with the SSRI fluoxetine, although treatment of depression with fluoxetine (up to 80 mg for 12 weeks) in one study was not found to result in increased prolactin levels (Salzman *et al.*, 1993). However, in a separate study, the administration of 60 mg of fluoxetine daily for a total of six days in six healthy post-menopausal women was found to increase mean 24-hour prolactin secretion significantly (Urban & Veldhuis, 1991). Similarly, in an open-label study conducted by our group, 2 (4.5%) of 44 men and 8 (22.2%) of 36 women with normal prolactin levels at baseline developed hyperprolactinemia following treatment of their MDD with fluoxetine (up to 60 mg for 12 weeks) (Papakostas *et al.*, 2006b).

There are also reports of galactorrhea with paroxetine (Bonin *et al.*, 1997; Davenport & Velamoor, 2002; Gonzalez *et al.*, 2000; Morrison *et al.*, 2001). In addition, in one naturalistic study, the rate of breast enlargement among women who received treatment with paroxetine appeared to be significantly higher than that of women treated with venlafaxine, while there was a trend for higher rates of breast enlargement with paroxetine than the other SSRIs (Amsterdam *et al.*, 1997). These findings could be attributed both to the greater weight gain with paroxetine, and an increase in prolactin levels with paroxetine reported in that study. Estradiol and human chorionic gonadotropin (hCG) levels were not influenced by the SSRIs in that study. However, paroxetine was not reported to result in significant increases in prolactin levels in two studies of depressed patients (Muck-Seler *et al.*, 2002; Salzman *et al.*, 1993) and one study of healthy volunteers (Schlosser *et al.*, 2000), although a significant increase in serum prolactin levels was reported in a separate study of healthy volunteers (Cowen & Sargent, 1997).

Citalopram was found to increase prolactin levels in one study of healthy volunteers (Laine *et al.*, 1997). There is one report of galactorrhea with fluvoxamine (Bonin *et al.*, 1994), while a small study of healthy volunteers suggests a weak ($p = 0.05$) effect of daily fluvoxamine for one month on prolactin levels (increased), with a substantial increase in 2/8 subjects (Spigset & Mjorndal, 1997). Finally, there are reports of galactorrhea (Bronzo & Stahl, 1993; Lesaca, 1996) and breast enlargement (Hall, 1994) with sertraline, although studies show no effect of sertraline on prolactin (Gordon *et al.*, 1998; Sagud *et al.*, 2002).

There are case reports of abnormalities in thyroid function tests in patients treated with sertraline (Harel *et al.*, 1995; McCowen *et al.*, 1997), and paroxetine (Takahashi *et al.*, 2007). Sagud *et al.* (2002), however, reported no change in thyroid stimulating hormone (TSH) or thyroxine (T4) levels in 15 MDD patients treated with sertraline (100 mg) from 4 to 24 weeks. In addition, in that study, while there was no change in T3 levels in the first four weeks of treatment, triiodothyronine (T3) levels were significantly increased after 24 weeks of treatment compared to baseline.

Administration of fluoxetine (up to 60 mg) in a study of 20 MDD patients for six weeks did not result in changes in TSH, free T4, total T4, T3 or thyroid binding globulin (TBG) levels (Shelton *et al.*, 1993). Similarly, treatment with fluvoxamine for four weeks did not alter T3, T4 or TSH levels in a separate study (Moreau *et al.*, 2000). Finally, administration of paroxetine (20 mg) to 25 MDD patients for a total of 24 weeks did not appear to result in changes in TSH or T3 levels, but did result in a significant decrease in T3 levels (Konig *et al.*, 2000).

Even less is known regarding the effects of SSRIs on the gonadal hormones or melatonin. Daily administration of paroxetine for four weeks in healthy volunteers did not seem to alter testosterone levels, melatonin secretion, or growth-hormone (GH) secretion in one study (Schlosser *et al.*, 2000). Similarly, there was no statistically significant increase in testosterone levels among men with MDD treated with open-label fluoxetine in a separate trial (60 mg up to 12 weeks — Papakostas *et al.*, 2006b). Treatment of panic disorder with fluvoxamine, however, did appear to increase melatonin levels (Den Boer & Westenberg, 1990). In fact, it has been proposed that, of all the SSRIs, fluvoxamine is a potent inhibitor of peripheral melatonin degradation (Hartter *et al.*, 2001). The potential clinical significance of such a relationship is, however, unclear. Finally, treatment of seasonal affective disorder (Childs *et al.*, 1995), but not OCD (Monteleone *et al.*, 1995) with fluoxetine has also been found to result in a statistically significant reduction in melatonin levels.

Until recently, the effects of the SSRIs on bone mineral density had not been systematically explored (Misra *et al.*, 2004). However, recent reports suggest a possible association between SSRI use and an increased risk of bone fractures (Ginsburg & Rosero, 2009; Richards *et al.*, 2007; Schneeweiss *et al.*, 2004; Vestergaard *et al.*, 2008; Ziere *et al.*, 2008), as well as decreased bone density in men (Haney *et al.*, 2007) and women (Diem *et al.*, 2007). The underlying mechanism for this has yet to be elucidated.

To date, there have been no reports published of amenorrhea during SSRI monotherapy. On the contrary, two female patients with Prader–Willi syndrome (PWS) who had primary amenorrhea developed vaginal bleeding believed to be menses following at least six months of treatment with fluoxetine (Warnock *et al.*, 1995).

2.2.4.6 *Metabolic*

The effects of the SSRIs on metabolism are variable. Weight gain in antidepressant trials is most often reported in one of two ways: either as a change in weight, or as the proportion of patients who gain 7% or more in weight. Many MDD patients (de Jonghe *et al.*, 1991; Michelson *et al.*, 1999; Sussman *et al.*, 2001) may experience reduced appetite and weight loss during the acute phase of treatment with

SSRIs. For example, reports in the literature suggest that short-term fluoxetine treatment is responsible for a decrease in food intake assessed by self-reported food diary (Greeno *et al.*, 1996), and this may account for the greater weight loss observed during diet plus fluoxetine treatment compared to placebo in overweight subjects (Visser *et al.*, 1993). There are also some reports that fluoxetine augmentation of a dietary program improves weight loss with respect to diet therapy alone in overweight or obese subjects (Ferguson *et al.*, 1987; Levine *et al.*, 1987), and that this improvement is dose dependant (Levine *et al.*, 1989).

However, there is a paucity of data regarding the long-term effects of SSRI treatment on body weight, with several studies providing conflicting results. The results of a large, cross-sectional study based on the General Electric Medical Records Database (a database containing de-identified patient information from a consortium of 5,000 physicians using General Electric Healthcare's CPO Electronic Medical Records which documents care for about four million patients) involving patients treated for a unipolar depressive episode with an antidepressant (monotherapy) for at least one year suggested differences in the proportion of patients who gained 7% or more in weight during treatment: mirtazapine was associated with the highest percentage of patients with weight gain (26%), followed by the SSRIs and venlafaxine (anywhere from 16%–19%), with bupropion and nefazodone demonstrating the lowest rates of weight gain (12%) (Papakostas, 2007) (Fig. 2.8).

Unfortunately, only a subset of randomized, long-term, controlled studies of SSRIs have reported weight data. Several studies suggest that long-term weight changes during treatment with the SSRIs fluoxetine, sertraline and escitalopram are similar to those seen during treatment with placebo (Davidson *et al.*, 2001; Emslie *et al.*, 2004; Gilaberte *et al.*, 2001; Koran *et al.*, 2002; Kornstein *et al.*, 2006; Michelson *et al.*, 1999; Rapaport *et al.*, 2001), although there is also evidence to suggest modest weight gain over placebo for escitalopram-treated patients with MDD in one study (Pigott *et al.*, 2007). In a separate trial, paroxetine was shown to be associated with a significantly higher rate of weight gain (25.5%) than sertraline

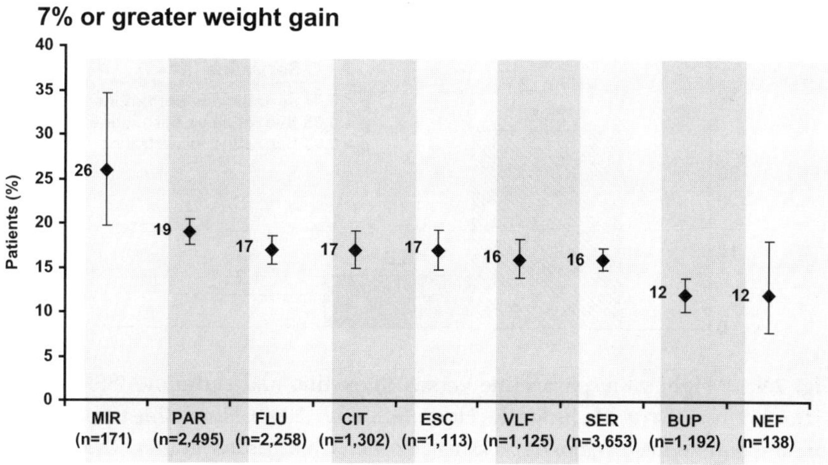

Fig. 2.8 Weight gain following one year of treatment. *Notes*: MIR: mirtazapine; FLU: fluoxetine; SER: sertraline; PAR: paroxetine; CIT: citalopram; ESC: escitalopram; VLF; venlafaxine; NEF: nefazodone; BUP: bupropion. [Data extracted from: Papakostas, G.I. (2007). Current limitations of antidepressant monotherapy: Tolerability. *Journal of Clinical Psychiatry*, 68 Suppl 10, 11–17.]

(4.2%) or fluoxetine (6.8%) (Fava *et al.*, 2000) (Fig. 2.9). Similarly, long-term treatment of social anxiety disorder with paroxetine was associated with a greater proportion of patients who experienced clinically significant weight gain than placebo (23% versus 9%; Stein *et al.*, 2002).

Regrettably, most long-term, placebo-controlled SSRI studies do not report relevant data with regards to weight gain (Allgulander *et al.*, 2005; Davidson *et al.*, 2005; Doogan *et al.*, 1992; Fineberg *et al.*, 2007; Gorwood *et al.*, 2007; Hochstrasser *et al.*, 2001; Hollander *et al.*, 2003; Kamijima *et al.*, 2006; Keller *et al.*, 1998; Klysner *et al.*, 2002; Lepine *et al.*, 2004; Martenyi *et al.*, 2002; Martenyi & Soldatenkova, 2006; McGrath *et al.*, 2006; Michelson *et al.*, 1999; Montgomery & Dunbar, 1993; Montgomery *et al.*, 1988, 1993, 1995, and 2005; Rapaport *et al.*, 2002 and 2004; Robert *et al.*, 1995; Romano *et al.*, 2001; Schmidt *et al.*, 2000; Stein *et al.*, 1996; Terra *et al.*, 1998; Walker *et al.*, 2000). As a result, in light of the paucity of relevant data, it is difficult to accurately estimate the potential risk for weight gain during

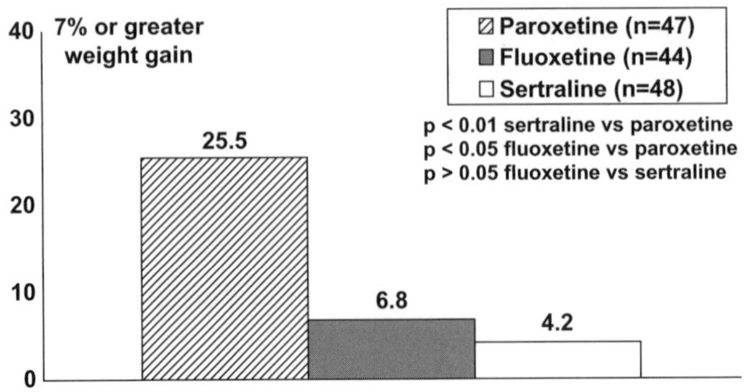

Fig. 2.9 Weight gain: paroxetine versus fluoxetine and sertraline (SSRIs).[Data extracted from: Fava, M., Judge, R., Hoog, S.L., *et al.* (2000). Fluoxetine versus sertraline and paroxetine in major depressive disorder: Changes in weight with long-term treatment. *Journal of Clinical Psychiatry*, 61, 863–867.]

the long-term treatment of MDD with the SSRIs. More recently, results from the Hordaland health study, a large population-based cross-sectional study in Norway, suggest an association between long-term SSRI use and abdominal obesity as well as hypercholesterolemia (Raeder *et al.*, 2006).

The mechanism underlying SSRI-related changes in weight is unclear, partly because many of the mechanistic studies focus on the short-term effects of SSRIs on biological factors related to weight. For example, although paroxetine (Hinze-Selch *et al.*, 2000) and fluoxetine (Moosa *et al.*, 2003) consistently do not appear to alter serum leptin levels in humans, there was a positive correlation between leptin levels after treatment with fluoxetine and body mass index in one study of women with depression (Moosa *et al.*, 2003). Sertraline was reported to decrease cerebrospinal fluid (CSF) hypocretin-1 (orexin-A) levels in MDD in one study (Salomon *et al.*, 2003). Fluoxetine has also been reported to increase metabolism (Bondi *et al.*, 2000), by enhancing thermogenesis (Bondi *et al.*, 2000; Bross *et al.*, 1995; Stinson *et al.*, 1992) in humans.

Other studies report some beneficial effects of SSRIs on metabolic parameters in obese or diabetic patients. In obese diabetic patients, fluoxetine has been noted to ameliorate mean blood glucose levels, daily insulin requirements, and glycohemoglobin levels (Chiasson *et al.*, 1989; Gray *et al.*, 1992; Kutnowski *et al.*, 1992; O'Kane *et al.*, 1994; Wise, 1992) by improving insulin sensitivity (Maheux *et al.*, 1997; Potter van Loon *et al.*, 1992). Similarly, in diabetic patients, SSRIs have also been reported to reduce weight, fasting plasma glucose, and glycosylated hemoglobin (HbA1c) levels (Goodnick, 2001).

In parallel, the SSRIs appear to possess anti-hyperlipidemic effects (Bailey and LeMelledo, 2003; Peter *et al.*, 2000), although a study of healthy volunteers reported an increase in cholesterol levels after eight weeks of daily paroxetine (Lara *et al.*, 2003b). Finally, treatment of depression with a number of agents, including SSRIs, did not appear to alter iron levels or transferrin in one study (Maes *et al.*, 1996).

2.2.4.7 *Immunologic*

A growing number of studies also examine the immunologic effects of the SSRIs. Paroxetine did not appear to alter serum soluble tumor necrosis factor (TNF) receptor p75 plasma levels in one study (Hinze-Selch *et al.*, 2000). However, fluoxetine (Kubera *et al.*, 2001), and sertraline (Maes *et al.*, 1999) have been reported to decrease interleukin-10 (IL-10) levels, and the IL-10/interferon-γ (IFN-γ) ratio in depression. Fluoxetine was reported to decrease (Kubera *et al.*, 2001), and sertraline to increase (Maes *et al.*, 1999) IFN-γ levels in depression, although the results of a subsequent study suggest that sertraline decreases IFN-γ production in depressed patients with multiple sclerosis (Mohr *et al.*, 2001b). Sertraline did not appear to alter the production of interleukin-1β in dysthymia in one study (Anisman *et al.*, 1999).

2.2.4.8 *Dermatologic*

There are several reports of rashes developing during SSRI treatment (Charbonnier *et al.*, 1987; Gupta *et al.*, 2002; Koran *et al.*, 2003; Sannicandro *et al.*, 2002; Spigset, 1999; Thedenat *et al.*, 2001; Warnock & Azadian, 2002), with a recent study suggesting a weak yet statistically significant relationship between the use of sertraline and an increased risk of Stevens–Johnson syndrome (Mockenhaupt *et al.*, 2008). There are also case reports of alopecia in patients on SSRIs (Ghanizadeh, 2008; Mercke *et al.*, 2000), as well as toxic epidermal necrolysis during paroxetine treatment (Ahmed & Eagleton, 2008).

2.2.4.9 *Risk of malignancy*

The use of SSRIs does not appear to confer an increased risk of lung cancer (Toh *et al.*, 2007), prostate cancer (Tamim *et al.*, 2008), ovarian cancer (Coogan *et al.*, 2000; Dublin *et al.*, 2002; Moorman *et al.*, 2005), colorectal cancer (Xu *et al.*, 2006) or hematologic malignancies (Bahl *et al.*, 2004). The results of one study suggested an increased risk for certain types of breast cancer among women on SSRIs (progesterone-negative or estrogen-positive/progesterone-negative receptor tumors) (Chien *et al.*, 2006), while separate studies identified a link between the use of specific SSRIs (paroxetine and/or sertraline), and the duration of SSRI use with an increased risk of breast cancer among women (Cotterchio *et al.*, 2000; Moorman *et al.*, 2003; Steingard *et al.*, 2003). However, a similar relationship between SSRI use and an increase in the risk of breast cancer overall or receptor-specific tumors was not established in several other studies (Coogan *et al.*, 2005 and 2009; Fulton-Kehoe *et al.*, 2006; Hague *et al.*, 2005; Gonzalez-Perez & Garcia-Rodriguez, 2005; Kelly *et al.*, 1999; Lash *et al.*, 2008; Wang *et al.*, 2001).

2.2.4.10 *Risk of teratogenicity*

There is accumulating information regarding the use of SSRIs early (first trimester) in pregnancy, although the bulk of available data focuses on fluoxetine (Addis & Koreng, 2000; Chambers *et al.*, 2006; Goldstein *et al.*, 1997; Loebstein & Koren, 1997; Nonacs & Cohen, 2003). For example, one prospective study of 128 pregnant women who took fluoxetine (Pastuszak *et al.*, 1993) 10 to 80 mg daily (mean 25.8 mg) during their first trimester did not report elevated rates of major malformations compared with matched groups of women taking TCAs or drugs thought not to be teratogenic. There was a higher, albeit not statistically significant, rate of miscarriages in the fluoxetine (13.5%) and TCA (12.2%) groups compared with the women exposed to known non-teratogenic drugs (6.8%). Whether this increased rate of miscarriages is biologically significant and, if so, whether it relates to the drugs or to the depressive disorder could not be determined from this study.

A large registry of fluoxetine exposure during pregnancy is consistent with generally reassuring data from the TCA era that antidepressant agents are not evidently teratogens. Emerging evidence involving the newer SSRIs is in accordance with existing data on fluoxetine (increased risk of miscarriages or preterm births, no evidence for a major role in contributing to teratogenicity) (Davis *et al.*, 2007; Einarson & Einarson, 2005; Hemels *et al.*, 2005; Hendrick *et al.*, 2003; Kulin *et al.*, 1998; Louik *et al.*, 2007; Pearson *et al.*, 2007; Sivojelezova *et al.*, 2005; Wichman *et al.*, 2006), with the exception of paroxetine where some studies suggest a small yet statistically significant dose-related increase in the risk for congenital heart malformations among infants born to mothers exposed during the first trimester of pregnancy (Berard *et al.*, 2007; Cole *et al.*, 2007; Kallen *et al.*, 2007; Louik *et al.*, 2007) as well as sertraline, which has been linked to a small increase in the risk for omphalocele and septal defects (Louik *et al.*, 2007). However, subsequent studies failed to confirm a relationship between paroxetine use during the first trimester and an increased risk of congenital heart malformations in the offspring (Diav-Citrin *et al.*, 2008; Einarson *et al.*, 2008). A recent study also failed to demonstrate a major association between early SSRI use during pregnancy and an increased risk of teratogenicity, although there was a small increase in the risk of three specific birth defects: anencephaly, cranisynostosis, and omphalocele (Alwan *et al.*, 2007). This study has yet to be replicated (data documenting the relative risk for each individual SSRI was not available in this study).

On the other hand, infants exposed to SSRIs during late-pregnancy may be at increased risk of a number of adverse events including serotonergic CNS adverse effects (Anbu & Theodore, 2006; Boucher *et al.*, 2008; Condon, 2003; Costei *et al.*, 2002; Davis *et al.*, 2007; Knooppert *et al.*, 2006; Koren & Boucher, 2009; Laine *et al.*,

2004; Moses-Kolko *et al.*, 2005; Santos & Pergolizzi, 2004), neonatal abstinence syndrome (Levinson-Castiel *et al.*, 2006), neonatal withdrawal syndrome (Dahl *et al.*, 1997; Nordeng *et al.*, 2001; Sanz *et al.*, 2005), and poor adaptation (Oberlander *et al.*, 2004; Sivojelezova *et al.*, 2005), although the incidence of these events has not been well established. Whenever present, the majority of these symptoms are often mild, and resolve within one to two weeks, although rarely (1 in 313 cases) a more severe syndrome consisting of seizures, dehydration, hyperpyrexia, weight loss has also been observed among infants born to mothers exposed to SSRIs during the third trimester (Moses-Kolko *et al.*, 2005).

Persistent pulmonary hypertension has also been reported among infants born to mothers exposed to an SSRI during the third trimester of pregnancy (Andrade *et al.*, 2009; Chambers *et al.*, 2006; Koren & Boucher, in press). More recently, evidence has emerged suggesting an increased risk of hypertension and pre-eclampsia among pregnant women who continue to take SSRIs beyond their first trimester of pregnancy (Toh *et al.*, 2009). This report has yet to be replicated.

In summary, decisions on continuing antidepressant drugs during pregnancy must be individualized, but it must be recalled that the effects of severe untreated depression on maternal and fetal health may be far worse than the unknown risks of fluoxetine or tricyclic drugs. Recently, the FDA has issued a warning for all SSRIs, reporting an increased risk for neonatal toxicity and recommending cessation of treatment prior to delivery. However, in clinical practice, the risk of post-partum depression often warrants continued treatment and close monitoring of the newborn. Whenever possible, unnecessary exposure to any drug should be minimized, and thoughtful planning of pre-pregnancy treatment and consideration of alternative interventions such as psychotherapies [e.g., cognitive-behavior therapy (CBT)] are to be recommended.

The FDA has defined the SSRIs as drugs belonging to pregnancy category C (either studies in animals have revealed adverse effects on the fetus and there are no controlled studies in women, or studies in women and animals are not available) with the exception of paroxetine which has been defined as belonging to pregnancy category D (there is positive evidence of human fetal risk, but the benefits from use in pregnant women may be acceptable despite the risk).

2.2.4.11 *Risk of transmission during breastfeeding*

To various degrees, SSRIs are secreted in breast milk of lactating women treated with the agents. A pooled analysis of antidepressant levels among nursing infants suggests that fluoxetine and citalopram produce the highest levels while paroxetine and sertraline usually produce undetectable levels in infants (Weissman *et al.*, 2004). It does not appear that short-term exposure of infants to SSRI levels typically present in breast milk results in a significant increase in serotonin-related adverse events (Berle *et al.*, 2004; Kristensen *et al.*, 2002; Lee *et al.*, 2004; Misri *et al.*, 2000; Piontek *et al.*, 2001; Rampono *et al.*, 2000; Taddio *et al.*, 1996; Wisner *et al.*, 1996 and 1998). However, the long-term effects of infant exposure to the breast milk containing various levels of SSRIs on infant growth and development are unknown. Small, naturalistic studies have suggested somewhat slower growth among infants breast-fed by mothers who take fluoxetine (Chambers *et al.*, 1999), but not paroxetine (Merlob *et al.*, 2004), consistent with data showing fluoxetine but not paroxetine to be detectable among infants breast-fed by mothers treated with either agent (Weissman *et al.*, 2004).

2.2.4.12 *Discontinuation syndrome*

A number of reports also describe discontinuation-emergent adverse events upon abrupt cessation of SSRIs. The events include dizziness, insomnia, nervousness, irritability, nausea, agitation (Bogetto *et al.*, 2002; Hindmarch *et al.*, 2000; Kreider *et al.*, 1995; Markowitz *et al.*, 2000; Rosenbaum *et al.*, 1998; Zajecka *et al.*, 1998), and electric shock-like sensations (Prakash & Dhar, 2008). The SSRIs prolong sleep-onset latency, reduce sleep efficiency, increase WASO, and they suppress REM sleep and prolong REM latency (Armitage 2000) — such abrupt discontinuation may result in the emergence of nightmares/ vivid dreaming (Pace-Schott *et al.*, 2001).

The risk of such withdrawal-related adverse events occurring seems to be inversely related to the plasma half-life of the SSRI, with escitalopram reported as having a lower risk than paroxetine (Baldwin *et al.*, 2006), and fluoxetine reported as having a significantly lower risk than paroxetine in three studies (Judge *et al.*, 2002; Michelson *et al.*, 2000a; Rosenbaum *et al.*, 1998). In fact, when patients with fluoxetine or paroxetine-remitted MDD underwent placebo substitution of their SSRI for three days, there was a greater drug level decrease in the CNS of paroxetine-treated group (88% decrease) than the fluoxetine-treated group (38%), with withdrawal-related adverse events correlating with CNS drug level in the paroxetine group (Henry *et al.*, 2000). An increase in plasma insulin-like growth factor-1 (IGF-1) levels during abrupt discontinuation of SSRIs has also been reported (Michelson *et al.*, 2000b).

For severe discontinuation-related adverse events, re-institution of the SSRI and slow taper may be necessary to alleviate these symptoms (Rosenbaum & Zajecka, 1997). There is also anecdotal evidence to support the use of ginger root (one or two 550-mg capsules t.i.d.) for disequilibrium and nausea associated with SSRI-discontinuation (Schechter, 1998).

2.2.5 *Dosing*

2.2.5.1 *Initial and optimal dose*

Although several individual placebo-controlled trials suggest that the SSRIs demonstrate a "flat" dose-response curve (i.e., higher starting doses of an SSRI do not necessarily improve outcome), the results of a meta-analysis of randomized, double-blind, placebo-controlled, fixed-dose SSRI studies in MDD suggest a modest increase in response rates with higher starting doses (Papakostas *et al.*, in press). However, the tolerability of higher starting SSRI doses was significantly worse, supporting the practice of initiating treatment with 10 mg for escitalopram (Lexapro), 20 mg for fluoxetine

(Prozac), paroxetine (Paxil), citalopram (Celexa), 25 mg for paroxetine CR (Paxil CR), and 50 mg for sertraline (Zoloft) and fluvoxamine (Luvox) (these doses also appear to be the minimally effective doses). Starting at lower doses, and increasing the doses shortly thereafter (i.e., after one to two weeks) may further improve tolerability.

2.2.5.2 *Serotonin transporter occupancy as a function of dose*

5HTT occupancy studies offer some insights into the relationship between SSRI dosing and clinical response. Specifically, *in vivo* serotonin transporter occupancy during treatment with low doses of SSRIs has been reported to range between 76.2–85% for fluoxetine (20 mg; Meyer *et al.*, 2004), 72.9–76% for fluvoxamine (25–50 mg; Suhara *et al.*, 2003; Takano *et al.*, 2006), 74.7–93.4% for paroxetine (20 mg; Meyer *et al.*, 2001 and 2004), and 77% for citalopram (20 mg; Meyer *et al.*, 2001), with higher doses yielding somewhat greater 5HTT occupancy for fluvoxamine (79%–93%; 200–400 mg; Suhara *et al.*, 2003), sertraline (85%; 150–200 mg; Voineskos *et al.*, 2007), citalopram (85%; 60–80 mg; Voineskos *et al.*, 2007), and paroxetine (92%–100%; 30–40 mg; Kent *et al.*, 2002). A recent, large study examining the role of dose and *in vivo* 5HTT occupancy confirms previous data, suggesting that usual starting doses of the SSRIs result in approximately 80% occupancy, with higher doses resulting in greater occupancy (Meyer *et al.*, 2004).

However, small and possibly underpowered studies conducted to date have not found a relationship between 5HTT occupancy and antidepressant response (Cavanagh *et al.*, 2006; Meyer *et al.*, 2004). In addition, a double-blind study randomized MDD patients, who failed to experience sufficient symptom improvement on 20 mg of paroxetine for six weeks, to either continue on 20 mg of paroxetine or undergo a dose-increase to 30–50 mg of paroxetine. The results did not demonstrate a difference in 5HTT occupancy between the two treatment groups (Ruhe *et al.*, 2009a). Recent studies also suggest that serotonin transporter polymorphisms may influence the relationship between 5HTT occupancy and clinical response during

SSRI treatment (Ruhe *et al.*, 2009b). Thus, at the present time, the inter-relationship between SSRI dosing, 5HTT occupancy and symptom improvement in MDD requires further clarification.

Sertraline, which possesses affinity for the dopamine transporter *in vitro*, appears to result in very low DAT occupancy *in vivo* (11% at 50–100 mg; Argelyan *et al.*, 2006).

2.2.5.3 *Plasma levels and clinical efficacy*

Contrary to the TCAs, SSRI plasma levels do not appear to be useful in guiding dosing in clinical practice. Specifically, there appears to be great variability from one patient to the next in terms of SSRI plasma levels for each given dose, while plasma levels also do not appear to correlate with the likelihood of response (Mauri *et al.*, 2002), or relapse (Brunswick *et al.*, 2000), although the results of a small ($n = 22$), four-week, open-label trial of citalopram for MDD indicate a significant correlation between the resolution of depressive symptoms and CSF levels of the s-stereoisomer of citalopram (Nikisch *et al.*, 2004).

Several factors may account for the lack of correlation between dose, plasma SSRI levels, and clinical response. SSRIs often take longer to achieve steady-state levels in the CNS than plasma (up to 30 days in one study — Strauss *et al.*, 1997), while rapid decreases in CNS concentrations ranging from 38% (fluoxetine) to 88% (paroxetine) only three days after discontinuation have been reported in one study (Henry *et al.*, 2000). In addition, mean CNS levels at steady state appear to be much higher than plasma steady-state levels (Karson *et al.*, 1993; Renshaw *et al.*, 1992), reported as high as 24 to 1 for fluvoxamine in one study (Strauss *et al.*, 1997). Furthermore, CNS and plasma elimination half-life may differ for some SSRIs. The CNS elimination half-life for the SSRI fluvoxamine (58–79 hours), for instance, was reported to be longer than its respective plasma elimination half-life (26–35 hours) in two studies (Bolo *et al.*, 2000; Strauss *et al.*, 1998). However, the CNS elimination half-life of fluoxetine combined with norfluoxetine in the latter study was not statistically different from the plasma elimination half-life (406 hours).

Finally, variability from patient to patient in the fraction of fluoxetine bound to CNS structures other than the 5HTT transporter (i.e., proteins and lipids) has recently been proposed as an additional factor that may contribute to the lack of correlation between SSRI dose, CNS drug level, and clinical response (Strauss & Dager, 2001).

2.2.5.4 *Cytochrome enzyme genotype and plasma levels*

There is growing evidence to suggest that genotype may also influence the relationship between dose and SSRI levels. For instance, certain mutations of the CYP2C19 (*2, *3) have been associated with increased metabolism of fluoxetine (Liu *et al.*, 2001), sertraline/N-desmethyl sertraline (Rudberg *et al.*, 2008a), escitalopram/citalopram (Rudberg *et al.*, 2006 and 2008b), but not fluvoxamine metabolism (Jan *et al.*, 2002), while others (*17) have been associated with ultra-rapid metabolism of escitalopram (Rudberg *et al.*, 2008c). In other studies, CYP2C19 but not 3A4 genotype was found to influence the plasma levels of citalopram and its major metabolite (desmethylcitalopram) (Yin *et al.*, 2006; Yu *et al.*, 2003).

In parallel, certain mutations of the CYP2D6 (i.e., *5, *10) have been associated with decreased metabolism of fluvoxamine (Gerstenberg *et al.*, 2003a; Watanabe *et al.*, 2008), paroxetine (Yoon *et al.*, 2000) and fluoxetine (Llerena *et al.*, 2004; Yu *et al.*, 2002). There are also reports of ultra-rapid metabolism of paroxetine in patients with CYP2D6 gene duplication (Charlier *et al.*, 2003; Guzey & Spigset, 2006). Other studies, however, did not find a correlation between the presence of CYP2D6*10 alleles and plasma fluvoxamine concentration/dose ratio in Japanese subjects (Gerstenberg *et al.*, 2003b; Ohara *et al.*, 2003). In parallel, CYP2D6 genotype does not appear to influence the likelihood of responding or developing side effects to fluoxetine in MDD (Gerstenberg *et al.*, 2003b; Roberts *et al.*, 2004). The results of one study also suggest CYP2D9 (*1) genotype to influence fluoxetine metabolism and plasma levels (Scordo *et al.*, 2005).

2.2.5.5 *P-glycoprotein interactions*

Citalopram (Uhr *et al.*, 2003b), paroxetine (Uhr *et al.*, 2003a), but not fluoxetine (Uhr *et al.*, 2000) also appear to be substrates for p-glycoprotein (p-GP), although it is unclear how p-GP substrate status influences the relationship between SSRI serum levels and the likelihood of clinical response *in vivo*. Furthermore, sertraline/desmethylsertraline and paroxetine are potent inhibitors, fluoxetine and fluvoxamine are intermediate inhibitors, while citalopram is a weak inhibitor of p-GP activity (Weiss *et al.*, 2003; Wang *et al.*, 2008), although concentrations required for this inhibition to occur are much higher than plasma levels typically achieved during the treatment of MDD with these agents (Weber *et al.*, 2005).

2.2.6 *Drug interactions*

Perhaps with the exception of citalopram and its stereo-isomer escitalopram (Hemeryck & Belpaire, 2002), SSRIs may inhibit cytochrome P450 isoenzymes to varying degrees, potentially causing substrate levels to rise, or reducing conversion of a substrate into its active form (Appendix A). As discussed above, the augmentation and combination of SSRIs with other serotonergic agents, tryptophan, 5HTP, or MAOIs may also result in the serotonin syndrome (Beasley *et al.*, 1993; Feighner *et al.*, 1990; Lane & Baldwin, 1997). Clinicians treating patients with such combinations should be aware of this potential, particularly in prescribed SSRIs with a longer half-life such as fluoxetine, and in polypharmacy where the potential for cross-inhibition of the cytochrome p450 isoenzymes is greatly increased.

2.3 Serotonin Receptor Antagonists and Agonists

2.3.1 *Trazodone and nefazodone*

2.3.1.1 *Neuropharmacology*

Both trazodone (Desyrel) and nefazodone (Serzone) primarily block serotonin 5HT2A receptors (Haria *et al.*, 1994; Hemrick-Luecke *et al.*,

1994; Meyer *et al.*, 1999; Taylor *et al.*, 1995), although the *in vivo* effects of nefazodone at the 5HT2A receptor appear to be modest: the 5HT2 occupancy after a single dose of 200 mg was 39% (Meyer *et al.*, 1999); it was less than 50% after six weeks of treatment with an average dose of approximately 450 mg (Mischoulon *et al.*, 2002). Trazodone and nefazodone also share an active metabolite, m-chlorophenylpiperazine (mCPP), which acts as a serotonin 5HT2C agonist and appears to be able to release serotonin presynaptically (Rothman *et al.*, 2002). In addition, serotonin 5HT2C receptors, when activated (Marcoli *et al.*, 1998; Maura *et al.*, 2000), may also inhibit the N-methyl-D-aspartate (NMDA)-emergent cyclic GMP elevation. Nefazodone also appears to act as non-competitive antagonists of nicotinic acetyl cholinergic receptors (Fryer and Lukas, 1999), while trazodone also appears to stimulate the μ1- and μ2-opioid receptors (Schreiber *et al.*, 2000). Trazodone is also a weak inhibitor of serotonin reuptake. As a result, the overall effect of trazodone is to increase the extra cellular levels of serotonin in the brain (Pazzagli *et al.*, 1999). This effect explains the fact that trazodone monotherapy has been associated with the occurrence of serotonin syndromes (Rao, 1998).

Trazodone is also a potent blocker of the α-1 adrenergic receptor. It has been associated with orthostatic hypotension, and is very sedating. In fact, in one controlled trial the incidence of asthenia and/or sedation with trazodone was almost double than that of fluoxetine (42.6% versus 21.5%) (Beasley *et al.*, 1991b). For this reason, lower doses of trazodone are more commonly used in clinical practice than standard antidepressant doses (25–150 mg at bedtime), most often for the treatment of insomnia secondary to antidepressant use (Dording *et al.*, 2002) (see Chap. 10). Nefazodone also has a significant affinity for the α-1 adrenergic receptors, but is considered to be less likely to cause orthostatic hypotension, and is less sedating than trazodone.

2.3.1.2 *Efficacy*

Although as effective as the SSRIs in the treatment of MDD (Papakostas & Fava, 2007) (Fig. 2.10), trazodone and nefazodone

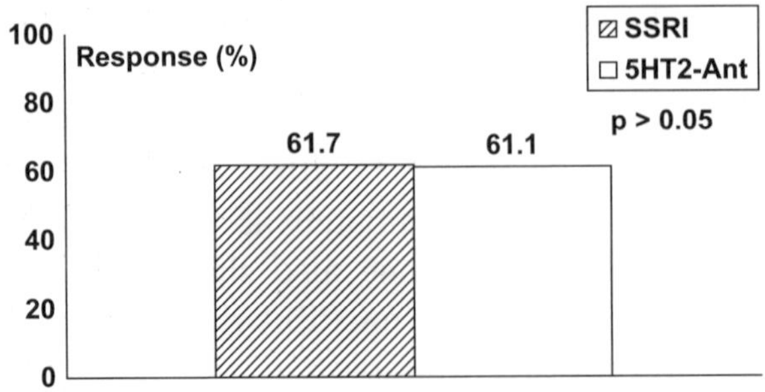

Fig. 2.10 Comparative efficacy of 5HT2-receptor antagonists (trazodone and nefazodone) versus SSRIs: Meta-analysis of 9 RCTs ($n = 988$). RCT: Randomized, Controlled Trial. [Data extracted from: Papakostas, G.I., & Fava, M. (2006). A meta-analysis of clinical trials comparing moclobemide with selective serotonin reuptake inhibitors for the treatment of major depressive disorder. *Canadian Journal of Psychiatry*, 51(12), 783–790.]

are used less commonly in first-line therapy (Petersen *et al.*, 2002). Placebo-controlled trials focusing on the use of nefazodone in elderly patients with MDD, in children/adolescents with MDD, or in patients with bipolar depression, dysthymic disorder, seasonal affective disorder or minor depression have not been published to date. There is evidence from a randomized, double-blind, placebo-controlled trial supporting the use of nefazodone for the treatment of MDD with comorbid alcohol use disorders (Roy-Byrne *et al.*, 2000). A single placebo-controlled study demonstrates superior efficacy for trazodone- than placebo-treated elderly patients with MDD (Gerner *et al.*, 1980). Placebo-controlled trials focusing on the use of trazodone in children/adolescents with MDD, or in patients with bipolar depression, dysthymic disorder, seasonal affective disorder or minor depression have not been published to date.

There is evidence from randomized, double-blind, placebo-controlled trial(s) to support the use of trazodone in psychiatric disorders often found comorbid in patients with MDD, including GAD (Rickels *et al.*, 1993), and bulimia nervosa (Pope *et al.*, 1989). Similarly, there is evidence from randomized, double-blind, placebo-controlled trials to support the use of nefazodone in PTSD (Davis *et al.*, 2000). Randomized, double-blind, placebo-controlled trials supporting the use of either agent for panic disorder, SAD, OCD, anorexia nervosa, or AD(H)D have yet to be published.

A small double-blind study reported nefazodone to be as effective as fluoxetine in the treatment of depression in outpatients with Parkinson's disease, with fewer motor side effects (Avila *et al.*, 2003). There are also open trials of nefazodone for the treatment of depression in HIV+ patients (Elliott *et al.*, 1999), patients with congestive heart failure (Lesperance *et al.*, 2003), and patients with chronic headaches (Saper *et al.*, 2001). There is one case report of remission of cancer chemotherapy-induced emesis during treatment of depression with nefazodone (Khouzam *et al.*, 1998).

The results of small trials support the use of trazodone in the treatment of HIV-positive subjects with adjustment disorders (De Wit *et al.*, 1999) or adjustment disorders in cancer patients (Razavi *et al.*, 1999), or in patients with depression and Parkinson's disease (Werneck *et al.*, 2009).

2.3.1.3 *Side effect profile*

Common side effects of trazodone include sedation, orthostatic hypotension, and headaches. A rare but serious side effect of trazodone is that of priapism of both the penis and the clitoris (Bardin *et al.*, 2002; Thompson *et al.*, 1990), which requires immediate medical attention. Priapism has been attributed to the α-adrenoreceptor blocking properties of trazodone by interference with the sympathetic control of penile detumescence (Saenz de Tejada *et al.*, 1991).

Rare cases of hepatotoxicity have been associated with the use of trazodone (Fernandes *et al.*, 2000; Longstreth & Hershman, 1985; Rettman & McClintock, 2001), and fatal cases of trazodone overdose have also been reported (de Meester *et al.*, 2001). Trazodone-associated hepatic toxicity may be due to trazodone-inducted mitochondrial toxicity (Dykens *et al.*, 2008).

There have been several reports of cardiac conduction changes and/or arrhythmias in patients taking trazodone (Aronson & Hafez, 1986; Chung *et al.*, 2008; Dattilo & Nordin, 2007; Himmelhoch *et al.*, 1984; Irwin & Spar, 1983; Janowsky *et al.*, 1983a and 1983b; Levenson,

1999; Lippmann *et al.*, 1983; McCracken & Cosanin, 1984; Rausch *et al.*, 1984; Service & Waring, 2008; van de Merwe *et al.*, 1984; Vitullo *et al.*, 1990; Vlay and Friedling, 1983; White & Wong, 1985), which may be due to the ability of trazodone to inhibit potassium channels (Casis *et al.*, 1998). There is also a risk of serotonin syndrome when trazodone is combined with serotonergic agents such as nefazodone (Margolese & Chouinard, 2000), TCAs (Nisijima *et al.*, 1996), SSRIs (George & Godleski, 1996; Reeves & Bullen, 1995), venlafaxine (McCue & Joseph, 2001), and buspirone (Goldberg & Huk, 1992).

Trazodone has been reported to increase prolactin levels (Otani *et al.*, 1995; Roccatagliata *et al.*, 1982). In one review trazodone was reported to carry one of the lowest risks for seizure of all antidepressants examined (Pisani *et al.*, 2002), although there have been reports of hyponatremia and seizure during trazodone overdose (Balestrieri *et al.*, 1992; Vanpee *et al.*, 1999). There are reports of adverse reactions (Menza, 1986; Montalbetti & Zis, 1988; Peabody, 1987) following the abrupt discontinuation of trazodone.

Common side effects of nefazodone include somnolence, dizziness, dry mouth, nausea, constipation, headache, amblyopia and blurred vision (Cyr and Brown, 1996). Treatment with nefazodone has the advantage of a lower risk of long-term weight gain than the SSRIs or TCAs (Papakostas, 2007; Sussman *et al.*, 2001), perhaps because of the appetite-reducing effects of mCPP (Sargent *et al.*, 1997). Nefazodone also has the advantage of a lower risk of sexual side effects than the SSRIs (Clayton *et al.*, 2002; Ferguson *et al.*, 2001; Montejo *et al.*, 2001).

Unlike the TCAs, MAOIs and SSRIs, nefazodone does not appear to suppress REM sleep (Rush *et al.*, 1998). In fact, an eight-week study comparing the effects of nefazodone and fluoxetine on sleep disturbances in outpatients with non-psychotic depression and insomnia found that fluoxetine was associated with approximately a 30% increase in the number of nocturnal awakenings, whereas nefazodone was associated with about a 15% decrease, a net difference of 45% (Rush *et al.*, 1998).

A rare but serious side effect of nefazodone is that of priapism of both the penis and the clitoris (Brodie-Meijer *et al.*, 1999; Toofanny &

Maddens, 1999), which requires immediate medical attention. In addition, an increasing number of reports (DeSanty & Amabile, 2007) suggest that treatment with nefazodone may be associated with hepatotoxicity (approximately 29 cases per 100,000 patient years; Carvajal *et al.*, 2002), which is often severe (more than 80% of cases), and appears during the first six months of treatment (Stewart, 2002). To date, there has even been one reported death due to such hepatotoxicity (Ehrentraut *et al.*, 2002). As a result, nefazodone was removed from the market in Canada, Europe, and the U.S. (on May 20th, 2004). Nefazodone-associated hepatic toxicity may be due to nefazodone-inducted mitochondrial toxicity (Dykens *et al.*, in Press). Nefazodone should be avoided in patients with current or a history of liver abnormalities, while liver enzymes should be checked periodically in patients on nefazodone.

There is also a report of nefazodone-emergent hypoglycemia in a patient with diabetes and MDD (Warnock & Biggs, 1997), and a single case report of nefazodone-associated torsades de pointes (Siddiqui & Khan, 2004). The combination of nefazodone with the SSRIs may result in serotonin syndrome (John *et al.*, 1997; Smith & Wenegrat, 2000). Nefazodone has also been reported to inhibit CYP3A4 (DeVane *et al.*, 2004), and co-administration of nefazodone with 3A4-metabolized drugs has been reported to result in increased drug levels (DeVane *et al.*, 2004; Lam *et al.*, 2003) (Appendix A). The abrupt discontinuation of nefazodone has been reported to result in adverse reactions (Benazzi, 1998; Kotlyar *et al.*, 1999; Lauber, 1999; Rajagopalan & Little, 1999).

The risk of abnormal mood elevation during the treatment of bipolar depression with either agent has not been systematically studied, nor has the risk of the emergence or worsening of suicidal ideation during the treatment of MDD with either agent. Although the data are limited compared to the SSRIs, the use of trazodone and nefazodone during pregnancy appears to be relatively safe, and not associated with a large increase in the risk for teratogenicity (Einarson *et al.*, 2003; Einarson & Einarson, 2005). Both agents belong to the FDA pregnancy category C. The use of either agent during breastfeeding has not been systematically studied.

2.3.1.4 *Dosing*

The minimal effective dose in MDD for trazodone is, usually, 300 mg daily, with 600 mg daily being the optimal dose. The minimal effective dose for nefazodone is usually 300 mg daily, with 600 mg daily being the optimal dose. Nefazodone, but not trazodone, is an inhibitor of p-glycoprotein activity (Stormer *et al.*, 2001). Finally, the presence of certain polymorphism for the gene coding for the CYP2D6 enzyme (Mihara *et al.*, 1997), or the CYP1A2 enzyme (Mihara *et al.*, 2001) does not appear to influence trazodone levels.

2.3.2 *Other 5HT-2 active agents*

2.3.2.1 *Ritanserin*

Ritanserin, a serotonin 5HT2A and 5HT2C antagonist, is not FDA-approved, but is available in Europe. One placebo-controlled study revealed ritanserin to be effective in the treatment of dysthymic disorder (Bersani *et al.*, 1991), although a second study found imipramine to be more effective than ritanserin in the treatment of dysthymia (Bakish *et al.*, 1994). In a separate study, ritanserin was reported to be as effective as amitriptyline in patients with depression and chronic headaches (Nappi *et al.*, 1990). Ritanserin appears to be effective for depression at doses above 5 mg.

2.3.2.2 *Fenfluramine and dexfenfluramine*

Fenfluramine (Pondimin) and dexfenfluramine (Redux) are substituted amphetamines that, similarly to mCPP, act to release 5HT presynaptically (Rothman & Baumann, 2002). Metabolites of these two agents also act as 5HT2C agonists, a property that may explain their anorectic effect, as well as 5HT2B receptor agonists, a property that may explain their adverse effects on cardiac valve function (Rothman & Baumann, 2002). Initially developed and FDA-approved as anti-obesity drugs, a number of double-blind studies reported greater reductions in depressive symptoms in fenfluramine- or dexfenfluramine-treated than placebo-treated patients (Blouin *et al.*, 1988; Brzezinski *et al.*, 1990; Galletly *et al.*, 1996; O'Rourke *et al.*, 1989). Both fenfluramine and dexfenfluramine were withdrawn from the market by the FDA in September of 1997 due to reports of cardiac valvulopathy, estimated in as many as one in eight patients treated for at least 90 days (Sachdev *et al.*, 2002). The use of these agents was also linked to the development of primary pulmonary hypertension and serotonergic neurotoxicity (Rothman & Baumann, 2002).

2.3.2.3 *Agomelatine*

Agomelatine, a newer agent, is a selective 5HT2C antagonist and also an agonist at various melatonergic receptors. The 5HT2C antagonism properties of agomelatine have been thought to be responsible for increases in frontocortical dopaminergic and adrenergic activity in animals during administration of agomelatine (Millan *et al.*, 2003). Placebo-controlled trials have found agomelatine to be effective in the treatment of MDD (Kennedy & Emslie, 2006; Loo *et al.*, 2002; Montgomery *et al.*, 2006; Olie & Kasper, 2007). Agomelatine also appears to be as effective as the SSRIs paroxetine (Loo *et al.*, 2002), and the SNRI venlafaxine (Kennedy *et al.*, 2008; Lemoine *et al.*, 2007) in the treatment of MDD, although the results of a recent study suggest agomelatine (25–50 mg) to be more effective than the SSRI sertraline (50–100 mg) in MDD (Kasper *et al.*, 2008). Treatment of MDD with agomelatine has been shown to improve the quality of sleep (increase sleep efficiency, time awake after sleep onset and the total amount of slow-wave sleep), while not influencing rapid eye movement (REM) latency, the amount of REM sleep, or REM density (Salva *et al.*, 2007). In fact, the treatment of MDD with agomelatine appears to result in a better quality of sleep than treatment with venlafaxine (Lemoine *et al.*, 2007), and a lower incidence of sexual dysfunction (Rasmussen *et al.*, 2006) than the SSRIs and the SNRI venlafaxine. The results of one study also suggest the rapid discontinuation of agomelatine to be well tolerated (Montgomery *et al.*, 2004).

There is an open-label study supporting the use of agomelatine in seasonal affective disorder (Pjrek *et al.*, 2007), and in the treatment of depressive episodes in patients with bipolar disorder (Calabrese *et al.*, 2007). Finally, there is evidence from a randomized, double-blind, placebo-controlled trial to support the use of agomelatine in the treatment of GAD, a psychiatric disorder often present in patients with MDD (Stein *et al.*, 2008). The usual starting dose for agomelatine is 25 mg daily (can be as low as 12.5 mg), with 25 mg daily appearing to be the minimally effective dose (usual dose range 25–50 mg).

On February 20th, 2009 the Committee for Medical Products for Human Use (CHMP) of the European Medicines Agency (EMEA) recommended the marketing authorization of agomelatine. The results of an application for agomelatine to be used in the treatment for MDD in the U.S. are pending with the FDA.

2.3.3 *5HT-1 active agents*

2.3.3.1 *Agonists*

Buspirone (Buspar) and gepirone (Ariza) act as full agonists at serotonin 5HT1A auto-receptors and are generally, but not exclusively, partial agonists at postsynaptic serotonin 5HT1A receptors (Blier & Ward, 2003). Buspirone and gepirone show weak α-1 adrenoreceptor affinity, but significant and selective α-1 adrenoreceptor intrinsic affinity, which was expressed in a tissue- and species-dependent manner (Rimele *et al.*, 1987). They also show weak dopamine D-2 antagonism properties (Piercey *et al.*, 1994). The latter effect is thought to lead to excitation of noradrenergic cell firing (Piercey *et al.*, 1994), antagonizing primarily presynaptic inhibitory dopamine D2 autoreceptors at dopaminergic neurons (Lechin *et al.*, 1998). Buspirone has also potent α-2-adrenoceptor antagonist properties via its principal metabolite, 1-(2-pyrimidinyl)-piperazine (Astier *et al.*, 2003; Gobert *et al.*, 1999).

A number of double-blind trials report buspirone (Fabre, 1990; Feiger, 1996; Feiger *et al.*, 2003; Rickels *et al.*, 1990 and 1991; Robinson *et al.*, 1990) and gepirone (Jenkins *et al.*, 1990; McGrath *et al.*, 1994;

Wilcox *et al.*, 1996; Bielski *et al.*, 2008) to be more effective than placebo in the treatment of MDD. Gepirone also appears to be more effective than placebo in the treatment of anxious depression (Alpert *et al.*, 2003). In addition, there is evidence from randomized, double-blind, placebo-controlled trials to support the use of buspirone in the treatment of GAD, a psychiatric disorder often present in patients with MDD (Sramek *et al.*, 1996). Gepirone's "new drug application" (NDA) for the treatment of MDD was reviewed by the FDA in November of 2007 (Gepirone received a non-approvable letter). Buspirone is not FDA approved for MDD.

One advantage of gepirone and perhaps buspirone is that their use does appear not to be related to a greater incidence of weight gain or sexual side effects than placebo, at least during the acute phase of treatment of depression (Feiger *et al.*, 2003). Effective daily doses for buspirone and gepirone for depression range between 30–90 mg and 40 mg–80 mg, respectively. Side effects are similar for these two agents and include headache, dizziness, light-headedness, nausea, vomiting, paresthesias, palpitations, tremor, tinnitus, sedation, anxiety, blurred vision, bradycardia, and insomnia (Newton *et al.*, 1986; Feiger *et al.*, 2003). The extended-release (ER) formulation of gepirone was designed for better tolerability when compared to the immediate release (IR) formulation, but was never approved by the FDA.

Tandospirone (Sediel) is another serotonin 5HT1A partial agonist. The use of adjunct tandospirone was not found to significantly hasten the antidepressant effects of clomipramine in one study (Yamada *et al.*, 2003), although dosages used in that study were not found to achieve significant 5HT1A-receptor occupancy *in vivo* (Nakayama *et al.*, 2002).

Other 5HT1A agonists are also being developed, with ipsapirone (Stahl *et al.*, 1998), and zalospirone (Rickels *et al.*, 1996) reporting greater effectiveness than placebo in controlled trials, while a second trial of ipsapirone showed efficacy over placebo only for core depressive symptoms (Lapierre *et al.*, 1998). For the serotonin 5HT1A partial agonist flesinoxan, there is only a small open trial in patients with treatment-resistant depression (Grof *et al.*, 1993). Finally, a double-blind, randomized, placebo-controlled trial focusing on the use of a new 5HT1A agonist (PRX-00023) as monotherapy for MDD is currently underway (clinicaltrials.gov; NCT00448292).

Finally, there is also no evidence to support the use in depression of selective 5HT1D-receptor agonists FDA-approved for the acute treatment of migraines, such as sumatriptan (Imitrex), rizatriptan (Maxalt), almotriptan (Axert), eletriptan (Revpax), naratriptan (Amerge), zolmitriptan (Zomig), and frovatriptan (Frova) (Ferrari *et al.*, 2002), although treatment of headaches with the triptans in one study was shown to result in concomitant reduction in depressive symptoms in outpatients with comorbid migraines and depression (Miranda *et al.*, 2001).

2.3.3.2 *Antagonists*

Pindolol (Barbloc, Vypen Visken in the U.S.), a β-adrenergic receptor antagonist and serotonin 5HT1A-receptor antagonist (Andree *et al.*, 1999), is FDA approved for hypertension. Due to its 5HT1A agonist activity, it has been hypothesized that pindolol may accelerate the onset of antidepressant action when co-administered with SSRIs (see Chap. 5).

2.3.4 *Agents acting on 5HT-3 and 5HT-4*

To date, there is no evidence to support the use in depression of selective 5HT3-receptor antagonists FDA-approved for the prevention of nausea and vomiting including ondansetron (Zofran), granisetron (Kytril), and tropisetron (Navoban) (Morrow *et al.*, 1995), although there is preliminary evidence to support the use of ondansetron for the treatment of anxiety (Freeman *et al.*, 1997; Hewlett *et al.*, 2003; Schneier *et al.*, 1996).

Finally, there is no evidence to support the use of the 5HT4-selective agonist and cholinergic enhancer cisapride (Propulsid), or mosapride (available only in Austria as Mosaro and Japan as Gasmotin) for depression. Cisapride carries a high risk for potentially lethal drug-interactions with a number of pharmacologic agents, including many antidepressants (Michalets *et al.*, 2000), and is no longer available due to its potential for arrhythmogenesis (Wysowski *et al.*, 2001). However, the approval of newer and safer 5HT4-selective agonists for the treatment of GI conditions, including tegaserod (Zelnorm) (Wagstaff *et al.*, 2003), could potentially help alleviate antidepressant-emergent nausea and upper-GI upset, the most commonly reported adverse event of the SSRIs, present in as many as one in four patients treated with 20 mg of fluoxetine in one study (Papakostas *et al.*, 2003). Tegaserod is commonly used at doses of 2.6 mg b.i.d. for the treatment of GI conditions. Side effects include diarrhea, abdominal pain, flatulence, headaches, and fatigue.

2.4 Serotonin Reuptake Enhancers

Tianeptine (Stablon) acts to *increase* rather than decrease the synaptic reuptake of serotonin and is typically considered a serotonin reuptake enhancer (De Simoni *et al.*, 1992; Wilde *et al.*, 1995). Tianeptine targets the phosphorylation state of glutamate receptors at the CA3 c/a synapse (Kole *et al.*, 2002), and has neuroprotective effects against hypoxia in tissue culture and against the deleterious effects of cytokines in cortex and white matter (Plaisant *et al.*, 2003). Tianeptine is available in France for the treatment of depression (but not the U.S.). Open trials have suggested its efficacy (Sonawalla *et al.*, 2003), and double-blind trials have demonstrated tianeptine to be superior to placebo (Costa e Silva *et al.*, 1997), and equivalent to the SSRIs (Kasper & Olie, 2002; Lepine *et al.*, 2001; Loo *et al.*, 1999 and 2001; Novotny & Faltus, 2002; Oral *et al.*, 2001; Waintraub *et al.*, 2002) and the TCAs (Invernizzi *et al.*, 1994) in the treatment of MDD. Tianeptine also appears to result in earlier improvement in concentration than fluoxetine (Novotny & Faltus, 2003). There is also evidence from an open-label trial supporting the use of tianeptine for the treatment of depression in patients with Parkinson's disease (Levin, 2007).

Treatment with tianeptine may result in a lower incidence of sexual side effects than the SSRIs or TCAs (Bonierbale *et al.*, 2003). Common side effects include dry mouth, constipation, dizziness, drowsiness, postural hypotension, insomnia, and nightmares (Costa e Silva *et al.*, 1997). Tianeptine does not appear to prolong cardiac conduction (Delalleau *et al.*, 1988). The daily dose most commonly found to be effective is 37.5 mg, given in t.i.d. dosing.

2.5 α-2 Adrenergic Receptor Agonists and Antagonists

The immediate action of yohimbine is to block the α-2 adrenergic inhibitory auto-receptor. Yohimbine is FDA approved for the treatment of sexual impotence (brand name: Yocon), and does not have a depression indication. Guanfacine (Tenex) also inhibits the α-2 adrenergic auto-receptor (Sorkin & Heel, 1986), while having no affinity for the serotonergic receptors. Guanfacine is FDA approved for the treatment of hypertension. To date, there is no evidence to support the use of guanfacine in depression, although both guanfacine (Taylor & Russo, 2001), and yohimbine (Connor *et al.*, 1999) appear to be effective for the treatment of AD(H)D, a psychiatric disorder which is often present in patients with MDD. Common daily doses for AD(H)D range between 0.25–2 mg. A single open trial reported decreases in depressive symptoms during treatment with the α-2 selective *agonist* clonidine (Catapres) in outpatients with comorbid MDD and post-traumatic stress disorder (PTSD) (Kinzie *et al.*, 1989).

2.6 Norepinephrine Reuptake Inhibitors (NRIs)

2.6.1 *Reboxetine*

Reboxetine (Wong *et al.*, 2000) acts by selectively inhibiting the norepinephrine transporter, thereby increasing synaptic norepinephrine levels. Reboxetine also appears to act as an antagonist of nicotinic acetyl cholinergic receptors (Miller *et al.*, 2002). Reboxetine has not received FDA-approval for the treatment of depression (the FDA declined Pharmacia's license application for the U.S. market in May 2001), but is available in Europe for the treatment of depression

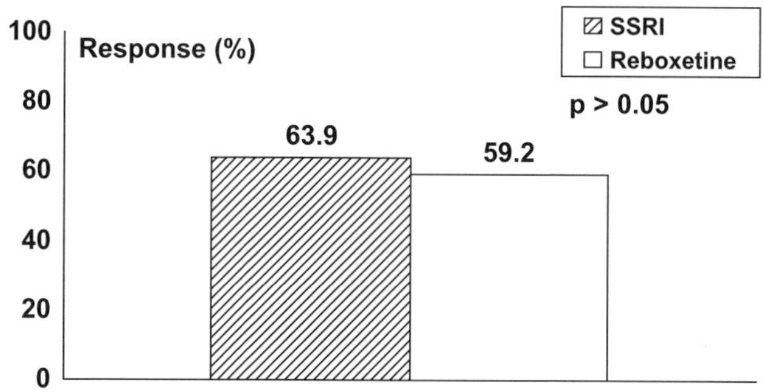

Fig. 2.11 Comparative efficacy of Reboxetine (NRI) versus SSRIs: Meta-analysis of 9 RCTs ($n = 2,641$). RCT: Randomized, Controlled Trial. [Papakostas, G.I., Nelson, J.C., Kasper, S., *et al.* (2008). A meta-analysis of clinical trials comparing reboxetine, a norepinephrine reuptake inhibitor, with selective serotonin reuptake inhibitors for the treatment of major depressive disorder. *European Neuropsychopharmacology*, 18(2), 122–127.]

(brand name: Edronax). Double-blind, placebo-controlled trials suggest reboxetine to be more effective than placebo (Andreoli *et al.*, 2002; Massana, 1998; Montgomery *et al.*, 2003; Versiani *et al.*, 2000), and as effective as the SSRIs (Papakostas *et al.*, 2008) and venlafaxine (Schwartz *et al.*, 2002) in the treatment of MDD (Fig. 2.11). There is also evidence from randomized, double-blind, placebo-controlled trials to support the use of reboxetine in the treatment of panic disorder, a psychiatric condition often present in patients with MDD (Versiani *et al.*, 2002). Results of placebo-controlled trials focusing on the use of reboxetine in elderly patients, children or adolescents with MDD, in dysthymic disorder, bipolar depression, seasonal affective disorder or minor depressive disorder have not yet been published.

There are open trials supporting the use of reboxetine in patients with comorbid depression and Parkinson's disease (Lemke, 2002), comorbid depression and epilepsy (Kuhn *et al.*, 2003), comorbid depression and HIV (Carvalhal *et al.*, 2003), and in the treatment of MDD in breast-cancer patients (Grassi *et al.*, 2004).

Controlled studies have suggested that reboxetine may be particularly effective in the treatment of cognitive disturbance in depression (Ferguson *et al.*, 2002), and more effective than the SSRIs in the treatment of cognition and attention in depression (Ferguson *et al.*, 2003). Although an earlier double-blind clinical trial had suggested reboxetine to be more effective than the SSRI fluoxetine in improving psychosocial functioning in depression (Dubini *et al.*, 1997; Massana, 1998; Massana *et al.*, 1999), this was not confirmed by a recent, large meta-analysis comparing reboxetine and the SSRIs for the treatment of MDD (Papakostas *et al.*, 2008).

The starting daily dose is usually 8 mg but can be as low as 4 mg, with effective daily doses ranging between 8–10 mg given in divided doses (twice a day). Common side effects include insomnia, headache, dry mouth, diaphoresis, urinary hesitancy, and constipation (Andreoli *et al.*, 2002). The incidence of nausea (Papakostas, 2007), headache, fatigue (Andreoli *et al.*, 2002; Papakostas, 2007), and sexual dysfunction (Clayton *et al.*, 2003) appears to be more common during treatment with the SSRIs than reboxetine, while the incidence of insomnia appears to be more common during treatment with reboxetine than with the SSRIs (Papakostas, 2007). In addition, long-term treatment with reboxetine does not appear to result in greater weight gain than placebo (Thase & Bartlett, 2001).

There are reports of hyponatremia during treatment with reboxetine (Abdelrahman *et al.*, 2003; Koelkebeck *et al.*, in press; Ranieri *et al.*, 2000). Reboxetine does not appear to alter cardiac conduction (Fleishaker *et al.*, 2001). Treatment with reboxetine may result in increased blood pressure in some patients. In fact, a genetic variant of the norepinephrine transporter (SCL6A2) has been found to confer an increased risk of developing higher blood pressure during treatment with reboxetine (Ono *et al.*, 2003).

The risks of exposure with reboxetine during pregnancy and breastfeeding have not been systematically studied. The risks of abnormal mood elevation during the treatment of bipolar depression, or the risk of the emergence or worsening of suicidal ideation during the treatment of MDD with reboxetine have also not been systematically studied. Reports of a "reboxetine withdrawal syndrome" have not been published to date.

Reboxetine possesses intermediate potency for p-GP inhibition (Weiss *et al.*, 2003). Reboxetine possesses two chiral centers and is available in a form containing two of its four enantiomers, but there is a paucity of information available regarding the individual properties of its isomers (Baker & Prior, 2002).

2.6.2 *Atomoxetine*

Atomoxetine also selectively inhibits the reuptake of norepinephrine (Preti, 2002). Atomoxetine is an FDA-approved treatment for AD(H)D (brand name: Strattera), a psychiatric disorder often present in patients with MDD. Until recently, there was only a single published report (open-label trial) focusing on the use of atomoxetine as monotherapy in MDD involving a total of 10 patients, with daily doses ranging from 40 mg to 70 mg (Chouinard *et al.*, 1984). More recently, the results of a double-blind, placebo-controlled trial of atomoxetine as monotherapy for MDD with comorbid ADHD in adolescents were published (Bangs *et al.*, 2007). Atomoxetine was found to be more effective than placebo in resolving symptoms of ADHD but not MDD in that study. In addition, there are data regarding the use of atomoxetine as adjunctive treatment in MDD (see Chaps. 6 and 9).

2.6.3 *Viloxazine*

Viloxazine (Vivalan) is also a selective norepinephrine reuptake inhibitor (Richelson & Nelson, 1984). However, there are no data focusing on the use of viloxazine for the treatment of MDD. Finally, a double-blind, randomized, placebo-controlled study focusing on a new norepinephrine reuptake inhibitor (LY2216684) as monotherapy for MDD is currently under way (clinicaltrials.gov; NCT00420004).

2.7 Selective *β* Adrenergic Receptor Agonists

At the present time, no such agents are available for clinical use in MDD either in the U.S., the E.U. or elsewhere. However, several randomized, double-blind, placebo-controlled studies focusing on the use of a novel, α-3-selective adrenergic receptor agonist (SR58611A) as monotherapy for MDD (clinicaltrials.gov; NCT00252330; NCT00252356; NCT00385307; NCT00345098), or elderly patients with MDD (clinicaltrials.gov; NCT00319709) are currently under way.

2.8 Dopamine-Selective Agents

2.8.1 *Receptor agonists*

Piribedil (Trivastal, Trivastan) is a non-ergot dopamine D2/D3 receptor agonist with a significant antagonist action on α-2A and α-2C adrenergic receptor subtypes (Ziegler *et al.*, 2003). Bromocriptine, cabergoline and pergolide are dopamine receptor agonists. Piribedil is not FDA-approved, but is available in Europe for the treatment of Parkinson's disease. Bromocriptine (Parlodel) is FDA-approved for the treatment of Parkinson's disease, hyperprolactinemia, and acromegaly, while amantadine (Symmetrel) and pergolide (Permax) are FDA-approved for the treatment of Parkinson's disease. Cabergoline (Dostinex, Cabaser) is FDA-approved for the treatment of hyperprolactinemia.

The use of older dopaminergic agents such as piribedil, amantadine, pergolide, bromocriptine, and cabergoline in depression is limited due to three principal reasons: (1) the paucity of supporting data, (2) the high incidence of side effects, particularly nausea (with the exception of amantadine), and (3) the development of newer dopaminergic agents discussed in further sections. Nevertheless, given the limited number of dopamine-selective agents available, studies focusing on the treatment of depression with these older agents are important in that they suggest an antidepressant role for dopamine that is independent of serotonin or norepinephrine. Specifically, open trials suggest monotherapy with the dopaminergic agent piribedil (Post *et al.*, 1978), and the D2-receptor agonist bromocriptine (Nordin *et al.*, 1981) to be effective in alleviating depression. Three double-blind studies show bromocriptine to be as effective as TCAs in the treatment of depression (Bouras *et al.*, 1982; Theohar *et al.*, 1982; Waehrens *et al.*, 1981). Bromocriptine also appears to decrease depressive symptoms in patients with Parkinson's disease (Jouvent *et al.*, 1983), and hyperprolactinemia (Mattox *et al.*, 1986). Treatment of hyperprolactinemia (Mattox *et al.*, 1986) and Parkinson's disease (Rektorova *et al.*, 2003) with pergolide also appears to result in a decrease in depressive symptoms. Only anecdotal evidence supports the use of cabergoline in depression (Takahashi *et al.*, 2003).

Pramipexole (Mirapex) and ropinirole (Requip) are selective dopamine D2/D3 receptor agonists (Gerlach *et al.*, 2003; Maggio *et al.*, 2003; Piercey *et al.*, 1998), and are FDA-approved for the treatment of Parkinson's disease. Small case series support the use of pramipexole in unipolar (Sporn *et al.*, 2000), and of both pramipexole and ropinirole in bipolar depression (Perugi *et al.*, 2001; Sporn *et al.*, 2000). Finally a large ($n = 174$) double-blind study comparing pramipexole to fluoxetine and to placebo found pramipexole to be as effective as fluoxetine and more effective than placebo (Corrigan *et al.*, 2000).

Treatment of Parkinson's disease with pramipexole also appears to result in decreases in depression severity (Lemke *et al.*, 2002; Rektorova *et al.*, 2003 and 2005) and anhedonia (Lemke *et al.*, 2002; Reichmann *et al.*, 2003) in some patients. The usual daily dose range for pramipexole is 0.5–3 mg, given in divided doses (twice or three times a day). The usual daily dose range for ropinirole is 0.75–3 mg, given in divided doses (twice or three times a day).

2.8.2 *Reuptake inhibitors*

Amineptine (Survector) is a TCA-derivative that predominantly inhibits dopaminergic reuptake, with minimal noradrenergic and no serotonergic activity (Garattini & Mennini, 1989; Garattini, 1997). Although amineptine is no longer in use due to its potential for abuse, reviewing studies of amineptine in depression is useful for two reasons: (1) such studies further establish an antidepressant role for dopamine and (2) such studies may provide further insights into the potential advantages for agents with predominantly dopaminergic activity in depression. The use of amineptine as an antidepressant is supported by a number of open trials (Boral *et al.*, 1989; Paes de Sousa & Tropa, 1989; Scarzella *et al.*, 1985), as well as placebo-controlled trials (Alevizos *et al.*, 1989; Boyer *et al.*, 1999). Amineptine also appears to be as effective as the TCAs (Borstein, 1979; Lemoine *et al.*, 1981; Mendis *et al.*, 1989; Rampello *et al.*, 1995; Van Amerongen *et al.*, 1979; Vauterin and Bazot, 1979), the MAOIs (Macher *et al.*, 1992), and the SSRIs (Dalery *et al.*, 1997) in MDD. In addition, the results of one controlled trial also report an earlier improvement in depressive symptoms with amineptine than the TCAs (Van Amerongen, 1979).

Similar to the MAOIs (see Chap. 4), several studies suggest the dopaminergic agent amineptine to be particularly effective in the treatment of fatigue and psychomotor retardation. Rampello *et al.* (1995) reported amineptine to be more effective than minaprine, clomipramine or placebo in patients affected by "retarded depression," which they described as exhibiting anergia, but also other symptoms including hypokinesia, reduction of speech, hypersomnia, reduced sexual activity, psychomotor slowness, hypomimia, and drowsiness. Dalery *et al.* (1997) found amineptine to be equally effective as fluoxetine in the overall treatment of MDD, but superior to fluoxetine on the retardation pole of the mood, anxiety, retardation, and danger scale. Vauterin and Bazot (1979) reported amineptine to be superior to the TCA trimipramine in depressed outpatients with respect to the treatment of sadness (depressed mood), psychomotor retardation, and social withdrawal.

Similar to amineptine, medifoxamine (Cledial) is a dopamine-selective reuptake inhibitor. Medifoxamine was briefly available in France for the treatment of depression, but was withdrawn from the market due to reports of hepatic enzyme elevations during treatment (Dumortier *et al.*, 2002; Marnata *et al.*, 1991).

The psychostimulants dextoamphetamine, pemoline, and methylphenidate have been, traditionally, regarded as presynaptic releasers of dopamine and as blockers of dopamine reuptake (Cardenas *et al.*, 2004; Saunders *et al.*, 2000; Volkow *et al.*,

2002). Dextroamphetamine (Dexedrine) is FDA-approved for the treatment of narcolepsy, exogenous obesity, and AD(H)D, a psychiatric disorder often present in patients with MDD. Pemoline (Cylert) is FDA-approved for AD(H)D, and methylphenidate (Ritalin, Concerta) is FDA-approved for the treatment of AD(H)D and narcolepsy.

The use of dexedrine (Kaufmann *et al.*, 1984; Little, 1993; Olin & Masant, 1996; Woods *et al.*, 1986), and methylphenidate (Askinazi *et al.*, 1986; El-Mallakh, 2000; Kauffman *et al.*, 1984; Lazarus *et al.*, 1994 and 1992; Lingam *et al.*, 1988; Little, 1993; Masand *et al.*, 1991b and c; Pickett *et al.*, 1990; Rothenhausler *et al.*, 2000; Stoll *et al.*, 1996; Woods *et al.*, 1986) in depression, particularly in depressed patients with comorbid medical illness, is supported by large chart reviews and small open trials cumulatively containing hundreds of patients. Wagner and Rabkin (2000), for instance, reported significant improvement in mood and energy among HIV+ depressed patients treated with double-blind dexedrine but not placebo. Similarly, methylphenidate was found to be as effective as desipramine in the treatment of MDD in HIV+ patients in one double-blind trial (Fernandez *et al.*, 1995), while both methylphenidate and pemoline were found to be more effective than placebo for the treatment of depression and fatigue in HIV+ patients (Breitbart *et al.*, 2001). A small placebo-controlled trial also found pemoline to be more effective than placebo in the treatment of some symptoms of depression, including depressed mood, fatigue, concentration, and memory (Elizur *et al.*, 1979). In summary, although promising, the widespread use of these agents is limited by their abuse potential (Drug Enforcement Agency Schedule II drugs) and paucity of supporting data from controlled trials.

2.8.3 *Receptor antagonists*

The antipsychotic amisulpride, a selective antagonist for D2 and D3 dopamine receptors, acts preferentially on presynaptic receptors, increasing dopaminergic transmission at low doses (Boyer *et al.*, 1999). Amisulpride was first reported to result in greater improvements in anergia and loss of interest in non-psychotic/non-depressed outpatients (Lecrubier *et al.*, 1988). Although amisulpride has not been FDA-approved [it is available in Europe (brand name: Solian) for the treatment of psychotic disorders], a number of studies suggest that it may have antidepressant effects. Specifically, the antidepressant potential of amisulpride has been suggested in open (Rocca *et al.*, 2002), and placebo-controlled trials (Boyer *et al.*, 1999; Lecrubier *et al.*, 1997). Amisulpride also appears to be as effective as the TCAs (Lecrubier *et al.*, 1997), and the SSRIs (Amore *et al.*, 2001; Cassano *et al.*, 2002; Smeraldi, 1998) in the treatment of depression. In fact, Amore *et al.* (2001) reported amisulpride to result in earlier improvement in depressive symptoms than sertraline in the treatment of dysthymic disorder and double depression, the latter condition defined as MDD and comorbid dysthymic disorder.

Chapter 3

Monoaminergic-Based Strategies: "Dual-Acting" Agents

3.1 Tricyclic Antidepressants (TCAs)

3.1.1 *Neuropharmacology*

Tricyclic antidepressants (TCAs), referred to as such because they share a chemical structure with two joined benzene rings, have been in use for almost half a century. With the exception of clomipramine, which has been reported to achieve anywhere from 83–100% *in vivo* 5HTT occupancy (20–210 mg daily; Suhara *et al.*, 2003), TCAs inhibit the reuptake of norepinephrine more potently than the reuptake of serotonin. Although the mechanism of the TCAs can range from combined serotonergic-noradrenergic reuptake inhibition to relatively selective noradrenergic reuptake inhibition, these agents will be discussed together in this chapter for the following reason: their safety and tolerability profile renders them more alike than not compared to most other antidepressants.

A variety of additional pharmacologic effects have been described for the TCAs. For example, doxepin, amitriptyline and nortriptyline inhibit glycine uptake by blocking the glycine transporter 1b (GLYT1b) and 2a (GLYT2a). Amoxapine displays a selective inhibition of GLYT2a, behaving as a 10-fold more efficient inhibitor of this isoform than of GLYT1b (Nunez *et al.*, 2000). Amoxapine is also a dopamine D2 receptor antagonist (Kapur *et al.*, 1999). Trimipramine and clomipramine also have some affinity for the dopamine D2 receptor *in vitro* (Richelson & Nelson, 1984).

TCAs, to varying degrees, are also fairly potent blockers of histamine H-1 receptors, serotonin 5-HT2 receptors, muscarinic acetylcholine receptors, and α-1 adrenergic receptors (Richelson & Nelson, 1984). Imipramine also appears to act as a neurokinin receptor inhibitor (Iwashita *et al.*, 1992). Finally, all TCAs also inhibit the sodium (Pancrazio *et al.*, 1998) and potassium channels (Casis *et al.*, 1998; Dreixler *et al.*, 2000; Grunnet *et al.*, 2001; Jo *et al.*, 2000; Teschemacher *et al.*, 1999).

3.1.2 *Classification*

The TCAs may be subdivided into tertiary amines and secondary amines. Tertiary amine TCAs include amitriptyline (Elavil, Adepril), imipramine (Tofranil, Antidepril), trimipramine (Surmontil, Herphonal), clomipramine (Anafranil, Clopress), and doxepin (Sinequan, Deptran). Secondary amine TCAs include nortriptyline (Pamelor, Aventyl), desipramine (Norpramin, Metylyl), protriptyline (Vivactil, Concordin), and amoxapine (Ascendin, Defanyl). In addition, maprotiline (Ludiomil), which is classified as a tetracyclic antidepressant, is commonly grouped with the TCAs due to similarities in dosing, mechanism of action, and side effects.

3.1.3 *Efficacy*

Although their overall efficacy in treating MDD is equivalent to that of the SSRIs (Anderson, 2000), TCAs are rarely chosen as first-line treatment for MDD (Petersen *et al.*, 2002). This is due to their inferior safety and tolerability profile compared to almost all newer agents. However, there is some evidence to suggest that TCA treatment may possess some advantages over SSRI treatment. For example, although the results of a large meta-analysis suggest no difference in efficacy between the TCAs and SSRIs in the treatment of MDD, there was a greater advantage for the tertiary amine TCAs over the SSRIs among inpatients. In addition, several studies also suggest TCAs may be more effective than the SSRIs in the treatment of melancholic depression, or in the treatment of depressed patients with certain comorbid medical conditions (Danish University Antidepressant Group, 1986 and 1990; Menza *et al.*, 2009; Navarro *et al.*, 2001; Robinson *et al.*, 2000; Roose *et al.*, 1994; Wermuth *et al.*, 1998), although not all studies support this finding (Mulsant *et al.*, 1999; Nelson *et al.*, 1999; Sandor *et al.*, 1998). Taken together, these studies indirectly suggest that treatment with agents that inhibit the reuptake of serotonin and norepinephrine may result in greater efficacy than treatment with serotonin-specific agents (i.e., the SSRIs) in severe depression, melancholic depression, or in MDD with significant MDD comorbidity (Figs. 3.1 and 3.2).

In addition, perhaps due to their ability to inhibit the reuptake of both serotonin and norepinephrine, as well as their ability to block sodium channels and potassium channels (Galeotti *et al.*, 1997 and 2001), TCAs appear to be more effective in treating neuropathic pain than the SSRIs (Sindrup *et al.*, 1999). In fact, the results of a meta-analysis reveal the TCAs to be superior to the SSRIs in the treatment of a number of somatic/pain disorders often diagnosed in patients with chronic depression, including headaches, fibromyalgia, irritable bowel disorder, idiopathic pain, tinnitus, and chronic fatigue

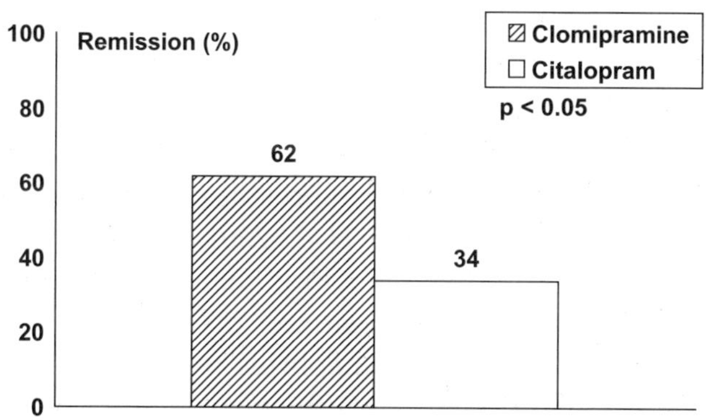

Fig. 3.1 Comparative efficacy of clomipramine (TCA) versus citalopram (SSRI) in endogenous MDD: A randomized, double-blind study ($n = 75$). [Data extracted from: Danish University Antidepressant Group (1986). Citalopram: Clinical effect profile in comparison with clomipramine. A controlled multicenter study. *Psychopharmacology*, 90, 131–138.]

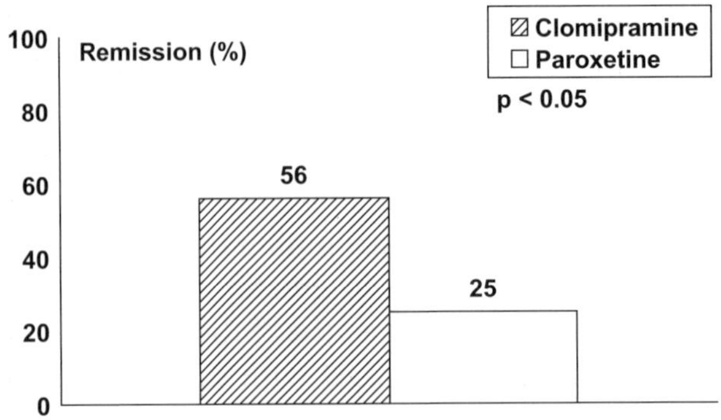

Fig. 3.2 Comparative efficacy of clomipramine versus paroxetine (SSRI) in endogenous MDD: A randomized, double-blind study ($n = 76$). [Data extracted from: Danish University Antidepressant Group (1990). Paroxetine: A selective serotonin reuptake inhibitor showing better tolerance, but weaker antidepressant effect than clomipramine in a controlled multicenter study. *Journal of Affective Disorders*, 18, 289–299.]

(O'Malley *et al.*, 1999). For this reason, TCAs and other agents which combine noradrenergic as well as serotonergic activity have been regarded by some researchers as being more effective than the SSRIs in the treatment of certain somatic symptoms of depression such as pain and headaches, and in the treatment of depression with comorbid medical illness.

Finally, it should also be pointed out that several studies suggest gender- and age-based differences in patient response to the TCAs versus the SSRIs. Martenyi *et al.* (2001), for instance, reported a greater resolution of depressive symptoms among women younger than 44 years of age during the treatment of MDD with the SSRI fluoxetine than the selective norepinephrine reuptake inhibitor (NRI) tetracyclic agent maprotiline. No difference in efficacy between these two treatments was reported for women older than 44 years of age, or for men. Kornstein *et al.* (2000) demonstrated greater response rates among women with MDD treated with the SSRI sertraline than the TCA imipramine, and greater response rates for men treated with imipramine than sertraline (Fig. 3.3).

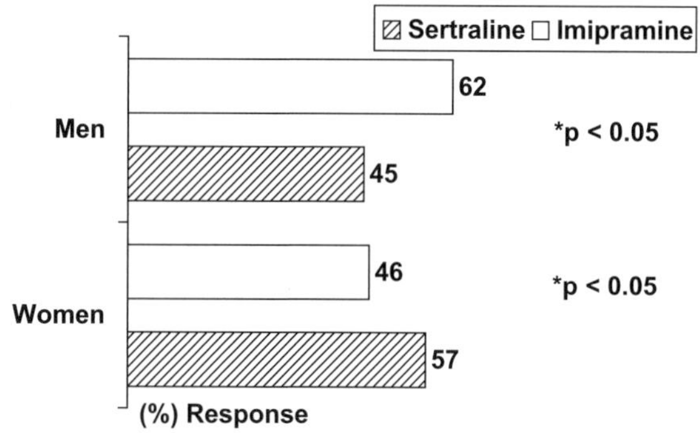

Fig. 3.3 Comparative efficacy of sertraline (SSRI) versus imipramine (TCA) among men and women with MDD ($n = 635$). *= pair-wise, within-gender comparisons. [Data extracted from: Kornstein, S.G., Schatzberg, A.F., Thase, M.E., *et al.* (2000). Gender differences in treatment response to sertraline versus imipramine in chronic depression. *American Journal of Psychiatry*, 157, 1445–1452.]

Interestingly, further analysis of the dataset revealed that sertraline was superior to imipramine in pre-menopausal but not post-menopausal women. However, it is also important to note that not all studies have found significant gender-based differences in antidepressant response. In a retrospective analysis of 11 trials, Lewis-Hall *et al.*, (1997) found no difference in response rates among women treated with either fluoxetine ($n = 427$) or a TCA ($n = 423$). Similarly, Hildebrandt *et al.* (2003) found no difference in response rates among women ($n = 196$) or men ($n = 96$) treated with clomipramine compared to citalopram, paroxetine, or moclobemide. Neither of these two studies, however, reported sub-analyses within specific age groups.

3.1.4 *Side effect profile*

Due to their ability to block the sodium (Pancrazio *et al.*, 1998) and potassium channels (Casis *et al.*, 1998; Dreixler *et al.*, 2000; Grunnet *et al.*, 2001; Jo *et al.*, 2000; Teschemacher *et al.*, 1999), TCAs are often arrythmogenic (Harrigan & Brady, 1999) and epileptogenic (Wedin *et al.*, 1986) when taken in very large (supra-therapeutic) quantities.

In general, TCAs are also less well tolerated than most newer antidepressants. In fact, the considerable side effect burden of TCAs accounts for higher dropout rates than the SSRIs (Anderson & Tomenson, 1995). The side effect profile of the TCAs can be subcategorized in terms of their relative affinity for a number of monoamine receptors and transporters. Overall, secondary amine TCAs tend to cause fewer anticholinergic, antihistaminergic and anti-α-1–related side effects than tertiary amine TCAs.

Amoxapine is the only TCA with documented, significant dopamine D-2 receptor antagonism. (Kapur *et al.*, 1999). There have been case reports of tardive dystonia and dyskinesia associated with amoxapine treatment (Hayashi *et al.*, 2000; Huang, 1986), and amoxapine should be avoided in patients with comorbid depression and Parkinson's disease (Sa *et al.*, 2001).

Anticholinergic-related side effects result from the affinity of TCAs for muscarinic cholinergic receptors and typically include sedation, dry mouth, blurred vision (Oshika, 1995), constipation, urinary hesitancy, tachycardia, memory difficulties, and ejaculatory difficulties. Finally, due to their anticholinergic effects, TCAs should be avoided in patients with narrow angle glaucoma (Oshika, 1995) and prostatic hypertrophy, as symptoms related to these conditions may worsen because of such anticholinergic effects. In elderly depressed patients, the presence of allele E4 of the apolipoprotein E (APOE) gene was found to confer an increased risk of developing anticholinergic cognitive side effects in one study (Pomara *et al.*, 2004).

Antihistaminergic-related side effects result from histaminergic H-1 receptor blockade and typically include increased appetite, weight gain, sedation, and fatigue. Weight gain with TCAs can be substantial. For example, in a double-blind extension study involving the treatment of MDD with either the TCA amitriptyline, mirtazapine or placebo, amitriptyline (22%) was associated with higher rates of weight gain, defined as a 7% or greater increase in weight compared to baseline, than mirtazapine (12.7%) or placebo (2.6%) (Montgomery *et al.*, 1998). As a result, TCAs may complicate the management of diabetes and worsen glycemic control (Lustman *et al.*, 1997; True *et al.*, 1987), and should be avoided whenever possible in diabetics (Goodnick, 2001). TCAs may also have hyperlipidemic effects, thus complicating their long-term use in patients with hyperlipidemia (Olusi *et al.*, 1996; Pollock *et al.*, 1994). TCAs-induced changes in soluble TNF receptor p75 (Hinze-Selch *et al.*, 2000), and leptin levels (Hinze-Selch *et al.*, 2000; Moosa *et al.*, 2003), have recently been proposed as potential underlying mechanisms contributing to TCA-related weight gain.

Xerostomia secondary to anticholinergic and antihistaminergic effects may also increase the risk of oral pathology, particularly dental caries (Peeters *et al.*, 1998).

Perhaps due to their sedative effects, a positive relationship between TCAs and an increased risk of a motor vehicle accident occurring in the elderly has been suggested by one epidemiologic study (Ray *et al.*, 1992). The sedative potential of various antidepressants is also a serious consideration for younger depressed patients, as they may increase the risk of mortality from automobile accidents. In fact, in one literature review (Ramaekers, 2003), sedating antidepressants (dothiepin, amitriptyline, imipramine, doxepin, mianserin) were found to result in driving impairments on a standardized road test comparable to impairments found in drivers with a blood alcohol level of 0.8 mg/ml (considered driving under the influence in most US states), while non-sedating antidepressants (moclobemide, fluoxetine, paroxetine, venlafaxine, nefazodone) were not found to affect driving performance. Subsequent studies have confirmed the relationship between sedating effects seen following TCA treatment and impaired driving ability (Brunnauer *et al.*, 2006; Iwamoto *et al.*, 2008). Treatment with TCAs has also been reported to worsen some aspects of memory, including immediate recall (Meyers *et al.*, 1991).

Despite pronounced sedative effects at therapeutic doses, and reports of TCA-related ventilatory suppression in patients with chronic obstructive sleep apnea (COPD; Greenberg *et al.*, 1993), the use of TCAs to treat depression among COPD patients with baseline hypercapnia appears to be effective (Borson *et al.*, 1992), and does not appear to result in worsening hypercapnia, spirometry, or ventilatory control (Gordon *et al.*, 1985).

Orthostatic hypotension and reflex tachycardia may result from α-1 adrenergic receptor antagonism. Antidepressant-emergent postural hypotension in the elderly may increase the risk of falls (Leipzig *et al.*, 1999) and fractures (i.e., hip fractures — Ray *et al.*, 1991). Nortriptyline is generally thought to be less likely to cause orthostatic hypotension than tertiary amine TCAs such as imipramine (Roose *et al.*, 1987a; Thayssen *et al.*, 1981). However, the affinity of nortriptyline for the α-1 adrenergic receptor, although less than the affinity of most TCAs, is actually greater (e.g., more than twice) than the affinity of desipramine and protriptyline (Richelson & Nelson, 1984). Homozygosity for the 3435T allele of the abcb1 gene, the multi-drug resistance gene that encodes a p-GP, appears to be a risk factor for occurrence of nortriptyline-emergent postural hypotension (Roberts *et al.*, 2002), which may be due to decreased CNS and, therefore, increased peripheral concentrations of the drug.

The ability of TCAs to inhibit the sodium channel may also result in electrocardiographic changes in susceptible individuals (for instance in post-myocardial infarction patients, in patients with bi-fascicular heart block, left bundle branch block or a prolonged QT interval), even at therapeutic doses (Nelson *et al.*, 1999) and, given that contemporary psychopharmacologists have access to a multitude of alternative treatment options, should be avoided in these patients. As mentioned previously, due to the inhibition of sodium channels and cholinergic receptors, the TCAs also carry a risk of seizure. Maprotiline and clomipramine are considered the TCAs with the greatest risk of seizures (Pisani *et al.*, 2002), particularly at higher doses. This combined risk of seizure and arrhythmia renders the TCAs as the least safe during overdose (Henry *et al.*, 1995; White *et al.*, 2008).

The TCAs appear to have variable effects on sleep physiology. For example, certain TCAs (e.g., amitriptyline, trimipramine) shorten sleep-onset latency, improve sleep efficiency and decrease wake time after sleep onset (WASO), while other TCAs (e.g., desipramine or protriptyline) prolong sleep-onset latency, reduce sleep efficiency and increase WASO (Winokur *et al.*, 2001). With the exception of trimipramine, all TCAs suppress rapid eye movement (REM) sleep

(Winokur *et al.*, 2001). Patients that receive a bedtime-only dose of TCAs are more likely to report nightmares than patients who divided their TCA regimen throughout the day (Flemenbaum, 1976; Strayhorn & Nash, 1978).

The endocrinologic effects of the TCAs are highly variable and, at times, appear contradictory. There are several case reports of TCA-emergent hyponatremia or syndrome of inappropriate antidiuretic hormone secretion (SIADH) (Adlakha *et al.*, 1991; Liskin *et al.*, 1984; Madhusoodanan & Osnos, 1981; Parker, 1984). There are also case reports of galactorrhea with imipramine (Klein *et al.*, 1964), and clomipramine (Anand, 1985; Fowlie & Burton, 1987), suggesting that an increase in prolactin levels, due to increased serotonergic turnover, may underlie such phenomenon (Hanna *et al.*, 1991). Amitriptyline and imipramine, however, do not appear to increase prolactin levels (Meltzer *et al.*, 1977; Sonntag *et al.*, 1996; Steiger *et al.*, 1997).

Linnoila *et al.* (1981) found no changes in total T3 or T4 in depressed outpatients treated with amitriptyline, imipramine, or desipramine. In a subsequent study, however, although administration of desipramine (up to 300 mg) in 19 MDD patients for six weeks did not result in changes in thyroid stimulating hormone (TSH), free thyroxine (T4), triiodothyronine (T3), or thyroid binding globulin levels, desipramine administration was found to result in increased total T4 levels (Shelton *et al.*, 1993). In contrast, administration of amitriptyline in MDD outpatients for six weeks was reported to result in decreased T4 and free T4 levels (Kusalic *et al.*, 1993). Finally, administration of imipramine for four weeks in MDD patients was not found to result in changes in testosterone levels (Sonntag *et al.*, 1996).

Clomipramine did not appear to alter follicle stimulating hormone (FSH), luteotropic hormone (LH), testosterone, prolactin, estradiol, and gonadotropin-releasing hormone (GnRH) levels in depressed men in one study (Maier & Koinig, 1994). Similarly, in a study involving administration of clomipramine or nortriptyline to six healthy volunteers for six days, there were no significant changes in TSH, growth hormone (GH), or prolactin levels reported (Widerlov *et al.*, 1978). Nordgren and von Scheele (1981) also found no effect of 28 days of nortriptyline therapy on T3, T3 reuptake, T4 or TSH in 20 MDD outpatients. Schlienger *et al.* (1980), however, reported reductions in T3, free T3 and TSH levels during clomipramine treatment. Treatment of endogenous depressives with nortriptyline for four weeks was also found to result in increases in prolactin levels (Nielsen, 1980). Doxepin, due to its antidopaminergic effects, also appears to increase prolactin levels during treatment (Nielsen *et al.*, 1980).

Chronic treatment with imipramine has been reported to result in hyperpigmentation of the face, arms, and back of hands (Ming *et al.*, 1999) requiring laser treatment (Atkin & Fitzpatrick, 2000).

Adverse events thought related to the inhibition of norepinephrine reuptake include tremors (Beasley *et al.*, 2000), as well as cases of "occult" pheochromocytoma "unmasked" by TCAs (Achong & Keane, 1981; Birkebaek & Perrild, 1986; Brown *et al.*, 2003; Ferguson, 1994; Johnson *et al.*, 1979; Korzets *et al.*, 1997; Kuhs, 1998; Mok & Swann, 1978).

Treatment with the TCAs appears to carry an increased risk of emergence of manic symptoms in the treatment of bipolar depression than the SSRIs paroxetine (Nemeroff *et al.*, 2001) and fluoxetine (Cohn *et al.*, 1989), and the NDRI bupropion (Sachs *et al.*, 1994). Finally, symptoms of gastrointestinal discomfort, sleep disturbance, movement disorders and mania have been temporally linked to abrupt discontinuation of TCAs (Garner *et al.*, 1993).

3.1.5 *Dosing*

There is a wide range of effective doses for the TCAs. Typical TCA antidepressant doses are 100–300 mg/day, with the exception of nortriptyline and protriptyline, which require lower doses. Due to their poor tolerability at higher doses, treatment with the TCAs is typically initiated at lower than therapeutic doses (e.g., 10 mg/day for imipramine) in order to minimize the risk of adverse events and premature treatment discontinuation. There is evidence to suggest a relationship between serum levels of TCAs and clinical response. Perry *et al.* (1994) pooled and analyzed all available studies examining the relationship between TCA blood levels and clinical response with the use of receiver operating characteristics curves. The relationship between clinical response and blood levels for desipramine was linear, with the threshold concentration in plasma for therapeutic response being greater than or equal to 116 ng/ml (response rates: 51% versus 15% for patients with levels above or below that threshold, respectively). The remaining TCAs exhibited a curvilinear (inverse "U" shaped curve) relationship between blood level and clinical response. The optimal range for nortriptyline, "total" imipramine (imipramine plus desipramine), and "total" amitriptyline (amitriptyline plus nortriptyline) (with their corresponding response rates within versus outside the level range) were: 58–148 ng/ml (66% versus 26%), 175–350 ng/ml (67% versus 39%), and 93–140 ng/ml (50% versus 30%), respectively.

Genotype may also influence the relationship between dose and TCA levels. Duplication of the CYP2D6L allele of the CYP2D6 enzyme, for instance, present in 2–7% of Caucasians (Agundez *et al.*, 1995) and up to 9% of Ethiopians and 25% of Tanzanians (Aklillu *et al.*, 1996), has been associated with ultra-rapid metabolism of nortriptyline (Bertilsson *et al.*, 1985), imipramine (Brosen *et al.*, 1986a and 1986b), and desipramine (Bergmann *et al.*, 2001; Spina *et al.*, 1984). There is also a single case report of ultra-rapid metabolism of maprotiline not resulting from 2D6 duplication (Vormfelde *et al.*, 1997).

Finally, some TCAs including doxepin (Uhr *et al.*, 2003a), amitriptyline (Uhr *et al.*, 2000), trimipramine (Uhr *et al.*, 2003b), and nortriptyline (Roberts *et al.*, 2002), are also substrates for p-glycoprotein (p-GP), which is expressed by the abcb gene in blood-brain barrier cells and acts as an extrusion pump for various xenobiotic compounds (Schinkel *et al.*, 1995 and 1996), including some antidepressants. The clinical relevance of these relationships remains unclear, although it is possible that p-GP status may influence the relationship between serum levels and CNS levels of TCAs.

3.2 Serotonin-Norepinephrine Reuptake Inhibitors (SNRIs)

Venlafaxine, desvenlafaxine, duloxetine and milnacipran share the property of being relatively potent reuptake inhibitors of serotonin and norepinephrine and are therefore considered SNRIs.

3.2.1 *Venlafaxine*

3.2.1.1 *Neuropharmacology*

Venlafaxine (Effexor) was the first SNRI to gain FDA approval for the treatment of MDD. At daily doses greater than 150 mg (Sanchez & Hytell, 1999), venlafaxine inhibits the reuptake of both serotonin and norepinephrine, while mostly inhibiting the reuptake of serotonin at lower doses (Harvey *et al.*, 2000; Roseboom & Kalin, 2000). Venlafaxine also appears to act as non-competitive antagonists of nicotinic acetyl cholinergic receptors (Fryer & Lukas, 1999).

3.2.1.2 *Efficacy*

Venlafaxine, along with the SSRIs and bupropion, is commonly chosen as first-line treatment for MDD (Petersen *et al.*, 2002). Similar to clomipramine, a TCA with robust "dual" serotonergic-noradrenergic effects, emerging evidence suggest that the treatment of MDD with venlafaxine results in greater remission rates than SSRI treatment (Nemeroff *et al.*, 2008; Papakostas *et al.*, 2007a; Rudolph, 2002; Smith *et al.*, 2002; Stahl *et al.*, 2002; Thase *et al.*, 2001a and 2005a), particularly among patients with severe MDD (Schmitt *et al.*, 2009) (Fig. 3.4).

In fact, to some degree, this finding can also be generalized to all antidepressants that simultaneously influence the serotonergic and noradrenergic systems versus the SSRIs (Papakostas *et al.*, 2007a) (Fig. 3.5).

However, contrary to the argument that noradrenergic-serotonergic agents are superior to the SSRIs in MDD, it should also be pointed out that studies have demonstrated the efficacy

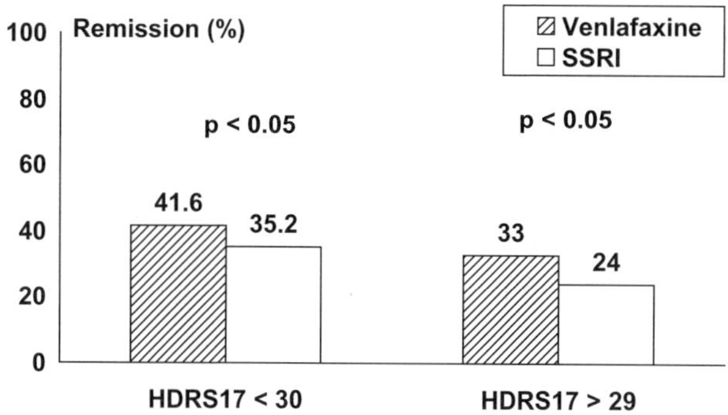

Fig. 3.4 Comparative efficacy of venlafaxine (SNRI) versus SSRIs: Pooled analysis of 31 RCTs ($n = 6{,}492$). RCT: Randomized, Controlled Trial. HDRS17 = 17-item Hamilton Depression Rating Scale. [Data extracted from: Schmitt, A.B., Bauer, M., Volz, H.P., *et al.* (2009). Differential effects of venlafaxine in the treatment of major depressive disorder according to baseline severity. *European Archives of Psychiatry and Clinical Neurosciences*, 259, 329–339.]

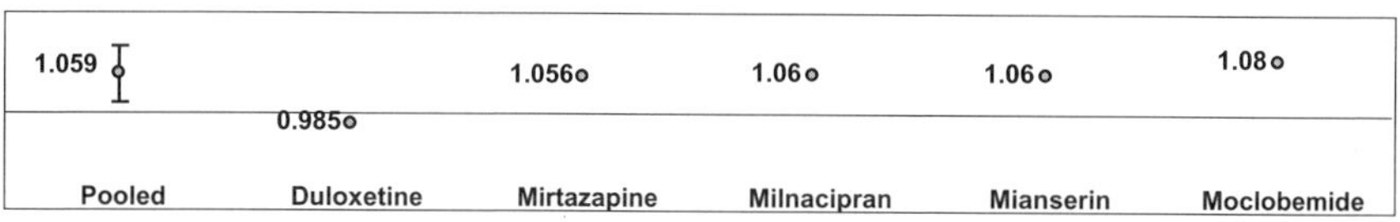

Fig. 3.5 Pooled risk ratio and individual risk ratios for response to a 5HT + NE versus an SSRI antidepressant in MDD. Error bars represent 95% CI of the pooled risk ratio: Treatment with a serotonergic-noradrenergic agent (*5HT + NE antidepressant) is more effective than the SSRIs ($p < 0.05$). Risk ratios for each individual serotonergic-noradrenergic agent within the pooled 95% CI (not significantly different; $p > 0.05$). [Data extracted from: Papakostas, G.I., Thase, M.E., Fava, M., *et al.* (2007). Are antidepressant drugs that combine serotonergic and noradrenergic mechanisms of action more effective than the selective serotonin reuptake inhibitors in treating major depressive disorder? A meta-analysis of studies of newer agents. *Biological Psychiatry*, 62(11), 1217–1227.]

of venlafaxine and the SSRI escitalopram to be, relatively, equivalent (Montgomery & Andersen, 2006), with escitalopram potentially being more advantageous for severe MDD (Kornstein *et al.*, 2009) (Fig. 3.6).

In addition, several reports suggest that improvement in depressive symptoms during treatment with venlafaxine may occur sooner

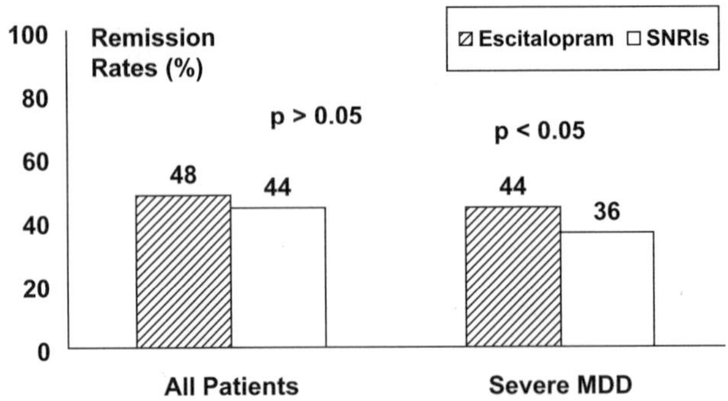

Fig. 3.6 Comparative efficacy of escitalopram versus the SNRIs duloxetine and venlafaxine in MDD: Pooled analysis of 4 RCTs. [Data extracted from: Kornstein, S.G., Li, D., Mao, Y., *et al.* (2009). Escitalopram versus SNRI antidepressants in the acute treatment of major depressive disorder. *CNS Spectrums*, 14(6), 326–333.]

than those of the SSRIs (Davidson *et al.*, 2002; Entsuah *et al.*, 2001), a phenomenon that some ascribe to the dual effects of venlafaxine on the serotonergic as well as the noradrenergic system. Contrary to this argument, venlafaxine was also found to result in earlier improvement than the TCA imipramine in one study (Benkert *et al.*, 1996). Venlafaxine also appears to be effective in treating somatic symptoms of depression (Bradley *et al.*, 2003).

Thase *et al.* (2005b) pooled eight randomized, controlled trials comparing the serotonin-norepinephrine reuptake inhibitor (SNRI) venlafaxine with an SSRI for MDD. They found that the probability of remission during treatment with venlafaxine was influenced by neither age or gender, while women older than 50 were less likely to respond to an SSRI than women younger than 50 (Fig. 3.7). This effect appeared to be ameliorated by the presence of hormone-replacement therapy.

The results of double-blind, placebo-controlled trials do not support the use of venlafaxine in the treatment of MDD in the elderly (Schatzberg & Roose, 2006), for children/adolescents (Courtney, 2004; Emslie *et al.*, 2007; Mandocki *et al.*, 1997; Whittington *et al.*, 2004), or for the treatment of depression in dementia (de Vasconcelos

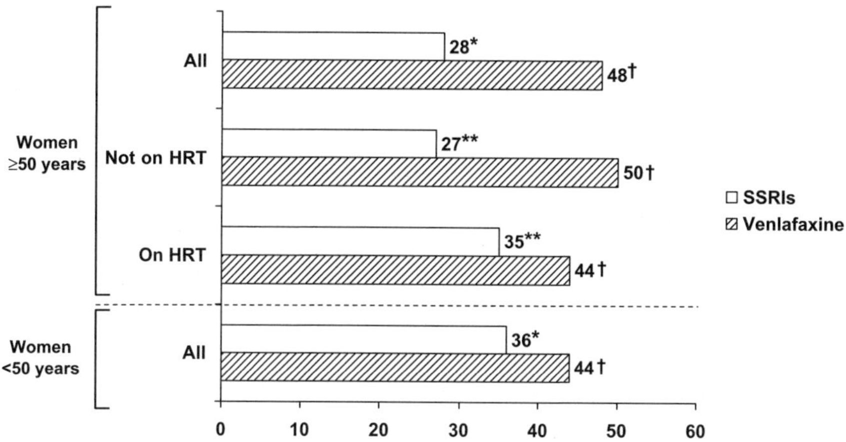

Fig. 3.7 Comparative efficacy (remission) of venlafaxine (SNRI) versus SSRIs among women with MDD (8 RCTs; $n = 744$). $^{*}p < 0.05$; $^{**}p < 0.01$; $^{\dagger}p > 0.05$ pair-wise venlafaxine–venlafaxine or SSRI–SSRI comparisons; Venlafaxine > SSRIs overall ($p < 0.05$). [Data extracted from: Thase, M.E., Entsuah, R., Cantillon, M., & Kornstein, S.G. (2005). Relative antidepressant efficacy of venlafaxine and SSRIs: Sex–age interactions. *Journal of Women's Health*, 14, 609–616.]

Cunha *et al.*, 2007). The results of a double-blind study also suggest venlafaxine to be superior to placebo as an augmentor of quetiapine in psychotic MDD (Wijkstra *et al.*, in press). Double-blind, placebo-controlled trials focusing on the use of venlafaxine for the treatment of major depression in patients with bipolar disorder (as an adjunct to mood stabilizers), or for the treatment of dysthymic disorder, seasonal affective disorder or in patients with post-partum depression or minor depressive disorder have not been published to date. However, double-blind, randomized studies suggest equivalent efficacy between venlafaxine and the SSRIs as adjuncts to mood stabilizer treatment for patients with bipolar depression (Post *et al.*, 2006; Vieta *et al.*, 2002), although higher rates of abnormal mood elevations (mania or hypomania) during venlafaxine- than SSRI- or bupropion-treatment were also reported in those studies.

Only open-label studies have focused on the use of venlafaxine in dysthymic disorder (Devanand *et al.*, 2004; Ravindran *et al.*, 1998). There is also anecdotal evidence for the use of venlafaxine as monotherapy in patients with MDD and comorbid ADHD (Hornig-Rohan & Amsterdam, 2002), or for the treatment of post-stroke depression (Cravello *et al.*, 2009; Kucukalic *et al.*, 2007). Finally, there is evidence from randomized, double-blind, placebo-controlled trial(s) to support the use of venlafaxine in the treatment of psychiatric disorders often present in patients with MDD including generalized anxiety disorder (GAD) (Katz *et al.*, 2002), panic disorder (Pollack *et al.*, 2007), social anxiety disorder (SAD) (Liebowitz *et al.*, 2005), post-traumatic stress disorder (PTSD) (Davidson *et al.*, 2006), but not obsessive-compulsive disorder (OCD), eating disorders, or attention deficit (hyperactivity) disorder [AD(H)D].

3.2.1.3 *Side effect profile*

Common side effects of venlafaxine include nausea, insomnia, sedation, sexual dysfunction, headache, sweating, tremor, palpitations, and dizziness.

Treatment-emergent nausea with venlafaxine appears to be more common than with the SSRIs, although the use of the extended form of venlafaxine (Effexor XR) is associated with lower rates of nausea than the immediate release form (Papakostas, 2007). Rates of insomnia or somnolence/fatigue appear to be equivalent between SSRI and venlafaxine treatment (Papakostas, 2007). Venlafaxine, however, appears to be less sedating than the TCAs (Shrivasta *et al.*, 1994), or trazodone (Cunningham *et al.*, 1994), while the potential for sexual dysfunction appears comparable to the SSRIs (Clayton *et al.*, 2002; Montejo *et al.*, 2001). Nearly 2–6% of venlafaxine-treated patients may also experience an increase in diastolic blood pressure (Rudolph & Derivan, 1996; Feighner, 1995), which appears to be dose-related (Thase, 1998). In fact, as many as 12% of patients treated with high doses (mean dose approximately 350 mg) of venlafaxine were reported to have developed hypertension in one study (Mbaya *et al.*, 2007).

There is a paucity of data regarding the long-term effects of treatment with venlafaxine on weight. Epidemiologic studies suggest the incidence of weight gain following one year of treatment of depression with venlafaxine (16%) to be equivalent to SSRI treatment

(16–19%), less than treatment with mirtazapine (26%), and greater than treatment with either nefazodone or bupropion (12%) (Papakostas, 2007). However, until recently, data on weight from long-term, placebo-controlled studies focusing on the use of venlafaxine for the treatment of mood or anxiety disorders had not been published (Entsuah *et al.*, 1996; Montgomery *et al.*, 2002a, 2002b and 2004a; Simon *et al.*, 2004). More recently, the results of a two-year study comparing venlafaxine with placebo for MDD did not reveal greater weight gain for venlafaxine- than placebo-treated patients (Keller *et al.*, 2007). Venlafaxine does not appear to alter TNF-α, soluble TNF-α receptor p55 and p75 levels, or leptin levels in MDD (Kraus *et al.*, 2002), biomakers thought to be relevant in antidepressant-associated weight gain (see relevant section for the TCAs).

There are case reports of venlafaxine-emergent hyponatremia (Bourgeois, 2005; Degner *et al.*, 2004; Egger *et al.*, 2006; Gupta & Saravay, 1997; Kirby *et al.*, 2002; Meynaar *et al.*, 1997; Ranieri *et al.*, 1997; Romero *et al.*, 2007; Roxanas *et al.*, 2007), hyperprolactinemia/galactorrhea (Sternbach, 2003; Wichman & Cunningham, 2008; Yang *et al.*, 2009), hypokalemia (Shang *et al.*, 2002), and hypogonadism (Bell & Shipman, 2000). In one naturalistic study, the rate of breast enlargement was lower with venlafaxine than with the SSRIs, while venlafaxine did not appear to alter serum prolactin, or estradiol levels (Amsterdam *et al.*, 1997).

As with the SSRIs, patients treated with venlafaxine may also experience bruxism (Jaffee & Bostwick, 2000; Brown & Hong, 1999; Alonso-Navarro *et al.*, 2009). There are also reports of abnormal bleeding or bruising (Kohn & Labbate, 1997; Linnebur *et al.*, 2002; Sarma & Horne, 2006), alopecia (Pitchot & Ansseau, 2001; Pereira & Goldman-Levine, 2007), hepatitis (Degner *et al.*, 2004; Phillips *et al.*, 2006), and hypersensitivity pneumonitis (Borderias *et al.*, 2008) associated with venlafaxine use.

The abrupt discontinuation of venlafaxine also carries a risk of withdrawal-related adverse events similar to those described for the SSRIs (Fava *et al.*, 1997; Stone *et al.*, 2007; Taylor *et al.*, 2006). However, the discontinuation syndrome seen with venlafaxine, a compound with a half-life of only a few hours, is more severe than that associated with the abrupt discontinuation of either escitalopram (Montgomery *et al.*, 2004b), or sertraline (Sir *et al.*, 2005).

There are also reports of serotonin syndrome in patients treated with venlafaxine alone (Kolecki, 1997a; Pan & Shen, 2003), or in combination with trazodone (McCue & Joseph, 2001), SSRIs (Bhatara *et al.*, 1998), mirtazapine (Dimellis, 2003), TCAs (Dougherty *et al.*, 2002; Perry, 2000), dextroamphetamine (Prior *et al.*, 2002), MAOIs (Brubacher *et al.*, 1996; Diamond *et al.*, 1998; Gitlin, 1997; Heisler *et al.*, 1996; Hodgman *et al.*, 1997; Kolecki, 1997b; Roxanas & Machado, 1998; Weiner *et al.*, 1998), and lithium (Mekler & Woggon, 1997), as well as reports of rhabdomyolysis during venlafaxine treatment (Wilson *et al.*, 2007).

Venlafaxine does appear to block myocardial sodium channels in animals (Khalifa *et al.*, 1999). In one uncontrolled study, 4 of 13 patients treated with venlafaxine experienced asystole during ECT (Gonzalez-Pinto *et al.*, 2002). Although the authors noted that this serious adverse event only occurred in patients on daily doses of venlafaxine greater than 300 mg and in patients anesthetized with propofol, in the absence of further data the use of venlafaxine in patients requiring ECT and perhaps even general anesthesia should be avoided. Similar cases have been reported since then (Lyons & Symon, 2008). There are also several reports of increased QTc intervals (Combes *et al.*, 2001; Howell *et al.*, 2007; Johnson *et al.*, 2006; Letsas *et al.*, 2006; Mbaya *et al.*, 2007) and a reduction in heart rate variability (Davidson *et al.*, 2005) in patients treated with venlafaxine, as well as a report of fatal cardiotoxicity following venlafaxine overdose (Hojer *et al.*, 2008). In fact, the results of one epidemiologic study suggested higher mortality rates (due to causes including seizures, serotonin syndrome, rhabdomyolysis, renal failure, and hepatic failure) following a venlafaxine versus an SSRI overdose (Flanagan, 2008).

Similar to the SSRIs, venlafaxine increases wake time after sleep onset and suppresses REM sleep (Salin-Pascual *et al.*, 1997).

Compared with the SSRIs, little is known regarding the effects of venlafaxine on pregnancy. As with the SSRIs, transient symptoms probably linked to increased serotonin activity or serotonin withdrawal have been reported among infants born to mothers who were exposed to venlafaxine during the third trimester of pregnancy (Ferreira *et al.*, 2007; Levinson-Castiel *et al.*, 2006; Boucher *et al.*, 2009). Also similar to the SSRIs, a link between venlafaxine exposure during the first trimester and an increased rate of fetal malformations has not been established for venlafaxine (Einarson *et al.*, 2001 and 2009; Einarson & Einarson, 2005). Venlafaxine has been labeled as belonging to the FDA pregnancy category C. Among the few studies conducted, considerable venlafaxine levels were found in the milk of mothers treated with venlafaxine, as well as detectible serum venlafaxine levels among breast-fed infants of mother treated with venlafaxine (Ilett *et al.*, 1998 and 2002; Berle *et al.*, 2004; Newport *et al.*, 2009). Any clinical relevance has yet to be determined.

Pooled data from placebo-controlled studies focusing on the risk of emergence or worsening of suicidal ideation during the treatment of adults with MDD with venlafaxine have not been published to date.

3.2.1.4 *Dosing*

Venlafaxine is generally effective at daily doses at or above 75 mg, and is often started at 75 mg or even 37.5 mg, typically in its extended release (XR) formulation (Wellington & Perry, 2001) (usual dose range 75–300 mg). The degree of serotonin transporter occupancy achieved with a 75 mg daily dose of venlafaxine is, roughly, 80%, which is equivalent to 20 mg fluoxetine, 50 mg sertraline, and 20 mg of paroxetine (Meyer *et al.*, 2004). At higher doses (225–450 mg), serotonin transporter occupancy is approximately 85% (Voineskos *et al.*, 2007).

Venlafaxine is a substrate for p-GP (Uhr *et al.*, 2003a), and is a weak inhibitor of p-GP activity (Weiss *et al.*, 2003). Venlafaxine has been shown to also induce the expression of p-glycoprotein *in vitro* (Ehret *et al.*, 2007). Finally, certain mutations for the CYP2D6 (Fukuda *et al.*, 2000a; Grasmader *et al.*, 2004; Hermann *et al.*, 2008; Lessard *et al.*, 1999; Preskorn *et al.*, 2009; Shams *et al.*, 2006; Whyte *et al.*, 2006), as well as mutations for the CYP2C19 enzyme (Fukuda *et al.*,

2000b) have been linked to increased venlafaxine levels, although the sum of serum concentration of venlafaxine and desvenlafaxine (active metabolite) appears to be constant regardless of patient CYP2D6 genotype (Hermann *et al.*, 2008). There is also a report of ultra-rapid metabolism of venlafaxine in patients with CYP2D6 gene duplication (Shams *et al.*, 2006; Veefkind *et al.*, 2000). Venlafaxine is marketed as a racemate of both enantiomers, with S(−) venlafaxine being a more potent inhibitor of CYP2D6 *in vitro* than the R(+) isomer (Otton *et al.*, 1996).

Little is known regarding the relationship between plasma venlafaxine levels and clinical response in MDD. The results of a small, unreplicated study suggest higher venlafaxine+O-desmethylvenlafaxine levels and a lower R(+)/R(−) venlafaxine plasma ratio in early sustained (first two weeks) versus late sustained responders to venlafaxine (Gex-Fabry *et al.*, 2004).

3.2.2 *Desvenlafaxine*

Desvenlafaxine (Pristiq), a major active metabolite of venlafaxine, is an SNRI with little affinity for muscarinic, histaminic, or adrenergic receptors (Deecher *et al.*, 2006). Desvenlafaxine has been approved by the FDA for the treatment of MDD.

Desvenlafaxine has been found to be more effective than placebo in the treatment of MDD in several randomized, double-blind clinical trials (Boyer *et al.*, 2008; DeMartinis *et al.*, 2007; Feiger *et al.*, 2009; Liebowitz *et al.*, 2008; Septein-Velez *et al.*, 2007; Tourian *et al.*, 2009), although not all studies demonstrate the superiority of desvenlafaxine over placebo for MDD (Lieberman *et al.*, 2008; Liebowitz *et al.*, 2007). Pooling nine ($n = 2{,}913$) randomized, double-blind, placebo-controlled trials of desvenlafaxine for depression reveals remission rates of 32% and 23% for desvenlafaxine- and placebo-treated patients, respectively (Thase *et al.*, 2009).

Two studies also report desvenlafaxine to be as effective as venlafaxine in the treatment of MDD (Lieberman *et al.*, 2008). Desvenlafaxine was also found to be more effective than placebo in reducing painful (somatic) symptoms (Brisard *et al.*, 2007), and anxiety (Tourian *et al.*, 2007) symptoms of depression. Desvenlafaxine has also been found to resolve menopausal hot flashes, a potential advantage for menopausal women with MDD (Archer *et al.*, 2009a and 2009b).

Side effects reported in those studies include nausea, dry mouth, sweating, somnolence, anorexia, constipation, asthenia, vomiting, tremor, nervousness, abnormal vision, sexual dysfunction, and an elevation of liver enzymes in some patients (Clayton *et al.*, 2009; DeMartinis *et al.*, 2007). As with other SNRIs and SSRIs, the abrupt discontinuation of desvenlafaxine may result in withdrawal symptoms (Montgomery *et al.*, 2009). The results of a double-blind, six-month trial do not suggest any difference in long-term weight gain during desvenlafaxine- than placebo-treatment of MDD (Petroneva *et al.*, 2007).

One major advantage of desvenlafaxine is that its metabolism does not appear to involve the hepatic cytochrome enzyme system (Schilling *et al.*, 2005). CYP2D6 genotype does not appear to influence desvenlafaxine concentrations in humans (Preskorn *et al.*, 2009). The results of one study suggest desvenlafaxine to accumulate in maternal breast milk (Newport *et al.*, 2009). Desvenlafaxine is generally effective at daily doses at or above 50 mg (100–200 mg), and is often started at 50 mg.

3.2.3 *Duloxetine*

3.2.3.1 *Efficacy*

Duloxetine (Cymbalta), more so than its negative enantiomer (LY248685 — Wong *et al.*, 1993), is an inhibitor of serotonin and norepinephrine reuptake (Bymaster *et al.*, 2001). Duloxetine is FDA-approved for the treatment of MDD.

Double-blind studies reveal duloxetine to be superior to placebo and as effective as the SSRIs fluoxetine, paroxetine (Lee *et al.*, 2007; Thase *et al.*, 2007b), and the SNRI venlafaxine (Perahia *et al.*, 2008) in the treatment of MDD, although duloxetine appears to be more effective than the SSRIs fluoxetine and paroxetine in the treatment of severe MDD (Thase *et al.*, 2007b) (Fig. 3.8).

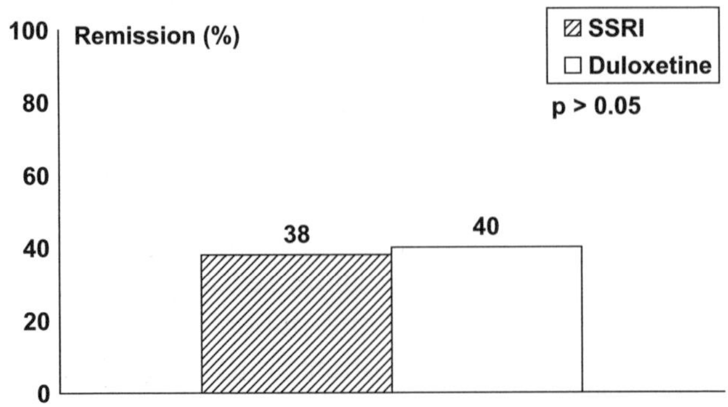

Fig. 3.8 Comparative efficacy of duloxetine (SNRI) versus SSRIs: Pooled analysis of 6 RCTs ($n = 1{,}140$). RCT: Randomized, Controlled Trial. [Data extracted from: Thase, M.E., Pritchett, Y.L., Ossanna, M.J., *et al.* (2007b). Efficacy of duloxetine and selective serotonin reuptake inhibitors: Comparisons as assessed by remission rates in patients with major depressive disorder. *Journal of Clinical Psychopharmacology*, 27(6), 672–676.]

The efficacies of duloxetine and escitalopram appear to be relatively equivalent overall (Khan *et al.*, 2007; Nierenberg *et al.*, 2007; Pigott *et al.*, 2007; Wade *et al.*, 2007), with escitalopram potentially being more advantageous for severe MDD (Kornstein *et al.*, 2009).

In addition to depressive symptoms, it has also been demonstrated that duloxetine is more effective than placebo in resolving painful symptoms in MDD patients (Krebs *et al.*, 2008). In fact, duloxetine also appeared to be more effective than the SSRI paroxetine in the treatment of somatic symptoms of MDD such as pain in one randomized, double-blind trial (Goldstein *et al.*, 2004), although other published trials do not show a difference in efficacy between duloxetine and paroxetine in the treatment of somatic/painful symptoms of depression (Detke *et al.*, 2004; Perahia *et al.*, 2006a; Eli Lilly Clinical Trial F1J-MC-HMAT-A). More recently, the results of a meta-analysis do not support greater analgesic effects for duloxetine than paroxetine in MDD (Krebs *et al.*, 2008). Finally, the results of a pooled analysis of clinical trials focusing on the use of duloxetine for MDD suggest a greater antidepressant effect following treatment with duloxetine among patients with anxious MDD defined using the dichotomous approach (see Chap. 1 for details) (Fava *et al.*, 2007).

The results of a double-blind, randomized placebo-controlled trial also support the use of duloxetine for elderly patients with MDD (Raskin *et al.*, 2007). There is also evidence from an open-label trial supporting the use of duloxetine for dysthymic disorder (Koran *et al.*, 2007) or seasonal affective disorder (Pjrek *et al.*, 2008). Double-blind, placebo-controlled trials focusing on the use of duloxetine for children/adolescents with MDD, or for the treatment of bipolar depression, dysthymic disorder, post-partum depression, seasonal affective disorder or minor depression have not been published to date. However, a double-blind, placebo-controlled trial focusing on the use of duloxetine for the treatment of dysthymic disorder is currently underway (clinicaltrials.gov; NCT00360724). Finally, there is evidence from randomized, double-blind, placebo-controlled trials to support the use of duloxetine in GAD (Allgulander *et al.*, 2007 and 2008), and fibromyalgia (Arnold *et al.*, 2004, 2005, and 2007; Choy *et al.*, 2009; Russell *et al.*, 2008), disorders often encountered in patients with MDD.

3.2.3.2 *Side effect profile*

Common side effects associated with duloxetine include dry mouth, headache, nausea, somnolence, sweating, insomnia, sexual dysfunction, and fatigue. Nausea and insomnia appear to be more common during duloxetine than SSRI treatment (Lam *et al.*, 2008), while somnolence/fatigue are equally prevalent during treatment with either duloxetine or an SSRI. Nausea appears to be more common during duloxetine than venlafaxine treatment (Perahia *et al.*, 2008; Allgulander *et al.*, 2008). Sexual dysfunction is more common with duloxetine than placebo (Detke *et al.*, 2004; Goldstein *et al.*, 2002 and 2004; Perahia *et al.*, 2006a), although less common than with the SSRIs paroxetine (Delgado *et al.*, 2005; Nelson *et al.*, 2006), or escitalopram (Clayton *et al.*, 2007b). Long-term weight gain with duloxetine appears to be similar to placebo at daily doses of 60 mg (Perahia *et al.*, 2006b; Wise *et al.*, 2006), and greater than placebo at daily doses above 60 mg (i.e., 80 mg or 120 mg — Nelson *et al.*, 2006; Wise *et al.*, 2006), although the results of one trial involving the use of 60 mg of duloxetine versus 10 mg of escitalopram or placebo for eight months in MDD patients did demonstrate statistically-significant greater weight gain among patients treated with duloxetine than placebo, as well as less weight gain during treatment with duloxetine than escitalopram ($p < 0.05$) (Pigott *et al.*, 2007).

Duloxetine does not appear to increase diastolic blood pressure (Thase *et al.*, 2005c; Wernicke *et al.*, 2007), or to have any clinically meaningful effect on electrocardiogram profiles in humans (Thase *et al.*, 2005c). Cases of SIADH/hyponatremia (Dirks & Van Hyfte, 2007; Kruger & Lindstaedt, 2007; Maramattom, 2006; Müssig *et al.*, 2009; Safdieh & Rudominer, 2006), cardiomyopathy (Bergman *et al.*, 2008; Colucci & Berry, 2006), eosinophilic pneumonia (Espeleta *et al.*, 2007), abnormal bleeding (Balhara *et al.*, 2007), and liver inflammation (Hanje *et al.*, 2006; Perahia *et al.*, 2007; Strombom *et al.*, 2008; Wernicke *et al.*, 2008a and 2008b) with duloxetine have been described. Duloxetine increases Stage 3 sleep and suppresses rapid eye movement (REM) sleep in patients with major depression (Kluge *et al.*, 2007).

Treatment of adults with MDD using duloxetine does not appear to result in the emergence or worsening of suicidal ideation (Acharya *et al.*, 2006). As with other SNRIs and SSRIs, the abrupt discontinuation of duloxetine may result in withdrawal symptoms (Perahia *et al.*, 2005).

The potential for abnormal mood elevations during the treatment of bipolar depression with duloxetine has not been systematically studied, nor have the effects of duloxetine treatment on pregnancy and breast-feeding. Duloxetine has been labeled as belonging to the FDA pregnancy category C.

3.2.3.3 *Dosing*

Duloxetine is commonly used at daily doses of 60–120 mg. Sixty milligrams of duloxetine a day appears to be the minimally effective (Pritchett *et al.*, 2007 also clinical trials F1J-MC-HMAG, F1J-MC-HMAH, and F1J-MC-HMAI) — this dosage is required in order to obtain 80% occupancy of serotonin transporter sites *in vivo* (Takano *et al.*, 2006). Starting at 30 mg daily or starting at 60 mg daily combined with food has been shown to improve tolerability versus starting at 60 mg without food (Whitmyer *et al.*, 2007). Duloxetine may inhibit the activity of CYP 2D6 (Wernicke *et al.*, 2005). Habitual smoking appears to reduce duloxetine plasma levels by about 15% (Fric *et al.*, 2008).

3.2.4 *Milnacipran*

A number of studies also demonstrate the norepinephrine and serotonin-reuptake inhibitor milnacipran (Mochizuki *et al.*, 2002) to be superior to placebo (Lecrubier *et al.*, 1996; Macher *et al.*, 1989), and equivalent to the SSRIs (Chang *et al.*, 2008; Papakostas & Fava, 2007) (Fig. 3.9), and TCAs (Kasper *et al.*, 1996 and 1997) in the treatment of MDD.

Treatment with milnacipran has also been reported to result in a faster onset of clinical response, as early as day seven, than fluvoxamine in MDD (Clerk *et al.*, 2001). Double-blind, placebo-controlled trials focusing on the use of milnacipran for elderly patients or children/adolescents with MDD, or for the treatment of bipolar

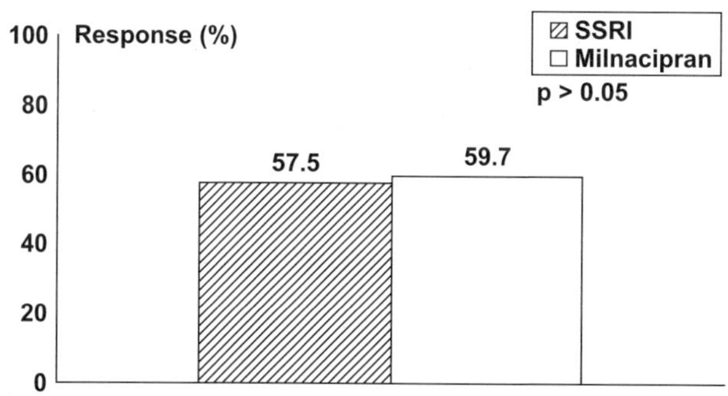

Fig. 3.9 Comparative efficacy of milnacipran (SNRI) versus SSRIs: Meta-analysis of 6 RCTs (n = 1,082). RCT: Randomized, Controlled Trial. [Data extracted from: Papakostas, G.I., & Fava, M. (2007). A meta-analysis of clinical trials comparing milnacipran, a serotonin-norepinephrine reuptake inhibitor, with a selective serotonin reuptake inhibitor for the treatment of major depressive disorder. *European Neuropsychopharmacology*, 20(17), 32–36.]

depression, dysthymic disorder, post-partum depression, seasonal affective disorder or minor depression have not been published to date. There is evidence to support the use of milnacipran for the treatment of fibromyalgia, a disorder often found comorbid with MDD (Clauw *et al.*, 2008; Gendreau *et al.*, 2005; Vitton *et al.*, 2004). In addition, there is anecdotal evidence for the use of milnacipran for comorbid MDD and diabetes mellitus (Abrahamian *et al.*, 2009).

Common side effects reported during treatment with milnacipran include nausea, sexual dysfunction, headaches, dry mouth, dysuria, tremor, tachycardia, weight gain, insomnia, and sedation, although the incidence of weight gain and sedation with milnacipran is lower than the TCAs (Annseau *et al.*, 1989). One major advantage of milnacipran is that its metabolism does not appear to require nor does it appear to influence the hepatic cytochrome enzyme system (Delini-Stula, 2000).

The potential for abnormal mood elevations following the treatment of bipolar depression with milnacipran has not been systematically studied, nor has the potential for the emergence or worsening of suicidal ideation during the treatment of MDD with milnacipran. The effects of milnacipran on pregnancy and breast-feeding are not known.

Milnacipran is available in Europe for the treatment of depression (brand name: Dalcipran, Ixel); it does not have FDA approval. Daily doses range form 50–200 mg, often divided in b.i.d. dosing (usual starting dose is 50 mg daily or 25 mg twice-daily).

3.3 5HT-2 and α-2 Adrenergic Receptor Antagonists

3.3.1 *Mirtazapine*

3.3.1.1 *Neuropharmacology*

Mirtazapine, particularly its (+) isomer (de Boer *et al.*, 1988), is an antagonist of the inhibitory α-2 adrenergic auto- and hetero-receptors (de Boer, 1996). For this reason, it is thought that the acute administration of mirtazapine produces a rapid increase in both noradrenalin and 5-HT neurotransmission, resulting in an enhanced tonic activation of postsynaptic 5-HT receptors (Haddjeri *et al.*, 1995). Mirtazapine was the first α-2 adrenergic receptor antagonist to be approved by the FDA for depression (brand name: Remeron). Since mirtazapine appears to be a blocker of serotonin 5HT2 and 5HT3 receptors as well, it is thought to enhance the release of norepinephrine and also enhance 5HT1A-mediated serotonergic transmission (Antilla *et al.*, 2001). Mirtazapine is also a potent histaminergic H-1 receptor antagonist.

3.3.1.2 *Efficacy*

Mirtazapine has been shown to be as effective as the SSRIs (Papakostas *et al.*, 2008a) (Fig. 3.10), TCAs (Marttila *et al.*, 1995; Richou, 1995; Zivkov *et al.*, 1995), and venlafaxine (Benkert *et al.*, 2006; Guelfi *et al.*, 2001; Lee *et al.*, 2007) in the treatment of MDD.

Similar to other dual serotonergic/noradrenergic antidepressants, mirtazapine has also been reported to result in an earlier onset

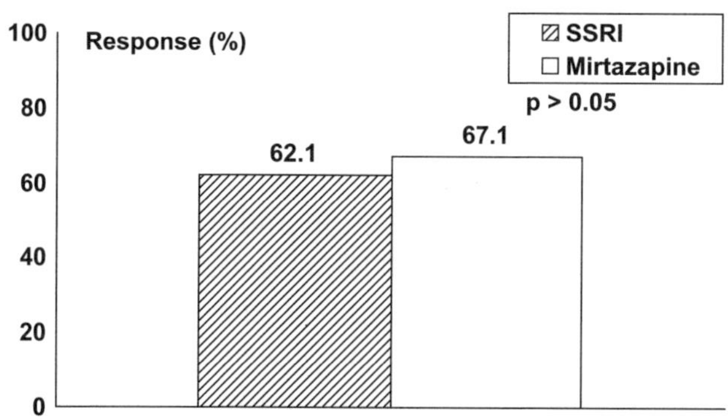

Fig. 3.10 Comparative efficacy of mirtazapine versus SSRIs: Meta-analysis of 10 RCTs (n = 1,904). RCT: Randomized, Controlled Trial. [Data extracted from: Papakostas, G.I., Homberger, C.H., & Fava, M. (2008a). A meta-analysis of clinical trials comparing mirtazapine with a selective serotonin reuptake inhibitor for the treatment of major depressive disorder. *Journal of Psychopharmacology*, 22(8), 843–848.]

of antidepressant action than the SSRIs (Benkert *et al.*, 2000; Behnke *et al.*, 2003; Leinonen *et al.*, 1999; Schatzberg *et al.*, 2002; Thase *et al.*, 2001b; Wade *et al.*, 2003), or venlafaxine (Benkert *et al.*, 2006).

Treatment with mirtazapine also appears to result in a better quality of sleep than SSRI treatment. Specifically, treatment with mirtazapine but not fluoxetine was found to result in a decreased sleep latency, increased sleep time, increased sleep efficiency (total time asleep/total time in bed), and decreased wake time after sleep onset in a small double-blind trial of MDD patients with insomnia (Winokur *et al.*, 2003). In fact, the results of a large meta-analysis of randomized clinical trials comparing mirtazapine with an SSRI for MDD suggested a greater resolution of symptoms of insomnia among mirtazapine than SSRI-treated patients (Winokur *et al.*, 2005). There are also encouraging preliminary reports of mirtazapine being more effective than the SSRIs in the treatment of somatic anxiety (Schatzberg *et al.*, 2002).

The results of a double-blind, placebo-controlled study also support the use of mirtazapine in elderly patients with MDD (Halikas *et al.*, 1995), but not in children and adolescents with MDD (http://www.clinicalstudyresults.org/documents/company-study_51_0.pdf). Double-blind, placebo-controlled trials focusing on the use of mirtazapine for treatment of bipolar depression, dysthymic disorder, post-partum depression, seasonal affective disorder or minor depression have not been published to date.

The results of double-blind, placebo-controlled trials support the use of mirtazapine for the prevention and treatment of post-stroke depression (Niedermaier *et al.*, 2004), as well as depression occurring after myocardial infarction (Honig *et al.*, 2007). The results of small open trials support the use of mirtazapine in depressed patients with epilepsy (Kuhn *et al.*, 2003), in HIV+ patients (Blanch *et al.*, 2001), and in menopausal women with depression unresponsive to estrogen replacement therapy (Joffe *et al.*, 2001). There is also anecdotal evidence for mirtazapine in treating interferon-associated depression (Russo *et al.*, 2003), for depression in patients with Parkinson's disease (Mizukami *et al.*, 2009), or depression in patients with cancer (Ersoy *et al.*, 2008; Raji *et al.*, 2007). Finally, there is evidence from randomized, double-blind, placebo-controlled trials to support the use of mirtazapine in the treatment of SAD (Muehlbacher *et al.*, 2005), and PTSD (Davidson *et al.*, 2003), psychiatric disorders often encountered in patients with MDD.

3.3.1.3 *Side effect profile*

Common side effects associated with mirtazapine include sedation, weight gain, insomnia, nausea, sexual dysfunction, dizziness, dry mouth, constipation, and orthostatic hypotension.

Treatment with mirtazapine is more likely to result in excessive daytime sedation and fatigue, and less likely to result in insomnia than SSRI treatment (Papakostas, 2007). Mirtazapine appears to have no effect on REM sleep (Winokur *et al.*, 2000). Studies regarding the impact of mirtazapine on driving ability present conflicting results, with one study suggesting worse driving performance with mirtazapine than SSRI treatment (Wingen *et al.*, 2005), while other studies suggesting equivalent driving ability between mirtazapine and the SSRIs (Brunnauer *et al.*, 2006), or reboxetine (Brunnauer *et al.*, 2008).

Due to blockade of 5HT2 and 5HT3 receptors, mirtazapine is associated with a lower risk of headaches (Den Braber *et al.*, 2003; Hong *et al.*, 2003), and nausea (Benkert *et al.*, 2000; Den Braber *et al.*, 2003; Hong *et al.*, 2003; Leinonen *et al.*, 1999; Papakostas, in press; Wade *et al.*, 2003) than the SSRIs.

Treatment with mirtazapine can result in significant long-term weight gain. Epidemiologic studies suggest the incidence of weight gain following one year of treatment of depression with mirtazapine (26%) to be significantly greater than treatment with SSRIs/venlafaxine (16–19%), and bupropion/nefazodone (12%) (Papakostas, 2007). Data comparing changes in weight during the long-term administration of mirtazapine- or placebo-treatment of MDD are in accordance with epidemiologic data (Thase *et al.*, 2001c), although weight gain seen during the long-term treatment of MDD with the TCA amitriptyline was considerably greater than weight gain during mirtazapine treatment in one trial (Montgomery *et al.*, 1998). The results of a small trial report increased TNF-α, soluble TNF-α receptors p55 and p75, and increased leptin levels during treatment of MDD with mirtazapine (Kraus *et al.*, 2002). Mirtazapine also appears to increase cholesterol levels (Nicholas *et al.*, 2003).

Only a subset of mirtazapine-SSRI comparator studies involve the use of a specific tool employed to measure sexual dysfunction. As a result, it is not possible to accurately estimate the relative likelihood of developing sexual dysfunction during the treatment of MDD with mirtazapine versus the SSRIs. In addition, there are few studies comparing mirtazapine with an SSRI that do involve the use of a specific instrument to measure sexual functioning. Conflicting results have been reported, with the SSRIs demonstrating higher rates of sexual dysfunction than mirtazapine in some (Benkert *et al.*, 2000; Philipp *et al.*, 2000) but not other trials (Wade *et al.*, 2003; Versiani *et al.*, 2002).

There are also reports of mirtazapine-emergent hyponatremia (Baybek *et al.*, 2006; Cheah *et al.*, 2008; Ladino *et al.*, 2003; Roxanas, 2003), akathisia (Girishchandra *et al.*, 2002), dystonia (Lu *et al.*, 2002), restless leg syndrome (Bonin *et al.*, 2000), hepatitis (Degner *et al.*, 2004), pancreatitis (Hussain & Burke, 2008; Sommer *et al.*, 2001), and serotonin syndrome (Hernandez *et al.*, 2002; Ubogu & Katirji, 2003), as well as serotonin syndrome when mirtazapine was combined with an SSRI (Benazzi, 1998a; Demers & Malone, 2001), venlafaxine (Dimellis, 2002), or 5HT3 antagonists (Turkel *et al.*, 2001).

Thrombocytopenia has also been reported with mirtazapine, thought to occur due to the formation of auto-antibodies to a glycoprotein complex (IIb/IIIa) (Liu & Sahud, 2003), as well as neutropenia (Aghelescu *et al.*, 2002; Ahmed, 2002; Kasper *et al.*, 1997), and bone marrow suppression (Biswas *et al.*, 2003; Hutchison, 2001). Mirtazapine does not appear to be a substrate for p-GP (Uhr *et al.*, 2003a).

The risk for abnormal mood elevations following the treatment of bipolar depression, or the risk for the emergence or worsening of suicidal ideation following the treatment of MDD with mirtazapine has not been systematically studied. A few reports have been published describing "withdrawal-like" reactions during the abrupt discontinuation of mirtazapine (Benazzi, 1998b; Berigan, 2001; McCall & Callender, 1999).

Similar to the SSRIs, mirtazapine treatment during early pregnancy appears to increase the risk of spontaneous abortions but not the baseline rate of major malformations (Djulus *et al.*, 2006; Einarson & Einarson, 2005). Mirtazapine has been labeled as belonging to the FDA pregnancy category C. Only a small study has been published focusing on the effects of mirtazapine-treatment of mothers on breast-fed infants (Kristensen *et al.*, 2007). Mirtazapine was detected in the serum of one in four infants tested. However, no adverse events were reported.

3.3.1.4 *Dosing*

Effective daily doses range between 30 and 60 mg/day. The starting daily dose is often 15 mg, but potentially it can be as low as 7.5 mg in the elderly.

3.3.2 *Mianserin*

Mianserin, an α-2 noradrenergic receptor antagonist and a serotonin 5HT2 antagonist, is available in Europe (brand name: Lantanon), but is not FDA-approved. Similar to mirtazapine, the (+) isomer appears to be more potent (six-fold) at inhibiting the α-2 receptors than the (−) isomer (de Boer *et al.*, 1988).

Double-blind studies report the efficacy of mianserin in the treatment of MDD to be equivalent to the TCAs (Moller *et al.*, 1991 and 1995; Wilcox *et al.*, 1994), and the SSRIs (Ahlfors *et al.*, 1988; Dalery *et al.*, 2001; Dorman, 1992; Karllson *et al.*, 2000; La Pia *et al.*, 1992; Malt *et al.*, 1999; Mertens & Pintens, 1988; Moon & Jesinger, 1991; Muijen *et al.*, 1988; Perez & Ashford, 1990; Phanjoo *et al.*, 1991).

Common side effects during mianserin treatment include somnolence, weight gain, dry mouth, sleep problems, tremor, and headaches. Effective daily doses for mianserin range from 30–60 mg, usually given at bedtime.

3.4 Norepinephrine-Dopamine Reuptake Inhibitors

3.4.1 *Bupropion*

3.4.1.1 *Neuropharmacology*

The mechanism of action of bupropion (Wellbutrin) has not been fully elucidated, although it appears to primarily block the reuptake of both dopamine and norepinephrine (Ascher *et al.*, 1995). Bupropion and its metabolites have been shown to be able to inhibit striatal uptake of the selective DAT-binding radioligand (11)C-β-CIT-FE *in vivo*, achieving DAT occupancy ranging from approximately 14% (Meyer *et al.*, 2002) to 26% (Learned Coughlin *et al.*, 2003; Szabo *et al.*, 2003) at therapeutic doses. This degree of DAT occupancy appears to be equivalent to that achieved after a single oral dose of methylphenidate 5–10 mg in human volunteers (Volkow *et al.*, 1998). However, when comparable methylphenidate doses were given intravenously to healthy volunteers (0.025–0.1 mg/Kg), significant increases in synaptic dopamine were not observed (Volkow *et al.*, 1999 and 2003), suggesting that additional mechanisms other than DAT inhibition may be involved.

Bupropion has also been reported to have mild affinity for the norepinephrine transporter (Foley *et al.*, 2002), although some researchers have argued that the effect of bupropion on norepinephrine is primarily through an increase in presynaptic norepinephrine release (Dong & Blier, 2001). Regardless of the exact mechanism, the overall effect of bupropion appears to be a dose-dependent increase in brain extra-cellular dopamine and norepinephrine concentrations (Li *et al.*, 2002; Nomikos *et al.*, 1989). Bupropion also appears to non-competitively inhibit the $\alpha 3\beta 2$-, $\alpha 3\beta 4$-, and $\alpha 4\beta 2$-nicotinic acetyl cholinergic receptors *in vitro* (Bondarev *et al.*, 2003; Fryer & Lucas, 1999; Miller *et al.*, 2002; Slemmer *et al.*, 2000). At least four stereo isomers of two major metabolites of bupropion (S,S-, R,R-hydroxybupropion, R,R-threohydrobupropion) were also reported to noncompetitively inhibit $\alpha 3\beta 4$-nicotinic acetyl cholinergic receptors *in vitro*, although not as potently as bupropion (Bondarev *et al.*, 2003).

Bupropion is commercially available as a racemate, but there is a paucity of information available about the individual properties of its enantiomers (Baker & Prior, 2002). Bupropion has two major (hydroxybupropion and threohydrobupropion) and one minor metabolite (erythrohydrobupropion) (Bondarev *et al.*, 2003). At steady state, the plasma levels of hydroxybupropion are approximately 45 to 50 times higher than the parent compound bupropion, while plasma levels of erythro- and threo-hydrobupropion are 3.5–6 and 18–26 times higher, respectively (Cooper *et al.*, 1984; Golden *et al.*, 1988; Learned-Coughlin *et al.*, 2003; Meyer *et al.*, 2002). Although each of these three compounds has four stereoisomers, only a subset of these eight potential compounds are detectable in human plasma after treatment with bupropion (Bondarev *et al.*, 2003). In addition, of the four stereoisomers tested in one study [(S, S)-, (R, R)-threohydrobupropion; (S, S)-, (R, R)-hydroxybupropion], only one (S, S-hydroxybupropion) had affinity comparable to bupropion for the DAT (K_i = 1295 versus 1020 nM, respectively) (Bondarev *et al.*, 2003). However, at steady state in humans, 96% of hydroxybupropion is predominantly in the form of R, R-isomer, with the remaining 4% in the S, S-form (Suckow *et al.*, 1997).

3.4.1.2 *Efficacy*

Bupropion appears to be as effective as the SSRIs (Papakostas, 2006; Thase *et al.*, 2005d) (Fig. 3.11) and venlafaxine (Hewett *et al.*, 2009; Thase *et al.*, 2006) in the overall treatment of MDD, as well as across various age groups among men and women (Papakostas *et al.*, 2007b). In addition, the rapidity of antidepressant effects of bupropion is comparable to those of the SSRIs overall, or of escitalopram specifically (Papakostas *et al.*, 2007c). Bupropion is also as effective as the SSRIs in the treatment of anxious symptoms of depression (Papakostas *et al.*, 2008b; Trivedi *et al.*, 2001). As a result, it is often used as a first-line treatment for MDD.

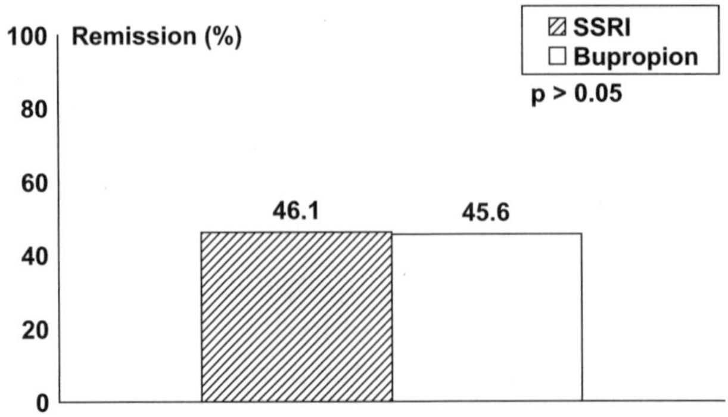

Fig. 3.11 Comparative efficacy of bupropion (NDRI) versus SSRIs: Pooled analysis of 10 RCTs ($n = 2{,}123$). RCT: Randomized, Controlled Trial. [Data extracted from: Papakostas, G.I. (2006). Dopaminergic-based pharmacotherapies for depression. *European Neuropsychopharmacology*, 16, 391–402.]

In addition, perhaps due to its dual noradrenergic and dopaminergic activity, bupropion appears to be more effective than the SSRIs in the treatment of lethargic symptoms of MDD, including somnolence and fatigue (Papakostas *et al.*, 2006) (Figs. 3.12–3.14). However, the treatment of patients with anxious depression (depression with high levels of comorbid anxiety symptoms) with the SSRIs appears to be more effective than treatment with bupropion (Papakostas *et al.*, 2008c) (Fig. 3.15).

The results of a double-blind, placebo-controlled trial do not support the use of bupropion in elderly patients with MDD (Hewett *et al.*, in press). However, the results of another double-blind, placebo-controlled trial support the use of bupropion in seasonal affective disorder (Modell *et al.*, 2005). Double-blind, placebo-controlled trials focusing on the use of bupropion for depression in children/adolescents, or for the treatment dysthymic disorder, postpartum depression or minor depression have not been published to date. The results of double-blind studies suggest comparable efficacy as well as lower rates of abnormal mood elevations among patients with bipolar depression treated with adjunctive (to mood stabilizers) bupropion than adjunctive desipramine (Sachs *et al.*, 1994), or venlafaxine (Post *et al.*, 2006). In the latter trial, adjunctive

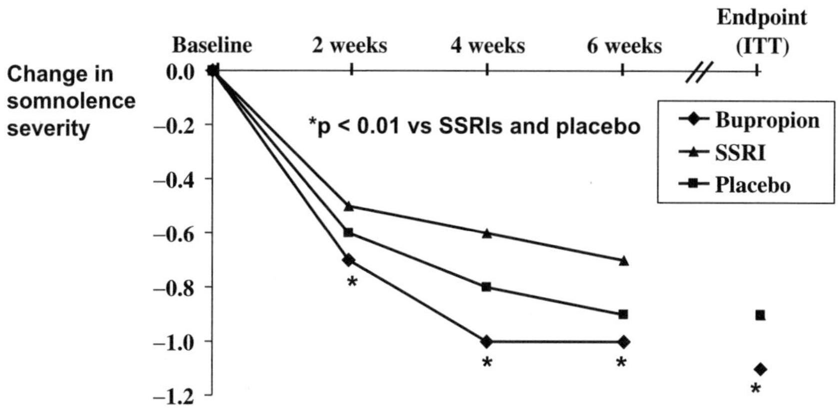

Fig. 3.12 Efficacy of bupropion (NDRI) versus SSRIs in treating somnolence in MDD: Pooled analysis of 6 RCTs ($n = 1{,}317$). RCT: Randomized controlled trial. [Data extracted from: Papakostas, G.I., Nutt, D.J., Hallett, L.A., *et al.* (2006). Resolution of sleepiness and fatigue in the treatment of major depressive disorder: A comparison of bupropion and the selective serotonin reuptake inhibitors. *Biological Psychiatry*, 16, 1350–1355.]

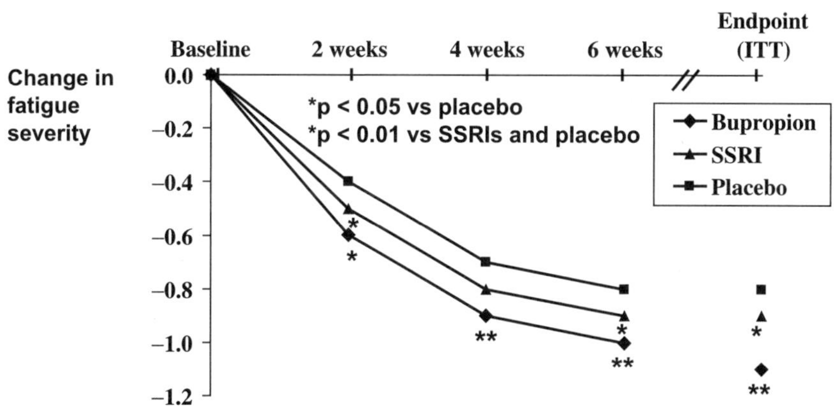

Fig. 3.13 Efficacy of bupropion (NDRI) versus SSRIs in treating fatigue in MDD: Pooled analysis of 6 RCTs ($n = 1{,}317$). RCT: Randomized controlled trial. [Data extracted from: Papakostas, G.I., Nutt, D.J., Hallett, L.A., *et al.* (2006). Resolution of sleepiness and fatigue in the treatment of major depressive disorder: A comparison of bupropion and the selective serotonin reuptake inhibitors. *Biological Psychiatry*, 16, 1350–1355.]

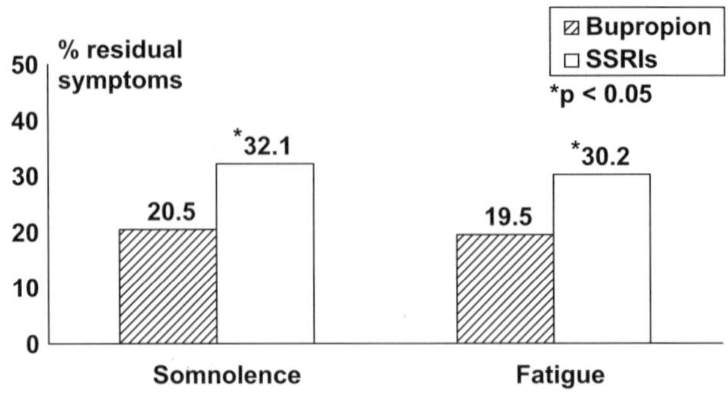

Fig. 3.14 Residual somnolence and fatigue in bupropion (NDRI) and SSRI remitters: Pooled analysis of 6 RCTs ($n = 1{,}317$). RCT: Randomized controlled trial. [Data extracted from: Papakostas, G.I., Nutt, D.J., Hallett, L.A., *et al.* (2006). Resolution of sleepiness and fatigue in the treatment of major depressive disorder: A comparison of bupropion and the selective serotonin reuptake inhibitors. *Biological Psychiatry*, 16, 1350–1355.]

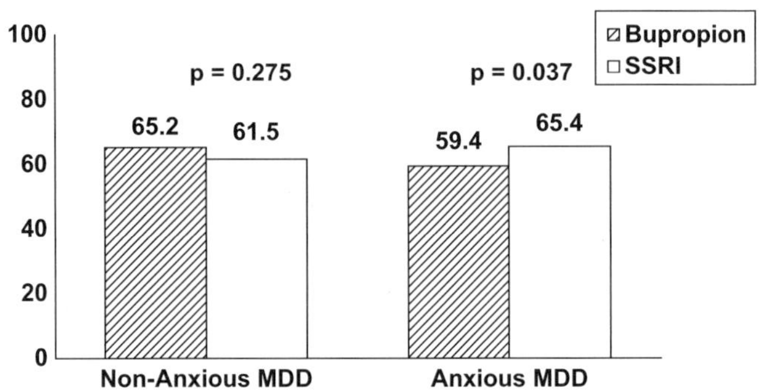

Fig. 3.15 Comparative efficacy (response rates) of bupropion (NDRI) versus SSRIs in anxious versus non-anxious MDD: Pooled analysis of 10 RCTs ($n = 2{,}122$). RCT: Randomized, controlled trial. [Data extracted from: Papakostas, G.I., Stahl, S.M., Krishen, A., *et al.* (2008c). Efficacy of bupropion and the selective serotonin reuptake inhibitors in the treatment of major depressive disorder with high levels of anxiety (anxious depression). *Journal of Clinical Psychiatry*, 69(8), 1287–1292.]

bupropion and sertraline were found to be equivalent with regards to their antidepressant efficacy as well as their risk for inducing abnormal mood elevations in patients with bipolar depression. However, the results of a subsequent, placebo-controlled trial do not show greater efficacy for bupropion than placebo when used as an adjunct to mood stabilizers in the treatment of bipolar depression (Sachs *et al.*, 2007).

There are also open-label trials focusing on the use of bupropion for the treatment of post-partum depression (Nonacs *et al.*, 2005), or for the treatment of MDD in patients with comorbid asthma (Brown *et al.*, 2007). In addition, in a small open trial, bupropion was found to alleviate depressive symptoms in 5 of 12 patients with Parkinson's disease (Goetz *et al.*, 1984). There are also open-label trials of bupropion for the treatment of depression in HIV+ patients (Currier *et al.*, 2003), or for the treatment of depression in breast-cancer patients (Mago *et al.*, 2008). Finally, there is also evidence from randomized, double-blind, placebo-controlled trials to support the use of bupropion in the treatment of AD(H)D, a psychiatric disorder often encountered in patients with MDD (Wilens *et al.*, 2005).

3.4.1.3 *Side effect profile*

One advantage of treatment with bupropion compared to the SSRIs and venlafaxine is the lower risk of sexual dysfunction (Clayton *et al.*, 2006; Papakostas, 2007; Thase *et al.*, 2005d and 2006). Treatment with bupropion is also associated with a lower incidence of nausea, and somnolence/sedation than the SSRIs (Papakostas, 2007). The rates of treatment-emergent insomnia are comparable between bupropion and SSRI treatment (Papakostas, 2007).

An additional advantage of bupropion is that it appears to decrease weight more so than placebo during the acute phase of treatment of depression (Settle *et al.*, 1999), and also in obesity (Gadde *et al.*, 2001; Jain *et al.*, 2002). The anti-obesity effects of bupropion also appear to be sustained during longer treatment periods (48–52 weeks) (Anderson *et al.*, 2002; Croft *et al.*, 2002). In addition, long-term (52 week) treatment of depression with bupropion did not appear to result in weight changes that are different from those seen during placebo-treatment in one randomized, double-blind trial (Weihs *et al.*, 2002). Although a difference in terms of weight changes in bupropion and SSRI-treated depressed patients is not immediately apparent during the acute phase of treatment in randomized trials (Coleman *et al.*, 1999; Croft *et al.*, 1999; Feighner *et al.*, 1991; Kavoussi *et al.*, 1997; Settle *et al.*, 1999; Weighs *et al.*, 2000), there is evidence to suggest that any beneficial effects of SSRIs in terms of weight reduction during the acute phase are not sustained during the continuation and maintenance phases (Michelson *et al.*, 1999; Sussman *et al.*, 2001). In fact, long-term treatment with some SSRIs may also result in long-term weight gain (Fava *et al.*, 2000). Thus, long-term treatment with bupropion may carry a lower risk of weight gain than long-term treatment with the SSRIs. Although this hypothesis has never been directly tested, the results of an epidemiologic study suggest a 12% incidence of 7% or greater weight gain following one year of bupropion treatment, compared to a 16–19% incidence of weight gain following one year of SSRI treatment (Papakostas, 2007). Unlike sertraline, bupropion does not alter CSF hypocretin-1 (Orexin-A) levels in depression (Salomon *et al.*, 2003).

Other common side effects of bupropion include dry mouth, headache, constipation, and tremor (Settle *et al.*, 1999). There is also a report of bupropion-emergent dystonia (Detweiler & Harpold, 2002), and hepatotoxicity (Humayun *et al.*, 2007). Although bupropion may elevate blood pressure in some patients (Kiev *et al.*, 1994; Roose *et al.*, 1991), it does not appear to consistently do so, even in hypertensive patients (Thase *et al.*, 2003). Several studies show no effect of bupropion on cardiac conduction (Kiev *et al.*, 1994; Roose *et al.*, 1991; Wenger *et al.*, 1983), orthostatic blood pressure (Kiev *et al.*, 1994; Roose *et al.*, 1991), or left ventricular ejection fraction in patients with congestive heart failure (Roose *et al.*, 1987b), although conduction delays or cardiogenic shock may occur in patients who overdose on bupropion (Isbister & Balit, 2003; Morazin *et al.*, 2007; Paris & Saucier, 1998; Wills *et al.*, 2009). The risk of mortality following an overdose of bupropion appears to be higher than that associated with an overdose of SSRIs (White *et al.*, 2008).

Caution is warranted when combining bupropion and paroxetine in the elderly, especially in those with memory impairments and orthostasis, as combining these two agents in the elderly was found to increase the risk of falls (Joo *et al.*, 2002). Treatment with bupropion does not appear to affect prolactin and growth hormone levels (Whiteman *et al.*, 1982 and 1983), or bone mineral density (Gadde *et al.*, 2001). Short-term administration of bupropion also did not appear to worsen diabetic control (Rowland *et al.*, 1997).

The major medically important adverse event associated with bupropion is seizure. Bupropion was first marketed in the U.S. in 1984, but temporarily withdrawn from the market from 1986–1989 due to concerns about seizure risk following an unexpectedly high seizure rate among women enrolled in a clinical trial evaluating the efficacy, safety, and tolerability of bupropion monotherapy for the treatment of bulimia nervosa. (Horne *et al.*, 1988). With the immediate-release formulation, the rate is 0.4% (4/1000) at doses up to 450 mg/day (Johnston *et al.*, 1991). Patients should only be administered to bupropion with extreme caution if a predisposition to seizure is present. For this reason, the maximum daily dose for bupropion SR and bupropion XL is 400 and 450 mg, respectively, with no single dose above 200 mg for the SR formulation. In addition, bupropion may be more likely to induce seizures in patients with eating disorders and histories of head trauma and should not be used in these patients. Since the risk of seizure appears to be related to dose as well as to the peak plasma concentrations, the SR and XL formulations are thought to be associated with a somewhat lower seizure risk, estimated at 0.1% for daily doses of 300 mg or less (Dunner *et al.*, 1998).

There are also several reports of bupropion-related hypersensitivity reactions (Bagshaw *et al.*, 2003; Benson, 2001; Chiaverini *et al.*, 2003; Conners *et al.*, 1996; Davis *et al.*, 2001; De Santiago Hernando *et al.*, 2002; Fabre *et al.*, 1983; Fays *et al.*, 2003; Glod *et al.*, 2003; Gonzales *et al.*, 2006; Knowles *et al.*, 2003; Lineberry *et al.*, 2001; Loo *et al.*, 2003; Malesker *et al.*, 1995; McCollom *et al.*, 2000; Peloso & Baillie, 1999; Tackett & Smith, 2008; Tripathi & Greenberger, 1999; Woolторton, 2002; Yolles *et al.*, 1999).

Unlike most other antidepressants (Winokur *et al.*, 2001), bupropion appears to *increase* rather than decrease REM sleep (Nofzinger *et al.*, 1995), which may explain reports of somnambulism (Khazaal *et al.*, 2003), or nightmares and vivid dreams (Becker & Dufresne,

1982) during treatment with bupropion. There have been no reports of bupropion worsening cataplexy or of new-onset cataplexy during treatment with bupropion, while there is a single case report of reduction in sleepiness and REM-sleep propensity in a woman with atypical depression and comorbid narcolepsy treated with bupropion (Rye *et al.*, 1998).

In double-blind trials (Griffith *et al.*, 1983; Miller and Giffith, 1983), substance abusers were unable to distinguish bupropion from placebo, but were able to distinguish amphetamine from placebo, suggesting low abuse potential. Studies also suggest that a minimum of 47% DAT occupancy is required for cocaine to produce euphoric effects (Volkow *et al.*, 1997), much less than the DAT occupancy during therapeutic doses of bupropion.

A pooled data analysis demonstrated that bupropion treatment of MDD did not result in the emergence or worsening of suicidal ideation more often than placebo in adults (http://ctr.gsk.co.uk/Summary/bupropion/IV_suicide_observational.pdf). As mentioned above, the risk of an abnormal mood elevation during the treatment of bipolar depression with bupropion is lower than the risk associated with desipramine or venlafaxine treatment, and equivalent to the risk seen with sertraline treatment.

There are also case reports describing "withdrawal-like" symptoms following the abrupt discontinuation of bupropion (Berigan & Harazin, 1999; Berigan, 2002), as well as a case report of hyponatremia during bupropion treatment (Bagley & Yaeger, 2005).

Similar to the SSRIs, bupropion treatment during early pregnancy appears to increase the risk of spontaneous abortions or pre-term births, but not the baseline rate of major malformations (Cole *et al.*, 2007; Chun-Fai-Chan *et al.*, 2005; Einarson & Einarson, 2005; Einarson *et al.*, 2009; also see GSK study EPIP083 part 2 at http://ctr.gsk.co.uk/Summary/paroxetine/studylist.asp). Bupropion has been labeled as belonging to the FDA pregnancy category C. The effects of bupropion-treatment of mothers on breast-fed infants have not been systematically studied. The results of a small study suggest that bupropion accumulates in human breast milk in concentrations much higher than in maternal plasma.

However, neither bupropion nor its metabolites were detected in the infant's plasma, indicating that accumulation did not occur in this infant (Briggs *et al.*, 1993). There is one report of a seizure in a breast-feeding infant of a mother on bupropion (Chaudron & Schoenecker, 2004).

3.4.1.4 *Dosing*

The dose range for the immediate (Wellbutrin) and sustained release formulation of bupropion (Wellbutrin SR) is 150–450 mg and 150–400 mg, respectively, in b.i.d. or t.i.d. dosing, with 100 mg or 150 mg being a common starting dose (can be as low as 75 mg with the immediate release formulation). The maximum single dose of Wellbutrin is 150 mg, and for Wellbutrin SR 200 mg. A once-daily dose formulation (Wellbutrin XL), available in 150 mg and 300 mg doses, was introduced in 2003 (usual starting dose is 150 mg). Recently, the use of the Wellbutrin XL formulation was shown to result in better treatment adherence than the Wellbutrin SR formulation (McLaughlin *et al.*, 2007; Stang *et al.*, 2007a and 2007b). The maximum daily dose for Wellbutrin SR is 400 mg, and for Wellbutrin and Wellbutrin XL is 450 mg.

Plasma levels derived for each respective dose of bupropion at steady state have been reported to vary as much as 10-fold between patients (Preskorn, 1983). The results of a small, unreplicated study suggest poor response to bupropion [immediate release (IR) formulation] for patients with trough levels lower than 25 ng/ml (Preskorn, 1983). CYP2B6 appears to be primarily responsible for the hydroxylation of bupropion (Hesse *et al.*, 2000), although elevated plasma level/dose rations for hydroxybupropion, but not bupropion or its two metabolites, have been reported in patients who are poor 2D6 metabolizers (Pollock *et al.*, 1996). Recently, an allele coding for the CYP2B6 enzyme (*4) has been associated with increased clearance of bupropion (increased hydroxybupropion concentrations) (Kirchheiner *et al.*, 2003). Neither bupropion nor its major metabolites appear to influence p-glycoprotein function (Wang *et al.*, 2008).

3.4.2 *Nomifensine*

Nomifensine (Merital) is a tricyclic antidepressant derivative that blocks the reuptake of norepinephrine (Kinney, 1985) and dopamine (Mercuri *et al.*, 1992). Although briefly available for the treatment of MDD in the US and EU, nomifensine is no longer available for the treatment of depression due to the risk of hemolytic anemia (Giers *et al.*, 1991).

Chapter 4

Monoaminergic-Based Strategies: "Triple-Acting" Agents

4.1 Monoamine Oxidase Inhibitors (MAOIs)

4.1.1 *Neuropharmacology*

MAOIs act by inhibiting monoamine oxidase (MAO), an enzyme found on the outer membrane of mitochondria, where it catabolizes a number of monoamines including dopamine, norepinephrine, and serotonin. After reuptake, norepinephrine, serotonin, and dopamine are either reloaded into vesicles for subsequent release or broken down by the enzyme MAO. MAO is present in two forms (MAO-A and MAO-B), which differ in their substrate preferences, inhibitor specificities, tissue expression, and cell distribution. MAO-A preferentially oxidizes serotonin and is irreversibly inactivated by low concentrations of the acetylenic inhibitor clorgyline. MAO-B preferentially oxidizes phenylethylamine (PEA) and benzylamine and is irreversibly inactivated by low concentrations of pargyline and deprenyl. Dopamine, tyramine, and tryptamine are substrates for both forms of MAO (Fava & Rosenbaum, 1995).

More recently, additional pharmacologic properties for the MAOIs have been revealed. MAOIs, for instance, also appear to inhibit the binding of [3H] quinpirole, a dopamine agonist with high affinity for D2 and D3 dopamine receptors (Levant *et al.*, 1996 and 1998). In addition, two of the MAOIs, selegiline and tranylcypromine, have methamphetamine and amphetamine as metabolites (Baker *et al.*, 1999; Slawson *et al.*, 2002). Phenelzine also elevates brain γ-aminobutyric acid (GABA) levels (Baker *et al.*, 1999). R[−] — but not S[+] — selegiline also appears to induce dopamine release by directly modulating ATP-sensitive potassium channels in the striatum (Neusch *et al.*, 1997). Finally, the (−) enantiomer of tranylcypromine also appears to more potently inhibit catecholamine uptake, while the (+) enantiomer appears to more effectively inhibit MAO (Baker & Prior, 2002).

Older MAOIs, including phenelzine (Nardil), tranylcypromine (Parnate), and isocarboxazid (Marplan), *irreversibly* inhibit the enzymatic activity of *both* MAO-A and MAO-B. Newer ones, such as brofaromine (Consonar) and moclobemide (Manerix), are relatively selective and preferentially inhibit MAO-A. Selegiline (Eldepryl), at least at oral doses of 10 mg daily, selectively inhibits MAO-B (Fowler *et al.*, 2001) (75–90% occupancy of brain MAO-B is achieved at daily doses of 10 mg — Hirvonen *et al.*, 2009). Finally, while older MAOIs result in irreversible inhibition of MAO, some newer ones such as moclobemide and brofaromine, result in reversible inhibition.

In addition to its oral formulation, selegiline is also available in a trans-dermal form (patch), designed to minimize the inhibition of the MAO enzymes found in the lining of the gastrointestinal (GI) tract (Mawhinney *et al.*, 2003). For instance, in one animal study, the inhibition of MAO in gastrointestinal tissue with transdermal selegiline appeared to be less than that in brain, with doses that produced maximal MAO-A and -B inhibition in brain inhibiting only 30–40% of gastrointestinal MAO-A (Wecker *et al.*, 2003). The transdermal form of selegiline has been approved by the FDA for the treatment of major depressive disorder (MDD) in 2006 (brand name: EmSam).

4.1.2 *Efficacy*

Although the overall efficacy of MAOIs for the treatment of MDD does not differ from that of other commonly used antidepressants including the SSRIs (Pande *et al.*, 1996; Papakostas & Fava, 2006) and TCAs (Thase *et al.*, 1995), their use is considerably limited by the risk

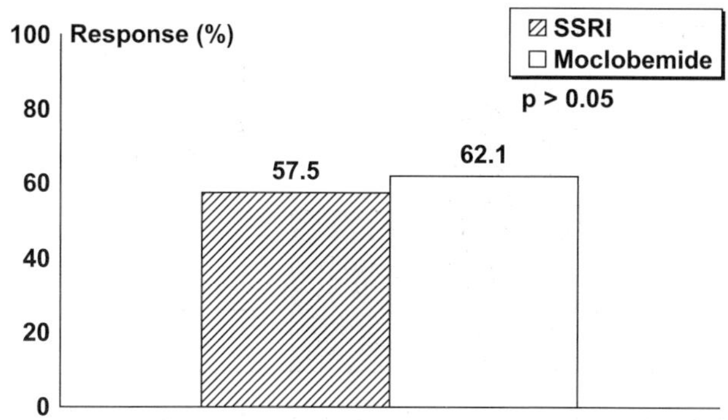

Fig. 4.1 Comparative efficacy of moclobemide (MAOI) versus SSRIs: Meta-analysis of 12 RCTs ($n = 1{,}207$). RCT: Randomized, Controlled Trial. [Data extracted from: Papakostas, G.I., & Fava, M. (2006). A meta-analysis of clinical trials comparing moclobemide with selective serotonin reuptake inhibitors for the treatment of major depressive disorder. *Canadian Journal of Psychiatry*, 51, 783–790.]

of potentially lethal adverse events such as hypertensive crises and serotonin syndromes (Fig. 4.1).

As a result, they are rarely chosen as first-line agents in the treatment of depression (Petersen *et al.*, 2002a). As mentioned above, a transdermal form of selegiline (EmSam) was approved by the FDA in 2006 for the treatment of MDD. Treating MDD with trans-dermal selegiline appears to be effective (Amsterdam *et al.*, 2003; Bodkin & Amsterdam, 2002; Feiger *et al.*, 2006), but also relatively safe (Robinson & Amsterdam, 2008), even in the absence of a tyramine-restricted diet (Amsterdam *et al.*, 2003), although the FDA requires a tyramine-free diet at the higher doses of the patch.

Of the newer MAOIs, moclobemide (a reversible inhibitor relatively selective for the MAO-A isoenzyme) has been shown to be effective in the treatment of dysthymic disorder (Lingjaerde *et al.*, 1993), as well as social anxiety disorder (Nutt & Montgomery, 1996). There is also preliminary evidence from an open-label trial to support the potential utility of moclobemide for the treatment of patients with Parkinson's disease and MDD (Giménez-Roldán *et al.*, 1997). Moclobemide has not been found to be effective in the treatment of seasonal affective disorder (Versiani *et al.*, 1997).

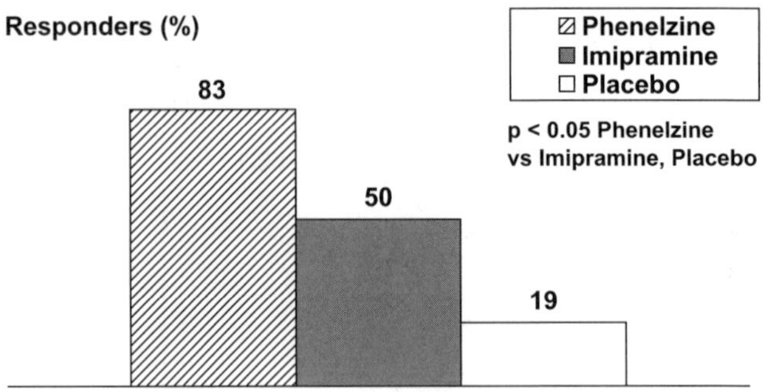

Fig. 4.2 Phenelzine (MAOI) versus imipramine (TCA) for atypical MDD: A randomized, double-blind study ($n = 90$). [Data extracted from: Quitkin, F.M., McGrath, P.J., Stewart, J.W., *et al.* (1990). Atypical depression, panic attacks, and response to imipramine and phenelzine. A replication. *Archives of General Psychiatry*, 47, 935–941.]

Perhaps due to their ability to inhibit the reuptake of dopamine in addition to serotonin and norepinephrine, the MAOIs appear to be more effective than TCAs (Liebowitz *et al.*, 1988; Quitkin *et al.*, 1990 and 1991; Stewart *et al.*, 2002; Thase *et al.*, 1995) in the treatment of patients with atypical depression characterized by mood reactivity in addition to symptoms such as hypersomnia, hyperphagia, extreme fatigue and rejection sensitivity, although not all studies support this finding (Larsen *et al.*, 1991; Paykel *et al.*, 1982; Robinson *et al.*, 1985) (Figs. 4.2 and 4.3). In addition, the results of one double-blind trial also report treatment with the MAOI moclobemide to be more effective that treatment with SSRIs in atypical depression (Lonnqvist *et al.*, 1994). However, two subsequent double-blind trials did not demonstrate the superiority of the MAOIs phenelzine (Pande *et al.*, 1996) and moclobemide (Sogaard *et al.*, 1999) versus the SSRIs in atypical MDD.

In parallel, while the MAOIs also seem to be effective in the treatment of fatigue in fibromyalgia, and chronic fatigue syndrome (Hannonen *et al.*, 1998; Hickie *et al.*, 2000; Natelson *et al.*, 1996 and 1998; White *et al.*, 1997), four out of five studies do not show any effect of the SSRIs on fatigue in these disorders (Cantini *et al.*, 1994; Goldenberg *et al.*, 1996; Norregaard *et al.*, 1995; Vercoulen *et al.*, 1996; Wolfe

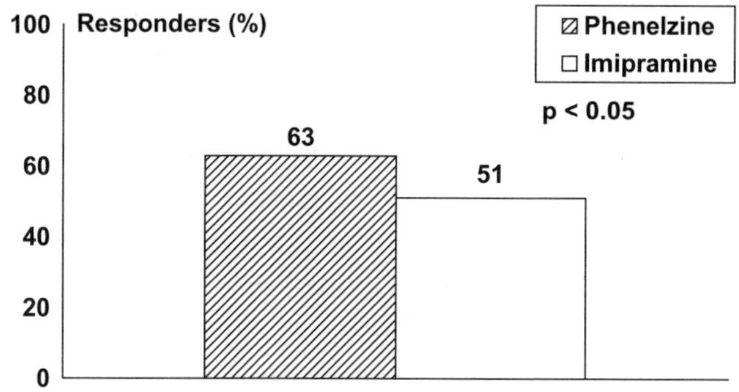

Fig. 4.3 Phenelzine (MAOI) versus imipramine (TCA) for atypical MDD: A randomized, double-blind study. [Data extracted from: Quitkin, F.M., Harrison, W., Stewart, J.W., *et al.* (1991). Response to phenelzine and imipramine in placebo nonresponders with atypical depression. A new application of the crossover design. *Archives of General Psychiatry*, 48, 319–323.]

et al., 1994). In conclusion, although to date there are no double-blind studies comparing the relative efficacy of MAOIs versus the SSRIs or TCAs in the treatment of fatigue in depression, the above studies suggest a potential advantage for MAOIs over SSRIs in the treatment of lethargic symptoms in MDD.

4.1.3 *Side effect profile*

In the GI tract and the liver, MAO catabolizes a number of dietary pressor amines, such as dopamine, tyramine, tryptamine and phenylethylamine (Hasan *et al.*, 1988). For this reason, consumption of foods containing high levels of dietary amines while on an MAOI or the combination of catecholaminergic agents and MAOIs may precipitate an adrenergic crisis, characterized by hypertension, hyperpyrexia, tachycardia, tremulousness and cardiac arrhythmias (Lavin *et al.*, 1993). Co-administration of MAOIs with antidepressants that potentiate serotonin could result in serotonin syndrome, characterized by alterations in cognition (disorientation, confusion), behavior (agitation, restlessness), autonomic nervous system function (fever, shivering, diaphoresis, diarrhea), and neuromuscular activity (ataxia, hyperreflexia, myoclonus) (Beasley *et al.*, 1993;

Feighner *et al.*, 1990; Lane & Baldwin, 1997). Since MAO enzymatic activity requires approximately 14 days to be restored, such food or medications should be avoided for two weeks after the discontinuation of an irreversible MAOI ("MAOI washout period"). Serotonergic and dopaminergic antidepressants are typically discontinued two weeks before the initiation of an MAOI, with the exception of fluoxetine, which needs to be discontinued five weeks in advance due to its relatively longer half-life.

Reversible MAO-A–selective inhibitors were designed to minimize the risk of hypertensive crises, and patients on conventional doses of moclobemide do not need to strictly adhere to the low tyramine diet, although at very high doses (i.e., 900 mg/day or more of moclobemide), inhibition of MAO-B also occurs (Bonnet, 2003). Similarly, transdermal selegiline, at doses that produced maximal MAO-B inhibition, was reported to also inhibit MAO-A in several brain regions tested (Wecker *et al.*, 2003). The use of transdermal selegiline does not appear to require the institution of a low tyramine diet when prescribed at 6 mg/day or less, although the FDA indicates that a diet is required for higher doses.

Although a number of studies have reported the absence of serious adverse events (i.e., hypertensive crisis or serotonin syndrome) during the combination of moclobemide with an SSRI (Dingemanse *et al.*, 1998; Ebert *et al.*, 1995; Joffe & Bakish, 1994), there have been a number of non-fatal (Dardennes *et al.*, 1998; Hilton *et al.*, 2000) and fatal reports of serotonin syndrome involving the co-ingestion of moclobemide and an SSRI/SNRI (Dams *et al.*, 2001; Finge *et al.*, 1997; Hojer *et al.*, 2002; Isbister *et al.*, 2001; Klys *et al.*, 2009; Rogde *et al.*, 1999; Singer & Jones, 1997). For these reasons, the concomitant use of moclobemide and serotonergic agents should be avoided. In addition, the co-ingestion of moclobemide and SSRIs in overdose may result in death, which needs to be taken into account when prescribing for patients at high risk for suicide (Isbister *et al.*, 2001).

As mentioned earlier, treating MDD with trans-dermal selegiline appears to be relatively safe at lower doses, even in the absence of a tyramine-restricted diet (Amsterdam *et al.*, 2003). However, although rare, serotonin syndrome may occur when oral selegiline is combined with serotonergic agents, particularly the SSRIs (Richard *et al.*, 1997). The risk of such drug interactions with the trans-dermal formulation of selegiline has not been studied. At the present time, it is recommended that such combinations should be avoided. In addition, it is important to keep in mind that, while relatively selective for the MAO-B enzyme, selegiline is an irreversible inhibitor for that enzyme and there is a lag time between discontinuation of selegiline and recovery in MAO-B activity (Fowler *et al.*, 1994).

The most common side effects of MAOIs include postural hypotension, insomnia, agitation, and sedation. Analyses of large prospective studies containing over 20,000 patients (Coulter & Pillans, 1995; Delini-Stula *et al.*, 1999) report the risk of hypertension or hypotension with moclobemide at, approximately, 0.11% and 0.05%, respectively. In a separate study, the use of moclobemide with pre-existing hypertension was not found to result in significant increases in blood pressure (Moll *et al.*, 1994). The MAOIs do not appear to prolong cardiac conduction (Georgotas *et al.*, 1987; McGrath *et al.*, 1987; O'Brien *et al.*, 1991).

Sexual dysfunction can sometimes occur with the MAOIs, although the incidence of sexual dysfunction is thought to be lower than with the SSRIs (Philipp *et al.*, 2000). In fact, the incidence of sexual dysfunction during the treatment of MDD with selegiline transdermal system has been reported as comparable to placebo (Amsterdam *et al.*, 2006; Clayton *et al.*, 2007).

Other side effects include weight change, dry mouth, constipation, and urinary hesitancy (Fava & Rosenbaum, 1995). There are reports of rare but serious hepatotoxicity with phenelzine (Bonkovsky *et al.*, 1986; Gomez-Gil *et al.*, 1996), as well as a report of acute myocarditis following an overdose of phenelzine (Waring & Wallace, 2007). One case of fatal intrahepatic cholestasis related to the use of moclobemide has also been reported (Timmings & Lamont, 1996). Peripheral neuropathies have also been reported, and may be prevented by concomitant therapy with pyridoxine (Harrison *et al.*, 1983; Stewart *et al.*, 1984). There are also several reports of thrombocytopenia during tranylcypromine abuse or overdose (Davids *et al.*, 2000; Chatterjee & Tosyali, 1995; O'Grady & Carney, 1997; Pennings *et al.*, 1997; Szelenyi & Albrecht, 1998), as well as a report of phenelzine-related leukopenia (Tipermas *et al.*, 1984). Finally, some cases of MAOI abuse have been reported (Ben-Arie O & George, 1979; Brady *et al.*, 1991; Davids *et al.*, 2000; Griffin *et al.*, 1981; Szelenyi & Albrecht, 1998).

The endocrinologic effects of treatment with the MAOIs are less well characterized. Joffe and Singer (1987) found no effect of treatment with phenelzine on thyroxine (T4), free T4, triiodothyronine (T3), T3 resin uptake, or thyroid stimulating hormone (TSH) in 16 outpatients with MDD. Moclobemide does not appear to alter growth hormone (GH), prolactin (Markianos *et al.*, 1988 and 1991; Steiger *et al.*, 1994), luteinizing hormone (LH), follicle-stimulating hormone (FSH) (Markianos *et al.*, 1991; Steiger *et al.*, 1994), total T4, or free T4 (Kusalic *et al.*, 1993) levels in humans. Similarly, brofaromine does not appear to alter prolactin, testosterone, FSH or LH levels in humans (Steiger *et al.*, 1987). Phenelzine (Stewart & Halbreich, 1989), tranylcypromine, but not selegiline (Murphy *et al.*, 1986) do appear to increase melatonin levels. In addition, in a separate study involving 12 depressed patients who were administered 400–600 mg of moclobemide orally for four weeks, significantly increases in testosterone levels were reported (Markianos *et al.*, 1991). There is only one case report of MAOI-related syndrome of inappropriate secretion of anti-diuretic hormone (SIADH) (Peterson *et al.*, 1978). MAOIs must be used with caution in patients with diabetes due to the possibility of worsening of hypoglycemia (Adnitt *et al.*, 1966 and 1968; Bressler *et al.*, 1968; Cooper *et al.*, 1966; Potter *et al.*, 1969; Rowland *et al.*, 1994).

Similar to the TCAs, the MAOIs have also been shown to alter sleep physiology (Winokur *et al.*, 2001). Irreversible MAOIs, for instance, prolong sleep-onset latency, reduce sleep efficiency, increase waking time after sleep onset (WASO), and suppress random eye movement (REM) sleep (Landolt *et al.*, 2001; Winokur *et al.*, 2001).

4.1.3.1 *Dietary restrictions and drug interactions*

As discussed above, treatment with MAOIs carries a risk of hypertensive crisis. To minimize this risk, patients on MAOIs need to adhere to a strict dietary regimen which excludes foods and beverages that have a high content of dietary amines including: all aged cheeses, sour cream, yogurt, fermented or dried meats (sausages, basderma, pastrami, pepperoni, louza, linguiça, chorizo), offal (liver, sweetbread, kidney, tripe, brains), fava and broad bean pods (lima, lentils, snow-peas), marmite yeast extract, sauerkraut, soy sauce and other soy products, overripe bananas and avocado, eggplant, spinach, pickled, dried or salted fish, caviar, fish-roe (tarama), and foods containing monosodium glutamate (MSG). Patients should also avoid consumption of caffeinated drinks, and most alcoholic beverages, especially tap beer, red wine, but also certain white wines including those that are resinated (retsina), botrytized (sauternes, montbazillac, tokaji aszú, beerenauslese, trockenbeerenausle, ausbruch, amarone, grasa de cotnari), aged (sherry), and others (riesling, vermouth).

Sympathomimetics, both prescribed and over-the-counter (including pseudoephedrine, ephedrine, oxymetazoline, dextroamphetamine, methylphenidate), potent noradrenergic or dopaminergic antidepressants, dextramethorphan and meperidine (Demerol) may also precipitate a hypertensive crisis. In addition, as mentioned above, combining MAOIs with potent serotonergic agents such as the TCAs, SSRIs, and others carries a risk of serotonergic syndrome.

There are reports of adverse reactions (Absher & Black, 1988; Curtin *et al.*, 2002; Halle & Dilsaver, 1993; Joyce & Walshe, 1983; Palladino, 1983), and worsening of mood and anxiety (Tyrer, 1984) following the abrupt discontinuation of MAOIs.

4.1.4 *Dosing*

Optimal dosages vary from agent to agent. Optimal doses for phenelzine range between 45 and 90 mg/day, doses of tranylcypromine and isocarboxazid generally range between 30 and

60 mg/day, while doses for moclobemide range from 300 mg to 900 mg daily. For oral selegiline, the minimal reported effective dose seems to be 30 mg/day, while for trans-dermal selegiline, the minimal effective dose reported is 6 mg/day. CYP2C19 and CYP2D6 genotypes do not appear to influence selegiline plasma levels (Laine *et al.*, 2001; Scheinin *et al.*, 1998).

4.2 Serotonin-Norepinephrine-Dopamine Reuptake Inhibitors

Sibutramine (Meridia) is a triple-acting, serotonin-, dopamine-, and norepinephrine-reuptake inhibitor (Glick *et al.*, 2000; Heal *et al.*, 1998) that is FDA-approved for the treatment of obesity. The antidepressant potential of sibutramine is suggested by its activity in animal models for depression (Glick *et al.*, 2000), but there are no published placebo-controlled studies in humans. However, the results of a small open trial of sibutramine in obese patients with binge-eating disorder indicate a significant reduction in depressive symptoms during treatment (Appolonario *et al.*, 2002). Doses commonly used for the treatment of obesity are 10–20 mg. The most commonly reported adverse effects of sibutramine are headache, constipation, and nausea. Dizziness, dry mouth, and insomnia have also often been reported by patients receiving sibutramine. Increases in blood pressure and heart rate require regular monitoring, especially in obese hypertensive patients. Neither left-sided cardiac valve disease nor primary pulmonary hypertension have been associated with the use of sibutramine (Nisoli & Carruba, 2003). Sibutramine does appear to decrease serum and cerebrospinal fluid (CSF) leptin levels (Rodrigues *et al.*, 2002), and the decrease in leptin levels during treatment with sibutramine was reported to be proportional to the reduction in total body fat in one study (Rodrigues *et al.*, 2002).

Randomized, double-blind, placebo-controlled studies focusing on the use of a new (GSK 372475) serotonin-norepinephrine-dopamine reuptake inhibitor (SNDRI) as monotherapy for MDD are currently under way (clinicaltrials.gov; NCT00420641 and NCT00448058).

4.3 Catechol-O-Methyltransferase (COMT) Inhibitors

The COMT enzyme is found throughout the human body and, similar to MAO, is involved in the catabolism of the monoamines. Tolcapone (Tasmar) and entacapone (Comtan) are two inhibitors of the COMT enzyme that have been approved by the FDA for the treatment of Parkinson's disease.

Inhibitors of the COMT enzyme have shown activity in animal models of depression, while administration of COMT inhibitors in humans has been reported to result in decreased COMT activity *in vivo* (Ceravolo *et al.*, 2002). While the results of a single open trial of tolcapone for MDD were suggestive of potential antidepressant effects, hepatotoxicity, diarrhea, and elevated liver function tests emerged in a large proportion of treated patients (Fava *et al.*, 1999), rendering its use in MDD unfeasible. Nevertheless, compounds with COMT inhibiting activity that are able to cross the blood–brain barrier and are better tolerated than tolcapone should be investigated as potential treatments for MDD.

Chapter 5

Polypharmacy from the Onset of Treatment

5.1 Adjunctive Treatment with Monoaminergic Agents

5.1.1 *Tryptophan*

Tryptophan is the precursor of 5-hydroxy tryptophan (5HT), otherwise known as serotonin. Tryptophan was the first agent to be studied as co-initiation therapy for depression when, in 1963, Coppen, Shaw and Farrell reported greater improvements in depressive symptoms among patients treated with tranylcypromine and tryptophan than tranylcypromine alone. To date, eight double-blind, placebo-controlled studies of tryptophan co-initiation with monoamine oxidase inhibitors (MAOIs) (Auyso *et al.*, 1971; Coppen *et al.*, 1963; Glassman *et al.*, 1969), tricyclic antidepressants (TCAs) (Chouinard *et al.*, 1979; Lopez-Ibor *et al.*, 1973; Shaw *et al.*, 1975; Thomson *et al.*, 1982), and fluoxetine (Levitan *et al.*, 2000) for depression have been published (Table 5.1). While all three MAOI studies report greater changes in depressive symptoms for patients that received co-therapy with tryptophan than placebo, four out of four TCA studies do not. However, the practice of combining tryptophan with an MAOI is not feasible from a safety perspective, due to the risk for serious adverse events including serotonin syndrome (see Chap. 4 for further details). Finally, a single study reported greater symptom improvement for fluoxetine-treated patients who received co-initiation therapy with tryptophan than placebo at week 1 but

Table 5.1 Double-blind studies of tryptophan co-initiation in major depression.

Study	*n*	Dose/Duration	Adjunct Agent	Result[a]
Coppen *et al.* 1963	25	N/A 3 weeks	Tranylcypromine	Tryptophan > Pbo
Glassman *et al.* 1969	20	12–18 g 3 weeks	Phenelzine	Tryptophan > Pbo
Ayuso *et al.* 1971	30	6 g 3 weeks	Nialamide	Tryptophan > Pbo
Lopez-Ibor *et al.* 1973	30	3 g 4 weeks	Amitriptyline	Tryptophan = Pbo
Shaw *et al.* 1975	54	6 g 4 weeks	Clomipramine Desipramine	Tryptophan = Pbo
Chouinard *et al.* 1979	25	6 g 4 weeks	Imipramine	Tryptophan = Pbo
Thompson *et al.* 1982	115	3 g 12 weeks	Amitriptyline	Tryptophan = Pbo
Levitan *et al.* 2000	30	2–4 g 8 weeks	Fluoxetine 20 mg	Tryptophan > Pbo week 1 but not thereafter

[a]All outcomes represent difference in the change in Hamilton Depression Rating Scale or Beck Depression Inventory.
Abbreviations: Pbo = Placebo, N/A = Information not available.

not thereafter. This finding has yet to be replicated. Side effects reported with this treatment combination from randomized, double-blind, placebo-controlled trials include somnolence, fatigue, insomnia, nausea, and sexual dysfunction.

5.1.2 *Pindolol*

During the mid-1990s, a number of case series and open-label trials were published, suggesting the rapid relief of depressive symptoms in the vast majority of patients with MDD, including many with treatment-resistant depression (TRD), during treatment with the serotonin 1A (5HT1A) and β-adrenergic receptor antagonist pindolol as an adjunct (either as co-initiation or augmentation therapy) to a number of antidepressants (Artigas *et al.*, 1994; Bakish *et al.*, 1997; Blier & Bergeron, 1995; GSK trial #29060/524). These were soon followed by 11 double-blind, placebo- or active comparator-controlled trials involving co-initiation of pindolol with either a selective serotonin reuptake inhibitor (SSRI), trazodone or milnacipran for the treatment of MDD (Table 5.2). Only two of these studies show pindolol co-initiation to be superior to placebo or an active comparator at endpoint (Perez *et al.*, 1997; Zanardi *et al.*, 1997), while three show pindolol co-initiation to result in greater symptom improvement than placebo early-on (during first two weeks of therapy), but not thereafter (Tome *et al.*, 1997; Bordet *et al.*, 1998; Isaac *et al.*, 2003). A recent meta-analysis of pindolol adjunctive studies for MDD (Ballestros & Callado, 2004) concluded that outcome favored pindolol over placebo at two weeks' time (odds ratio 2.8, 95%CI: 1.4–5.7) but not at six weeks' time (odds ratio 1.4, 95% CI: 0.8–2.7). Thus, the sum of the evidence focusing on the use of this strategy in MDD suggests a more rapid improvement in depressive symptoms, but not necessarily a greater resolution of depressive symptoms at endpoint.

Some have argued that pindolol is often under-dosed in adjunctive randomized-controlled trials in MDD, which may explain the overall modest effect over placebo seen in these studied (Fig. 5.1). For example, the results of one positron emission tomography (PET) study indicate that augmenting SSRIs or venlafaxine with a 5-mg t.i.d. regimen achieved modest (19%) but significant occupancy of the 5HT1A auto-receptor, while the augmenting with the regimen used in the vast majority of clinical trials (2.5 mg t.i.d.) did not achieve significant 5HT1A receptor occupancy (Rabiner *et al.*, 2001). Increased irritability can sometimes be a limitation of this treatment strategy (Blier & Bergeron, 1995). Side effects reported with this treatment combination from randomized, double-blind, placebo-controlled trials include headache, nausea, fatigue, and somnolence.

Table 5.2 Double-blind studies of pindolol co-initiation in MDD.

Study	*n*	Dose/Duration	Adjunct Agent	Result[a]
Berman *et al.* 1997	43	7.5–10 mg 6 weeks	Fluoxetine 20 mg	Pindolol = Pbo
Perez *et al.* 1997	111	7.5 mg 6 weeks	Fluoxetine 20 mg	Pindolol > Pbo at endpoint
Tome *et al.* 1997	80	7.5 mg 6 weeks	Paroxetine 20 mg	Pindolol > Pbo day 14 but not thereafter
Zanardi *et al.* 1997	63	7.5 mg 1 or 4 weeks[b]	Paroxetine 20 mg	Pindolol > Pbo all time points[b]
Bordet *et al.* 1998	100	15 mg 6 weeks	Paroxetine 20 mg	Pindolol > Pbo day 10 but not thereafter
Berman *et al.* 1999	86	7.5–10 mg 6 weeks	Fluoxetine 20 mg	Pindolol = Pbo
Isaac *et al.* 2003	78	2.5 mg 6 weeks	Milnacipran 100 mg	Pindolol > Pbo day 7 only
Berney *et al.* 2008	8	7.5 mg 3 weeks	Citalopram 20 mg	Pindolol = Pbo all time points
Geretsegger *et al.* 2008	53	7.5 mg 4 weeks	Paroxetine 20 mg	Pindolol = Pbo
GSK 29060/518	154	7.5 mg 6 weeks	Paroxetine 20 mg	Pindolol = Desipramine monotherapy
GSK 29060/512	160	7.5 mg 6 weeks	Paroxetine 20 mg	Pindolol = Pbo all time points

[a]All outcomes represent difference in the change in Hamilton Depression Rating Scale or Montgomery-Asberg Depression Rating Scale, baseline to endpoint.

[b]Pindolol was administered in either of two parallel groups, 1 week duration followed by 3 weeks of placebo (double-blind substitution), or 4 weeks duration. Pindolol was superior to placebo for both groups at all time points during which it was administered.

Abbreviations: Pbo = Placebo.

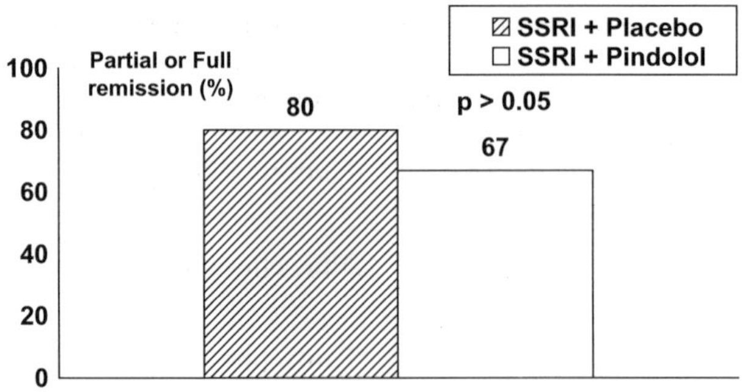

Fig. 5.1 SSRI plus pindolol (5HT1A antagonist) as initial treatment for MDD: A randomized, double-blind study ($n = 86$). [Data extracted from: Berman, R.M., Anand, A., Cappiello, A., *et al.* (1999). The use of pindolol with fluoxetine in the treatment of major depression: Final results from a double-blind, placebo-controlled trial. *Biological Psychiatry*, 45, 1170–1177.]

5.1.3 *Typical antipsychotic agents*

The potential utility of co-initiating standard antidepressant therapy with typical antipsychotic agents in order to alleviate symptoms of depression and anxiety was first described in several case reports, chart reviews, and open-label or uncontrolled trials (Browne, 1966; Chacon & Downham, 1967; Coffee, 1964; Dorfman, 1966; Faleni & Cia, 1972; Krakowski, 1962; Kris & Gerst, 1964; Mattey, 1963; Pollack, 1962; Ravn, 1961; Shubin & Mandel, 1967; Smith E Incas, 1965; Vann, 1959). These reports were soon followed by several double-blind studies comparing the co-initiation of TCAs and typical neuroleptics versus TCA monotherapy for the treatment of depression and anxiety (Anderson *et al.*, 1972; Bennett *et al.*, 1984; Bennie & Schiff, 1974; Beber, 1971; Davis, 1968; Desilverio *et al.*, 1970; Diamond, 1966; Feet *et al.*, 1985; Feldman, 1965; Hollister *et al.*, 1966 and 1967; Lowney *et al.*, 1969; Moller *et al.*, 1986; O'Hara *et al.*, 1978; Ota *et al.*, 1970; Rickels *et al.*, 1967, 1972 and 1982; Sinclair *et al.*, 1975; Sussex Clinical Trials Group, 1985; Valle-Jones *et al.*, 1983).

However, many of these studies were conducted before the advent of DSM-III and, as a result, are difficult to interpret in the context of contemporary nosology. For example, the majority of these studies either selected patients on the basis of symptoms rather than diagnosis, or offered an insufficient description of the studied population (i.e., unclear if psychotic patients were excluded or what the primary diagnosis was) (Anderson *et al.*, 1972; Beber, 1971; Bennie & Schiff, 1974; Davis, 1968; Diamond, 1966; Hollister *et al.*, 1966; Lowney *et al.*, 1969; O'Hara *et al.*, 1978; Ota *et al.*, 1970; Sinclair *et al.*, 1975; Sussex Clinical Trials Group, 1985; Valle-Jones *et al.*, 1983). In addition, several of these studies either involved the enrollment of a significant proportion of patients with psychotic symptoms or with a diagnosis of bipolar disorder (Hollister *et al.*, 1967; Feldman, 1965). Finally, one study was limited due to very short duration of treatment [merely three weeks in duration, with adjunctive neuroleptic administered only during the first week of treatment (Moller *et al.*, 1986)].

The remaining six studies are summarized in Table 5.3. No difference in the degree of depressive symptom resolution at endpoint between treatment groups was found in any of the six trials, while only one of these studies reported greater efficacy early on (weeks 1–2) for patients treated with the combination of desipramine plus thioridazine versus patients treated with desipramine monotherapy (Bennett *et al.*, 1984). Thus, overall, the sum of the evidence does not support a potential role for combining antidepressants with typical antipsychotic agents from the onset of therapy for MDD. Side effects with this combination can vary from agent to agent, but may include sedation, fatigue, insomnia, somnolence, nausea, hyperprolactinemia, dyslipidemia, glucose dysregulation, weight gain, and extrapyramidal symptoms including akathisia, dystonic reactions, Parkinsonism, neuroleptic malignant syndrome, and tardive dyskinesia.

5.1.4 *5HT2 and α-2 adrenergic receptor antagonists*

Thus far, four double-blind, placebo-controlled studies of co-initiation therapy with the 5HT2 and α-2 antagonist mianserin or mirtazapine for MDD have been published (Table 5.4). All four studies consistently show a greater decrease in depression severity in

Table 5.3 Double-blind studies of typical antipsychotic co-initiation in major depression.

Study	*n*	Antipsychotic	TCA Duration	Result[a]
Rickels *et al.* 1967	131	Fluphenazine 1.5–3 mg	Amitriptyline 75–150 mg 4 weeks	TA = Pbo
Desilverio *et al.* 1970	138	Perphenazine 8 mg	Amitriptyline 100 mg 4 weeks	TA = Pbo
Rickels *et al.* 1972	100	Perphenazine 6–12 mg (+Amitriptyline 100–150 mg)[b]	Doxepin[b] 100–150 mg 4 weeks	TA + Amitriptyline = Doxepin[b]
Rickels *et al.* 1982	130	Perphenazine[b] 8–12 mg + (+Amitriptyline 100–150 mg)[b]	Doxepin[b] 100–150 mg 4 weeks	TA + Amitriptyline = Doxepin[b]
Bennett *et al.* 1984	14	Thioridazine 100 mg	Desipramine 200 mg 3 weeks	TA > Pbo day 7, 14 only
Feet *et al.* 1985	63	Dixyrazine 50 mg or 100–200 mg	Imipramine 8 weeks	TA = Pbo

[a]All outcomes represent difference in the change in depression severity using various scales.
[b]Patients were randomized to receive treatment with either Perphenazine plus Amitriptyline versus Doxepin monotherapy.
Abbreviations: TA = Typical neuroleptic, TCA = Tricyclic antidepressant, Pbo = placebo.

patients treated with mianserin co-therapy than those who received TCA or SSRI monotherapy. However, there is a paucity of studies focusing on combining either mirtazapine or mianserin with agents other than the SSRIs/TCAs. The results of three separate chart reviews had suggested a 50–60% response rate among patients treated with the combination of venlafaxine and mirtazapine for MDD (Chung *et al.*, 2007; Hannan *et al.*, 2007; Malhi *et al.*, 2008). More

Table 5.4 Double-blind, placebo-controlled studies of mianserin, T3, and Li co-initiation.

Study	*n*	Dose	Agent Augmented	Result[a]
Mianserin/Mirtazapine				
Lauritzen *et al.* 1992	40	30 mg 6 weeks	Imipramine	Mianserin > Pbo
Dam *et al.* 1998	34	30 mg 6 weeks	Fluoxetine 20 mg	Mianserin > Pbo
Maes *et al.* 1999	31	7.5 mg 5 weeks	Fluoxetine 20 mg	Mianserin > Pbo
Blier *et al.* 2009	61	30–45 mg 6 weeks	Paroxetine 20–30 mg	Mirtazapine > Pbo
T3				
Prange *et al.* 1969	20	25 mcg 3 weeks	Imipramine	T3 > Pbo day 4, 7, 9, 14 but not endpoint
Wilson *et al.* 1970	20	25 mcg 3 weeks	Imipramine	T3 > Pbo day 2, 4, 7, 11 but not endpoint
Wheatley *et al.* 1972	52	20 or 40 mcg 3 weeks	Amitriptyline	T3 40 mcg > Pbo w2 but not endpoint
Feighner *et al.* 1972	31	25 mcg 3 weeks	Amitriptyline	T3 > Pbo w1 but not endpoint
Appelhof *et al.* 2004	106	25 mcg 50 mcg 8 weeks	Paroxetine	T3 = Pbo all time points
Posternak *et al.* 2008	50	25 mcg 6 weeks	Various ADs[c]	T3 > Pbo weeks 1–3
Cooper *et al.* 2007	124	40–50 mcg 8 weeks	Sertraline	T3 > Pbo
Garlow *et al.* 2007	151	50 mcg 8 weeks	Sertraline	T3 = Pbo all time points

(Continued)

Table 5.4 (*Continued*)

Study	n	Dose	Agent Augmented	Result[a]
Li				
Shahal *et al.* 1996	22	0.80 mEq/L[b] 5 weeks	Imipramine	Li = Pbo
Cappiello *et al.* 1998	29	0.67 mEq/L[b] 4 weeks	Desipramine	Li > Pbo week 1, 2 but not week 4
Januel *et al.* 2003	62	0.5 mEq/L[b] 6 weeks	Clomipramine	Li > Pbo week 1 but not thereafter

[a]All outcomes represent difference in the change in Hamilton Depression Rating Scale scores, baseline to endpoint.
[b]Plasma level for lithium.
[c]Included SSRIs, venlafaxine, bupropion, mirtazapine.
Pbo = Placebo.

recently, the results of the fourth level of the Sequenced Alternatives to Treatment to Relieve Depression (STAR*D) trial suggest numerically but not statistically greater remission rates among patients with TRD treated with the combination of venlafaxine plus mirtazapine (13.7%), than patients who received tranylcypromine (MAOI) monotherapy (6.9%) (McGrath *et al.*, 2006). The lack of statistical significance of this finding could, quite possibly, be due to inadequate statistical power ($n = 109$). Although highly promising, this strategy has yet to be tested in non-TRD populations. Side effects reported with this treatment combination from randomized, double-blind, placebo-controlled trials include weight gain, dry mouth, headache, dizziness, nausea, fatigue, and somnolence.

5.1.5 *Other antidepressants*

A preliminary, small, open-label trial first reported on the use of TCAs desipramine combined with fluoxetine from the onset of treatment in MDD (Nelson *et al.*, 1991). That study had suggested

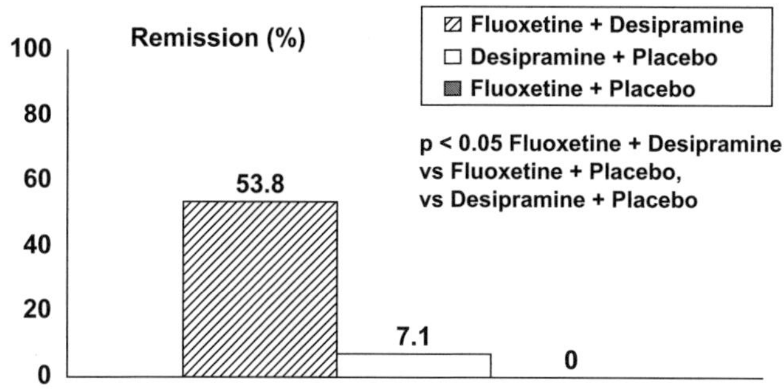

Fig. 5.2 Fluoxetine (SSRI) plus desipramine (TCA) as initial treatment for MDD: A randomized, double-blind study ($n = 38$). [Data extracted from: Nelson, J.C., Mazure, C.M., Jatlow, P.I., *et al.* (2004). Combining norepinephrine and serotonin reuptake inhibition mechanisms for treatment of depression: A double-blind, randomized study. *Biological Psychiatry*, 55, 296–300.]

the combined use of those two agents to result in particularly rapid antidepressant effects. Subsequently, a double-blind, placebo-controlled study examining the use of desipramine co-therapy with fluoxetine (20 mg) for a total of six weeks in a mixed population of MDD patients with or without TRD was published (Nelson *et al.*, 2004) (Fig. 5.2). Patients treated with a combination of the two agents had higher remission rates than patients treated with either monotherapy, which is in accordance with the notion that treatments influencing serotonergic- and noradrenergic-function may be more effective in relieving depression than agents acting on only one monoamine system (also see Chap. 3). This strategy has yet to be tested in strictly non-TRD populations. Potential limitations of this strategy include somnolence, weight gain, and fatigue, as well as the potential for drug–drug interactions as most TCAs are metabolized by cytochrome (CYT) P450 2D6.

Studies focusing on the co-initiation of antidepressants with other antidepressants are rare. Although preliminary, open-label trials suggested the potential utility of co-initiation therapy with escitalopram and bupropion XL in MDD (Leuchter *et al.*, 2008; Stewart *et al.*, 2009), the results of a randomized, double-blind, placebo-controlled, fixed-dose trial which compared escitalopram (4 mg), bupropion XL (150 mg), and their combination for MDD ($n = 534$) reported greater

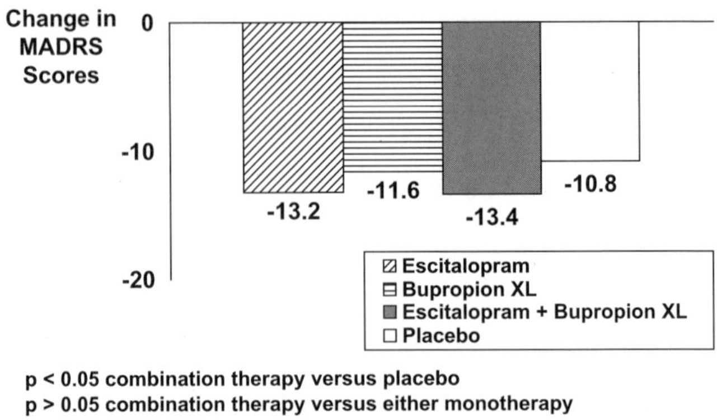

Fig. 5.3 Escitalopram (4 mg), bupropion XL (150 mg) or their combination for MDD: A randomized, double-blind, placebo-controlled study ($n = 534$). MADRS: Montgomery-Asberg Depression Rating Scale. [Data extracted from: Tsai, J., Tourkodimitris, S., & Bose, A. (2008). Low-dose combination of bupropion and escitalopram is an effective treatment combination for adult outpatients. APA Annual Meeting.]

efficacy for patients treated with the combination of the two drugs than placebo, but not when compared to either patients who received bupropion or escitalopram monotherapy (Tsai *et al.*, 2008) (Fig. 5.3).

Maes *et al.* (1996) reported greater improvement in depressive symptoms among MDD patients who received fluoxetine (20 mg) co-initiation therapy with, possibly, sub-therapeutic doses (100 mg) of trazodone versus patients who received treatment with fluoxetine monotherapy. Young *et al.* (1979) reported greater symptom improvement among MDD outpatients randomized to receive six weeks of treatment with trimipramine monotherapy, that patients treated with MAOI monotherapy (phenelzine or isocarboxazid) or MAOI and trimipramine combined. Finally, only anecdotal evidence supports the use of an SSRI–reboxetine combination for MDD (non-TRD) (Camarasa *et al.*, 2005).

5.1.6 *Atypical antipsychotic agents*

A rapidly growing literature is beginning to establish the use of the atypical antipsychotic agents as first-line therapy for the treatment of major depressive episodes in patients with bipolar disorder. Specifically, there is evidence from randomized, double-blind, placebo-controlled trials supporting the use of olanzapine either as monotherapy or combined with the SSRI fluoxetine (Tohen *et al.*, 2003), or quetiapine monotherapy (Calabrese *et al.*, 2005; McElroy *et al.*, 2008; Thase *et al.*, 2006; Vieta *et al.*, 2007; Young *et al.*, 2008) for the treatment of major depressive episodes in this patient population. However, far much less is known regarding the role of the atypical antipsychotic agents as first-line treatment for MDD.

Open-label trials have focused on the use of the atypical antipsychotic quetiapine (Baune *et al.*, 2006; Hussain *et al.*, 2006), risperidone (Hirose & Ashby, 2002), sulpiride (Uchida *et al.*, 2005), and olanzapine (Corya *et al.*, 2003) as co-initiation therapy with standard antidepressants in MDD. The olanzapine study also contained a significant proportion of TRD patients (approximately 25.9% of 560 patients). Remission rates reported in these trials range between, approximately, 60–90% for non-TRD patients.

To date, two double-blind, placebo-controlled studies examining the use of atypical antipsychotic co-initiation therapy for MDD have been published. In the first study, Parker *et al.* (2005) reported a greater resolution of depressive symptoms following two weeks of combined treatment with olanzapine and an SSRI than SSRI-treatment alone. However, in a subsequent, 8-week trial, Garakani *et al.* (2008) did not demonstrate greater antidepressant effects among MDD patients ($n = 114$) during treatment with fluoxetine plus quetiapine (25–100 mg) versus fluoxetine monotherapy, although a greater reduction in insomnia scores early-on (weeks 1–3) but not at endpoint was reported among quetiapine-treated patients. Side effects with this combination can vary from agent to agent, but may include sedation, fatigue, insomnia, somnolence, nausea, hyperprolactinemia, dyslipidemia, glucose dysregulation, weight gain, and extrapyramidal symptoms including akathisia, dystonic reactions, Parkinsonism, neuroleptic malignant syndrome, and tardive dyskinesia.

5.1.7 *Dopaminergic agents*

Small, open label-trials report on the use of methylphenidate co-initiation therapy with either a TCA (Gwirtsman *et al.*, 1994), or an SSRI (Lavretsky *et al.*, 2001 and 2003) for MDD. A small ($n = 9$), double-blind trial of methylphenidate versus placebo co-initiation of sertraline revealed no difference early-on (week 2) or at endpoint (week 9) in terms of depressive symptom resolution between the two groups (Postolache *et al.*, 1999), although a subsequent small trial ($n = 16$) of methylphenidate versus placebo co-initiation with citalopram demonstrated a trend towards statistical significance ($p = 0.05$) for a greater resolution of depressive symptoms following methylphenidate- than placebo-treatment (Lavretsky *et al.*, 2006). Potential adverse events of this treatment strategy may include headaches, vertigo, nausea, anorexia, weight loss, insomnia, irritability, and the risk for psychostimulant dependence and/or abuse. Finally, there is also a study focusing on co-initiation of antidepressants with the dopamine receptor agonist pramipexole for MDD (clinicaltrials.gov; NCT00086307).

5.1.8 *Other monoaminergic agents*

For the selective α-2 adrenergic *agonist* Clonidine, there is an open-label trial suggesting its potential utility when combined from the onset of treatment with imipramine in decreasing depressive symptoms among outpatients with comorbid MDD and PTSD (Kinzie & Leung, 1989). However, a double-blind, placebo-controlled trial of yohimbine (α-2 adrenergic *antagonist*) combined with fluoxetine from the onset of treatment demonstrated a more rapid improvement of depressive symptoms among patients who received adjunctive yohimbine versus those treated with fluoxetine monotherapy (Sanacora *et al.*, 2004). This finding is in line with the notion that combining serotonin or serotonin-norepinephrine reuptake inhibitors (i.e., SSRIs/TCAs) with agents which block the α-2 adrenergic receptor (i.e., mirtazapine and mianserin) from the onset of treatment may result in better outcome than SSRI or TCA monotherapy.

Studies focusing on the use of a new serotonin-2 receptor antagonist (M100907 — clinicaltrials.gov; NCT00070694), or a new selective agonist for the α-3 adrenergic receptor (SR58611A — clinicaltrials.gov; NCT00432614) combined with standard antidepressants from the onset of treatment of MDD are currently under way. Finally, a recent case report suggests the potential clinical usefulness of adding buspirone to bupropion from the outset of treatment (Fava, 2007).

5.2 Adjunctive Treatment with Neuroendocrine Agents

5.2.1 *Thyroid hormones*

Antidepressant effects for triiodothyronine (T3) were first reported in 1958 (Feldmesser-Reiss, 1958; Flach *et al.*, 1958). Ever since, four double-blind, placebo-controlled studies of co-initiation of T3 and TCAs in depressed patients have been published (Feighner *et al.*, 1972; Prange *et al.*, 1969; Wheatley, 1972; Wilson *et al.*, 1970) (Table 5.4). A greater improvement early-on (weeks 1–2) but not at endpoint for patients who received adjunctive T3 versus those who received TCA monotherapy was reported in all four studies. A meta-analysis of placebo-controlled trials concluded that T3 was significantly more effective than placebo in accelerating clinical response to TCAs in MDD (odds ratio: 0.58, 95%CI: 0.21–0.94) (Altshuler *et al.*, 2001).

For T3 co-initiation therapy with newer antidepressants, there are four double-blind studies (Table 5.4). Two studies (Appelhoff *et al.*, 2004; Garlow *et al.*, 2007) report no difference in depressive symptom resolution between T3 and placebo co-initiation with SSRIs at any time point during the study. A third study by Posternak *et al.* (2008) did demonstrate an acceleration of antidepressant response during adjunctive T3 than antidepressant monotherapy. Finally, a study by Cooper-Kazaz *et al.* (2007) reported a greater resolution of depressive symptoms at endpoint among patients treated with a combination of sertraline and T3, than patients who received sertraline

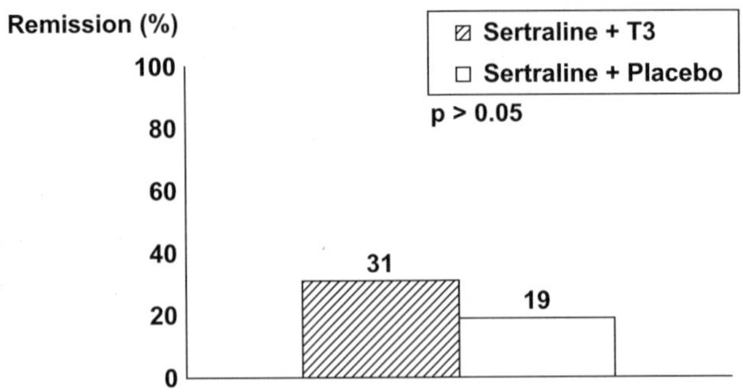

Fig. 5.4 Sertraline (SSRI) plus triiodothyronine (T3) as initial treatment for MDD: A randomized, double-blind study ($n = 124$). [Data extracted from: Cooper-Kazaz, R., Apter, J.T., Cohen, R., *et al.* (2007). Combined treatment with sertraline and liothyronine in major depression: A randomized, double-blind, placebo-controlled trial. *Archives of General Psychiatry*, 64(6), 679–688.]

monotherapy (Fig. 5.4). A meta-analysis of placebo-controlled trials concluded that T3 was not significantly more likely to accelerate or enhance clinical response to SSRIs in MDD (Papakostas *et al.*, 2009). Thus, at the present time, it remains unclear whether T3-SSRI co-initiation is an effective treatment strategy in MDD and, if so, for which subset of MDD patients. Reported side effects involving the use of T3 combined with antidepressants include palpitation, sweating, tremor, and nervousness as well as nausea, headache, somnolence, insomnia, and dry mouth.

Studies focusing on co-initiation with thyroxine (T4) for the treatment of depression have not been published. The results of a double-blind, placebo-controlled study suggest a more rapid improvement (first two weeks) in symptoms among 18 depressed outpatients randomized to receive intramuscular thyroid-stimulating hormone (TSH — 10 international units on days 1 and 8) in addition to imipramine (150 mg) than placebo plus imipramine (Prange *et al.*, 1970). This report has yet to be replicated. Finally, there is only a single, negative, double-blind, placebo-controlled co-initiation study of thyrotropin-releasing hormone (TRH — 600 mcg intravenously three times a week) with amitriptyline (150 mg) for depression (Coppen *et al.*, 1974).

5.2.2 *Estrogen*

Non-randomized studies focusing on the use of adjunctive estrogen with common antidepressants for MDD present conflicting results. For example, a post-hoc analysis of data from a double-blind, placebo-controlled trial of fluoxetine for the treatment of geriatric depression (age older than 60) revealed that fluoxetine was more effective than placebo only for patients who were on estrogen-replacement therapy at the time (Schneider *et al.*, 1997). However, this finding was not replicated in a subsequent post-hoc analysis for fluoxetine from a dataset involving patients 45 years of age or older (Amsterdam *et al.*, 1999).

With respect to prospective studies, Prange *et al.* (1972) did not find any difference in efficacy among younger (20–45 years of age) women with MDD randomized, in a double-blind fashion, to receive co-initiation treatment with imipramine and estrogen versus imipramine alone. Similarly, Dias *et al.* (2006) found no difference in efficacy among women with postmenopausal depression ($n = 72$) randomized in a double-blind fashion to receive treatment with venlafaxine either: (i) estrogen, metdroxyyprogesterone, and methyltestosterone, (ii) estrogen and medroxyprogesterone, or (iii) medroxyprogesterone. However, Rasgon *et al.* (2007) reported a greater resolution of depressive symptoms early on (weeks 2–4) but not at endpoint (week 10) among women with post-menopausal MDD treated with sertraline and estrogen than sertraline and placebo. Subsequent prospective, randomized, double-blind controlled studies have yet to be published. Side effects reported during treatment with this combination include headache, constipation, somnolence, sweating, and nausea.

5.2.3 *Other neuroendocrine agents*

A five-week, double-blind, placebo-controlled study involving co-initiation therapy with metyrapone, a steroid synthesis inhibitor, of either fluvoxamine or nefazodone demonstrated greater depressive symptom resolution among metyrapone- than placebo-treated patients at all time points (day 3, weeks 1–5) (Jahn *et al.*, 2004)

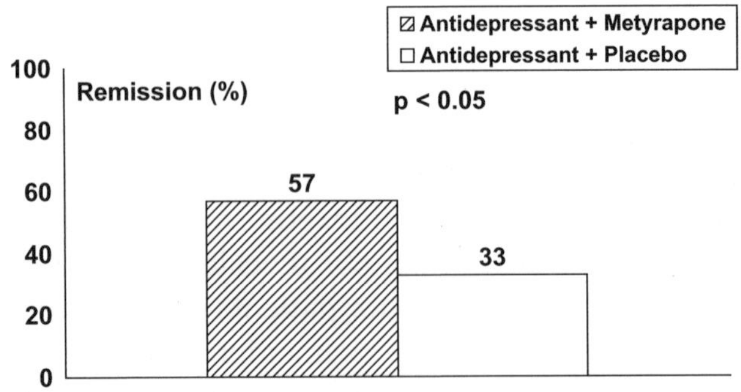

Fig. 5.5 Antidepressant plus metyrapone as initial treatment for MDD: A randomized, double-blind study ($n = 63$). [Data extracted from: Jahn, H., Schick, M., Kiefer, F., *et al.* (2004). Metyrapone as additive treatment in major depression: A double-blind and placebo-controlled trial. *Archives of General Psychiatry*, 61, 1235–1244.]

(Fig. 5.5). This study has yet to be replicated. Side effects reported include nausea, headaches, drowsiness, somnolence, dry mouth, and nervousness.

A double-blind, placebo-controlled study of co-initiation therapy of fluoxetine and tibolone, a gonadomimetic agent that has been found to stimulate estrogen receptors, did not show greater benefit for tibolone than placebo for the treatment of postmenopausal women with MDD (Berlanga *et al.*, 2003). Side effects reported include nausea and headaches.

Dexamethasone (0.75 mg) co-initiation of imipramine was not found to be more effective than placebo with respect to response rates at endpoint (3 weeks), although more patients responded to adjunctive dexamethasone than placebo at week 1 (Feighner *et al.*, 1972).

Finally, a double-blind, placebo-controlled trial of melatonin (5–10 mg, slow release formulation) co-initiation with fluoxetine for the treatment of sleep disturbance of MDD and/or insomnia resulting from fluoxetine use has been published (Dolberg *et al.*, 1998). Although melatonin significantly improved the quality of sleep in these patients, there was no difference in depressive symptom scores between the two groups throughout the study. Side effects reported include diarrhea, constipation, and headaches.

5.3 Other Agents

5.3.1 *Lithium*

The observation by De Montigny and colleagues (1981) of rapid (within 48 hours) relief of depressive symptoms among eight inpatients with MDD who had not experienced significant symptom improvement following a trial of TCAs sparked considerable interest in the further study of this promising treatment strategy over the next two decades. To date, the majority of adjunct lithium studies focus on the treatment of resistant depression. However, three double-blind, placebo-controlled trials of lithium co-initiation along with clomipramine (Januel *et al.*, 2003), imipramine (Shahal *et al.*, 1996) and desipramine (Cappiello *et al.*, 1998) for the treatment of MDD have been published (Table 5.4). Two studies showed greater efficacy for lithium than placebo at week 1 (Januel *et al.*, 2003; Cappiello *et al.*, 1998), with the study by Cappiello *et al.* also showing greater efficacy for lithium at week 2 (Fig. 5.6). The efficacy of lithium was equivalent to placebo thereafter for both studies. A third study did not reveal greater efficacy for adjunctive lithium than placebo at any time point (Shahal *et al.*, 1996).

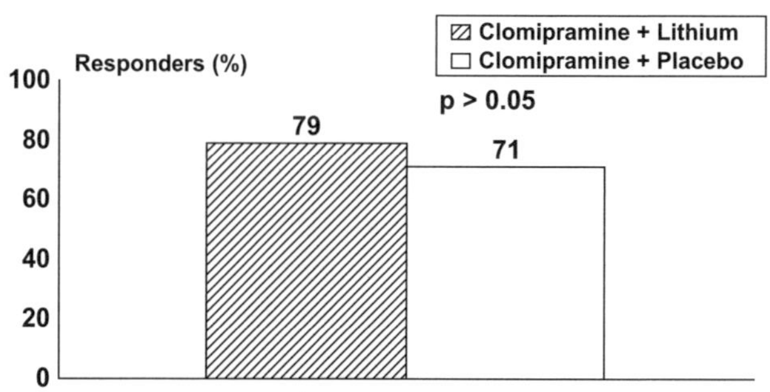

Fig. 5.6 Clomipramine (TCA) plus lithium as initial treatment for MDD: A randomized, double-blind study ($n = 149$). [Data extracted from: Januel, D., Poirier, M.F., D'alche-Biree, F., *et al.* (2003). Multicenter double-blind randomized parallel-group clinical trial of efficacy of the combination clomipramine (150 mg/day) plus lithium carbonate (750 mg/day) versus clomipramine (150 mg/day) plus placebo in the treatment of unipolar major depression. *Journal of Affective Disorders*, 76, 191–200.]

Thus, while the efficacy of lithium in the treatment of manic (Smith *et al.*, 2007), or depressive episodes (Goodnick, 2007), as well as in the prophylaxis of bipolar disorder (Geddes *et al.*, 2004) has been demonstrated in several randomized, double-blind, placebo-controlled trials, studies reviewed above do not suggest any potential utility of lithium as first-line, adjunctive therapy for MDD.

Potential side effects during treatment with adjunctive lithium may include tremor, somnolence, sedation, nausea, anorexia, abdominal pain, diarrhea, polyuria (via antagonism of antidiuretic hormone), edema, rash (including acne and psoriasis), leukocytosis, hypothyroidism, hyperthyroidism, ataxia, weight gain, renal insufficiency, electrocardiographic changes, arrhythmias, cardiac conduction abnormalities and, in rare cases, development of the nephritic syndrome. The use of lithium early during pregnancy is also associated with an increased risk of major birth defects.

5.3.2 *GABA-ergic agents*

The potential utility of co-therapy with standard antidepressants and benzodiazepines in order to alleviate symptoms of depression and anxiety has been described in numerous case reports, chart reviews, and open-label or uncontrolled trials (Bailey *et al.*, 1981; Grainger, 1972; Haider, 1967a; Wells *et al.*, 1988). In addition, numerous double-blind studies comparing the co-initiation of benzodiazepines and antidepressants versus antidepressant monotherapy for the treatment of depression and anxiety have been published (Beber, 1971; Calcedo Ordonez *et al.*, 1992; Dominguez *et al.*, 1984; Fawcett *et al.*, 1987; Feet *et al.*, 1985; Feighner *et al.*, 1979; General Practitioners Research Group, 1969; Haider, 1967b; Hare, 1971; Houck, 1970; Jacobson, 1978; James & Dean, 1985; Morakinyo, 1970; Nolen *et al.*, 1993; Rickels *et al.*, 1970; Smith, 1973; Smith *et al.*, 1998). However, many of these studies either select patients on the basis of symptoms rather than diagnosis, or offer an insufficient description of the studied population (i.e., diagnosis not stated) (Beber, 1971; Haider, 1967; Hare, 1971; Jacobson, 1978; James & Dean, 1985; Morakinyo, 1970; Smith, 1973). Details for the remaining 10 studies are presented in Table 5.5. A meta-analysis of placebo-controlled trials

Table 5.5 Double-blind, placebo-controlled studies of co-initiation with benzodiazepines or other GABA-ergic agents.

Study	*n*	Agent Duration	Antidepressant	Result[a]
General Pract. 1969	103	Chlordiazepoxide 30–60 mg 8 weeks	Amitriptyline 75–150 mg	Benzodiazepine = Pbo
Houck 1970	49	Chlordiazepoxide 20–40 mg 4 weeks	Amitriptyline 50–100 mg	Benzodiazepine > Pbo
Rickels *et al.* 1970	223	Chlordiazepoxide 4 mg 4 weeks	Amitriptyline 100 mg	Benzodiazepine = Pbo
Feighner *et al.* 1979	279	Chlordiazepoxide 50 mg 4 weeks	Amitriptyline 100–200 mg	Benzodiazepine > Pbo
Dominguez *et al.* 1984	63	Triazolam 0.5 mg 4 weeks	Imipramine 50–300 mg	Benzodiazepine = Pbo
Feet *et al.* 1985	63	Diazepam 10 mg 8 weeks	Imipramine 100–200 mg	Benzodiazepine = Pbo
Fawcett *et al.* 1987	69	Alprazolam 2–6 mg 6 weeks	Desipramine 100–300 mg	Benzodiazepine = Pbo
Calcedo Ord. *et al.* 1992	83	Bentazepam 75 mg 6 weeks	Clomipramine 100–150 mg	Benzodiazepine > Pbo at week 1 but not endpoint
Nolen *et al.* 1993	80	Lormetazepam 2 mg or Flunitrazepam 2 mg 4 weeks	Maprotiline or Nortriptyline[b]	Benzodiazepine >= Pbo[c]
Smith *et al.* 1998	80	Clonazepam 0.5–1 mg 3 weeks	Fluoxetine 20–40 mg	Benzodiazepine > Pbo weeks 1–3
Fava *et al.* 2006	545	Eszopiclone 3 mg 8 weeks	Fluoxetine 20–40 mg	Eszopiclone > Pbo

(*Continued*)

Table 5.5 (*Continued*)

Study	*n*	Agent Duration	Antidepressant	Result[a]
Ji *et al.* 2007	221	Zolpidem 10 mg 4 weeks	Paroxetine 10–20 mg	Zolpidem > Pbo
Fava *et al.* 2008	385	Zolpidem CR 12.5 mg 8 weeks	Escitalopram 10 mg	Zolpidem = Pbo

[a]All outcomes represent difference in the change in Hamilton Depression Rating Scale scores, baseline to endpoint, except for Nolen *et al.* where response rates were reported (defined as a 50% or greater decrease in HDRS-6 scores, baseline to endpoint), Feet *et al.* where a MADRS-based visual analogue scale was used, and General Practitioners 1969 where a scale developed by that group was used.
[b]Plasma-level used to guide dosage (optimal level: 100–150 ng/ml).
[c]Lormetazepam + TCA > TCA = Pbo but not flunitrazepam.
Abbreviations: Pbo = Placebo.

of benzodiazepine co-initiation for MDD (Furukawa *et al.*, 2001) revealed greater response rates for benzodiazepine- than placebo-treated patients at week 1 (odds ratio: 1.63, 95% CI: 1.18–2.27), week 2 (odds ratio: 1.41, 95% CI: 1.14–1.76), and week 4 (odds ratio: 1.38, 95% CI: 1.15–1.66), but not week 6 (odds ratio: 1.06, 95% CI: 0.76–1.99). Patients treated with adjunctive benzodiazepines were also less likely to discontinue treatment prematurely (odds ratio: 0.63, 95% CI: 0.49–0.82).

A subsequent, double-blind, placebo-controlled trial of eszopiclone and fluoxetine co-initiation in MDD, however, revealed higher remission rates following eight weeks of adjunctive treatment than fluoxetine monotherapy (42% versus 33%) (Fava *et al.*, 2006 — Table 5.5) (Fig. 5.7). This study is in the process of being replicated with the use of venlafaxine in place of fluoxetine (NCT00435279). More recently, a double-blind, placebo-controlled trial of zolpidem and paroxetine co-initiation in MDD also demonstrated higher remission rates for patients who received combination therapy than those who received paroxetine monotherapy (Ji *et al.*, 2007 — Table 5.5). However, a study examining the use of

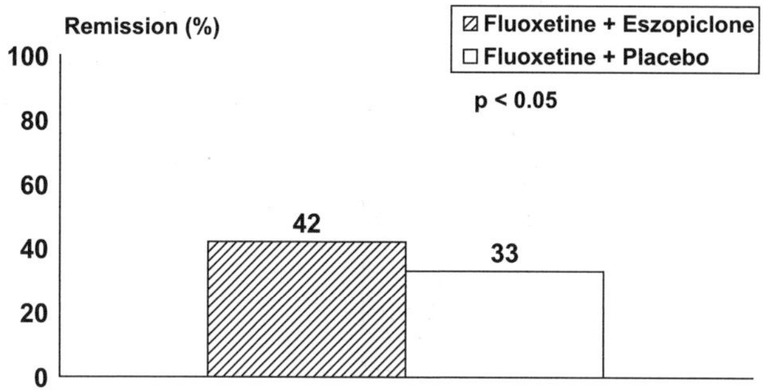

Fig. 5.7 Fluoxetine (SSRI) plus eszopiclone as initial treatment for MDD: A randomized, double-blind study ($n = 545$). [Data extracted from: Fava, M., McCall, W.V., Krystal, A., *et al.* (2006). Eszopiclone co-administered with fluoxetine in patients with insomnia coexisting with major depressive disorder. *Biological Psychiatry*, 59, 1052–1060.]

zolpidem-controlled release (CR) and escitalopram co-therapy versus escitalopram monotherapy in MDD did not demonstrate a statistically significant difference in the degree of resolution of depressive symptoms between the two treatment groups (Fava *et al.*, 2008). Preliminary evidence suggests that the combination of antidepressants and GABA-ergic agents may be particularly advantageous for patients with anxions MDD than those without (Papakostas *et al.*, in press). Potential disadvantages of the combination of antidepressants with GABA-ergic agents include sedation, somnolence, cognitive side effects, and the risk for abuse/dependence.

5.3.3 *Folates and s-adenosylmethionine (SAMe)*

Hypofolatemia has consistently been found to confer an increased risk of poorer response to pharmacotherapy in MDD, and a delayed onset of antidepressant response to the SSRIs (Chap. 1). To date, two studies explore whether the addition of folate to the psychopharmacologic regimen of MDD patients can improve outcome. Godfrey *et al.* (1990) randomized 24 hypofolatemic patients with MDD to receive co-therapy with antidepressants and folate versus antidepressant monotherapy, and reported a greater resolution

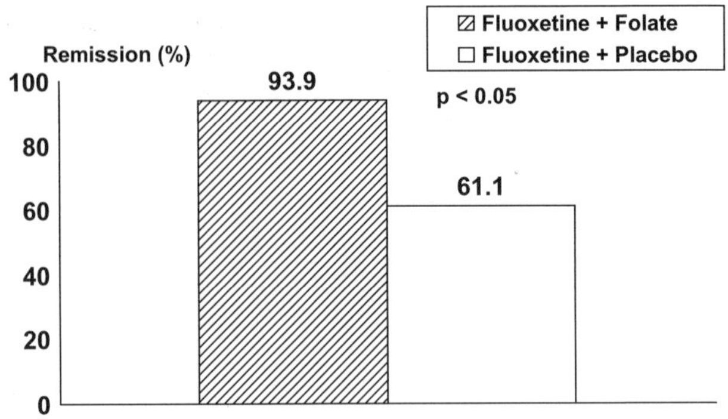

Fig. 5.8 Fluoxetine (SSRI) plus folate as initial treatment for women with MDD: A randomized, double-blind study ($n = 69$). [Data extracted from: Coppen, A., & Bailey, J. (2000). Enhancement of the antidepressant action of fluoxetine by folic acid: A randomised, placebo controlled trial. *Journal of Affective Disorders*, 60, 121–130.]

of depressive symptoms among patients who received combination therapy versus those who received monotherapy. In a subsequent, randomized, double-blind study, Coppen and Bailey (2000) reported a higher response rate among MDD patients treated with fluoxetine–folic acid (500 mcg) co-therapy versus patients who received fluoxetine monotherapy (Fig. 5.8). In fact, the advantage in efficacy for combination treatment versus monotherapy was more pronounced among women than men. A meta-analysis combining these two studies concluded that antidepressant monotherapy resulted in significantly lower response rates than antidepressant–folate co-therapy (odds ratio: 0.47, 95% CI: 0.24–0.92) (Taylor *et al.*, 2004).

More recently, a third, smaller ($n = 27$) randomized, double-blind study also demonstrated a greater resolution of depressive symptoms among MDD patients treated with the combination of fluoxetine (20 mg) plus folic acid (10 mg) than those treated with fluoxetine alone (Resler *et al.*, 2008).

SAMe is one of the metabolic end-products of folate (Papakostas *et al.*, 2003 — also see Chap. 13). In a double-blind, placebo-controlled study of SAMe co-initiation with imipramine in MDD patients, Berlanga *et al.* (2001) reported that depressive symptoms decreased earlier by the end of week 2 in the SAMe group than imipramine monotherapy group. Common side effects reported during the treatment of MDD with adjunct folates or SAMe include insomnia, nausea, anxiety, and headaches.

5.3.4 *Anticonvulsants*

Studies continue to emerge supporting the use of the anticonvulsants as first-line treatment for bipolar disorder. Specifically, evidence from randomized, double-blind, placebo-controlled trials support the use of valproate monotherapy (Bowden *et al.*, 1994 and 2006; Hirschfeld *et al.*, 2003; Pope *et al.*, 1991), adjunct valproate (Müller-Oerlinghausen *et al.*, 2000), and carbamazepine monotherapy (Weisler *et al.*, 2004 and 2005), for the treatment of manic episodes in patients with bipolar disorder. Similarly, evidence from double-blind, placebo-controlled trials also supports the use of lamotrigine monotherapy (Calabrese *et al.*, 1999; Geddes *et al.*, 2009; Frye *et al.*, 2000) for the treatment of major depressive episodes in patients with bipolar disorder.

However, the utility of the anticonvulsants when used adjunctively as first-line treatment for MDD is, largely, unknown. A small ($n = 40$), double-blind, placebo-controlled trial of lamotrigine cotherapy with paroxetine versus paroxetine monotherapy involving mostly MDD patients did not reveal a significant difference between the two groups with respect to depression severity at any time point (Normann *et al.*, 2002) (Fig. 5.9), although certain individual HAMD item mean scores including items No. 1 (depressed mood), 2 (guilt), and 7 (work and interest) were lower for the lamotrigine- than placebo-treated group early-on (from week 1 to week 4). However, paroxetine doses were increased for all patients from 20 mg to 40 mg during week 2, which may explain why there was no difference in the improvement in depressive symptoms at endpoint between the two treatment groups.

Side effects associated with the use of lamotrigine include headache, nausea, dizziness, ataxia, somnolence, insomnia, tremor, rash, diplopia, and blurred vision. Rare side effects include Stevens–Johnson syndrome, hypofolatemia, and leucopenia.

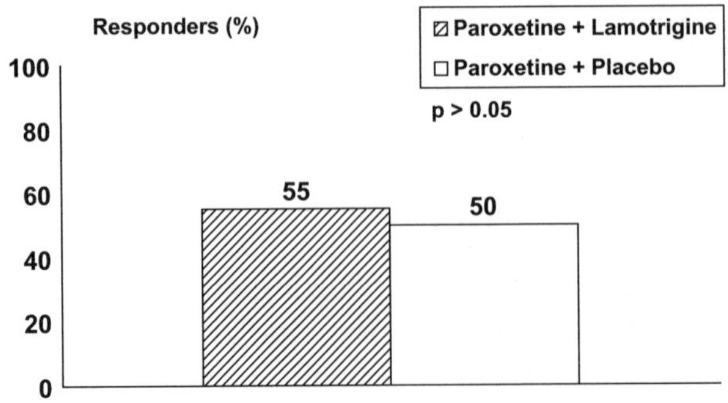

Fig. 5.9 Paroxetine (SSRI) plus lamotrigine as initial treatment for major depression: A randomized, double-blind study ($n = 40$). [Data extracted from: Normann, C., Hummel, B., Scharer, L.O., *et al.* (2002). Lamotrigine as adjunct to paroxetine in acute depression: A placebo-controlled, double-blind study. *Journal of Clinical Psychiatry*, 63, 337–344.]

Side effects associated with the use of valproate include somnolence, nausea, dizziness, tremor, nystagmus, insomnia, nervousness, blurred vision, weakness, fatigue, hirsutism, alopecia, and weight gain. Rare side effects include an elevation in liver enzymes, pancreatitis, hyperammonemia, thrombocytopenia, and teratogenicity if used during pregnancy.

Potential side effects during combined antidepressant–carbamazepine treatment may include nausea, diplopia, sedation, dizziness, ataxia, leukopenia (which may range from mild to severe) and rash (in rare cases Stevens–Johnson syndrome).

5.3.5 *Miscellaneous other agents*

Muller *et al.* (2006) recently reported the results of a double-blind, placebo-controlled trial of celecoxib (cyclogenase-2 selective inhibitor) co-initiation with reboxetine for MDD (Fig. 5.10). Greater resolution of depressive symptoms was reported among celecoxib- than placebo-treated patients, and a similar trend toward statistical significance for response rates in favor of adjunctive celecoxib treatment was observed ($p = 0.05$).

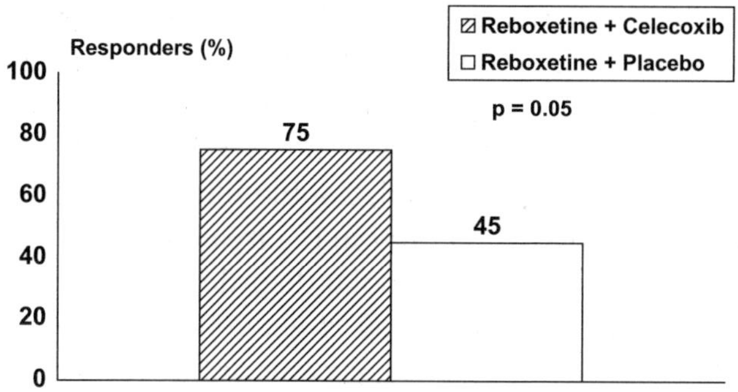

Fig. 5.10 Reboxetine (NRI) plus celcoxib as initial treatment for MDD: A randomized, double-blind study ($n = 40$). [Data extracted from: Muller, N., Schwarz, M.J., Dehning, S., *et al.* (2006). The cyclooxygenase-2 inhibitor celecoxib has therapeutic effects in major depression: Results of a double-blind, randomized, placebo controlled, add-on pilot study to reboxetine. *Molecular Psychiatry*, 11, 680–684.]

That celecoxib may possess antidepressant effects was also supported by the results of a randomized, double-blind, placebo-controlled trial focusing on the use of adjunctive celecoxib (to mood stabilizers) for the treatment of major depressive episodes in patients with bipolar disorder (Nery *et al.*, 2008).

A randomized, double-blind, placebo-controlled study focusing on the use of a new cyclogenase-2 selective inhibitor (Cimicoxib) combined with standard antidepressants from the onset of treatment of MDD is currently under way (NCT00510822).

The results of a randomized, double-blind, placebo-controlled trial of zinc-imipramine co-therapy in MDD did not demonstrate greater remission rates among imipramine-treated patients who received adjunctive zinc than those who received adjunctive placebo therapy (Siwek *et al.*, 2009).

Jazayeri *et al.* (2008) randomized MDD patients, in a double-blind fashion, to receive treatment with either fluoxetine (20 mg), EPA (1 gm) or the combination of fluoxetine (20 gm) and EPA (1 gm) for a total of eight weeks. There was no difference in the resolution of depressive symptoms among patients treated with either monotherapy. However, patients treated with the combination of the two agents demonstrated a greater resolution of depressive symptoms than patients treated with either monotherapy. Several other randomized, double-blind, placebo-controlled trials focusing on co-initiation of antidepressants with omega-3 fatty acids for MDD are also currently under way (NCT00289484; NCT00256412; NCT00067301). Two randomized, double-blind, placebo-controlled trial of EPA as adjunctive therapy in the treatment of major depressive episodes in patients with bipolar disorder have been conducted to date, with one study (Frangou *et al.*, 2006) but not the second (Keck *et al.*, 2006) demonstrating greater antidepressant effects for adjunctive EPA than placebo. However, a larger ($n = 240$) randomized, double-blind, placebo-controlled trial focusing on the use of ω-3 fatty acids as an adjunct in the treatment of major depressive episodes in patients with bipolar disorder is currently under way (NCT00001146).

There is only one negative double-blind, placebo-controlled study of inositol (12 g/day for 4 weeks) co-initiation with SSRIs in MDD (Levine *et al.*, 1999) (Fig. 5.11). Side effects may include nausea, headache, insomnia, and somnolence.

Similarly, two separate randomized, double-blind, placebo-controlled trials did not demonstrate statistically significant differences in symptom improvement for the treatment of major depressive episodes among patients with bipolar disorder who

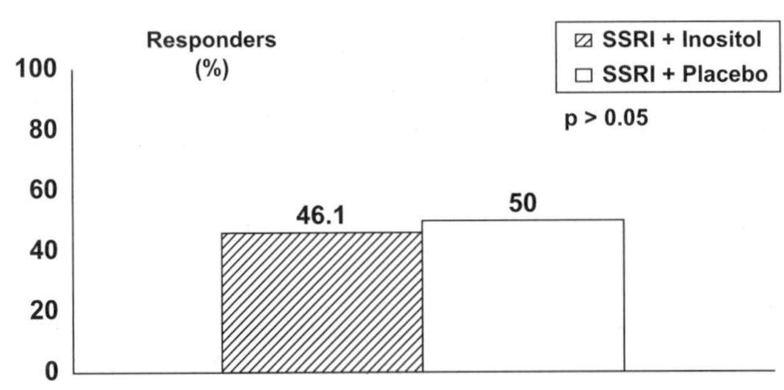

Fig. 5.11 SSRI plus inositol as initial treatment for MDD: A randomized, double-blind study ($n = 27$). [Data extracted from: Levine, J., Mishori, A., Susnosky, M., *et al.* (1999). Combination of inositol and serotonin reuptake inhibitors in the treatment of depression. *Biological Psychiatry*, 45, 270–273.]

received adjunctive inositol versus placebo (Chengappa *et al.*, 2000; Eden Evins *et al.*, 2006).

The results of a double-blind, randomized study suggest greater improvement in depressive symptoms and a similar trend towards statistical significance in remission rates ($p = 0.05$) among 84 patients with vascular depression treated with adjunctive nimodipine, a calcium channel blocker, than vitamin C, which was used as the inactive comparator (Taragano *et al.*, 2001) (Fig. 5.12). This finding has yet to be replicated. Side effects reported include hypotension, nausea, dizziness, bradycardia, vertigo, and insomnia.

An open-label trial had suggested the potential utility of modafinil co-initiation with SSRIs for the treatment of depression and fatigue in MDD outpatients with prominent fatigue and hypersomnia (Ninan *et al.*, 2004). However, a subsequent randomized, double-blind trial did not report a greater resolution of depressive symptoms, somnolence or fatigue among MDD patients treated with modafinil and an SSRI than those treated with an SSRI alone (Dunlop *et al.*, 2007) (Fig. 5.13). Side effects associated with the combination of modafinil and antidepressants include headache, nervousness, nausea, insomnia, diarrhea, dizziness, and dry mouth.

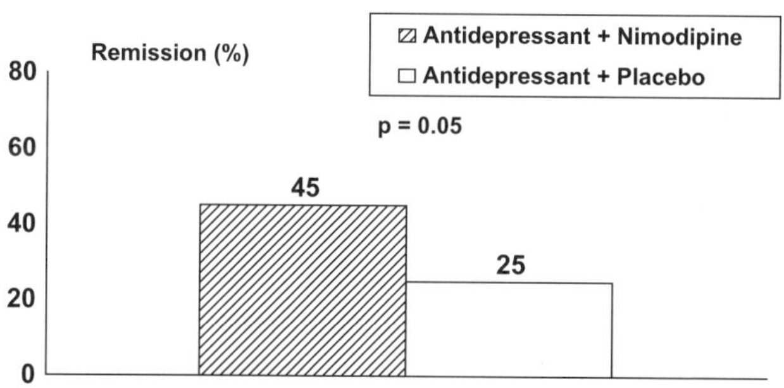

Fig. 5.12 Antidepressant plus nimodipine as initial treatment for vascular depression: A randomized, double-blind study ($n = 84$). [Data extracted from: Taragano, F.E., Allegri, R., Vicario, A., *et al.* (2001). A double blind, randomized clinical trial assessing the efficacy and safety of augmenting standard antidepressant therapy with nimodipine in the treatment of 'vascular depression'. *International Journal of Geriatric Psychiatry*, 16, 254–260.]

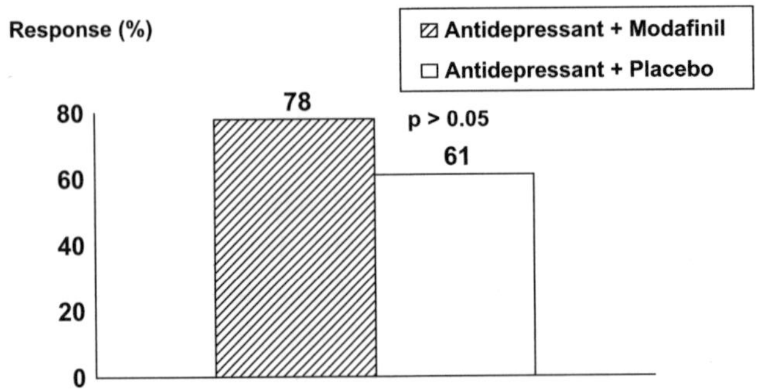

Fig. 5.13 SSRIs plus modafinil as initial treatment for MDD: A randomized, double-blind study ($n = 73$). [Data extracted from: Dunlop, B.W., Crits-Christoph, P., Evans, D.L., *et al.* (2007). Coadministration of modafinil and a selective serotonin reuptake inhibitor from the initiation of treatment of major depressive disorder with fatigue and sleepiness: A double-blind, placebo controlled study. *Journal of Clinical Psychopharmacology*, 27(6), 614–619.]

A randomized, double-blind, placebo-controlled study focusing on the use of a neurokinin-2 receptor antagonist (saredutant) combined with standard antidepressants from the onset of treatment of MDD is currently under way (NCT00531622).

Finally, the results of a small ($n = 38$), double-blind, randomized, placebo-controlled trial of galantamine (acetylcholinesterase inhibitor; see Chap. 11) co-initiation with the SNRI venlafaxine did not demonstrate a greater resolution of depressive symptoms or cognitive symptoms among elderly (age > 50) non-demented patients with MDD (Holtzheimer *et al.*, 2008) (Fig. 5.14).

However, a double-blind, randomized, placebo-controlled study examining the use of donepezil (acetylcholinesterase inhibitor; see Chap. 11) as an augmentation of antidepressants for elderly (age > 50 years) subjects with MDD who were cognitively impaired but not demented demonstrated a greater improvement in immediate recall ($p = 0.05$) but not targeted memory, attention, verbal fluency, processing speed, executive functioning, or depressive symptoms among patients treated with an antidepressant and donepezil than those treated with an antidepressant alone (Pelton *et al.*, 2008). Side effects reported during combined treatment with antidepressants

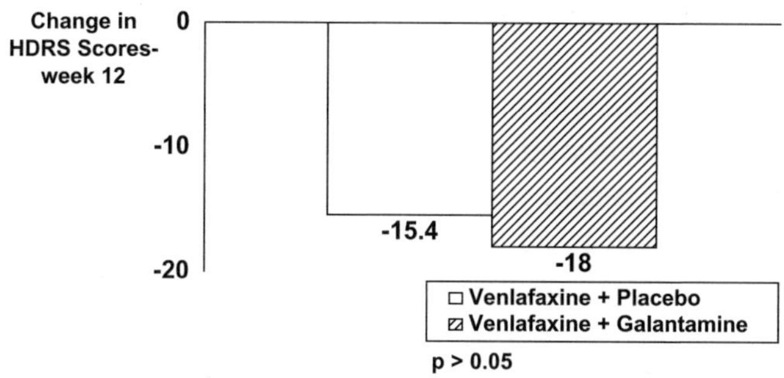

Fig. 5.14 Galantamine co-initiation with venlafaxine (SNRI): A randomized, double-blind, placebo-controlled study ($n = 38$). HDRS: Hamilton Depression Rating Scale [Data extracted from: Holtzheimer, P.E. 3rd., Meeks, T.W., Kelley, M.E., *et al.* (2008). A double blind, placebo-controlled pilot study of galantamine augmentation of antidepressant treatment in older adults with major depression. *International Journal of Geriatric Psychiatry*, 23(6), 625–631.]

and acetylcholinesterase inhibitors include headache, nausea, dizziness, and sweating. A larger, randomized, double-blind, placebo-controlled trial of donepezil co-initiation with antidepressants for the treatment of elderly non-demented patients with MDD is currently under way (NCT00177671).

Summary and Conclusion of Part I

Over the last few decades, the monoamine theory of depression has guided the discovery and development of dozens of new treatment for depression. In recent years, the rapid emergence of monoamine-based antidepressants which differ in terms of their effects on the noradrenergic, dopaminergic and serotonergic system is beginning to redefine depressive subtypes in ways that highlight their differential effects on the treatment of select depressive symptoms, symptom clusters and syndromes, allowing us to make generalizations as to the underlying neurophysiologic process of depression and recovery, as well as generalizations regarding the potential efficacy advantages of triple-acting agents over other contemporary antidepressant classes. In general, first-line antidepressant treatment choice in MDD should be guided by a combination of the following factors:

1. History of therapeutic success or failure,
2. History of poor tolerability or the occurrence of a serious adverse event,
3. Indication (with respect to comorbid axis-I disorders, if present),
4. Efficacy,
5. Tolerability,
6. Safety, and
7. Patient preference (selecting an agent that the patient believes is more likely to be successful over one that is believed to be inferior may enhance the chances of a placebo response).

As pointed out in Chap. 1, the use of antidepressants as monotherapy for MDD leaves much to be desired in terms of their overall efficacy. One approach to enhance treatment efficacy has been to simultaneously initiate treatment with two drugs (co-initiation therapy or co-therapy), usually involving an antidepressant and a non-antidepressant drug (or, in some cases, two antidepressants). In summary, a number of randomized, double-blind co-therapy studies consistently suggest that lithium or T3 may hasten the onset of clinical response of the TCAs, although antidepressant effects over placebo past 2 to 3 weeks of adjunctive treatment with these agents have never been demonstrated. For T3 co-initiation of the SSRIs, there is disagreement in the results of conducted trials, with one study reporting greater efficacy for combined T3-SSRI treatment than SSRI monotherapy, a second study reporting equivalent efficacy at endpoint between the two treatment groups with a more rapid improvement in depressive symptoms for T3-SSRI treated patients, and two studies suggesting no difference in the rapidity of symptom improvement or antidepressant efficacy between the two treatment groups. Controlled studies of co-initiation of the SSRIs with lithium have not been published.

Similarly, while the results of meta-analyses also suggest that adjunct pindolol or benzodiazepines may hasten the onset of antidepressant action of conventional antidepressants, greater symptom resolution for adjunctive pindolol or benzodiazepines than placebo has not been demonstrated past two (for pindolol) or four (for the benzodiazepines) weeks of treatment. However, two separate studies report that patients treated with the combination of an SSRI and a "newer" GABA-ergic agent (eszopiclone, zolpidem) were more likely to experience remission of MDD than patients treated with an SSRI alone.

Tryptophan co-initiation has consistently been shown to enhance the antidepressant effects of the MAOIs, and has been shown to accelerate the antidepressant effects of the SSRIs in one study. However, the use of this practice is limited due to the risk of serotonin syndrome (primarily when combined with MAOIs) as well as the risk of eosinophilia-myalgia syndrome. However, cotherapy of antidepressants with mianserin, a much safer strategy, appears to consistently enhance the antidepressant effects of the SSRIs or TCAs in all three studies published to date. A single trial of desipramine combined with fluoxetine from the onset of treatment also suggests greater efficacy (remission rates) during combination than monotherapy treatment. Folate, intravenous SAMe, yohimbine, metyrapone, nimodipine (for vascular depression), cox-2 inhibitors, and the atypical antipsychotic olanzapine also appear to be promising adjunctive treatments to either enhance or accelerate the antidepressant effects of conventional antidepressants. However, positive-controlled studies for these agents, with the exception of folate, have yet to be replicated. Finally, a number of promising pharmacotherapeutic strategies to enhance the rapidity of action or efficacy of antidepressants including oral SAMe, modafinil, and atypical antipsychotics other than olanzapine and quetiapine have yet to be subject to double-blind, controlled investigation.

At the present time, co-therapy is not practiced broadly, due to the relative paucity of studies examining its merits and limitations versus traditional antidepressant monotherapy. One possible exception is the use of anxiolytics and hypnotics to target insomnia and/or anxiety in MDD. Research focusing on this treatment approach is significantly lagging behind. An additional area that has not received adequate attention is the impact of differential antidepressant treatment strategies on comorbid axis-I disorders in patients with MDD. In particular, several antidepressants have not been adequately studied and, presently, do not have an indication with respect to a certain comorbid axis-I disorders (for example, the SSRIs/SNRIs and AD(H)D, or the NDRI bupropion and anxiety disorders). It would be interesting to examine whether co-therapy of antidepressants not indicated for the treatment of a comorbid axis-I disorders along with agents that have been found to be effective in treating that disorder can result in greater overall remission rates (with respect to MDD as well as the comorbid disorder), as well as a greater functional improvement than antidepressant monotherapy. An accelerated effort towards conducting yet more double-blind co-therapy studies in MDD will be required to further refine our ability to successfully treat MDD to remission.

Part II

Next-Step Treatment Strategies

As illustrated in Chap. 1, many patients with MDD fail to achieve full remission of symptoms despite treatment with a course of antidepressant monotherapy (first-line treatment). In the second part of this book, we will discuss treatment strategies for patients with MDD that do not respond to first-line treatment (treatment-resistant MDD or TRD). Specifically, in Chap. 6, we discuss the use of polypharmacy strategies for patients who have not experienced significant symptom improvement following adequate antidepressant treatment. These treatment strategies are termed augmentation (when a non-antidepressant drug is added to an antidepressant treatment regimen) and combination (when an antidepressant drug is added to the treatment regimen) therapy. The use of polypharmacy strategies for TRD can have several advantages over the monotherapy strategies (increasing the antidepressant dose or switching to a new antidepressant). For example, combining two agents with different mechanisms (i.e., serotonergic and noradrenergic mechanism) may result in a synergistic pharmacologic (dual- or triple-acting) effect. In addition, the risk for a potential loss of any partial benefit experienced during the first antidepressant trial inherent in switching (see Chap. 9 regarding the risk of symptom worsening following the discontinuation of an antidepressant) is minimized when choosing an augmentation or combination strategy, as is the risk of precipitating antidepressant withdrawal symptoms during switching (see Chaps. 2–4 for more details on the risk of precipitating adverse events following the discontinuation of antidepressants). Finally, augmentation/combination strategies may also be used to target side effects resulting from the initial antidepressant treatment in addition to improving overall outcome (see Chap. 10 for more details).

In Chap. 7, we then discuss the use of monotherapy strategies for TRD, which include either increasing the dose of an antidepressant or switching from one antidepressant to another. Several advantages for monotherapy over polypharmacy strategies have been suggested. For example, by increasing the dose of an antidepressant or switching from one antidepressant to another, one would avoid the potential for drug interactions inherent in the use of polypharmacy. In addition, monotherapy strategies may also prove advantageous with regards to compliance (it is easier to remember to take one pill than several). Lastly, monotherapy may also be associated with lower cost than polypharmacy (assuming one is not more likely to receive monotherapy than polypharmacy with a brand-name antidepressant).

Finally, in Chap. 8, we review a number of non-pharmacologic approaches that exist for the treatment of patients with TRD, including the use of electroconvulsive therapy, vagus nerve stimulation, transcranial magnetic stimulation, and the use of various psychotherapies.

Chapter 6

Polypharmacy Strategies for Treatment-Resistant Depression

6.1 Adjunctive Treatment with Monoaminergic Agents

6.1.1 *Pindolol*

During the mid-1990s, a number of case series and open-label trials reported a rapid relief of depressive symptoms in the majority of patients with TRD following adjunctive treatment with the serotonin 1A (5HT1A) and β-adrenergic receptor antagonist pindolol (Artigas *et al.*, 1994; Bakish *et al.*, 1997; Blier & Bergeron, 1995). These reports were soon followed by five double-blind studies of pindolol as an adjunct to antidepressants in TRD (Table 6.1). Two of these studies involve the adjunctive use of pindolol with either low-dose trazodone (100 mg — Maes *et al.*, 1996), or fluoxetine (Maes *et al.*, 1999), and report adjunctive pindolol to be superior to placebo in terms of depressive symptom reduction. Both of these studies, however, also contained a number of patients who were not treatment-resistant (12/52 or roughly 23% of the total sample). Subsequently, three double-blind, placebo-controlled studies have been published examining the use of pindolol augmentation in a combined population of selective serotonin reuptake inhibitor (SSRI) and tricyclic antidepressant (TCA) non-responders (Perez *et al.*, 1999) (Fig. 6.1), or SSRI-nonresponders alone (Perry *et al.*, 2004; Sokolski *et al.*, 2004). Only the smallest ($n = 9$) of the three trials reported greater symptom improvement over placebo among patients treated with adjunctive

Table 6.1 Double-blind studies of adjunct pindolol in TRD.

Study	*n*	Dose Duration	Antidepressant	Result[a]
Maes *et al.*, 1996	33	7.5 mg 4 weeks	Trazodone 100 mg	Pindolol > Pbo
Maes *et al.*, 1999	31	7.5 mg 5 weeks	Fluoxetine 20 mg	Pindolol > Pbo
Perez *et al.*, 1999	80	7.5 mg 4 weeks	SSRIs or TCAs	Pindolol = Pbo
Perry *et al.*, 2004	42	7.5 mg 3 weeks	SSRIs	Pindolol = Pbo
Sokolski *et al.*, 2004	9	7.5 mg 4 weeks	Paroxetine 40 mg	Pindolol > Pbo

[a]All outcomes represent difference in the change in Hamilton Depression Rating Scale or Montgomery-Asberg Depression Rating Scale during treatment.
Abbreviations: SSRIs = Selective Serotonin Reuptake Inhibitors, TCAs = Tricyclic Antidepressants, Pbo = placebo.

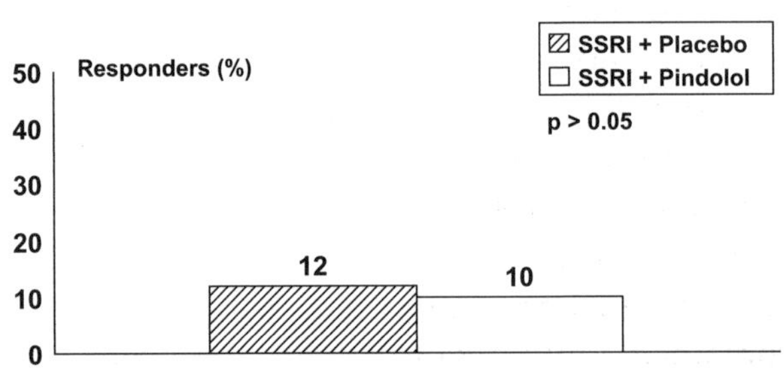

Fig. 6.1 Pindolol augmentation of SSRIs for TRD: A randomized, double-blind study ($n = 80$). [Data extracted from: Perez, V., Soler, J., Puigdemont, D., *et al.* (1999). A double-blind, randomized, placebo-controlled trial of pindolol augmentation in depressive patients resistant to serotonin reuptake inhibitors. Grup de Recerca en Trastorns Afectius. *Archives of General Psychiatry*, 56, 375–379.]

pindolol (Sokolski *et al.*, 2004). Thus, the sum of the evidence does not support the use of adjunctive pindolol for TRD. As mentioned in Chap. 5, it is possible that the dose of pindolol used in these studies may have not been adequate. Side effects reported with this treatment combination include somnolence, nausea, postural hypotension, sweating, and dry mouth.

6.1.2 *5HT2 and α-2 adrenergic-receptor antagonists*

Thus far, four double-blind, placebo-controlled studies of adjunct treatment with the combined 5HT2 and *α*-2 antagonists mirtazapine or mianserin for TRD have been published (Table 6.2). A combination study of mianserin along with fluoxetine (Maes *et al.*, 1999) revealed a greater decrease in depression severity in fluoxetine-mianserin than fluoxetine-treated patients. In a subsequent double-blind, placebo-controlled study, Ferreri *et al.* (2001) randomized fluoxetine (20 mg)-resistant patients with major depressive disorder (MDD) to continued fluoxetine (20 mg) versus mianserin augmentation of fluoxetine, versus switching to mianserin. Patients treated with mianserin augmentation of fluoxetine experienced greater improvement in depression symptom severity than patients who continued treatment with fluoxetine monotherapy, while the degree of symptom improvement for the mianserin switch group was numerically intermediate in magnitude than the other two groups (but not statistically different than either group). Similarly, Carpenter *et al.* (2002a) reported greater reduction in depression severity in TRD patients treated with mirtazapine augmentation than placebo (Fig. 6.2).

However, not all studies of adjunctive treatment with 5HT2 antagonists/*α*-2 antagonists have been "positive". Licht and Qvitzau (2003) randomized MDD outpatients with sertraline (100 mg)-resistant depression to receive treatment with mianserin augmentation of sertraline versus continued sertraline (100 mg) treatment, versus treatment with an increased sertraline dose (200 mg). No difference in outcome between the mianserin augmentation and continued sertraline (100 mg) group was found. However, it appears that sertraline non-responders had their sertraline dose increased from 50 mg to 100 mg only two weeks prior to randomization. Given the often-delayed time-course of clinical response to the SSRIs (Nierenberg *et al.*, 2000), this may explain the

Table 6.2 Double-blind studies of adjunct 5HT2/α-2 antagonists in TRD.

Study	*n*	Agent and Dose Duration	Antidepressant	Result[a]
Maes *et al.*, 1999	31	Mianserin 7.5 mg 5 weeks	Fluoxetine 20 mg	Mianserin > Pbo
Ferreri *et al.*, 2001	104	Mianserin 30 mg 6 weeks	Fluoxetine 20 mg	Combination > Fluoxetine[b]
Carpenter *et al.*, 2002a	26	Mirtazapine 15–30 mg 4 weeks	Mostly SSRIs	Mirtazapine > Pbo
Licht & Qvitzau, 2003	295	Mianserin 30 mg 6 weeks	Sertraline 100 mg	Mianserin = Pbo[c]

[a]All outcomes represent difference in the change in Hamilton Depression Rating Scale or Montgomery-Asberg Depression Rating Scale during treatment.
[b]Fluoxetine-resistant patients either continued on fluoxetine, or received adjunctive treatment with mianserin, or were switched to mianserin monotherapy. Result: mianserin augmentation > fluoxetine monotherapy. Mianserin switch = mianserin augmentation or paroxetine monotherapy.
[c]Sertraline-resistant patients either continued on same dose of sertraline (100 mg), or received adjunctive treatment with mianserin, or had their dose of sertraline increased to 200 mg (many patients had dose increase from 50 to 100 mg sertraline 2 weeks prior to randomization). Result: mianserin augmentation = sertraline 100 mg > sertraline 200 mg.
Abbreviations: TRD = treatment-resistant depression, SSRIs = selective serotonin reuptake inhibitors, Pbo = placebo.

lack of difference in outcome between these two groups. In support of this argument, patients who had a further dose-increase during randomization (200 mg) did poorer than patients randomized to continue on 100 mg.

Finally, as discussed in Chap. 5, the results of the fourth level of the Sequenced Alternatives to Treatment to Relieve Depression (STAR*D) trial suggest numerically but not statistically greater remission rates among patients with TRD treated

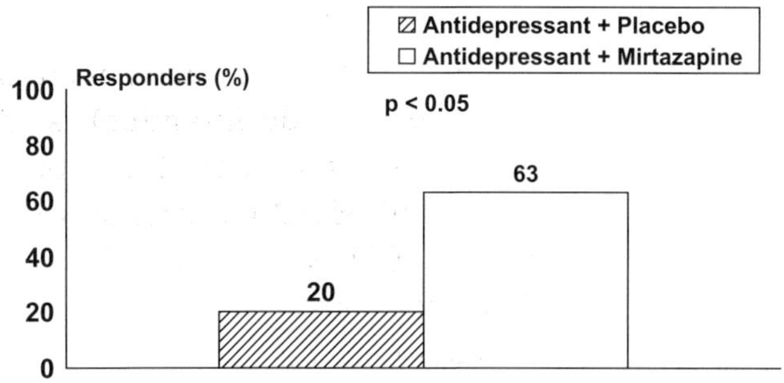

Fig. 6.2 Mirtazapine-antidepressant combination for TRD: A randomized, double-blind study ($n = 26$). [Data extracted from: Carpenter, L.L., Yasmin, S., & Price, L.H. (2002). A double-blind, placebo-controlled study of antidepressant augmentation with mirtazapine. *Biological Psychiatry*, 51, 183–188.]

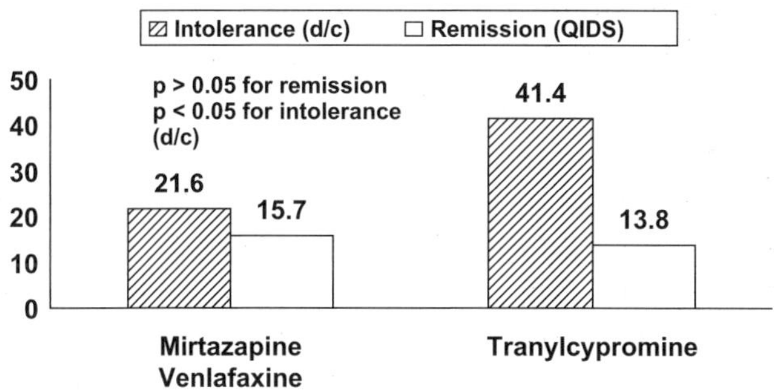

Fig. 6.3 STAR*D Level 4: Combined mirtazapine–venlafaxine versus tranylcypromine for TRD: A randomized study ($n = 109$). [Data extracted from: McGrath, P.J., Stewart, J.W., Fava, M., *et al.* (2006). Tranylcypromine versus venlafaxine plus mirtazapine following three failed antidepressant medication trials for depression: A STAR*D report. *American Journal of Psychiatry*, 163, 1531–1541.]

with the combination of venlafaxine plus mirtazapine (13.7%) than the monoamine oxidase inhibitor (MAOI) tranylcypromine (6.9%) (McGrath *et al.*, 2006) (Fig. 6.3). The lack of statistical significance of this finding could quite possibly be due to inadequate statistical power ($n = 109$). Although highly promising, this potential finding has yet to be confirmed in larger studies. Side effects reported with this treatment include weight gain, increased appetite, tinnitus, constipation, blurred vision, tremor, and somnolence.

6.1.3 *Tricyclic antidepressants*

Preliminary case reports, chart reviews, and small, open-label trials report on the use of the TCAs (usually desipramine) as adjuncts to other antidepressants (mostly SSRIs) for the treatment of treatment-resistant, as well as non-resistant MDD (Amsterdam *et al.*, 1997; Levitt *et al.*, 1999; Montes *et al.*, 2004; Rampello *et al.*, 2004; Zajecka *et al.*, 1995). However, only three controlled studies focusing on the use of adjunct TCAs in TRD have been published. Two of these studies compared desipramine augmentation of 20 mg of fluoxetine with lithium augmentation of 20 mg of fluoxetine versus an increase in fluoxetine dose (40–60 mg) among MDD outpatients with fluoxetine (20 mg)-resistant depression. In the first study, increasing the dose of fluoxetine was found to be more effective than desipramine or lithium augmentation (Fava *et al.*, 1994). In the second study, a similar trend towards statistical significance was found in favor of dose-increase versus the augmentation strategies (Fava *et al.*, 2002). However, as discussed in Chap. 5, a double-blind, placebo-controlled study examining the use of desipramine combined with fluoxetine from the onset of treatment (co-therapy) versus fluoxetine or desipramine monotherapy in a mixed TRD and non-TRD population reported greater remission rates among patients who received combination treatment than patients who received treatment with monotherapy (Nelson *et al.*, 2004). This study has yet to be replicated in strictly TRD populations. Potential limitations of this strategy include somnolence, weight gain, and fatigue, as well as the potential for drug–drug interactions as most TCAs are metabolized by cytochrome (CYT) P450 2D6.

6.1.4 *Selective 5HT1A agonists*

The augmentation of SSRIs or clomipramine with buspirone initially appeared to be a promising therapeutic strategy for TRD, and was supported by several open-label studies involving a total of 65 MDD outpatients, 20–68% of who responded following buspirone augmentation (20–50 mg, 3–4 weeks) (Dimitriou & Dimitriou, 1998;

Fischer *et al.*, 1998; Joffe & Schuller, 1993). These open-label trials were soon followed by two double-blind, placebo-controlled trials. In the first trial, Landen *et al.* (1998) randomized 119 outpatients with SSRI-resistant depression to receive buspirone augmentation (10–30 mg BiD) of SSRIs versus continued SSRI monotherapy for four weeks. In the second trial, Appelberg *et al.* (2001) randomized 102 MDD outpatients with SSR-resistant depression to receive buspirone augmentation of SSRIs (10–30 mg BiD) versus SSRI monotherapy for six weeks. No difference in terms of efficacy between the two groups was found for either study. However, in the latter of two trials, a greater reduction in depression severity in patients who received adjunctive buspirone than those who did not at the week 1 time-point was noted, suggesting that buspirone augmentation of SSRIs may hasten the onset of clinical response in TRD.

More recently, however, the results of the second level of the large, multicenter Sequenced Alternatives to Relieve Depression (STAR*D) trial reported no difference in remission rates among patients with citalopram-resistant depression who were subsequently randomized to receive either bupropion or buspirone augmentation (Trivedi *et al.*, 2006). In fact, adjunctive buspirone treatment was significantly less well tolerated than adjunctive bupropion (dropout rates due to intolerance were 12.5% versus 20.6%). Side effects reported with this treatment combination include somnolence, headache, nausea, and sweating. At the present time, only a single, open-label trial focuses on the use of the selective 5HT1A-agonist tandospirone as adjunctive treatment for SSRI/SNRI-resistant MDD (Sumiyoshi *et al.*, 2008). By the end of the four-week trial, 26.3% of 18 patients had remitted.

6.1.5 *Other antidepressants*

Studies focusing on augmentation of antidepressants with SSRIs for MDD are few. Small chart reviews and open-label trials report on the use of SSRI augmentation of citalopram (Bondolfi *et al.*, 1996 and 2000), and TCAs (Weilburg *et al.*, 1989). Interestingly enough, Maes *et al.* (1996) reported greater improvement in depressive symptoms over placebo among TRD patients during adjunctive treatment of trazodone with fluoxetine while Altamura *et al.* (2008a and b) suggest a greater resolution of depressive symptoms among patients with SSRI-resistant MDD who received augmentation with intravenous citalopram than placebo.

Augmentation with the selective norepinephrine and dopamine reuptake inhibitor (NDRI) bupropion has been reported as the most popular augmentation strategy for the treatment of MDD in one survey (Mischoulon *et al.*, 1999). However, until recently, supporting evidence has been limited to case reports (Clayton & Kaltsounis-Puckett, 2002; Fatemi *et al.*, 1999), retrospective chart reviews (Bodkin *et al.*, 1997; Papakostas *et al.*, 2006), and open-label trials (DeBattista *et al.*, 2003a; Eller *et al.*, 2009; Lam *et al.*, 2004; Maron *et al.*, 2009). As mentioned in the above section focusing on buspirone, the results of the second level of the large, multi-center, randomized clinical trial STAR*D reported no difference in remission rates among patients with citalopram-resistant depression who were subsequently randomized to receive either bupropion or buspirone augmentation (Trivedi *et al.*, 2006) (Fig. 6.4). However, adjunctive bupropion treatment was significantly better tolerated than adjunctive buspirone (dropout rates due to intolerance were 12.5% versus 20.6%). Double-blind, placebo-controlled studies focusing on

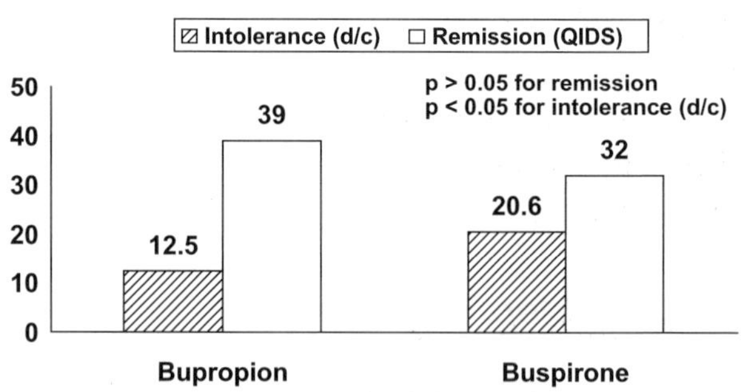

Fig. 6.4 STAR*D Level 2: Addition of bupropion versus buspirone to citalopram for TRD: A randomized study ($n = 565$). [Data extracted from: Trivedi, M.H., Fava, M., Wisniewski, S.R., *et al.* (2006). Medication augmentation after the failure of SSRIs for depression. *New England Journal of Medicine*, 354, 1243–1252.]

the use of adjunctive bupropion in TRD have yet to be published. However, at least one such study is under way (clinicaltrials.gov; NCT00296517). Side effects reported with this combination include headache, insomnia, dry mouth, nausea, anxiety, agitation, frequent urination, and constipation.

Numerous case reports/series (Lopez-Munoz *et al.*, 2006), and open-label trials (Hawley *et al.*, 2000; Jaracz *et al.*, 2004; Rapaport *et al.*, 2002; Rubio *et al.*, 2004; Tavormina *et al.*, 2002) involving a total of 225 MDD or bipolar depressed treatment-nonresponders who received reboxetine augmentation of the SSRIs (Devarjan & Dursun, 2000; Hawley *et al.*, 2000; Jaracz *et al.*, 2004; Lopez-Munoz *et al.*, 2007; Rapaport *et al.*, 2002; Rubio *et al.*, 2004; Tavormina *et al.*, 2002), or other agents including venlafaxine or mirtazapine (Lopez-Munoz *et al.*, 2006; Rubio *et al.*, 2004) have been published. These open-label studies report response rates ranging from 37.5–61%. Double-blind studies have yet to be reported. Side effects reported for this treatment combination include insomnia, nervousness, dry mouth, headaches, and restlessness.

For the norepinephrine-reuptake inhibitor atomoxetine, a single case-report (Berigan, 2004) and a small ($n = 15$), open-label trial (Carpenter *et al.*, 2005) have been published suggesting its potential utility when used as an adjunct treatment for TRD. Sixty percent of patients responded following adjunctive treatment with 40 mg of atomoxetine for a total of 8–10 weeks in the open-label trial. However, a subsequent, large ($n = 146$), double-blind, placebo-controlled trial of atomoxetine augmentation of sertraline for sertraline non-responders did not demonstrate any difference in efficacy between the two treatment groups (Michelson *et al.*, 2007). Side effects reported with this treatment include dry mouth, nervousness, insomnia, and constipation.

Only anecdotal evidence supports the use of the selective 5HT2 antagonist trazodone (Bertschy *et al.*, 2005; Nierenberg *et al.*, 1992; Zetin, 1984), and nefazodone (Taylor *et al.*, 2003), or the serotonin-norepinephrine reuptake inhibitor (SNRI) venlafaxine (Gomez Gomez & Teixido Perramon, 2000; Hornig-Rohan & Amsterdam, 2002) as augmentation strategies for antidepressant-resistant MDD.

There is only a single case series describing the use of the SNRIs milnacipran (Takahashi *et al.*, 2005), or duloxetine (Papakostas *et al.*, 2006) as an augmentation in patients with SSRI (Takahashi *et al.*, 2005) or bupropion- (Papakostas *et al.*, 2006) resistant depression.

Finally, periodically throughout the past few decades, case reports and small open trials have focused on the use of combining various monoamine oxidase inhibitors (MAOIs) with TCAs or carbamazepine in patients with TRD (Berlanga & Ortega-Soto, 1995; Hawley *et al.*, 1996; Ketter *et al.*, 1995; Konig & Westerford, 1997; Pestality *et al.*, 2003; Schmauss *et al.*, 1988). However, despite these reports and in light of the multitude of alternative augmentation options, the potential for serious adverse events such as hypertensive crises or serotonin syndrome has limited the use of this practice.

6.1.6 *Atypical antipsychotic agents*

Due to their unique receptor-affinity profile, the atypical antipsychotic agents have been subject to intense investigation as adjunctive therapies in TRD. Specifically, following a report by Ostroff and Nelson (1999) in which eight outpatients with SSRI-resistant MDD remitted within one week after the addition of low-dose risperidone, a number of case reports/series (Barbee *et al.*, 2004a & b; Detweiler & Trinkle, 2003; Fe-Bornstein *et al.*, 2002; Goforth & Carroll, 2007; Hellerstein, 2004; Hellerstein *et al.*, 2008; Jackson *et al.*, 2004; Kaplan, 2000; O'Connor & Silver, 1998; Pitchot & Ansseau, 2001; Sokolski, 2008; Sokolski & Brown, 2006; Stoll & Haura, 2000; Takahashi *et al.*, 2008; Viner *et al.*, 2003; Worthington *et al.*, 2005), and open-label trials (Adson *et al.*, 2004 and 2005; Anderson *et al.*, 2009; Beaune *et al.*, 2007; Bellino *et al.*, in press; Carta *et al.*, 2007; Corya *et al.*, 2003; Doree *et al.*, 2007; Dunner *et al.*, 2007; Levitt *et al.*, 2004; Mago *et al.*, 2004; Moeller *et al.*, 2004; Olver *et al.*, 2008; Pae *et al.*, 2007; Papakostas *et al.*, 2004 and 2005; Parker, 2002; Patkar *et al.*, 2006a; Rocca *et al.*, 2002; Sagud *et al.*, 2006; Sato *et al.*, 2009; Schwartz *et al.*, 2007; Sharpley *et al.*, 2005; Shelton & Addington, 2005; Simon & Nemeroff 2005; Takahaski *et al.*, in press; Tani *et al.*, 2004; Targum *et al.*, 2004; Zheng *et al.*, 2007) have focused on the use of the atypical antipsychotic agents clozapine, risperidone, olanzapine, ziprasidone, amisulpride, aripiprazole, perospirone, and quetiapine in TRD. Response rates for these open trials range from roughly 15–60%.

Until recently, a total of 10 randomized, double-blind, placebo-controlled trials had been conducted (Corya *et al.*, 2006; Keitner *et al.*, 2009; Khullar *et al.*, 2006; Mahmoud *et al.*, 2007; Mattingly *et al.*, 2006; McIntyre *et al.*, 2007; Shelton *et al.*, 2001 and 2005; Thase *et al.*, 2007) focusing on the use of either olanzapine, risperidone, or quetiapine in TRD (Table 6.3). A meta-analysis of these 10 trials suggested higher response (57.2% versus 35.4%), and remission rates (47.4%

Table 6.3 Double-blind studies of adjunct atypical antipsychotics in TRD.

Study	*n*	Atypical neuroleptic Duration	Antidepressant	Result[a]
Shelton *et al.*, 2001	28	Olanzapine 5–20 mg 8 weeks	Fluoxetine 20–60 mg	Olanzapine > Pbo
Shelton *et al.*, 2005	288	Olanzapine 6–12 mg 12 weeks	Fluoxetine 25–50 mg	Olanzapine = Pbo
Corya *et al.*, 2006	303	Olanzapine 1–12 mg 12 weeks	Fluoxetine 5–50 mg	Olanzapine = Pbo
Khullar *et al.*, 2006	15	Quetiapine 8 weeks	SSRI or SNRI	Quetiapine > Pbo
Mattingly *et al.*, 2006	40	Quetiapine 200–400 mg 8 weeks	SSRI or SNRI	Quetiapine > Pbo
Thase *et al.*, 2007 (study 1)	206	Olanzapine 6–18 mg 8 weeks	Fluoxetine 50 mg	Olanzapine = Pbo
Thase *et al.*, 2007 (study 2)	200	Olanzapine 6–18 mg 8 weeks	Fluoxetine 50 mg	Olanzapine > Pbo

(*Continued*)

Table 6.3 (*Continued*)

Study	*n*	Atypical neuroleptic Duration	Antidepressant	Result[a]
Mahmoud *et al.*, 2007	274	Risperidone 0.5–2 mg 6 weeks	Various	Risperidone > Pbo
McIntyre *et al.*, 2007	58	Quetiapine 50–600 mg 8 weeks	SSRI or SNRI	Quetiapine > Pbo
Berman *et al.*, 2007	362	Aripiprazole 2–20 mg 6 weeks	SSRI or SNRI	Aripiprazole > Pbo
Marcus *et al.*, 2008	381	Aripiprazole 2–20 mg 6 weeks	SSRI or SNRI	Aripiprazole > Pbo
El-Khalili *et al.*, 2008	446	Quetiapine 150 or 300 mg 6 weeks	SRI or SNRI	Quetiapine > Pbo (300 mg only)
Reeves *et al.*, 2008	24	Risperidone 0.25–2 mg 8 weeks	Various	Risperidone = Pbo
Berman *et al.*, 2009	349	Aripiprazole 2–20 mg 6 weeks	SSRI or SNRI	Aripiprazole > Pbo
Bauer *et al.*, 2009	493	Quetiapine 150 or 300 mg 6 weeks	SSRI or SNRI	Quetiapine > Pbo (150 mg and 300 mg)
Keitner *et al.*, 2009	97	Risperidone 0.5–3 mg 4 weeks	Various	Risperidone > Pbo

[a]Difference in mean change in Hamilton Depression Rating Scale or Montgomery–Asberg Depression Rating Scale scores during treatment except for Keitner *et al.* (difference in remission rates).

Abbreviations: SSRI = selective serotonin reuptake inhibitor, SNRI = serotonin-norepinephrine reuptake inhibitor, Pbo = placebo.

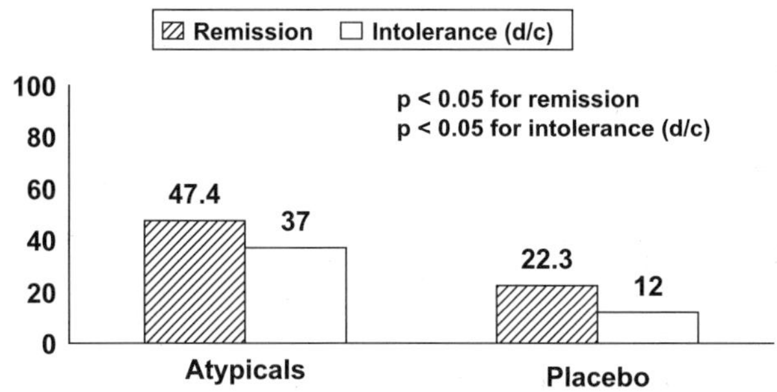

Fig. 6.5 Atypical antipsychotic augmentation for TRD: A meta-analysis of 10 RCTs* ($n = 1{,}500$). RCT: Randomized, controlled trial. [Data extracted from: Papakostas, G.I., Shelton, R.C., Smith, J., & Fava, M. (2007). Augmentation of antidepressants with atypical antipsychotic medications for treatment-resistant major depressive disorder: A meta-analysis. *Journal of Clinical Psychiatry*, 68, 826–831.]

versus 22.3%) among patients who received augmentation of antidepressants with an atypical antipsychotic than patients who continued on antidepressant monotherapy, although the rate of treatment discontinuation due to intolerance was nearly 3.5 times higher relative to placebo for patients treated with an atypical antipsychotic (Papakostas *et al.*, 2007) (Fig. 6.5).

More recently, the results of three double-blind, placebo-controlled trial also support the use of aripiprazole as an augmentation for SSRI-resistant MDD (Berman *et al.*, 2007 and 2009; Marcus *et al.*, 2008) (Fig. 6.6).

The results of a small ($n = 24$), pilot study also report a greater resolution of suicidal ideation (but not depressive symptoms according to the primary outcome measure) among patients with antidepressant-resistant MDD (Reeves *et al.*, 2008).

Finally, the results of two identical, large, randomized, double-blind, placebo-controlled studies focusing on the use of quetiapine augmentation of antidepressants for TRD also confirm the results of earlier studies of much smaller sample sizes (Bauer *et al.*, 2009; El-Khalili *et al.*, 2008) (Fig. 6.7). A recent metal-analysis pooling all 16 trials reported remission rates of 30.7% versus 17.2% in favor of treatment with adjunctive atypicals (Nelson & Papakostas, 2009).

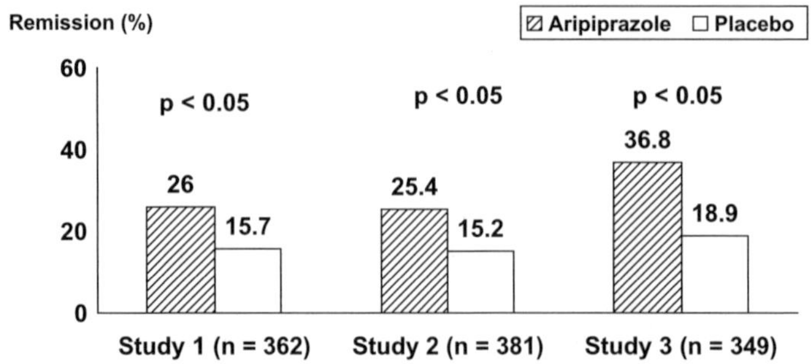

Fig. 6.6 Aripiprazole augmentation in TRD: Results of three randomized, double-blind, placebo-controlled trials. [Study 1: Berman, R.M., Marcus, R.N., Swanink, R., *et al.* (2007). The efficacy of aripiprazole as adjunctive therapy in major depressive disorder: A multicenter, randomized, double-blind, placebo-controlled study. *Journal of Clinical Psychiatry*, 68(6), 843–853. Study 2: Marcus, R.N., McQuade, R.D., Carson, W.H., *et al.* (2008). The efficacy and safety of aripiprazole as adjunctive therapy in major depressive disorder: A second multicenter, randomized, double-blind, placebo-controlled Study. *Journal of Clinical Psychopharmacol*, 28(2), 156–165. Study 3: Berman, R.M., Fava, M., Thase, M.E., *et al.* (2009). Aripiprazole augmentation in major depressive disorder. *CNS Spectrums*, 14(4), 197–206.]

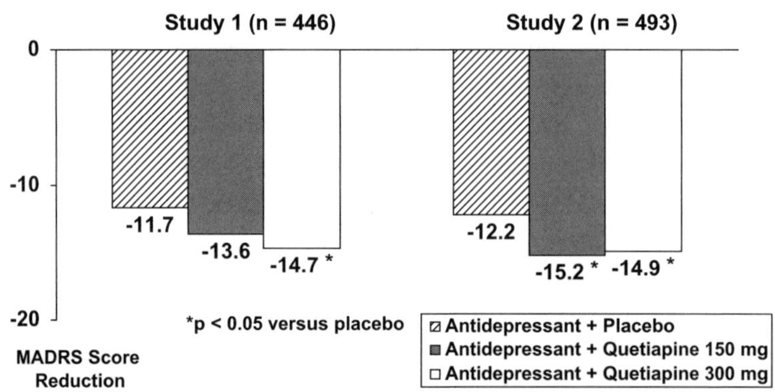

Fig. 6.7 Quetiapine augmentation in TRD: Results of two randomized, double-blind, placebo-controlled trials. MADRS: Montgomery-Asberg Depression Rating Scale. [Study 1: El-Khalili, N., Joyce, M., Atkinson, S., *et al.* (2008). Adjunctive extended release quetiapine fumarate (quetiapine XR) in patients with major depressive disorder and inadequate response. American Psychiatric Association Annual Meeting. Study 2: Bauer, M., Pretorius, H.W., Constant, E.L., *et al.* (2009). Extended release quetiapine as adjunct to an antidepressant in patients with major depressive disorder: Results of a randomized, placebo-controlled, double-blind study. *Journal of Clinical Psychiatry*, 70(4), 540–549.]

Side effects with this combination can vary from agent to agent, but may include sedation, fatigue, insomnia, somnolence, nausea, hyperprolactinemia, dyslipidemia, glucose dysregulation, weight gain, and extrapyramidal side effects including akathisia, restlessness, dystonic reactions, Parkinsonism, neuroleptic malignant syndrome, and tardive dyskinesia.

6.1.7 *Dopaminergic agents*

Several case reports (Bader *et al.*, 1998; Buhagiar & Cassar, 2007; Linet, 1989; Sekine *et al.*, 2000), and case series (Fawcett *et al.*, 1991; Feinberg, 2004; Masand *et al.*, 1998; Sovner, 1990) report on the use of adjunctive methylphenidate for SSRI- (Buhagiar & Cassar, 2007; Linet, 1989; Masand *et al.*, 1998), venlafaxine- (Bader *et al.*, 1998; Masand *et al.*, 1998), mianserin- (Sekine *et al.*, 2000), or MAOI- (Fawcett *et al.*, 1991; Feinberg, 2004; Sovner, 1990) resistant depression. However, while small open label-trials report on the use of methylphenidate augmentation in MAOI-, TCA- (Feighner *et al.*, 1985) or SSRI-resistant MDD (Rabkin *et al.*, 1994; Stoll *et al.*, 1996), the results of two double-blind, placebo-controlled trials of methylphenidate augmentation of standard antidepressants in TRD did not show greater resolution of depressive symptoms for the methylphenidate- than placebo-treated groups (Patkar *et al.*, 2006b; Ravindran *et al.*, 2008) (Fig. 6.8). The long acting methylphenidate formulation (Concerta) was used in both double-blind studies. Side effects reported when combining psychostimulants with antidepressants can include headache, insomnia, nausea, anxiety, and loss of appetite. Psychostimulants also carry a risk of physiological/psychological dependence and/or abuse.

Pramipexole and ropinirole are selective dopamine D2- and D3-receptor agonists. Although pramipexole appears to be effective as an adjunct (Goldberg *et al.*, 2004; Zarate *et al.*, 2004) for bipolar depression, only anecdotal evidence exists suggesting the potential utility of pramipexole and ropinirole as adjuncts in unipolar TRD (Cassano *et al.*, 2004 and 2005; Gupta *et al.*, 2006; Lattanzi *et al.*, 2002; Sporn *et al.*, 2000). Finally, case reports or open-label

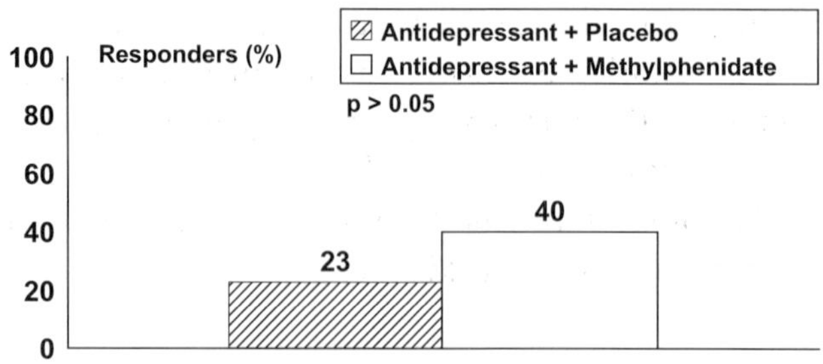

Fig. 6.8 Methylphenidate augmentation for TRD: A randomized, double-blind study ($n = 60$). [Data extracted from: Patkar, A.A., Masand, P.S., Pae, C.U., *et al.* (2006). A randomized, double-blind, placebo-controlled trial of augmentation with an extended release formulation of methylphenidate in outpatients with treatment-resistant depression. *Journal of Clinical Psychopharmacology*, 26, 653–656.]

trials of augmentation with various dopaminergic agents including bromocriptine (Inoue *et al.*, 1996), pergolide (Bouckoms & Mangini, 1993; Izumi *et al.*, 2000), and cabergoline (Shingo *et al.*, 2004; Takahashi *et al.*, 2003) in TRD have yet to be followed by controlled investigations. Side effects commonly reported during combined treatment with antidepressants and dopamine receptor agonists include headache, nausea, loss of appetite, and insomnia. A randomized, double-blind, placebo-controlled trial of pramipexole augmentation of SSRIs for SSRI-resistant MDD is currently under way (clinicaltrials.gov; NCT00231959).

6.1.8 *Other monoaminergic agents*

Case reports (Pollack & Hammerness, 1993), and uncontrolled clinical trials (Cappiello *et al.*, 1995; Schmauss *et al.*, 1988) provide mixed results for augmentation of antidepressants with the α-2 selective noradrenergic receptor *antagonist* yohimbine for TRD. However, the results of a double-blind, placebo-controlled trial do not support the efficacy of augmenting TCAs (Charney *et al.*, 1986) with yohimbine for TCA-resistant MDD.

Similarly, there is a single, negative, double-blind placebo-controlled trial of thioridazine augmentation of moclobemide for

TRD (Stabl *et al.*, 1995). Finally, the results of open-label trials do not support the use of the serotonergic agent fenfluramine (Price *et al.*, 1990), or reserpine (Price *et al.*, 1987), a naturally derived product with amine-depleting effects, as augmentation for TCA-resistant MDD.

6.2 Adjunctive Treatment with Neuroendocrine Agents

6.2.1 *Thyroid hormones*

Antidepressant effects for triiodothyronine (T3) were first reported in 1958 (Feldmesser-Reiss; 1958; Flach *et al.*, 1958). Ever since, a number of case studies (Berigan & Zeff, 2000; Browne *et al.*, 1990a; Cooke, 1990; Cooke *et al.*, 1992; Joffe, 1988 and 1992; Kan & Ho, 2001), and open-label trials (Abraham *et al.*, 2006; Agid & Lerer, 2003; Banki, 1977; Birkenhager *et al.*, 1997; Earle, 1970; Goodwin *et al.*, 1982; Iosifescu *et al.*, 2005; Kelly & Lieberman, 2009; Schwarcz *et al.*, 1984; Targum *et al.*, 1984; Thase *et al.*, 1989a; Tsutsui *et al.*, 1979) have been published reporting on the treatment of depressive disorders with the use of adjunctive T3. In addition to MDD, some of these trials also involved mixed depressed populations, including patients with psychotic features (Birkenhager *et al.*, 1997), or bipolar depression (Banki, 1977; Goodwin *et al.*, 1982). The majority of these open trials report on the augmentation of TCAs with T3 in TCA-resistant patients (Early, 1970; Banki, 1977; Birkenhager *et al.*, 1997; Goodwin *et al.*, 1982; Iosifescu *et al.*, 2005; Schwarcz *et al.*, 1984; Targum *et al.*, 1984; Thase *et al.*, 1989; Tsutsui *et al.*, 1979). One case report focuses on the use of T3 augmentation of trazodone (Browne *et al.*, 1990a), one on the use of T3 augmentation of mirtazapine (Berigan & Zeff, 2000), and one on the use of T3 augmentation of phenelzine (Joffe *et al.*, 1988), while two case series (Cook *et al.*, 1992; Joffe *et al.*, 1992), and two open trials ($n = 45$) report on the use of adjunctive T3 (25–50 mcg) in SSRI-resistant MDD (Agid & Lerer, 2003; Iosifescu *et al.*, 2005). Doses used in these studies range from 10 mcg to 50 mcg, with treatment durations of two to four weeks.

Table 6.4 Double-blind, randomized studies of adjunct T3 in TRD.

Study	*n*	T3 dose Duration	Agent Augmented	Result[a]
Coppen *et al.*, 1972	17	25 mcg 2 weeks	Imipramine[b]	T3 > Pbo
Steiner *et al.*, 1978	12	25 mcg 5 weeks	Imipramine	T3 = Pbo
Gitlin *et al.*, 1987	16	25 mcg 2 × 2 weeks[b]	Desipramine	T3 = Pbo
Joffe *et al.*, 1993	50	37.5 mcg 2 weeks	Desipramine or Imipramine	T3 > Pbo
Joffe *et al.*, 2006	36	37.5 mg 2 weeks	Several[c]	T3 = Pbo

[a]Greater decrease in Hamilton Depression Rating Scale Scores than placebo during treatment.
[b]Cross-over design.
[c]Either sertraline, venlafaxine, or bupropion.
Abbreviation: Pbo = placebo.

Response rates range, roughly, from 25% to 65% (with the exception of one study that reports a 0% response rate — Birkenhager *et al.*, 1997).

To date, four double-blind, placebo-controlled studies of T3 augmentation of TCAs in TCA-resistant depression have been published (Coppen *et al.*, 1972; Gitlin *et al.*, 1987; Joffe *et al.*, 1993; Steiner *et al.*, 1978). Details for these double-blind trials are reported in Table 6.4. In summary, both TCA studies of two-weeks duration report greater decrease in depression severity in the T3 than the placebo group (Coppen *et al.*, 1972; Joffe *et al.*, 1993). However, this was not replicated in both studies of longer duration (Gitlin *et al.*, 1987; Steiner *et al.*, 1978). A meta-analysis of randomized, placebo-controlled trials of T3 for TRD revealed a modest, non-statistically significant difference in efficacy between T3 and placebo (risk ratio 1.53, 95%CI: 0.7–3.35) (Aronson *et al.*, 1996).

A subsequent trial comparing lithium with T3 and placebo augmentation of antidepressants (including the SSRIs) did not report any difference in the degree of resolution of depressive symptoms between the three treatment groups (Joffe *et al.*, 2006). More recently, the results of the third level of STAR*D did not report any statistical difference in efficacy between T3 and lithium augmentation of antidepressants (sertraline, venlafaxine, or bupropion) for TRD ($n = 142$), although numerically greater remission rates were reported among T3 than lithium-treated patients (24.7% versus 15.9%), while T3 augmentation was significantly better tolerated (fewer participants in the T3 group left treatment because of side effects — 23.2% versus 9.6%) (Nierenberg *et al.*, 2006) (Fig. 6.9). Reported side effects include palpitation, sweating, tremor, nausea, headache, somnolence, insomnia, and dry mouth.

Open trials suggest the potential utility of thyroxine (T4) as an adjunct in TRD (Bauer *et al.*, 1998 and 2002; Lojko & Rybakowski, 2007; Rudas *et al.*, 1999). However, the results of a double-blind study ($n = 40$) report T3 (37.5 mcg) to be superior to T4 (150 mcg) as an adjunct to TCAs in TCA-resistant MDD (Joffe & Singer, 1990). Finally,

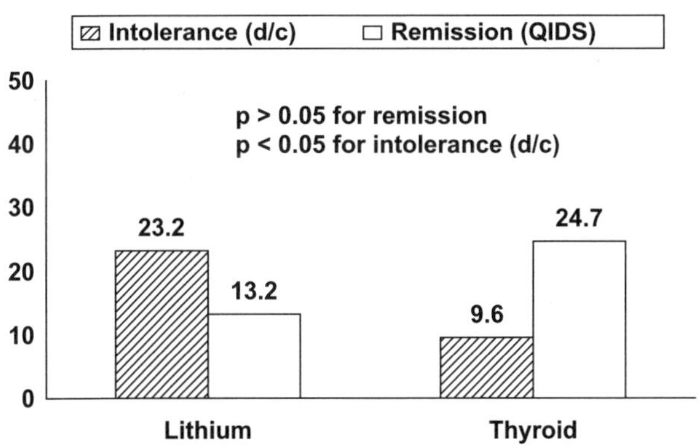

Fig. 6.9 STAR*D Level 3: Lithium versus T3 augmentation for TRD: A randomized study ($n = 142$). [Data extracted from: Nierenberg, A.A., Fava, M., Trivedi, M.H., *et al.* (2006). A comparison of lithium and T(3) augmentation following two failed medication treatments for depression: A STAR*D report. *American Journal of Psychiatry*, 163, 1519–1530.]

there is a negative double-blind, placebo-controlled augmentation study of one-week duration involving the use of intravenous thyrotropin-releasing hormone for TRD (Mountjoy *et al.*, 1974).

6.2.2 *Androgens*

Studies have also explored the potential utility of adjunctive testosterone therapy in TRD. Seidman and Rabkin (1998) reported that four of five hypogonadal outpatients with SSRI-resistant MDD remitted after receiving open-label testosterone for a total of eight weeks (400 mg intramuscular every two weeks). In a subsequent, double-blind study, 22 hypogonadal men with TRD received either adjunct testosterone (10 g of 1% testosterone gel daily) or placebo for eight weeks (Pope *et al.*, 2003) (Fig. 6.10). A greater reduction in depressive symptoms was reported in the testosterone than placebo group. However, more recently, a somewhat smaller ($n = 12$) double-blind, placebo-controlled study of testosterone gel (1%) augmentation for TRD did not show greater efficacy for testosterone than placebo (Orengo *et al.*, 2005).

A larger randomized, double-blind, placebo-controlled study is under way (NCT00304746). Potential disadvantages of this

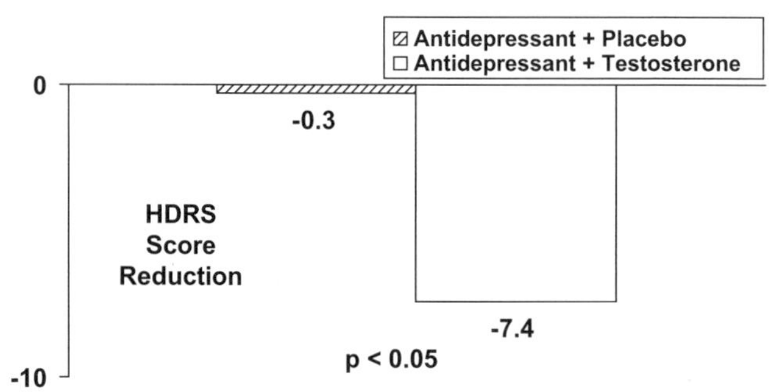

Fig. 6.10 Testosterone augmentation in men with TRD: A randomized, double-blind study ($n = 22$). HDRS: Hamilton Depression Rating Scale. [Data extracted from: Pope, H.G. Jr., Cohane, G.H., Kanayama, G., *et al.* (2003). Testosterone gel supplementation for men with refractory depression: A randomized, placebo-controlled trial. *American Journal of Psychiatry*, 160, 105–111.]

treatment strategy include hirsutism (among women), dysuria, prostatic hypertrophy and erythrocytosis.

6.2.3 *Estrogens*

A number of case reports and small, open-label trials suggest the potential utility of estrogen augmentation in TRD (Berlanga, 1988; Clayton & Kaltsounis-Puckett, 2002; Morgan *et al.*, 2007; Rasgon *et al.*, 2002). To date, two double-blind, placebo-controlled trials of estrogen augmentation for women with TRD have been published. The first study focuses on the use of estrogen for pre- and post-menopausal women with TRD (TCA-resistant) (Shapira *et al.*, 1985; Zohar *et al.*, 1985). This study did not reveal any difference in efficacy between estrogen and placebo. A second study, however, revealed greater resolution of depressive symptoms among perimenopausal women with TRD randomized to receive treatment with adjunctive estrogen than placebo (Morgan *et al.*, 2005). Side effects reported during treatment with this combination include headache, constipation, somnolence, sweating, and nausea.

The results of double-blind, placebo-controlled trial examining the adjunctive use of the selective estrogen receptor modulator raloxifene for TRD did not reveal any difference in antidepressant efficacy between the two treatment groups (Grigoriadis *et al.*, 2005).

6.2.4 *Steroids and steroid synthesis inhibitors*

Only two studies have examined the use of steroids as adjuncts for the treatment of depression. A response rate of 66.6% after four weeks of open-label treatment with adjunctive (to SSRIs) prednisone (7.5 mg daily) was reported in a small ($n = 6$) trial of outpatients with MDD resistant to a numerous- (anywhere from 3 to 13) antidepressant trials (Bouwer *et al.*, 2000). Similarly, Dinan *et al.* (1997) reported a 60% response rate at three weeks among 10 outpatients with SSRI-resistant MDD who received adjunct oral dexamethasone (3 mg $\times$ 4 days). Side effects reported with this treatment combination include nausea, insomnia, and anxiety.

The results of a small ($n = 6$) open-label study of augmentation of imipramine with the steroid synthesis inhibitor metyrapone for imipramine-resistant depression suggest a significant reduction in depressive symptoms following metyrapone augmentation (Rogoz *et al.*, 2004a). Double-blind adjunctive studies of steroids or steroid-synthesis inhibitors for TRD have yet to be published.

6.2.5 *Melatonin*

Dalton *et al.* (2000) studied nine outpatients with TRD who received open-label adjunct treatment (to a number of antidepressants including SSRIs, TCAs, venlafaxine and MAOIs) with melatonin for eight weeks (5 mg sustained release). Although there were no responders in that study, four patients experienced a 50% or more reduction in the sum of HAMD item No. 3, 4, 5 scores (early, middle, and late insomnia).

6.3 Other Agents

6.3.1 *Lithium*

The observation by De Montigny and colleagues (1981) of rapid (within 48 hours) relief of depressive symptoms among eight inpatients with MDD who had not experienced significant symptom improvement following a trial of tricyclic antidepressants sparked considerable interest in the further study of this promising treatment strategy over nearly two decades.

Specifically, numerous case reports/series and open-label trials involving over 200 patients report on the augmentation of TCAs with lithium for TRD (Birkenhager *et al.*, 2006; Dallal *et al.*, 1990; DeMontigny *et al.*, 1981, 1983 and 1985; Dinan, 1993; Finch & Katona, 1989; Flint & Rifat, 1994 and 1996; Fontaine *et al.*, 1991; Garbutt *et al.*, 1986; Kushnir, 1986; Lafferman *et al.*, 1988; Louie & Meltzer, 1984; Price *et al.*, 1986; Schrader & Levien, 1985; Sluzewska *et al.*, 1997; Thase *et al.*, 1989b; van Marwijk *et al.*, 1990; Zimmer *et al.*, 1991). 10 of these (Flint & Rifat, 1994 and 1996; Fontaine *et al.*, 1991; Kushnir, 1986; Lafferman *et al.*, 1988; Louie & Meltzer, 1984; Price *et al.*, 1986; Sluzewska *et al.*, 1997; van Marwijk *et al.*, 1990; Zimmer *et al.*, 1991) also report on lithium augmentation of other agents as well (SSRIs mostly but also MAOIs, bupropion, mianserin, trazodone). Response rates in open-label trials range from 24% to 100%.

In addition, several case reports/series (Camprubi & Puri, 1995; Howland, 1991; Manning & Connor, 1994) and several open-label trials involving over 100 patients report on the augmentation of SSRIs with lithium (Delgado *et al.*, 1988; Dinan, 1993; Flint & Rifat, 1994 and 1996; Fontaine *et al.*, 1991; Hawley *et al.*, 1994; Kok *et al.*, 2007; Price *et al.*, 1986; Schindler & Anghelescu, 2007; Sluzewska *et al.*, 1997; Whyte *et al.*, 2004). The duration of augmentation for these studies varies from 1 to 14 weeks. Response rates for open-label studies range from 26% to 60%.

There are, however, relatively fewer studies examining the use of lithium as an adjunct to antidepressants other than TCAs and SSRIs. As mentioned in above paragraphs, some studies also involved a considerable number of patients who had lithium added to other agents such as mianserin, trazodone, bupropion, adinazolam, or MAOIs. For studies in which separate outcomes for lithium augmentation of MAOIs are reported, there is only a small case series involving three patients (Nelson & Byck, 1982), and an open-label trial for older (60 years of age or more) MDD patients in which 53.6% of patients responded (Flint & Rifat, 1996). A case report (Zullino *et al.*, 2001), and two open-label trials of lithium augmentation for venlafaxine-resistant MDD have been published (Bertschy *et al.*, 2003; Hoencamp *et al.*, 2000). Approximately 32–39% of patients in these open-label trials responded following adjunctive treatment with lithium for four to six weeks. Finally, two case reports/series of lithium augmentation for trazodone-resistant depression have been published to date (Kushnir, 1986; Lafferman *et al.*, 1988).

There have been 10 double-blind studies of lithium augmentation of TCAs for TRD published to date (Browne M *et al.*, 1990b; Dinan & Bary, 1989; Heninger *et al.*, 1983; Hoencamp *et al.*, 1994; Joffe *et al.*, 1993; Kantor *et al.*, 1986; Nierenberg *et al.*, 2003; Schopf *et al.*, 1989; Stein & Bernadt, 1993; Zusky *et al.*, 1988) (Fig. 6.11).

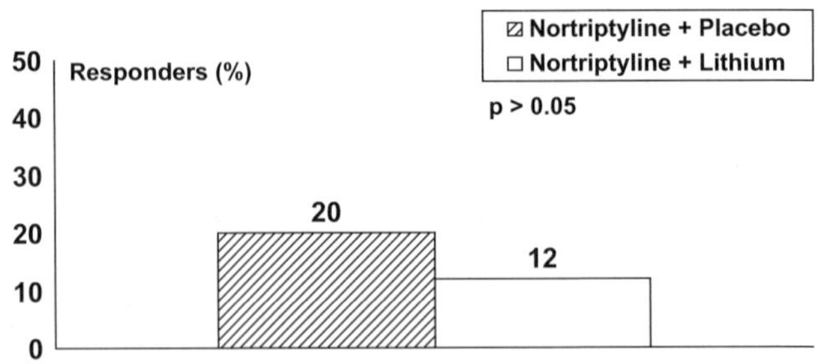

Fig. 6.11 Lithium augmentation of nortriptyline for TRD: A randomized, double-blind study ($n = 35$). [Data extracted from: Nierenberg, A.A., Papakostas, G.I., Petersen, T., *et al.* (2003). Lithium augmentation of nortriptyline for subjects resistant to multiple antidepressants. *Journal of Clinical Psychopharmacology*, 23, 92–95.]

All but two of these studies involve adjunctive placebo as a comparator. Dinan and Bary (1989) compared lithium augmentation of TCAs with ECT, while Hoencamp *et al.* (1994) compared lithium augmentation of TCAs with an MAOI (brofaromine). The study by Joffe *et al.* (1993) involved a placebo as well as an active comparator (triiodothyronine — T3). Details of these clinical trials are reported in Table 6.5. In summary, lithium was found to be more effective than placebo at week 1 in one study of one-week duration (Schopf *et al.*, 1989), and one study of three weeks duration (Dinan & Bary, 1989), and more effective than placebo at week 2 in two studies of two-weeks duration (Heninger *et al.*, 1983; Joffe *et al.*, 1993). In the study by Dinan and Bary (1989), lithium augmentation was not found to be more effective than ECT at endpoint (week 3). In the remaining five studies, lithium was not found to be more effective than placebo or active comparator at any given time point. The mean lithium level for studies showing greater efficacy for lithium at week 1 or 2 versus the remaining studies was 0.59 mEq/L versus 0.64 mEq/L, respectively.

Five double-blind studies of lithium augmentation of SSRIs have been published to date (Baumann *et al.*, 1995; Fava *et al.*, 1994 and 2002; Joffe *et al.*, 2006; Katona *et al.*, 1995). Two of these studies (Fava *et al.*, 1994 and 2002) involved the use of an active comparator rather

Table 6.5 Double-blind studies of adjunct Li in TRD.

Study	*n*	Li level (mean)	Antidepressant and Trial Duration	Result[a]
Augmentation of TCAs				
Heninger *et al.*, 1983	21	N/A	TCAs 2 weeks	Li > Pbo
Kantor *et al.*, 1986	7	N/A	TCAs 2 days	Li = Pbo
Zusky *et al.*, 1988	16	0.6 mEq/L	TCAs 3 weeks	Li = Pbo
Schopf *et al.*, 1989	27	0.5 mEq/L	TCAs 1 week	Li > Pbo
Dinan & Barry, 1989	30	N/A	TCAs 3 weeks	TCA + Li > ECT[c] week 1 but not week 3
Browne *et al.*, 1990b	17	N/A	TCAs 2 days	Li = Pbo
Stein & Bern, 1993	34	N/A	TCAs 3 weeks	Li = Pbo
Joffe *et al.*, 1993	50	0.68 mEq/L	TCAs 2 weeks	Li > Pbo
Hoencamp *et al.*, 1994	51	0.69 mEq/L	Mapritilline 6 weeks	Maprotiline + Li = Brofaromine[c]
Nierenberg *et al.*, 2003	35	0.62 mEq/L	Nortriptyline 6 weeks	Li = Pbo
Augmentation of SSRIs				
Fava *et al.*, 1994	41	0.21 mEq/L	Fluoxetine 20 mg 4 weeks	Fluoxetine 40–60 mg > Li[b]
Katona *et al.*, 1995	62	N/A	SSRIs or Lofepramine 6 weeks	Li = Pbo
Baumann *et al.*, 1996	24	0.75 mEq/L	SSRIs 1 week	Li > Pbo
Fava *et al.*, 2002	101	0.37 mEq/L	Fluoxetine 20 mg 4 weeks	Fluoxetine 40–60 mg > Li[b]

(*Continued*)

Table 6.5 *(Continued)*

Study	*n*	Li level (mean)	Antidepressant and Trial Duration	Result[a]
Augmentation of Agents from Multiple Antidepressant Classes				
Joffe *et al.*, 2006	36	N/A	2 weeks	Li = Pbo

[a]All outcomes represent difference in the change in Hamilton Depression Rating Scale scores.
[b]Fluoxetine dose-increase (40–60 mg/day) versus fluoxetine (20 mg) plus lithium.
[c]ECT (Dinan *et al.*), or brofaromine (Hoencamp *et al.*) as active comparator. No placebo.
Abbreviations: TCA = tricyclic antidepressant, ECT = electroconvulsive therapy, Pbo = placebo, N/A = Information not available.

than placebo (fluoxetine dose-increase versus lithium augmentation of fluoxetine versus desipramine augmentation of fluoxetine in outpatients with fluoxetine-resistant MDD), while the remaining involved placebo as a comparator. One study involved lofepramine in addition to fluoxetine as an augmented agent (Katona *et al.*, 1995). Details of these clinical trials are reported in Table 6.5. In summary, lithium was found to be more effective than placebo at week 1 in only one study (Baumann *et al.*, 1996). In the remaining three studies, lithium was not found to be more effective than placebo or an active comparator at any given time point.

More recently, Joffe *et al.* (2006) compared lithium with T3 and placebo augmentation of antidepressants (including but not limited to the SSRIs), and did not report any difference in the degree of resolution of depressive symptoms between the three treatment groups (Joffe *et al.*, 2006). Similarly, the results of the third level of STAR*D did not report any statistical difference in efficacy between T3 and lithium augmentation of antidepressants (sertraline, venlafaxine, or bupropion) for TRD ($n = 142$), although numerically lower remission rates were reported among lithium (15.9%) than T3-treated patients (24.7%), while lithium augmentation was also significantly less-well tolerated. (more participants in the lithium group left treatment because of side effects — 23.2% versus 9.6%) (Nierenberg *et al.*, 2006).

An older meta-analysis of placebo-controlled studies (Bauer & Dopfmer, 1999) had concluded that lithium was more effective than placebo as an adjunct in TRD (odds ratio 2.14, 95%CI: 1.23–3.70). However, no distinction was made in either of two analyses between studies of two-weeks duration and studies of longer duration. This is of great relevance, since advantages of lithium augmentation over placebo in TRD have not been demonstrated past two weeks of treatment in any individual trial (see Table 6.5 for details). A more recent meta-analysis by Bauer *et al.* (2003) also does not make a distinction between studies of short versus adequate duration. In addition, a relapse prevention trial involving the use of adjunctive lithium is included in the analysis along with studies focusing on the acute-phase of treatment with adjunctive lithium (Bauer *et al.*, 2000). Thus, the sum of the evidence presented here does not provide conclusive evidence in support of the use of lithium as an augmentation for TRD. Potential side effects during treatment with adjunctive lithium may include tremor, somnolence, sedation, nausea, anorexia, abdominal pain, diarrhea, polyuria (via antagonism of antidiuretic hormone), edema, rash (including acne and psoriasis), leukocytosis, hypothyroidism, hyperthyroidism, ataxia, weight gain, renal insufficiency, electrocardiographic changes, arrhythmias, cardiac conduction abnormalities and, in rare cases, development of the nephritic syndrome. The use of lithium early during pregnancy is also associated with an increased risk of major birth defects.

6.3.2 *ω-3 fatty acids*

To date, three double-blind studies have been published. A double-blind study involving 20 MDD outpatients resistant to SSRIs ($n = 17$), mirtazapine ($n = 2$), or moclobemide ($n = 1$) randomized to treatment with adjunctive omega-3 fatty acid (ethyl-eicosapentaenoic acid or E-EPA, 2 g daily) versus placebo for four weeks revealed greater decreases in depression severity at weeks 2, 3 and 4 (endpoint) in the E-EPA than placebo group (Nemets

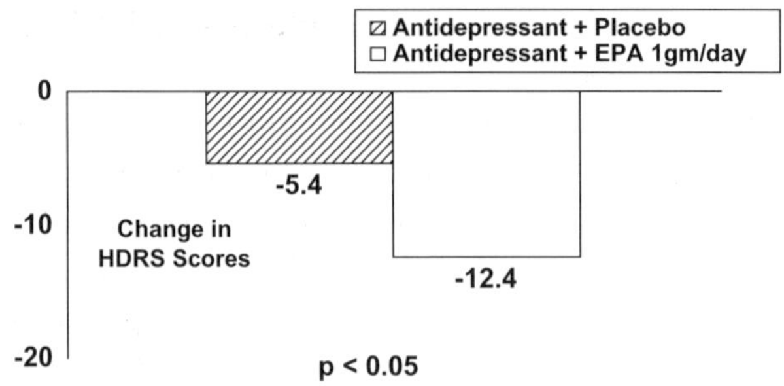

Fig. 6.12 Omega-3 fatty acid (EPA) augmentation for TRD: A randomized, double-blind study ($n = 35$). HDRS: Hamilton Depression Rating Scale. [Data extracted from: Peet, M., & Horrobin, D.F. (2002). A dose-ranging study of the effects of ethyl-eicosapentaenoate in patients with ongoing depression despite apparently adequate treatment with standard drugs. *Archives of General Psychiatry*, 59, 913–919.]

et al., 2002). Similarly, Peet and Horrobin (2002) reported greater improvement in depressive symptoms among TRD patients who received augmentation with 1 g/daily of ethyl-EPA than placebo (Fig. 6.12). However, no difference in outcome between placebo-treated patients and patients treated with 2 or 4 g/daily of ethyl-EPA was reported in that study. Finally, Su *et al.* (2003) reported greater improvements in depressive symptoms following eight weeks of adjunctive treatment with an ω-3 fatty acid combination (440 mg EPA plus 220 mg docosahexanoic-DHA acid) than placebo in TRD. Although a promising strategy, the relationship between ω-3 type (EPA versus DHA), dose and efficacy is not well understood.

6.3.3 *Modafinil*

Case reports/series (Berigan, 2001; Even *et al.*, 2004; Holder *et al.*, 2002; Keller-Ashton, 2004; Menza *et al.*, 2000; Nasr, 2004; Price *et al.*, 2005; Schwartz *et al.*, 2002; Xiong *et al.*, 2005), and open-label trials (De Battista *et al.*, 2004; Lundt, 2004; Markovitz & Wagner, 2003; Rasmussen *et al.*, 2005; Schwartz *et al.*, 2004; Thase *et al.*, 2006) have suggested the potential utility of modafinil augmentation for the treatment of MDD outpatients who experienced insufficient improvement and residual fatigue and hypersomnia following treatment with various antidepressants. However, double-blind, placebo-controlled studies present equivocal results. DeBattista *et al.* (2003b) studied 136 MDD outpatients with incomplete response to antidepressants who were also experiencing significant fatigue and/or hypersomnia who were randomized to receive therapy with adjunctive modafinil (100–400 mg) versus placebo for a total of six weeks. Overall, there was no difference between the two treatment groups at endpoint in terms of the change in depressive symptoms, global improvement, hypersomnia or fatigue. However, significantly greater improvement in hypersomnia and fatigue early-on (week 1–2) in modafinil than placebo-treated patients was reported.

Fava *et al.* (2005) studied 311 MDD outpatients with an incomplete response to an SSRI who were also experiencing significant fatigue and hypersomnia who were then randomized to receive modafinil augmentation (200 mg) versus placebo for eight weeks. Greater global improvement was reported at endpoint among modafinil than placebo-treated patients. There were no significant differences in reduction of depressive symptoms, hypersomnia or fatigue between the two groups. However, there was a greater reduction in depressive symptoms and hypersomnia in modafinil than placebo-treated patients who had a significant burden of depressive symptoms at baseline (at least moderate depression). More recently, a post-hoc analysis (Fava *et al.*, 2007) was conducted on a pooled dataset combining both randomized, double-blind, modafinil augmentation studies (DeBattista *et al.*, 2003b; Fava *et al.*, 2005). In that analysis, greater antidepressant efficacy for modafinil than placebo-augmentation of antidepressants for TRD was confirmed as well as greater efficacy in resolving somnolence but not fatigue (Fig. 6.13). A randomized, double-blind, placebo-controlled trial also demonstrated greater antidepressant effects among bipolar disorder patients experiencing a major depressive episode treated with adjunctive modafinil than placebo (Frye *et al.*, 2007).

Side effects reported during modafinil augmentation of antidepressants include headache, nervousness, irritability, nausea, insomnia, diarrhea, dizziness, and dry mouth.

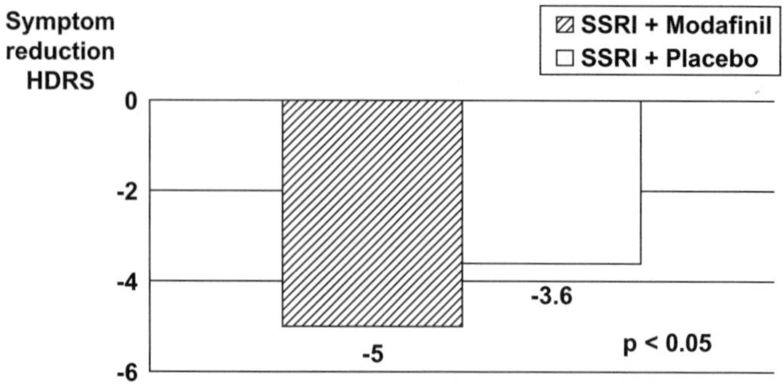

Fig. 6.13 Modafinil augmentation of SSRIs for TRD: A pooled-analysis of two clinical trials ($n = 348$). HDRS: Hamilton Depression Rating Scale. [Data extracted from: Fava, M., Thase, M.E., DeBattista, C., *et al.* (2007). Modafinil augmentation of selective serotonin reuptake inhibitor therapy in MDD partial responders with persistent fatigue and sleepiness. *Annals of Clinical Psychiatry*, 19(3), 153–159.]

6.3.4 *Glutamatergic agents*

Only case series and small open-label trials report on the use of adjunctive amantadine, a non-competitive N-methyl-D-aspartate (NMDA) receptor antagonist, in mixed MDD and bipolar depressed populations with TRD (Dietrich *et al.*, 2000; Rogoz *et al.*, 2004b; Stryjer *et al.*, 2003).

Similarly, there is only anecdotal evidence to support the use of the glutamate-modulating agent riluzole as adjunctive therapy in MDD (Sanacora *et al.*, 2007). More recently, however, Zarate *et al.* (2006) demonstrated a greater resolution of depressive symptoms over placebo in patients with TRD beginning approximately two hours after a single intravenous infusion of the NMDA-receptor antagonist ketamine; effects which, in many cases, lasted up to one week (Fig. 6.14). The main limitation of this treatment strategy involves the potential for uncomfortable cognitive side effects (mild hallucinations, temporary disorientation, concentration difficulties). In light of this pivotal work, studies examining whether such effects can be reproduced with the use of more tolerable NMDA-receptor antagonists, and whether such effects can be sustained for longer periods of time are warranted. However, it should also be noted

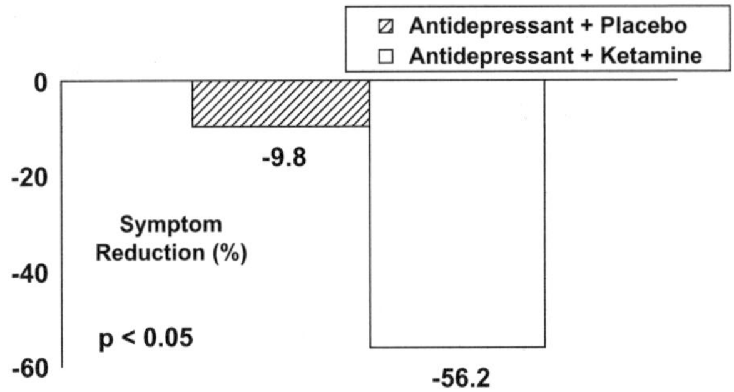

Fig. 6.14 A randomized, double-blind study of intravenous ketamine (Augmentation) for TRD: Antidepressant effects the following day ($n = 18$). [Data extracted from: Zarate, C.A. Jr., Singh, J.B., Carlson, P.J., *et al.* (2006). A randomized trial of an N-methyl-D-aspartate antagonist in treatment-resistant major depression. *Archives of General Psychiatry*, 63, 856–864.]

that a possibly underpowered ($n = 30$), randomized, double-blind, placebo-controlled trial of augmentation of paroxetine with a single, intravenous dose of a NMDA-receptor antagonist (CP-101,606) for paroxetine-resistant depression did not reveal a greater resolution of depressive symptoms (at the 0.05 level of significance) between the two treatment groups six weeks post-infusion (Preskorn *et al.*, 2008). Finally, a small ($n = 22$), double-blind, placebo-controlled, cross-over trial involving the use of the antibiotic d-cycloserine, an agonist at the glycine site of the NMDA receptor, as an augmentation for TRD did not reveal statistically significant therapeutic advantages of d-cycloserine versus placebo adjuvant treatment (Heresco-Levy *et al.*, 2006).

A randomized, double-blind, placebo-controlled trial of memantine augmentation of antidepressants for TRD is currently under way (NCT00344682).

6.3.5 *Anticonvulsants*

Only anecdotal evidence exists to support the use of older anticonvulsants such as carbamazepine (Ciusiani *et al.*, 2004; Cullen *et al.*, 1991; De la Fuente & Mendlewicz, 1992; Dietrich & Emrich,

1998; Hantouche *et al.*, 2005; Otani *et al.*, 1996; Pasquini *et al.*, 2007; Rybakowski *et al.*, 1999; Steinacher *et al.*, 2001), pregabalin (Showraki, 2007), and valproate (Corrigan, 1992; Hantouche *et al.*, 2005; Pasquini *et al.*, 2007), as adjunctive treatment in MDD patients who were antidepressant nonresponders.

Case series and retrospective chart reviews and small, open-label studies have suggested the potential usefulness of lamotrigine augmentation for MDD resistant to various antidepressants (Barbee & Jamhour, 2002; Gabriel *et al.*, 2006; Gutierrez *et al.*, 2005; Maltese, 1999; Rocha & Hara, 2003; Schindler & Anghelescu, 2007; Schindler & Anghelescu, 2007; Sloan Manning *et al.*, 2005). A double-blind, placebo-controlled study of lamotrigine (25–100 mg/day) when combined with fluoxetine (20 mg) in 23 TRD (MDD and bipolar depressed) patients did not reveal a greater reduction in depressive symptoms scores for lamotrigine- than placebo-treated patients (Barbosa *et al.*, 2003). Similarly, a double-blind, placebo-controlled trial of lamotrigine (50–200 mg) augmentation of antidepressants for 34 outpatients with antidepressant-resistant MDD did not reveal a difference in the degree of resolution of depressive symptoms between the two treatment groups (Santos *et al.*, 2008). However, a much larger trial ($n = 195$) did show greater efficacy for lamotrigine than placebo when added to the treatment of patients with paroxetine-resistant MDD although the magnitude of the treatment effect (lamotrigine–placebo difference in symptom reduction during treatment) was rather modest (mean difference in HDRS-17 score change of 0.3 units) and of questionable clinical significance (Barbee *et al.*, 2007) (Fig. 6.15). Side effects during combined lamotrigine-antidepressant treatment may include sweating, nausea, vertigo, headache, tremor, rash (in extreme cases, Stevens–Johnson syndrome), sedation, dry mouth, constipation, or leukopenia.

There are only case reports or chart reviews for gabapentin (Yasmin *et al.*, 2001), or topiramate (Barbee, 2003; Carpenter *et al.*, 2002b) augmentation in TRD. A small ($n = 25$), double-blind, placebo-controlled trial of phenytoin augmentation of SSRIs did not report any difference in the degree of resolution of depressive symptoms between the two groups (Shapira *et al.*, 2006). Finally, there

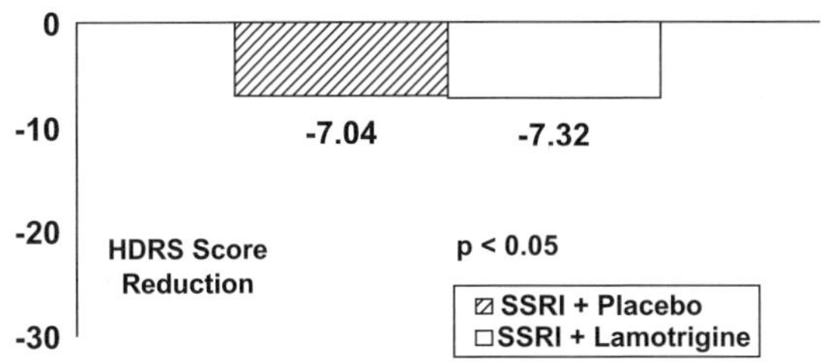

Fig. 6.15 Lamotrigine augmentation of paroxetine (SSRIs) for TRD: A randomized, double-blind study ($n = 96$). HDRS: Hamilton Depression Rating Scale [Data extracted from: Barbee, J.G., Jamhour, N.J., Stewart, J.W., *et al.* (2007). Lamotrigine as an antidepressant augmentation in treatment refractory unipolar depression. Presented at the 160th Annual Meeting of the American Psychiatric Association. San Diego, California.]

is preliminary evidence to suggest that adjunctive carbamazepine and perhaps gabapentin may be effective in the treatment of somatic symptoms of depression resistant to standard antidepressant treatment (Kudoh *et al.*, 1998; Maurer *et al.*, 1999).

6.3.6 *Inositol*

Antidepressant effects for adjunct inositol (12 g daily) were first reported in an open-label trial involving 12 patients with SSRI- and TCA-resistant MDD, nine of whom responded (Levine *et al.*, 1993). However, this report was soon followed by a negative double-blind, placebo-controlled study of inositol (12 g/day for four weeks) augmentation of SSRIs in SSRI-resistant MDD (Nemets *et al.*, 1999) (Fig. 6.16). Side effects may include nausea, headache, insomnia, and somnolence.

6.3.7 *Folates, s-adenosyl methionine (SAMe) and B-vitamins*

Hypofolatemia has consistently been found to confer an increased risk of poorer response to pharmacotherapy in MDD. This also pertains to the specific clinical scenario of augmentation of SSRIs (see Chap. 1). However, only one study explores whether the addition of

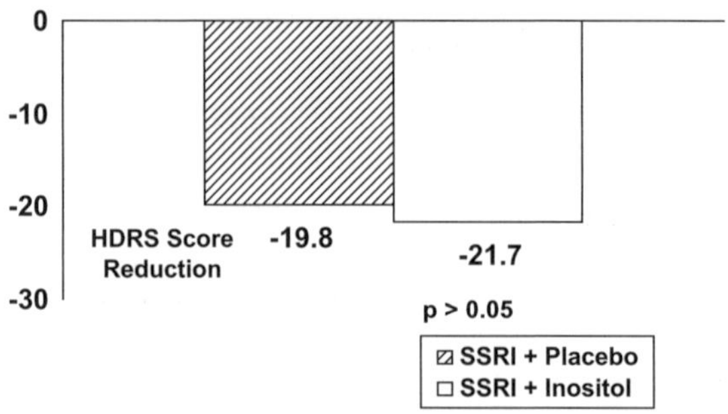

Fig. 6.16 Inositol augmentation of SSRIs for TRD: A randomized, double-blind study ($n = 36$). HDRS: Hamilton Depression Rating Scale. [Data extracted from: Nemets, B., Mishory, A., Levine, J., & Belmaker, R.H. (1999). Inositol addition does not improve depression in SSRI treatment failures. *Journal of Neural Transmission*, 106, 795–798.]

folate to the psychopharmacologic regimen of SSRI-resistant MDD patients can improve outcome. Among subjects with SSRI refractory depression, our group reported that folinic acid, a form of folate that enters the central nervous system as biologically active methyltetrahydrofolate, was associated with improved response in a proportion of subjects when added to the SSRI in an open trial (Alpert *et al.*, 2002). At present, our group is in the process of conducting a randomized, double-blind, placebo-controlled trial of methylfolate as an augmentation of SSRIs in SSRI-resistant MDD (clinicaltrials.gov: NCT00321152).

SAMe is one of the metabolic end-products of folate (Papakostas *et al.*, 2003; see Chap. 13 for details). The results of an open trial report a 50% response rate when SAMe (1600 mg/day) was added to the SSRI regimen of SSRI-nonresponders (Alpert *et al.*, 2004). Controlled trials for adjunctive folates or oral SAMe in TRD have yet to be published. At present, our group is in the process of conducting a randomized, double-blind, placebo-controlled trial of SAMe as an augmentation of antidepressants in TRD (clinicaltrials.gov: NCT00093847). Common side effects reported during the treatment of MDD with adjunct folates or SAMe include insomnia, nausea, anxiety, and headaches.

Finally, in a double-blind, randomized study, Bell *et al.* (1989) did find vitamin B augmentation (10 mg each of B1, B2 and B6) of TCAs to result in greater symptom resolution than placebo among 14 TRD (MDD) outpatients.

6.3.8 *Cholinergic agents*

Mecamylamine is a nicotinic-receptor antagonist ($\alpha 4\beta 2$, $\alpha 3\beta 2$, $\alpha 7$ — see Chap. 11 for a review of nicotinic receptors). The results of a double-blind, randomized, placebo-controlled trial demonstrate a greater resolution of depressive symptoms, particularly irritability, among outpatients with citalopram-resistant MDD (Dunbar *et al.*, 2007) (Fig. 6.17). This study was recently replicated, albeit on a smaller scale (George *et al.*, 2008).

The results of a small ($n = 20$), randomized, double-blind, placebo-controlled trial of galantamine augmentation of antidepressants for TRD did not demonstrate a difference in antidepressant effects between the two treatment groups that was statistically significant (Elgamal & MacQueen, 2008). There is also an open-label trial of verenicline ($\alpha 4\beta 2$ nicotinic partial agonist and $\alpha 7$ full agonist) augmentation for TRD (Philip *et al.*, 2009).

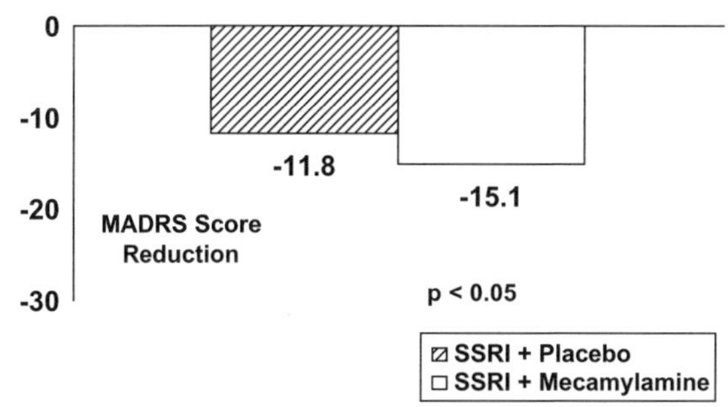

Fig. 6.17 Mecamylamine augmentation of citalopram (SSRI) for TRD: A randomized, double-blind study ($n = 184$). MADRS: Montgomery-Asberg Depression Rating Scale [Data extracted from: Dunbar, G., Kuchibhalta, R., & Kumar, R. (2007). Mecamylamine as an augmentation treatment for depressed patients who were non-responders to citalopram. *European Neuropsychopharmacology*, 17(s4), S348.]

6.3.9 *Miscellaneous other agents*

Only a small case report (Stoll & Rueter, 1999) and a small open-label trial (Varga *et al.*, 1982) have been published focusing on the use of adjunct opiates for the treatment of refractory depression, the latter study reporting a 0% response rate. For the opiate antagonist naltrexone, there is only a case report for its use as an adjunctive agent for TRD (Amiaz *et al.*, 1999). There is a small ($n = 12$) open-label trial of tramadol augmentation of SSRIs in SSRI-resistant MDD reporting a 50% response rate following three weeks of treatment (Fanelli & Montgomery, 1996). Tramadol, structurally similar to venlafaxine (Markowitz & Patrick, 1998), is a μ-opioid receptor agonist with relatively weak serotonin and norepinephrine reuptake inhibitor properties (Raffa *et al.*, 1992). Similarly, there are case reports (Deicken, 1987; Ries & Wittkowsky, 1986), and a small open-label trial (Morishita & Aoki, 1999 and 2002), but no controlled trials of benzodiazepine augmentation for TRD. In addition, there are open-label trials of chromium augmentation (McLeod *et al.*, 1999), creatinine monohydrate augmentation (Roitman *et al.*, 2007), augmentation with the phosphodiesterase inhibitor papaverine (Malison *et al.*, 1997) or the cycloxygenase-1 and -2 inhibitor acetylsalicylic acid (Mendlewicz *et al.*, 2006) for TRD but no controlled trials. Finally, the results of a randomized, double-blind, placebo-controlled trial support the use of N-acetyl cysteine (see Chap. 13 for details) as adjunctive therapy (to mood stabilizers) for the treatment of depressive symptoms among patients with bipolar I/II disorder who were either mildly depressed or in remission (Berk *et al.*, 2008). Studies focusing on patients with treatment-resistant MDD have yet to be published.

Chapter 7

Monotherapy Strategies for Resistant Depression

7.1 Increasing the Dose of Antidepressants

A number of uncontrolled reports suggest the potential efficacy of increasing the dose in antidepressant non-responders (Cantrell *et al.*, 1999; Fava *et al.*, 1992; Smith *et al.*, 1998; Wohlreich *et al.*, 2006). In addition, at least 11 randomized studies examining the potential efficacy of dose-increase strategies in TRD have been conducted to date (see Table 7.1). Nine of these 11 studies compare increasing the antidepressant dose versus continuing on the same dose for non-responders. None of these nine studies have demonstrated the superiority of increasing the dose versus continuing on the same dose, while, in fact, one of these studies reported that rapidly increasing the dose (i.e., from 100 mg to 200 mg of sertraline only two weeks following an increase from 50 mg to 100 mg) resulted in lesser improvements in depression severity than continuing on the same dose (100 mg) (Licht & Qvitzau, 2002). However, a major limitation of all but three of these trials (Heiligenstein *et al.*, 2002; Kornstein *et al.*, 2008; Ruhe *et al.*, 2009) is that the duration of treatment required in order to declare a depressive episode as treatment-resistant and, subsequently, randomize patients to continue with the same dose versus undergo a dose increase was four weeks or less. In light of the time-course of clinical response to SSRIs (Nierenberg *et al.*, 2000), it is quite possible that a delayed clinical response among patients randomized to continue on low-dose antidepressant may be responsible for the lack of difference in efficacy between the lower and

Table 7.1 Randomized dose-increase studies in TRD.

Study	*n*	Sample	Lead-in	High-dose	Comparator	Result[a]
Dornseif *et al.*, 1989	371	TRD[b]	3 weeks	Flx 60 mg 5 weeks	Fluoxetine 20 mg	20 mg = 60 mg
Schweitzer *et al.*, 1990	77	TRD[b]	3 weeks	Flx 60 mg 5 weeks	Fluoxetine 20 mg	20 mg = 60 mg
Fava *et al.*, 1994	41	TRD[c]	8 weeks	Flx 40–60 mg 4 weeks	Lithium versus desipramine augmentation	Flx > Li = DMI
Benkert *et al.*, 1997	86 AC	TRD[d]	3 weeks	Prx. 40 mg 3 weeks	Paroxetine 20 mg	20 mg = 50 mg
Benkert *et al.*, 1997	88 AC	TRD[e]	3 weeks	Maprot. 150 mg 3 weeks	Maprotiline 100 mg	100 mg = 150 mg
Fava *et al.*, 2002	101	TRD[c]	8 weeks	Flx 40–60 mg 4 weeks	Lithium versus desipramine augmentation	Flx = Li = DMI
Licht. & Qvitzau, 2002	295	TRD[f]	2 weeks	Sert. 200 mg 5 weeks	Sertraline 100 mg versus mianserin augmentation	Sert100 = Mian > Sert200 mg
Heiligenstein, 2002[g]	29	TRD[c]	9 weeks	Flx. 40–60 mg 10 weeks	Fluoxetine 20 mg	20 mg = 40–60 mg

(*Continued*)

Table 7.1 *(Continued)*

Study	*n*	Sample	Lead-in	High-dose	Comparator	Result[a]
Eli Lilly F1J-AY-HMCZ	202	TRD[h]	4 weeks	Dul. 90–120 mg 4 weeks	Duloxetine 60 mg	60 mg = 90–120 mg
Kornstein *et al.*, 2008	255	TRD[i]	6 weeks	Dul. 120 mg 8 weeks	Duloxetine 60 mg	60 mg = 120 mg
Ruhe *et al.*, 2009	107	TRD[j]	6 weeks	Prx. 30–50 mg	Paroxetine 20 mg	20 mg = 30–50 mg

[a]All outcomes represent difference in the change in Hamilton Depression Rating Scale (HDRS), baseline to endpoint.
[b]Insufficient improvement following 3 weeks of fluoxetine 20 mg.
[c]Insufficient improvement following 8 weeks of fluoxetine 20 mg.
[d]Insufficient improvement following 3 weeks of paroxetine 20 mg.
[e]Insufficient improvement following 3 weeks of maprotiline 100 mg.
[f]Insufficient improvement following 4 weeks of sertraline 50 mg followed by 2 weeks of sertraline 100 mg.
[g]Patients ages 9–17 years.
[h]Insufficient improvement following 4 weeks of duloxetine 60 mg. Study was open-label.
[i]Insufficient improvement following 6 weeks of duloxetine 60 mg.
[j]Insufficient improvement following 6 weeks of paroxetine 20 mg.
Abbreviations: Flx = fluoxetine, sert = sertraline, prx = paroxetine, dul = duloxetine, TRD = treatment-resistant depression, maprot = Maprotiline, mian = mianserin, Li = lithium augmentation, DMI = desipramine augmentation.

higher-dose groups in these studies. These methodological issues may therefore explain the failure to show the advantage of increasing the dose over continuing the same dose.

In contrast to these negative findings, two studies comparing increasing the SSRI dose versus augmenting with either lithium, or desipramine among patients who had not experienced sufficient symptom improvement following eight weeks of treatment with fluoxetine (20 mg) actually support the usefulness of increasing the dose. In fact, an increase in fluoxetine dose (from 20 mg to 40–60 mg) resulted in significantly higher remission rates than lithium or desipramine augmentation of fluoxetine (20 mg) in one study (Fava *et al.*, 1994). Similarly, a trend towards statistical significance for greater symptom improvement following an increase in fluoxetine dose (from 20 mg to 40–60 mg) when compared to the addition of either lithium or desipramine was also reported in a larger study of identical design (Fava *et al.*, 2002) (Fig. 7.1). When the

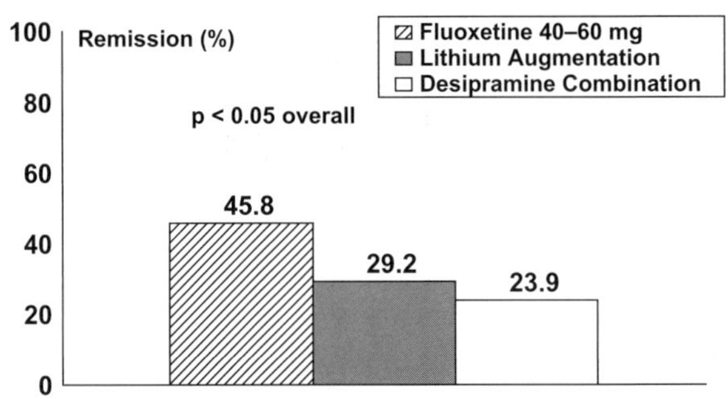

Fig. 7.1 Fluoxetine (SSRI) dose increase versus Li augmentation versus desipramine (TCA) combination for fluoxetine-resistant MDD: Pooled results from two randomized, double-blind studies. [Study 1: Data extracted from: Fava, M., Rosenbaum, J.F., McGrath, P.J., *et al.* (1994). Lithium and tricyclic augmentation of fluoxetine treatment for resistant major depression: A double-blind, controlled study. *American Journal of Psychiatry*, 151, 1372–1374. Study 2: Data extracted from: Fava, M., Alpert, J., Nierenberg, A., *et al.* (2002). Double-blind study of high-dose fluoxetine versus lithium or desipramine augmentation of fluoxetine in partial responders and nonresponders to fluoxetine. *Journal of Clinical Psychopharmacology*, 22, 379–387.]

data are pooled from both studies, a statistical significance advantage for increasing the dose is observed in terms of remission rates compared to the addition of lithium or desipramine to fluoxetine. Although further research is required in order to examine the relative efficacy of increasing the antidepressant dose versus other augmentation and switch strategies for TRD (particularly in the case of non-SSRI antidepressants), the sum of the evidence available to date suggests that, in the absence of intolerable side effects, increasing the dose of antidepressants from minimally effective to optimal is a reasonable if not preferred first step for patients who have not experienced full remission of symptoms despite four weeks of treatment.

7.2 Switching Antidepressants Due to Lack of Efficacy

7.2.1 *Switching from a TCA to an SSRI or MAOI and vice versa*

Numerous open-label trials report on the use of monoamine oxidase inhibitors (MAOIs) in TCA-resistant major depressive disorder (MDD) (Flint & Rifat, 1996; Thase *et al.*, 1992), or MDD resistant to a number of antidepressants (Amsterdam & Berwish, 1989; Amsterdam & Shults, 2005; Georgotas *et al.*, 1983; Nolen *et al.*, 1985 and 1988). Similarly, open-label trials also report on switching to TCAs (Flint & Rifat, 1996; Gervasoni *et al.*, 2009; Nierenberg *et al.*, 2003; Weintraub, 2001), or an SSRI (Amsterdam *et al.*, 1994; Beasley *et al.*, 1990; George *et al.*, 1999; Papakostas *et al.*, 2003) for patients resistant to antidepressants.

Four double-blind, randomized, crossover studies have been published focusing on switching from TCAs to MAOIs or SSRIs, and vice versa in TRD (i.e., SSRI- and TCA- non-responders crossed over to the alternative treatment, or TCA- and MAOI- non-responders crossed over to the alternative treatment). Specifically, Peselow *et al.* (1989) studied MDD outpatients who either did not experience sufficient improvement following a six-week, double-blind trial of imipramine ($n = 10$) versus paroxetine ($n = 25$), or could not tolerate treatment who were switched over to the alternative treatment (imipramine versus paroxetine). The results showed that 73% of paroxetine-resistant or intolerant patients responded to imipramine while 50% of imipramine-resistant or intolerant patients responded to paroxetine ($p < 0.05$). Thase *et al.* (2002) studied outpatients with chronic MDD who failed to respond to a 12-week, prospective trial of sertraline ($n = 117$, 50–200 mg) versus imipramine ($n = 51$, 50–300 mg), who were then crossed over to treatment with the alternative medication for 12 additional weeks. The outcome was such that 60% of imipramine-resistant patients responded to sertraline, while 44% of sertraline-resistant patients responded to imipramine ($p = 0.03$) (Fig. 7.2).

McGrath *et al.* (1987) reported a 29% response rate for phenelzine non-responders ($n = 14$) who were switched over to imipramine (up to 300 mg, 6 weeks), and a 65% response rate for imipramine non-responders ($n = 26$) who were switched over to phenelzine (up to 75 mg, 6 weeks) ($p < 0.05$). Finally, in a subsequent, larger study involving non-melancholic MDD outpatients with mood

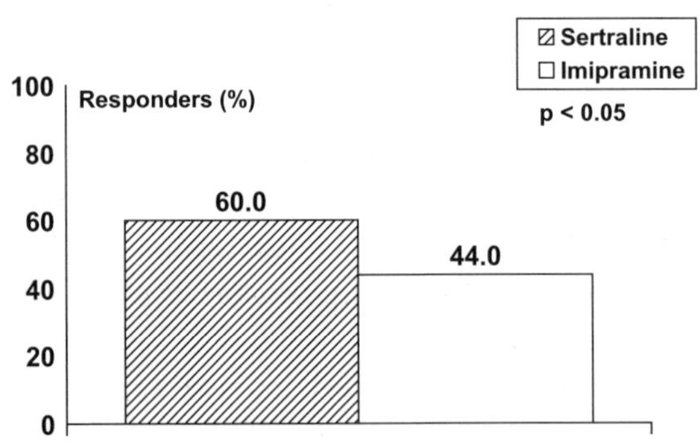

Fig. 7.2 Switching imipramine (TCA)-resistant MDD to sertraline (SSRI) and *vice versa* (cross-over design): A randomized, double-blind study ($n = 168$). [Data extracted from: Thase, M.E., Rush, A.J., Howland, R.H., *et al.* (2002). Double-blind switch study of imipramine or sertraline treatment of antidepressant-resistant chronic depression. *Archives of General Psychiatry*, 59, 233–239.]

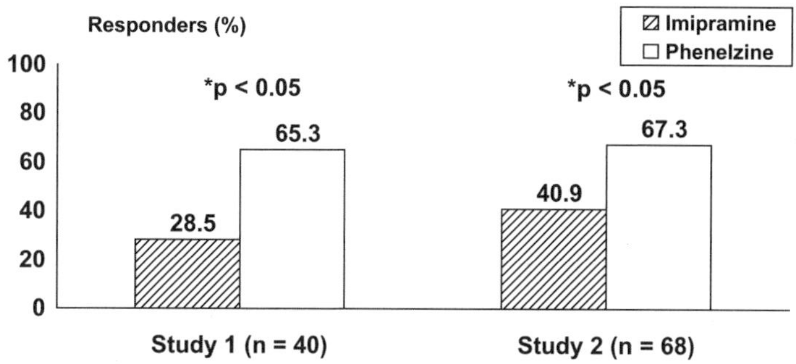

Fig. 7.3 Switching imipramine (TCA)-resistant MDD to phenelzine (MAOIs) and *vice versa* (cross-over): A randomized, double-blind study. [Study 1: Data extracted from: McGrath, P.J., Stewart, J.W., Harrison, W., & Quitkin, F.M. (1987). Treatment of tricyclic refractory depression with a monoamine oxidase inhibitor antidepressant. *Psychopharmacology Bulletin*, 23, 169–172. Study 2: Data extracted from: McGrath, P.J., Stewart, J.W., Nunes, E.V., *et al.* (1993). A double-blind crossover trial of imipramine and phenelzine for outpatients with treatment-refractory depression. *American Journal of Psychiatry*, 150, 118–123.]

reactivity, McGrath *et al.* (1993) reported a 67% response rate among imipramine non-responders ($n = 46$) who were treated with phenelzine (up to 90 mg, 6 weeks), and a 41% response rate among phenelzine non-responders ($n = 22$) who received imipramine (up to 300 mg, 6 weeks) ($p < 0.05$) (Fig. 7.3).

However, in light of their crossover design, the results of these four studies need to be interpreted with caution for the following reasons:

1. Even assuming that initial treatments, although different, are of equivalent efficacy, large sample sizes are required in order to ensure that non-significant differences in efficacy during the first treatment phase do not bias the second treatment phase (response rates between antidepressants in randomized controlled trials (RCTs) of MDD are almost always equivalent but almost never equal).
2. Differential treatment tolerability during the first phase may also bias the results of the second phase, since patients experiencing side effects are more likely to discontinue treatment in the case

of non-response than remission (thus, patients who complete a treatment that is less well tolerated would be more likely to have experienced a more robust response than those who complete a treatment that is better tolerated).

Four double-blind trials focusing on the use of the MAOIs in TCA- or SSRI-resistant MDD which employ a parallel (not cross-over) design have been published. Two of these double-blind studies compare the MAOIs brofaromine and tranylcypromine in TCA-resistant depression (MDD and major depression in the setting of bipolar illness — BPD) (Nolen *et al.*, 1993; Volz *et al.*, 1994). There was no difference in outcome between the two groups for either study. Birkenhager *et al.* (2004) compared switching to tranylcypromine versus phenelzine for TCA- or SSRI-resistant MDD, and reported equivalent response rates for both treatments (44% versus 47%, respectively). Finally, a study by Hoencamp *et al.* (1994) compared switching to brofaromine versus lithium augmentation of maprotiline for maprotiline-resistant depression (MDD and BPD), and reports no difference in outcome between the two groups.

7.2.2 Switching to a TCA or an MAOI following the failure of multiple antidepressants

In the third level of STAR*D, Fava *et al.* (2006) reported no difference in remission rates among patients with TRD switched to either mirtazapine or nortriptyline, although both treatments resulted in very modest remission rates (8–19.8%, depending on the definition used) (Fig. 7.4). No difference in tolerability between the two treatments was observed. Finally, the results of the fourth level of the STAR*D trial do not suggest any difference in efficacy among TRD patients switched to the MAOI tranylcypromine or the combination of mirtazapine and venlafaxine (McGrath *et al.*, 2006). However, tranylcypromine was significantly less well tolerated than the combination of mirtazapine and venlafaxine (41.4% versus 21.6% attrition rates).

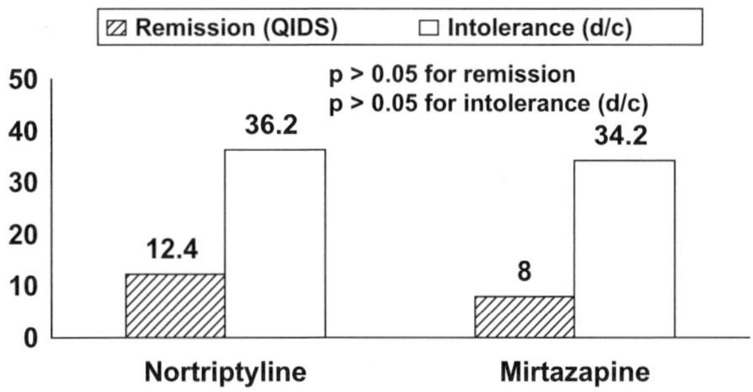

Fig. 7.4 STAR*D Level 3: Switching to mirtazapine versus nortriptyline for TRD: A randomized study ($n = 235$). QIDS: Quick Inventory of Depressive Symptomatology. [Data extracted from: Fava, M., Rush, A.J., Wisniewski, S.R., *et al.* (2006). A comparison of mirtazapine and nortriptyline following two consecutive failed medication treatments for depressed outpatients: A STAR*D report. *American Journal of Psychiatry*, 163, 1161–1172.]

7.2.3 *Switching from one SSRI to another, or to a non-SSRI antidepressant*

Although the SSRIs appear to be the most popular first-line treatment of choice among clinicians (Petersen *et al.*, 2002), a number of open-label trials suggest that switching from one SSRI to another due to lack of adequate response (Flint & Rifat, 1996; Joffe *et al.*, 1996; Thase *et al.*, 1997 and 2001a; Zarate *et al.*, 1996) may still be of benefit for many patients. Similarly, a number of open-label studies also examine switching from an SSRI to the α-2/5HT2 antagonist mirtazapine (Fava *et al.*, 2001), the norepinephrine-dopamine reuptake inhibitor (NDRI) bupropion (Fava *et al.*, 2003; Lam *et al.*, 2004; Walker *et al.*, 1993), the serotonin-norepinephrine–reuptake inhibitor (SNRI) venlafaxine (Baldomero *et al.*, 2005; de Montigny *et al.*, 1999; Kaplan, 2002; Mazeh *et al.*, 2007; Mbaya, 2002; Mitchell *et al.*, 2000; Montes *et al.*, 2004; Nierenberg *et al.*, 1994; Raynert-Dupuis *et al.*, 2002; Saiz-Ruiz *et al.*, 2002; Whyte *et al.*, 2004), or the SNRI milnacipran (Hoffman-La Roche clinical trial ML17259) for SSRI-resistant MDD. In addition, the results of a recent trial suggest no difference in efficacy between switching to standard (mean dose 148 mg/day) versus higher (mean dose 309 mg/day) doses of venlafaxine for patients who did not respond to, or could not tolerate treatment with an SSRI, although the standard-dose group tolerated better (Thase *et al.*, 2006).

Four double-blind, randomized, parallel clinical trials have compared the efficacy of switching to an SSRI versus a newer, non-SSRI antidepressant in adults with MDD. Poirier *et al.* (1999) studied 123 outpatients with MDD resistant to two antidepressants (mostly SSRIs and TCAs), who were then randomized to treatment with paroxetine (20–40 mg) versus venlafaxine (37.5–300 mg). Remission rates were statistically higher following the switch to venlafaxine than paroxetine (37% versus 18%, $p = 0.02$ in the intent-to-treat population). In a subsequent study, however, Lenox-Smith and Jiang (2008) examined 406 SSRI-nonresponders who were switched to venlafaxine versus citalopram. No differences in response or remission rates were reported between these two treatment groups (Fig. 7.5).

Thase *et al.* (2001b) studied 250 outpatients with MDD resistant to fluoxetine, paroxetine or citalopram, who were switched

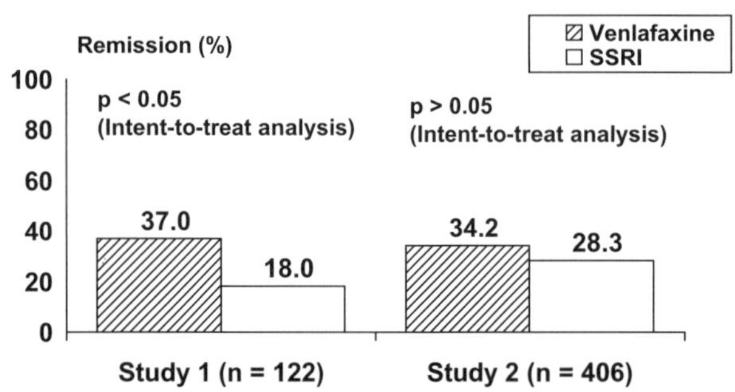

Fig. 7.5 Switching SSRI-resistant MDD to venlafaxine (SNRI) versus a 2nd SSRI (paroxetine or citalopram): Results from two randomized, double-blind studies. [Study 1: Poirier, M.F., & Boyer, P. (1999). Venlafaxine and paroxetine in treatment-resistant depression. Double-blind, randomised comparison. *British Journal of Psychiatry*, 175, 12–16. Study 2: Lenox-Smith, A.J., & Jiang, Q. (2008). Venlafaxine extended release versus citalopram in patients with depression unresponsive to a selective serotonin reuptake inhibitor. *International Clinical Psychopharmacology*, 23(3), 113–119.]

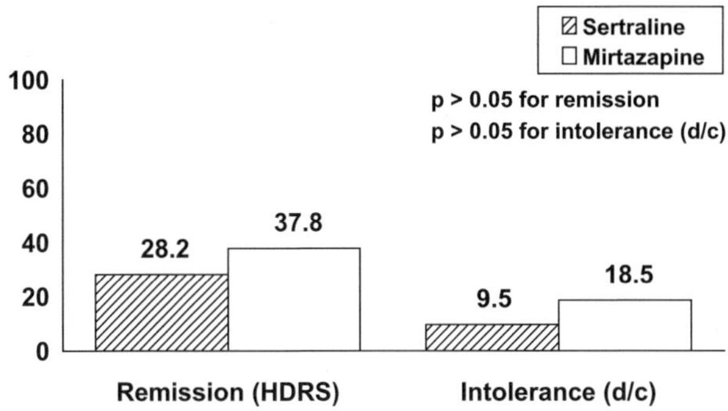

Fig. 7.6 Switching SSRI-resistant MDD to mirtazapine versus a 2nd SSRI (sertraline): A randomized, double-blind study ($n = 250$). [Data extracted from: Thase, M.E., Kremer, C., & Rodrigues, H. (2001). Mirtazapine versus sertraline after SSRI non-response. Presented at the 41st annual New Clinical Drug Evaluation Unit meeting, Boca Raton, Florida.]

to sertraline (50–200 mg) versus mirtazapine (15–45 mg) for eight weeks. Higher remission rates were reported in the mirtazapine than sertraline-treated group at week 2 (12.6% versus 4.8%), but not week 8 (37.8% versus 28.2%) (Fig. 7.6).

Ferreri *et al.* (2001) randomized outpatients with fluoxetine (20 mg)-resistant MDD to treatment with either adjunctive mianserin (60 mg), adjunctive placebo, or switching to mianserin (60 mg) for six weeks. Mianserin augmentation led to statistically greater remission rates (44%) than placebo (18%), but not mianserin switch (33%). The difference in response rates between continued fluoxetine plus placebo versus mianserin switch was also not statistically significant. Finally, the results of the second level of the Sequenced Alternatives to Relieve Depression (STAR*D) trial suggest no difference in remission rates among citalopram non-responders switched to sertraline, bupropion, or venlafaxine and treated for up to 14 weeks (Rush *et al.*, 2006). No difference in overall tolerability was observed between the three treatment groups.

More recently, a meta-analysis was conducted examining whether it is preferable to switch SSRI non-responders to a second SSRI versus a newer antidepressant (venlafaxine, bupropion, or mirtazapine)

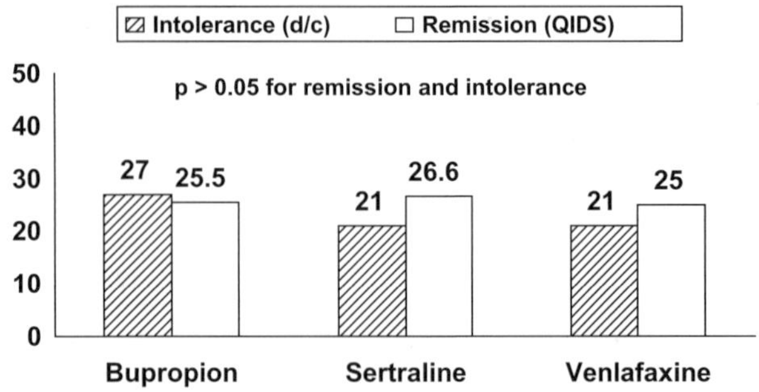

Fig. 7.7 STAR*D Level 2: Switching patients with citalopram (SSRI)-resistant MDD to venlafaxine (SNRI), bupropion (NDRI), or a 2nd SSRI (Sertraline): A randomized study (n = 727). [Data extracted from: Rush, A.J., Trivedi, M.H., Wisniewski, S.R., *et al.* (2006). Bupropion-SR, sertraline, or venlafaxine-XR after failure of SSRIs for depression. *New England Journal of Medicine*, 354(12), 1231–1242.]

(Papakostas *et al.*, 2008). Four randomized clinical trials were pooled (Lenox-Smith & Jiang, 2008; Poirier & Boyer, 1999; Rush *et al.*, 2006; Thase *et al.*, 2001) ($n = 1,496$). Patients randomized to switch to a non-SSRI antidepressant (bupropion, mirtazapine, venlafaxine) were more likely to experience remission ($p = 0.007$) than patients who were switched to a second SSRI (citalopram, paroxetine, or sertraline). The combined risk ratio for remission was 0.77, indicating a 23% relative advantage in remission rates in favor of switching to a non-SSRI than an SSRI antidepressant. There was also a non-significant trend ($p = 0.08$) in the rate of discontinuation due to intolerance favoring the within-class switch strategy. These results suggest a modest yet significant advantage in remission rates when switching patients with SSRI-resistant depression to a non-SSRI than to an SSRI antidepressant (Fig. 7.8).

Subsequent to the publication of the meta-analysis by Papakostas *et al.* (2008), the results of a randomized, double-blind, placebo-controlled trial were published focusing on switching adolescents with SSRI-resistant MDD to either a second SSRI or the SNRI venlafaxine (Brent *et al.*, 2008). No difference in efficacy outcome between the two treatment groups was reported.

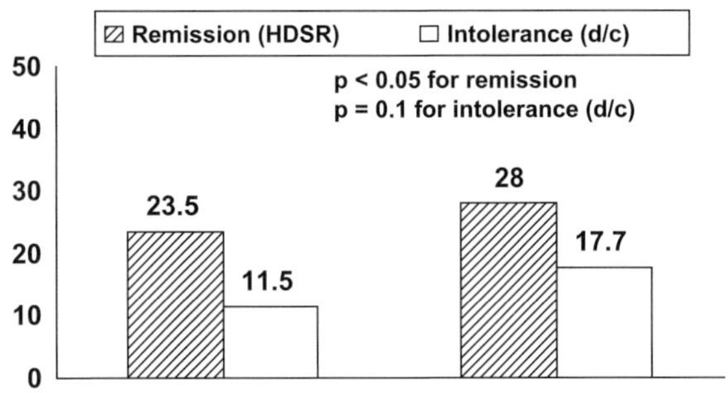

Fig. 7.8 Treatment of SSRI-resistant major depressive disorder: A meta-analysis of randomized controlled trials comparing within (2nd SSRI)- versus across (non-SSRI)-class switches (4 RCT; $n = 1{,}496$). RCT: Randomised controlled clinical trial. [Data extracted from: Papakostas, G.I., Fava, M., & Thase, M.E. (2008). Treatment of SSRI-resistant major depressive disorder: A meta-analysis of randomized controlled trials comparing within-versus across-class switches. *Biological Psychiatry*, 63(7), 699–704.]

7.2.4 *Other switch strategies*

More recently, the results of an open-label trial were published involving switching to duloxetine for MDD patients who either could not tolerate or did not experience sufficient symptom improvement following treatment with an SSRI or venlafaxine (Wohlreich *et al.*, 2005a and b). In parallel, a group of MDD patients not on an antidepressant were also treated with open-label duloxetine. The results showed that 50.9% of patients switched to duloxetine remitted following 12 weeks of treatment with duloxetine, which was comparable to remission rates following duloxetine-treatment among patients who were not switched from another antidepressant (54.5%). Directly switching from an SSRI to duloxetine (i.e., without a gradual taper of the SSRI) appears to be as well tolerated (with respect to discontinuation-related adverse events) as a tapered-switch (Perahia *et al.*, 2008). A recent open-label study of eight-weeks' duration reported a 48.8% remission rate among 88 outpatients with SSRI/venlafaxine-resistant MDD following a switch to duloxetine (Wohlreich *et al.*, 2006). There is also an open-label trial focusing on switching elderly MDD patients with SSRI-resistant MDD to duloxetine (Karp *et al.*, 2008).

Similarly, open-label trials describe the use of trazodone (Cole *et al.*, 1981), or nefazodone for patients with MDD resistant to SSRIs (Mischoulon *et al.*, 2004), or a number of antidepressants (Sajatovic *et al.*, 1999). Finally, Fava *et al.* (2003b) reported a 44.5% response rate among 128 outpatients with SSRI-resistant MDD switched to the NRI reboxetine and treated for up to eight weeks. However, double-blind comparator trials focusing on switching to these and other antidepressants for TRD are lacking.

Chapter 8

Non-pharmacologic Approaches for Resistant Depression

8.1 Device-Based Therapies

8.1.1 *Electroconvulsive therapy*

Electroconvulsive therapy (ECT), in use since the early 1930s for the treatment of mood disorders, is approved by the U.S. Food and Drug Administration (FDA) for treatment-resistant depression (TRD). To date, dozens of clinical trials have evaluated the efficacy of ECT as a treatment for major depressive disorder (MDD). A meta-analysis of such trials has recently concluded that (1) bilateral (more so than unilateral) ECT is more effective than sham ECT in MDD, (2) ECT is more effective than pharmacotherapy in MDD, and (3) "there is limited randomized evidence on the efficacy of ECT in the specific subgroups of patients who are presently more likely to receive it — e.g., older patients or those with treatment resistant depression" (UK ECT review group., 2003). Indeed, to date, randomized double-blind clinical trials comparing "real" versus sham ECT for patients with well-defined TRD have not been published. Similarly, while a handful of open-label, randomized studies have been published comparing ECT with pharmacotherapy for TRD (Davidson *et al.*, 1978; Dinan & Barry, 1989; Folkerts *et al.*, 1997; Steiner *et al.*, 1978), double-blind, randomized clinical trials comparing "real" ECT plus placebo with sham ECT plus antidepressants in populations with well-defined TRD have also not been published to date.

More recently, the results of a double-blind, randomized clinical trial comparing unilateral versus bilateral ECT for TRD (defined as non-remission following treatment with at least two agents of different mechanism of action) suggested no difference in efficacy between the two treatment groups (Eschweiler *et al.*, 2007). If fact, remission rates of 13–17% were reported in the latter study, which are comparable to those seen among MDD patients who did not experience sufficient symptom improvement following two antidepressant trials, who were either switched to mirtazapine or nortriptyline (12.3–19.8%), or received adjunctive treatment with lithium or triiodothyronine (T3) (15.9–24.7%) (see Chaps. 6 and 7 for details).

Even less is known regarding the long-term efficacy of continued ECT treatment in MDD. This is of particular concern for patients with TRD, since they appear to have higher relapse rates than non-TRD patients (see Chap. 9 for further details). Specifically, several double-blind, randomized studies have shown that continued treatment with imipramine (Seager & Bird, 1962; van den Broek *et al.*, 2006), nortriptyline (Sackeim *et al.*, 2001a), or paroxetine (Lauritzen *et al.*, 1996) is more effective in preventing a depressive relapse than continued treatment with placebo among ECT responders/remitters. In addition, the results of a double-blind, randomized, placebo-controlled trial suggest lower relapse rates among ECT-remitters (psychotic or non-psychotic MDD) following treatment with a combination of nortriptyline and lithium than nortriptyline alone (Sackeim *et al.*, 2001a). However, when Kellner *et al.* (2006) randomized ECT remitters (MDD) to continue treatment with maintenance ECT versus a combination of lithium and nortriptyline, no difference in relapse rates between the two treatment groups was observed (Fig. 8.1). The results of the latter trial suggest that continued ECT is not more effective than pharmacotherapy for the prevention of MDD relapse among ECT-remitters. On the other hand, in the same study, the remission rates reported with ECT prior to randomization were fairly impressive for a TRD population (suggesting that the population may not have been as refractory as originally thought), although the absence of a control does not allow us to draw firm conclusions. Side effects associated with ECT may

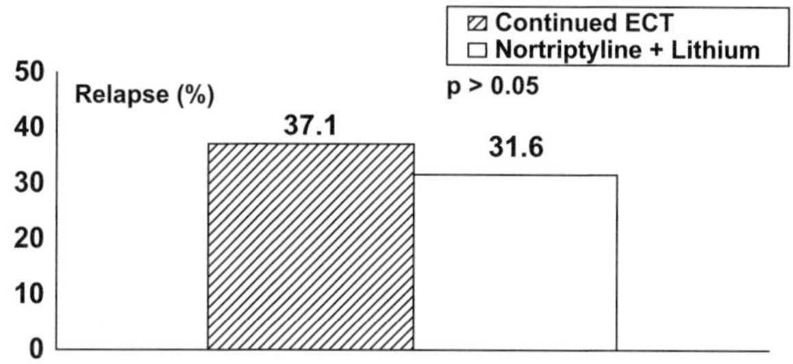

Fig. 8.1 Electroconvulsive therapy (ECT) versus pharmacotherapy for relapse prevention in major depression: A randomized study ($n = 201$). [Data extracted from: Kellner, C.H., Knapp, R.G., Petrides, G., *et al.* (2006). Continuation electroconvulsive therapy vs pharmacotherapy for relapse prevention in major depression: A multisite study from the Consortium for Research in Electroconvulsive Therapy (CORE). *Archives of General Psychiatry*, 63, 1337–1344.]

include headache, memory loss, confusion, cognitive impairment, insomnia, and somnolence. Recent evidence suggests that the combination of ECT with either nortriptyline or venlafaxine can enhance outcomes in TRD (Sackeim *et al.*, 2009).

8.1.2 *Vagus nerve stimulation*

Vagus nerve stimulation (VNS), in which the vagus nerve is stimulated by electrical impulses from an implanted pacemaker, was approved in July of 2005 by the FDA for the treatment of refractory depression. Interestingly enough, however, only two clinical trials have examined the efficacy of VNS during the short-term phase of MDD treatment. In the first such study, 60 patients with refractory depression (defined as non-response following treatment with at least two antidepressants of a different class) received VNS for a total of 10 weeks. Seventeen percent (17.3%) of patients remitted (Rush *et al.*, 2000; Sackeim *et al.*, 2001b). There is only a single randomized controlled trial focusing on the use of VNS during the acute-phase of treatment of MDD. More specifically, Rush *et al.* (2005a) randomized 235 outpatients with refractory MDD (did not experience significant symptom reduction following treatment with at least two antidepressants of a different class) ($n = 210$ MDD; $n = 24$ bipolar

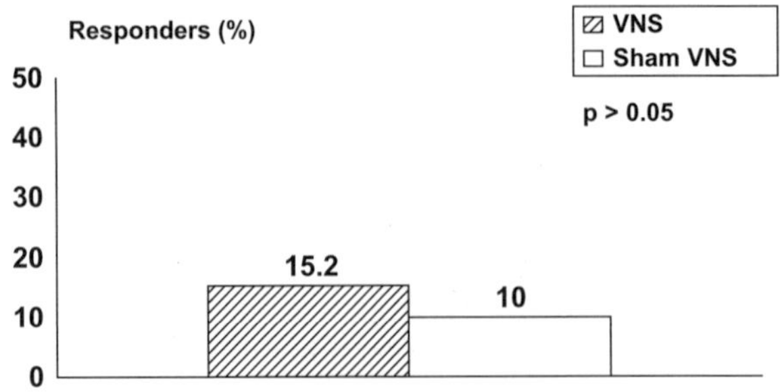

Fig. 8.2 VNS in TRD: A randomized, double-blind study ($n = 235$). [Data extracted from: Rush, A.J., Marangell, L.B., Sackeim, H.A., *et al.* (2005). Vagus nerve stimulation for treatment-resistant depression: A randomized, controlled acute phase trial. *Biological Psychiatry*, 58, 347–354.]

depression) to receive treatment with either VNS or sham VNS for 10 weeks. By the end of the trial period, 15.2% of patients who received VNS responded compared to 10% of patients who received sham VNS ($p > 0.05$ — remission rates not reported) (Fig. 8.2). Overall, the results of the latter study do not demonstrate acute antidepressant effects of VNS for TRD.

Three reports also focus on the long-term efficacy of VNS treatment. Nahas *et al.* (2005) reported on patients from the first of two acute-phase studies (Rush *et al.*, 2000; Sackeim *et al.*, 2001b) who continued to receive VNS for a total duration of two years. Roughly 22% of patients met criteria for remission at the end of the two-year follow-up period. Rush *et al.* (2005b) reported on patients from the second of two acute-phase studies (Rush *et al.*, 2005a). Patients who received VNS during the acute phase of treatment continued to receive VNS for nine additional months, while patients who received sham VNS during the acute phase of treatment received real VNS for 12 additional months. All patients received treatment as usual (options included pharmacotherapy, psychotherapy, somatic therapies or a combination). At study endpoint, 15.6% of patients met criteria for remission. When the latter group was compared with a cohort of depressed outpatients with TRD who received treatment as usual alone for 12 months, a significant difference in remission rates emerged in favor of the cohort who received VNS treatment (15.6% versus 5.6%) (George *et al.*, 2005). Subsequent studies on the use of VNS in MDD or TRD have not been published. Side effects associated with VNS may include incision site pain and/or infection, headache, neck pain, dysphagia, voice alteration, dyspepsia, nausea, dizziness, dyspnea, cough, and pharyngitis.

8.1.3 *Transcranial magnetic stimulation*

Transcranial magnetic stimulation (TMS) involves the use of magnetic pulses applied over the cranium with the use of a wand (non-invasive), in order to generate an electrical current in the underlying central nervous system (CNS). The results of several meta-analyses suggest that TMS treatment can result in a greater short-term (2–3 weeks) improvement than sham TMS in MDD (Loo *et al.*, 2005). In addition, more randomized-controlled trials (RCTs) specifically focusing on TRD have been published for TMS than all other somatic therapies combined (including ECT and VNS). A number of these studies report greater efficacy among patients with TRD who receive TMS over the left prefrontal area than those who receive sham TMS (Avery *et al.*, 2005; Berman *et al.*, 2000; Fitzgerald *et al.*, 2003; George *et al.*, 2000; Jorge *et al.*, 2004; Pascual-Leone *et al.*, 1996), although others do not (Loo *et al.*, 1999; Manes *et al.*, 2001; Minussi *et al.*, 2005; Padberg *et al.*, 1999 and 2002). In addition, the results of a randomized clinical trial suggest TMS over the left prefrontal cortex and ECT to result in equivalent response rates among 40 patients with TRD (Grunhaus *et al.*, 2003).

The frequency of TMS over the left prefrontal area (fast versus slow) does not appear to result in differential improvement in TRD (George *et al.*, 2000; Minuissi *et al.*, 2005; Padberg *et al.*, 1999). However, the intensity of TMS (high versus low intensity) does not appear to result in differential improvement in TRD in favor of high-intensity treatment (100% motor cortex threshold intensity) (Padberg *et al.*, 2002).

Until recently, a major limitation of these trials is the duration of treatment and follow-up, which does not exceed three weeks.

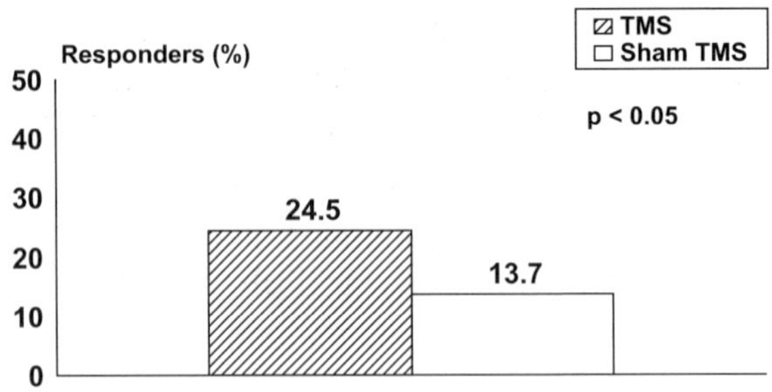

Fig. 8.3 TMS in TRD: A randomized, double-blind study ($n = 301$). [Data extracted from: O'Reardon, J.P., Solvason, H.B., Janicak, P.G., *et al.* (2007). Efficacy and safety of transcranial magnetic stimulation in the acute treatment of major depression: A multisite randomized controlled trial. *Biological Psychiatry*, 62(11): 1208–1216.]

Recently, however, O'Reardon *et al.* (2007) reported the results of a large ($n = 301$), six-week, sham TMS-controlled trial of TMS (left prefrontal cortex) for TRD. A greater resolution of depressive symptoms was reported among TMS- than sham-treated patients at endpoint (Fig. 8.3).

The results of a preliminary pilot study also suggest the use of magnetic resonance imagery to help focus rTMS (high frequency–10 Hz) to the left dorsolateral prefrontal cortex (junction area of Brodmann areas 46 and 9) to result in a greater reduction in depressive symptoms than non-MRI-guided rTMS (Fitzgerald *et al.*, 2009).

The results of one (Fitzgerald *et al.*, 2003), but not a second trial (Kauffmann *et al.*, 2004) also suggest low frequency TMS over the right prefrontal area to result in greater resolution of depressive symptoms in TRD than sham TMS (Fitzgerald *et al.*, 2003).

However, a subsequent, randomized, double-blind, sham-TMS and placebo pill-controlled study comparing low frequency (1 Hz) right prefrontal rTMS with venlafaxine for treatment-resistant depression did not demonstrate a difference in antidepressant efficacy between the two treatment groups (Bares *et al.*, 2009).

Bilateral (prefrontal cortex) TMS for TRD did not appear to be effective in one study (Loo *et al.*, 2003). Relapse-prevention studies of TMS have yet to be published. Side effects associated with TMS include headaches, dizziness, and scalp discomfort/numbness and/or pain.

8.1.4 *Deep brain stimulation*

Deep brain stimulation (DBS) is an invasive procedure, as it involves the placement of electrodes within the CNS. In an open-label trial, Mayberg *et al.* (2005) treated six TRD patients with DBS (electrodes placed in the subguenal cingulated cortex — Brodmann area 25). Four patients experienced a clinical response following six months of treatment.

In a separate open-label trial, Malone *et al.* (2009) treated 15 TRD patients with DBS (ventral capsule/ventral striatum), and reported remission rates of 33.3%, 26.6%, and 33.3% after 3, 6, and 12 months. No other studies have been published thus far focusing on the use of DBS in TRD or MDD.

8.1.5 *Transcranial direct current stimulation (tDCS)*

tDCS involves injecting low-amplitude direct currents into the brain via scalp electrodes. The results of a Phase II, randomized, double-blind, sham-tDCS controlled trial of dorsolateral prefrontal cortex (DLFPC) versus occipital cortex tDCS for MDD ($n = 40$) demonstrated a greater resolution of depressive symptoms among patients who received DLFPC than occipital or sham tDCS (Boggio *et al.*, 2008). This study has yet to be replicated.

8.1.6 *Bright light therapy*

White light, either of constant intensity or gradually increasing intensity to simulate dawn ("dawn simulation"), has been studied as a treatment for depression. In fact, a recent meta-analysis of RCTs comparing light therapy with "sham" light therapy for depression suggests that bright light therapy is (1) effective for the treatment of seasonal effective disorder, (2) effective for the treatment of non-seasonal affective disorders, and (3) not effective when used as an adjunct to standard antidepressants for non-seasonal depression (Golden *et al.*, 2005). Unfortunately, studies focusing on the use of light therapy in TRD have yet to be published [Neumister *et al.* (1999) studied bright light augmentation among MDD patients following non-response to three weeks of antidepressant treatment, which is too short a treatment duration in order to declare a depressive episode as treatment-resistant].

8.1.7 *Acupuncture*

Allen *et al.* (2006) randomized 151 patients with MDD to specific acupuncture (acupuncture points specific for depression as defined by traditional Chinese medicine), non-specific acupuncture (points non-specific for depression), or a waitlist (control) group for eight weeks. A greater resolution of depressive symptoms was reported among patients who received acupuncture than those who did not, although the two acupuncture groups did not differ with regards to their efficacy (Fig. 8.4). Similarly, disappointing results were reported in sham acupuncture-controlled adjunctive acupuncture trials for MDD (Zhang *et al.*, 2009) and bipolar disorder (Dennehy *et al.*, 2009). The efficacy of acupuncture in TRD remains to be studied.

8.2 Psychotherapy

Along with antidepressants, psychotherapy is a first-line treatment for MDD, with cognitive behavior therapy (CBT)/cognitive therapy (CT) having, by far, the most evidence from randomized clinical

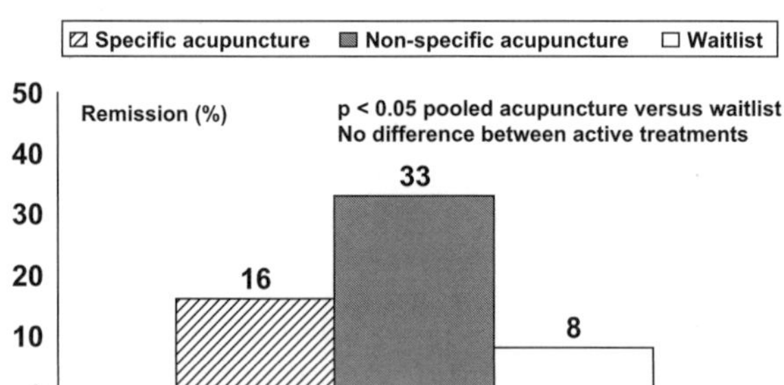

Fig. 8.4 Acupuncture in MDD: A randomized study ($n = 151$). [Data extracted from: Allen, J.J., Schnyer, R.N., Chambers, A.S., *et al.* (2006). Acupuncture for depression: A randomized controlled trial. *Journal of Clinical Psychiatry*, 67, 1665–1673.]

trials (RCTs) supporting their efficacy. Indeed, the results of a large meta-analysis have demonstrated that the efficacy of CBT is equivalent to that of pharmacotherapy for the treatment of depression (DeRubeis *et al.*, 1999). More recently, meta-analyses have also demonstrated greater efficacy for psychotherapy when combined with pharmacotherapy from the onset of treatment when compared to either pharmacotherapy (Pampallona *et al.*, 2004; Cuijpers *et al.*, 2009), or psychotherapy (Thase *et al.*, 1997) when administered separately.

Several open-label trials have been published exploring the use of CBT (Cooper, 1994; Fava *et al.*, 1997; Leykin *et al.*, 2007; Thase & Howland, 1994), CT (Scott, 1992; Fennel & Teasdale, 1982; Miller, 1985; Mirabel-Sarron *et al.*, 1993), psycho-educational group therapy (Antonuccio *et al.*, 1984), or intensive short-term dynamic therapy for TRD (Abbass, 2006). Interestingly enough, however, there is a relative paucity of controlled studies focusing on the use of psychotherapy for TRD. Specifically, only seven such trials have been published to date examining the efficacy of psychotherapy in TRD, all focusing on the use of cognitive behavioral therapy (CBT).

In the first such study, Harpin *et al.* (1982) compared CBT with a waiting list as a control among 12 patients with depression "unresponsive to antidepressants". CBT resulted in a greater resolution of depressive symptoms than the control group. Similarly, De Jong *et al.* (1986) studied a group of 30 chronically depressed patients who did not improve sufficiently following antidepressant treatment. Patients were randomized to receive either CBT, milieu therapy (control group), or wait list (control group). Patients treated with CBT had a better outcome that the other two groups. However, when Bristow and Bright (1995) compared CBT with the administration of a self-help manual (control group) among 10 patients who either refused, could not tolerate, or did not respond to antidepressant treatment, no difference in efficacy between the two groups was found. Shortly thereafter, Barker *et al.* (1987) randomized 20 patients who had not experienced sufficient symptom improvement following antidepressant treatment and were then switched to a different antidepressant to receive either adjunct CBT versus no CBT (no control for psychotherapy included in this trial). There

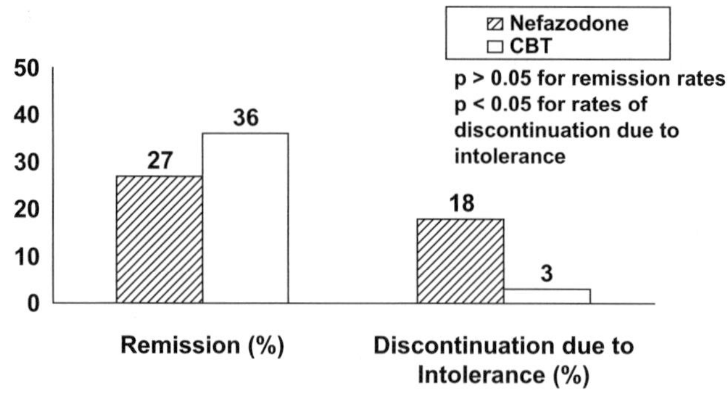

Fig. 8.5 CBT versus nefazodone in TRD ($n = 140$) (cross-over for CBT and nefazodone non-responders). [Data extracted from: Schatzberg, A.F., Rush, A.J., Arnow, B.A., *et al.* (2005). Chronic depression: Medication (nefazodone) or psychotherapy (CBASP) is effective when the other is not. *Archives of General Psychiatry*, 62, 513–520.]

was no difference in efficacy between the two treatment groups. More recently, Schatzberg *et al.* (2005) examined the efficacy of the alternative treatment (12-week cross-over design) among 140 patients with nefazodone- or psychotherapy- (cognitive behavioral system of psychotherapy — CBASP) resistant MDD. Both treatments demonstrated equivalent efficacy, although more nefazodone- than CBASP-treatment patients discontinued treatment due to intolerance (Fig. 8.5). In a separate study, Brent *et al.* (2008) randomized adolescents with SSRI-resistant MDD to switch to a second antidepressant with or without adjunctive CBT. Patients who received adjunctive CBT demonstrated higher rates of clinical response than those who did not.

Finally, Thase *et al.* (2007) reported the results of the second levels of sequenced treatment alternatives to relieve depression (STAR*D) trial involving the use of CBT. Specifically, citalopram non-responders either underwent a switch from citalopram to CBT versus antidepressants (sertraline, bupropion or venlafaxine), or an augmentation of citalopram with CBT versus bupropion or buspirone. Patients who received CBT had similar response and remission criteria than those assigned to medication strategies, although

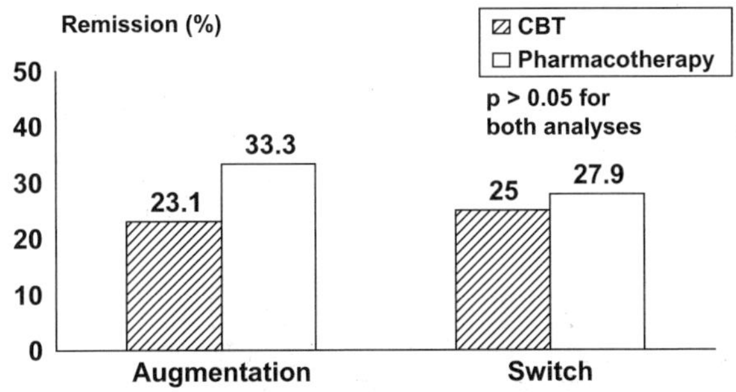

Fig. 8.6 CBT versus pharmacotherapy in TRD (STAR*D Level 2): A randomized study. [Data extracted from: Thase, M.E., Friedman, E.S., Biggs, M.M., *et al.* (2007). Cognitive therapy versus medication in augmentation and switch strategies as second-step treatments: A STAR*D report. *American Journal of Psychiatry*, 164, 739–752.]

patients who received drug augmentation, improved more rapidly than patients who received CBT augmentation, while patients switched to CBT experienced fewer side effects than patients switched to a second antidepressant (Fig. 8.6). No other controlled studies focusing on the use of psychotherapy in TRD have since been published.

8.3 Exercise

Using a 2 × 2 factorial study design, Dunn *et al.* (2005) randomized patients with mild to moderate MDD to receive treatment with aerobic-exercise treatment that varied in total energy expenditure (7 kcal/Kg per week or 17.5 kcal/Kg per week) or frequency (either three or five days a week), or to a control exercise group (three days a week of flexibility exercise). Patients randomized to two of the four exercise groups (17.5 kcal/Kg per week) had higher remission rates than the control group (31–41% versus 15%). More recently, Trivedi *et al.* (2006) reported a significant reduction in depressive symptoms following augmentation of antidepressants with exercise therapy for TRD. Randomized, controlled trials focusing on the use of exercise therapy in TRD have yet to be published.

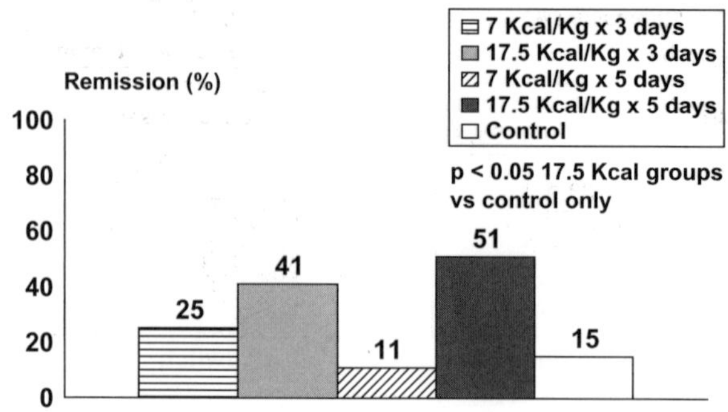

Fig. 8.7 Exercise treatment for depression: Efficacy and dose response from a randomized study ($n = 80$). [Data extracted from: Dunn, A.L., Trivedi, M.H., Kampert, J.B., *et al.* (2005). Exercise treatment for depression: Efficacy and dose response. *American Journal of Preventive Medicine*, 28, 1–8.]

8.4 Yoga and Meditation

A number of clinical trials have focused on the use of various forms of Yoga or meditation for the treatment of various mood disorders (Astin *et al.*, 2003; Janakiramaiah *et al.*, 2000; Sephton *et al.*, 2007; Sharma *et al.*, 2006). Studies in TRD have yet to be conducted.

Summary and Conclusion of Part II

Treatment-resistant major depressive disorder (TRD) is common (see Chap. 1). However, despite decades of research, no clear consensus has emerged regarding strategies to optimize the efficacy of antidepressants (either from the onset of treatment or following non-response to first-line treatment), largely owing to an insufficient number of randomized clinical trials (RCTs). Nevertheless, a number of strategies are available to help optimize treatment efficacy in MDD, including pharmacologic (augmentation, switching, dose-increase), as well as non-pharmacologic [psychotherapy, electroconvulsive therapy (ECT), vagus nerve stimulation (VNS), transcranial magnetic stimulation- (TMS)] treatment strategies.

With regards to adjunctive (augmentation and combination) pharmacotherapeutic strategies for TRD, the majority of studies published to date involve the use of lithium, the atypical antipsychotics, pindolol, psychostimulants, anticonvulsants T3, buspirone, modafinil, desipramine, ω-3 fatty acids or the 5HT2/ α-2 antagonists. In summary, antidepressant effects over placebo for adjunctive buspirone have never been demonstrated past week 1, and for adjunctive lithium or T3 past week 2. Although two studies suggest adjunctive pindolol to be effective in mixed treatment-resistant and non-resistant populations, two subsequent, larger placebo-controlled trials of pindolol augmentation for TRD patients were negative. Psychostimulants and anticonvulsants (lamotrigine and phenytoin) do not appear to be effective as adjuncts in TRD in placebo-controlled studies.

In contrast to these agents, antidepressant effects for adjunctive 5HT2/α-2 antagonists mianserin or mirtazapine in TRD have been demonstrated in three of four studies, while the one negative study has been criticized for methodological flaws. In addition, a meta-analysis of 16 randomized, placebo-controlled trials focusing on the use of the atypical neuroleptics as adjuncts in TRD suggest the potential efficacy of this treatment strategy for TRD, although tolerability appears to be a major limitation. Furthermore, three positive double-blind augmentation studies of ω-3 fatty acids for TRD have been published to date. Taken together, it appears that augmentation of the SSRIs with either combined 5HT2/α-2 antagonists such as mirtazapine and mianserin, the atypical antipsychotic agents, or ω-3 fatty acids are, at the present time, the adjunct strategies best supported by the existing literature for TRD. Testosterone, NMDA-receptor antagonists, mecamylamine, desipramine, and modafinil appear to be, to various extents, promising adjunctive treatments for TRD. However, positive controlled studies for these agents have yet to be replicated. Finally, a number of potentially successful augmentation strategies including bupropion, reboxetine, folates, SAMe, steroid synthesis inhibitors and steroids have yet to be subject to double-blind, placebo-controlled investigation.

In contrast to augmentation and combination strategies for TRD, only 13 RCTs have been published or presented at major scientific meetings focusing on the use of switch strategies for TRD. Of these, four involve the use of a crossover rather than a parallel design and, thus, yield limited information, while three compare switching TRD patients to two different MAOIs. Two studies compare augmentation with switching for TRD, while none compares switching with increasing the dose of an antidepressant in MDD. Thus, at the present time, the relative efficacy of switching versus augmentation/combination versus increasing the dose for TRD is unclear.

Four RCTs have compared switching to agents of different class in MDD (an SSRI, venlafaxine, bupropion, mirtazapine, or nortriptyline). Switching to venlafaxine was shown to be superior to switching to an SSRI in one but not two other trials. Results for the remaining trials/agents are equivocal. However, pooling these four trials suggests a slight efficacy advantage for switching to a newer, non-SSRI agent (venlafaxine, bupropion, or mirtazapine) than to a second SSRI. Therefore, at the present time, switching to a second SSRI versus a non-SSRI newer agent (bupropion, mirtazapine, venlafaxine) in SSRI-resistant MDD appears to be the strategy best supported by the literature. Double-blind switch studies focusing on newer agents including duloxetine, desvenlafaxine, reboxetine, selegiline transdermal system, or agomelatine have yet to be published.

With respect to increasing the dose in antidepressant non-responders, even less is known. In fact, double-blind studies published to date have yet to provide strong evidence to support this common treatment strategy. However, study design is an obvious limitation, with the duration of treatment required to declare a depressive episode as treatment-resistant being brief (three weeks), or doses escalated rapidly. In fact, one of two studies of adequate duration supports the use of higher doses of fluoxetine for TRD. Future controlled dose-increase studies involving patients who have not responded to an antidepressant of a given dose and for an adequate duration would greatly further our understanding of the relative utility of dose-increase strategies for TRD. Nevertheless, given the relative user-friendliness of this therapeutic approach (dose-increase), it is widely recommended particularly for patients who have demonstrated significant symptom improvement (short of remission) and reasonable tolerability at lower doses.

A number of non-pharmacologic strategies for TRD have been described as well. Of these, the use of ECT for TRD is best supported by the literature (although the long-term efficacy of ECT in preventing MDD relapse among ECT remitters remains in question). In addition, open-label, randomized studies suggest ECT to be more effective than pharmacotherapy for TRD. This has yet to be established in double-blind, placebo- and sham-ECT-controlled trials. The results of a randomized, double-blind, sham-TMS-controlled trial also support the use of TMS for TRD, while there is also data from randomized clinical trials supporting the use of specific psychotherapies (cognitive-behavioral therapy-CBT and cognitive behavioral system of psychotherapy — CBASP) either as monotherapy or as adjuncts to standard antidepressants for antidepressant-resistant MDD. Finally, the use of VNS in TRD has not been well established by the existing literature (one equivocal randomized, double-blind, sham-VNS-controlled trial).

At the present time, there is no clear consensus among experts regarding whether it is optimal to increase the dose, switch, or augment/combine in TRD. Several factors, however, appear to be very relevant with regards to influencing clinician/patient treatment decisions on the preferred next-step treatment choice. These include:

1. The trajectory of symptom improvement during first-line treatment. Partial improvement would favor increasing the dose or augmenting/combining while lack of improvement would favor switching.
2. The tolerability of the first-line treatment. Poor tolerability would favor switching while good tolerability would favor augmenting/combining or increasing the dose.
3. Treatment history. Patients who have a history of robust response with a specific dose of an agent, a specific agent, or a specific combination of agents may demonstrate as robust a response with the same treatment regimen during the present episode. This may influence the relative likelihood of increasing the dose versus switching versus augmenting/combining in TRD.
4. The potential for drug discontinuation-related adverse events. Such potential favors increasing the dose, or augmenting/combining, versus switching. Switching from a serotonergic- to a non-serotonergic agent carries the highest risk.
5. The potential for drug interactions. This potential favors dose increase or switching versus polypharmacy. It is compounded among patients with a greater burden of medical illness due to the greater number of concomitant medications.
6. The potential for poor treatment adherence due to forgetfulness. This favors dose/increase and switching versus polypharmacy.
7. The presence of treatment refractoriness (i.e., multiple failed medication and psychotherapy trials). Such presence may signal for the need to resort to somatic therapies.

Part III

Maintaining Treatment Gains

Introduction to Part III

Parts I and II of this book focus on reviewing treatment strategies that help bring about remission in Major Depressive Disorder (MDD). Equally important as achieving full remission of symptoms in MDD is helping maintain patients in a relatively symptom-free state on a long-term basis. In addition to preventing further suffering, maintaining remission over long periods of time is important in order to help restore psychosocial functioning (Kocsis *et al.*, 2002). In fact, a number of studies suggest that the risk of subsequent relapse increases with each successive major depressive episode, while the risk of recurrence progressively decreases as the duration of recovery increases (Lavori *et al.*, 1984; Solomon *et al.*, 2000). Therefore, in the third part of this book, our focus is to describe pharmacotherapies designed to help maintain treatment gains.

Chapter 9 is a review of studies focusing on the long-term use of pharmacologic treatments in order to help prevent a relapse/recurrence of MDD. As with studies examining the efficacy of antidepressants in treating a depressive episode, studies examining the role of pharmacotherapies in MDD prophylaxis vary in their design. Briefly, the most common design is one in which patients who responded or remitted following open-label treatment (lead-in phase) with a pharmacologic agent are randomized in a double-blind fashion to continue to receive treatment with that agent or are switched to placebo (double-blind placebo-substitution).

These studies are typically required by the U.S. Food and Drug administration (FDA) in order to approve a drug as a treatment for MDD (i.e., for drugs to be labeled as "antidepressants"). Less common are antidepressant "extension trials", in which MDD patients who have either responded or remitted to an antidepressant or placebo are continued on that treatment for an extended period of time. We then conclude Chap. 9 with a description of studies focusing on the treatment of MDD relapse/recurrence.

It is becoming increasingly clear that, in order to increase the likelihood of long-term adherence to pharmacologic treatment in MDD as well as minimize patient discomfort, it is important for physicians to identify and manage side effects that often arise during the course of pharmacotherapy. Chapter 10 is a review reporting on the use of adjunctive pharmacotherapeutic strategies for the treatment of antidepressant-associated side effects, followed by an overview of the studies describing switching from one antidepressant to another due to intolerance.

Chapter 9

Pharmacotherapy of Relapse/Recurrence Prevention and Treatment

9.1 Antidepressant Continuation and Maintenance Therapy Studies

9.1.1 *Tricyclic antidepressants* (*TCAs*)

Fourteen studies involve comparing the long-term efficacy of TCAs versus placebo in preventing depressive relapse (Table 9.1 and Claghorn *et al.*, 1993; Stewart *et al.*, 1997 from Table 9.5). Three focus on elderly patients with MDD (Alexopoulos *et al.*, 2000; Cook *et al.*, 1986; Reynolds *et al.*, 1999). None focus on either children or adolescents. All but two (Cook *et al.*, 1986; Stewart *et al.*, 1997) show continued treatment with TCAs to be superior to placebo-substitution in the prevention of depressive relapse/recurrence.

9.1.2 *Monoamine oxidase inhibitors* (*MAOIs*)

Relatively fewer studies examine the long-term prophylactic effects of the MAOIs as the TCAs. All four double-blind, placebo-substitution studies focusing on the long-term prophylactic effects of continued treatment with phenelzine in phenelzine-responders are positive (see Table 9.2; Stewart *et al.*, 1997 from Table 9.5). There is also one positive double-blind, placebo-substitution study for continued selegiline in selegiline-responders (Amsterdam & Bodkin, 2006).

Table 9.1 Double-blind, placebo-substitution of TCAs among TCA-responders/remitters.

Study	Lead-in AD Duration	Double-blind AD Duration	*N*	Results
Mindham *et al.*, 1972/73	AMI or IMI variable	AMI or IMI or Pbo 24 weeks	92	Relapse rate drug < Pbo (22% vs 50%)
Klerman *et al.*, 1974	AMI 6 weeks	AMI or Pbo 32 weeks	100	Relapse rate drug < Pbo (12% vs 30%)
Coppen *et al.*, 1978	AMI minimum 6 weeks	AMI or Pbo 52 weeks	32	Relapse rate drug < Pbo (0.0% vs 50%)
Stein *et al.*, 1980	AMI 8 weeks	AMI or Pbo 24 weeks	17	Relapse rate drug < Pbo (28% vs 69%)
Bialos *et al.*, 1982	AMI variable	AMI or Pbo 24 weeks	17	Relapse rate drug < Pbo (0% vs 80%)
Cook *et al.* 1986	TCAs (naturalistic) 1 year	TCA (same) or Pbo 32 weeks	15	Relapse rate drug = Pbo (0% vs 33.3%)

(Continued)

Table 9.1 (*Continued*)

Study	Lead-in AD Duration	Double-blind AD Duration	*N*	Results
Frank *et al.*, 1990	IMI minimum 20 weeks	IMI or Pbo 156 weeks	128	Relapse rate drug < Pbo (32% vs 78%)
Rouillon *et al.*, 1991 a/b	MAP 8 weeks	MAP or Pbo 52 weeks	733	Relapse rate drug < Pbo (16–23.8% vs 31.5–37.5%)
Kupfer *et al.*, 1992	IMI 3 years	IMI or Pbo 104 weeks	20	Relapse rate drug < Pbo (9% vs 66%)
Kocsis *et al.*, 1996	DMI 26 weeks	DMI or Pbo 104 weeks	129	Relapse rate drug < Pbo (11% vs 52%)
Reynolds *et al.*, 1999	NT minimum 16 weeks	NT or Pbo 156 weeks	53	Relapse rate drug < Pbo (43% vs 90%)
Alexopoulos *et al.*, 2000	NT minimum 16 weeks	NT or Pbo 104 weeks	43	Relapse rate drug < Pbo (18% vs 52%)

Abbreviations: TCA = tricyclic antidepressant, AD = antidepressant, IMI = imipramine, DMI = desipramine, MAP = maprotiline, N = nortriptyline, Pbo = placebo.

Table 9.2 Double-blind, placebo-substitution MAOIs among MAOI-responders/remitters.

Study	Lead-in AD Duration	Double-blind AD Duration	*N*	Results
Davidson & Raft, 1984	Phenelzine 12 weeks	Phenelzine vs Pbo 20 weeks	18	Relapse rate drug < Pbo (14% vs 100%)
Harrison *et al.*, 1986	Phenelzine minimum 6 weeks	Phenelzine vs Pbo 24 weeks	12	Relapse rate drug < Pbo (20% vs 100%)
Robinson *et al.*, 1991	Phenelzine minimum 22 weeks	Phenelzine vs Pbo 104 weeks	47	Relapse rate drug < Pbo (29% vs 81%)
Amsterdam & Bodkin, 2006	Selegiline (transdermal) 8 weeks	Selegiline vs Pbo 52 weeks	322	Relapse rate drug < Pbo (16.8% vs 30.7%)

Abbreviations: MAOI = monoamine oxidase inhibitor, AD = antidepressant, Pbo = placebo.

9.1.3 *Selective serotonin reuptake inhibitors (SSRIs)*

Twenty-four double-blind, long-term, placebo-substitution trials involving continued treatment of SSRI-responders with SSRIs have been published to date (Table 9.3; also Claghorn *et al.*, 1993 and Keller *et al.*, 2007a and b, Kocsis *et al.*, 2007 from Table 9.5). Four of these studies focus on elderly patients (Gorwood *et al.*, 2007; Klysner *et al.*, 2002; Reynolds *et al.*, 2006), and three on children/adolescents (Cheung *et al.*, 2008; Emslie *et al.*, 2004 and 2008). All studies but two show continued treatment with SSRIs to be superior to placebo in preventing depressive relapse/recurrence in MDD (Figs. 9.1 and 9.2).

9.1.4 *Newer antidepressants*

Double-blind, placebo-controlled studies have also been published for agomelatine, amineptine, bupropion, desvenlafaxine, duloxetine, gepirone, mianserin, milnacipran, mirtazapine, nefazodone, reboxetine, tianeptine, and venlafaxine (see Table 9.4 and also Keller *et al.*, 2007a and b, Kocsis *et al.*, 2007 from Table 9.5). None of these studies focus on the treatment of elderly patients, children or adolescents. All studies demonstrate lower relapse/recurrence rates among antidepressant than placebo-treated patients. However, the duration of follow-up for these studies varies widely, with the agomelatine and desvenlafaxine studies being shorter than nine months in duration, which is the length of time required for a patient in remission to be considered recovered (Nierenberg & DeCecco, 2001).

9.1.5 *Summary of continuation and maintenance trials*

Numerous controlled studies of pharmacotherapeutic agents for relapse prevention have been published to date. Although the amount of supportive data varies widely from agent to agent (especially for the elderly, children or adolescents), the sum of

Table 9.3 Double-blind, placebo-substitution of SSRIs among SSRI-responders/remitters.

Study	Lead-in AD Duration	Double-blind AD Duration	*N*	Results
Montgomery *et al.*, 1988	Fluoxetine 24 weeks	Fluoxetine vs Pbo 52 weeks	220	Relapse rate drug < Pbo (26% vs 57%)
Montgomery *et al.*, 1992/93	Citalopram 6 weeks	Citalopram vs Pbo 24 weeks	147	Relapse rate drug < Pbo (8–12% vs 31%)
Doogan & Caillard, 1992	Sertraline 8 weeks	Sertraline vs Pbo 44 weeks	295	Relapse rate drug < Pbo (13% vs 45.7%)
Montgomery & Dunbar, 1993	Paroxetine 8 weeks	Paroxetine vs Pbo 52 weeks	135	Relapse rate drug < Pbo (16% vs 43%)
Robert & Montgomery, 1995	Citalopram 8 weeks	Citalopram vs Pbo 24 weeks	226	Relapse rate drug < Pbo (13.8% vs 24.3%)
Keller *et al.*, 1998	Sertraline 28 weeks	Sertraline vs Pbo 76 weeks	161	Relapse rate drug < Pbo (6% vs 23%)
Reimherr *et al.*, 1998	Fluoxetine 12–14 weeks	Fluoxetine vs Pbo 50 weeks	395	Relapse rate drug < Pbo Variable[a]
Terra & Montgomery, 1998	Fluvoxamine 24 weeks	Fluvoxamine vs Pbo 52 weeks	204	Relapse rate drug < Pbo (12.7% vs 35.1%)
Schmidt *et al.*, 2000	Fluoxetine 13 weeks	Fluoxetine vs Pbo 25 weeks	501	Relapse rate drug < Pbo (26% vs 37% vs 50%)

(Continued)

Table 9.3 (*Continued*)

Study	Lead-in AD Duration	Double-blind AD Duration	*N*	Results
Gilaberte *et al.*, 2001	Fluoxetine 32 weeks	Fluoxetine vs Pbo 48 weeks	140	Relapse rate drug < Pbo (20% vs 40%)
Hochstrasser *et al.*, 2001	Citalopram 22 weeks	Citalopram vs Pbo 48 weeks	269	Relapse rate drug < Pbo (18.1% vs 41.5%)
Klysner *et al.*, 2002	Citalopram 22 weeks	Citalopram vs Pbo 48 weeks	121	Relapse rate drug < Pbo (23.3% vs 67.2%)
Rapaport *et al.*, 2004	Escitalopram 8 weeks	Escitalopram vs Pbo 36 weeks	274	Relapse rate drug < Pbo (26% vs 40%)
Emslie *et al.*, 2004	Fluoxetine 19 weeks	Fluoxetine vs Pbo 32 weeks	40	Relapse rate drug < Pbo (34% vs 60%)
Kamijima *et al.*, 2005	Sertraline 8 weeks	Sertraline vs Pbo 16 weeks	235	Relapse rate drug < Pbo (8.5% vs 19.5%)
Kornstein *et al.*, 2006	Escitalopram 16 weeks	Escitalopram vs Pbo 52 weeks	139	Relapse rate drug < Pbo (30% vs 62%)
McGrath *et al.*, 2006	Fluoxetine 12 weeks	Fluoxetine vs Pbo 52 weeks	292	Relapse rate drug < Pbo (45.9% vs 72%)
Reynolds *et al.*, 2006	Paroxetine Variable	Paroxetine vs Pbo 108 weeks	116	Relapse rate drug < Pbo (36% vs 63%)

(*Continued*)

Table 9.3 (*Continued*)

Study	Lead-in AD Duration	Double-blind AD Duration	*N*	Results
Gorwood *et al.*, 2007	Escitalopram 12 weeks	Escitalopram vs Pbo 24 weeks	305	Relapse rate drug < Pbo (9% vs 33%)
Emslie *et al.*, 2008	Fluoxetine 12 weeks	Fluoxetine vs Pbo 24 weeks	102	Relapse rate drug < Pbo (42% vs 69.2%)
Cheung *et al.*, 2008	Sertraline 36 weeks	Sertraline vs Pbo 52 weeks	22	Relapse rate drug + Pbo (0% vs 38%, respectively)
Petersen *et al.*, in press	Fluoxetine 12 weeks + 28 weeks with or without CBT	Fluoxetine vs Pbo 24 weeks	30	Relapse rate drug = Pbo (29% vs 50%, respectively)

[a]Patients randomized to 4 groups: 1) continued fluoxetine 20 mg for 50 weeks, 2) continued fluoxetine 20 mg for 14 weeks followed by a switch to placebo for 36 weeks, 3) continued fluoxetine 20 mg for 38 weeks followed by a switch to placebo for 12 weeks, 4) switching to placebo during randomization and continued treatment with placebo for 50 weeks.
Results: 1) Relapse rate for patients who received 12 weeks of continuation treatment with fluoxetine < relapse rate for patients who did not receive any continuation treatment with fluoxetine (26.4% vs 48.6%). 2) Relapse rate for patients who received 26 weeks of continuation treatment with fluoxetine < relapse rate for patients who received 14 weeks of continuation treatment with fluoxetine (9.0% vs 32.2%). 3) Relapse rate for patients who received 50 weeks of continuation treatment with fluoxetine = relapse rate of patients who received 38 weeks of continuation treatment with fluoxetine (10.7% vs 16.2%).
Abbreviations: Pbo = placebo; SSRI = selective serotonin reuptake inhibitor.

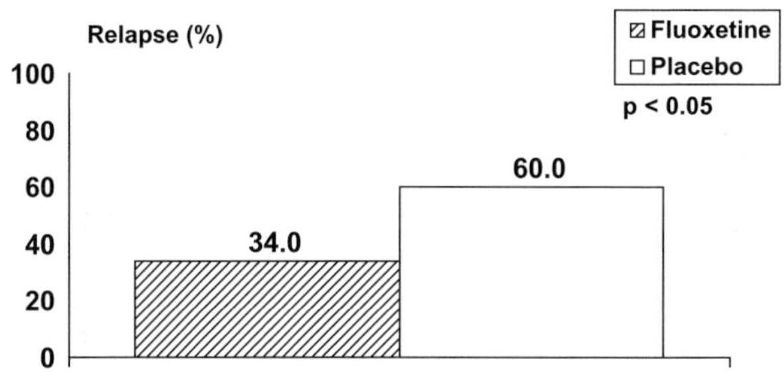

Fig. 9.1 A randomized, double-blind, relapse prevention study of fluoxetine (SSRI) for MDD in children and adolescents ($n = 40$). [Data extracted from: Emslie, G.J., Heiligenstein, J.H., Hoog, S.L., *et al.* (2004). Fluoxetine treatment for prevention of relapse of depression in children and adolescents: A double-blind, placebo-controlled study. *Journal of the American Academy of Child and Adolescent Psychiatry*, 43, 1397–1405.]

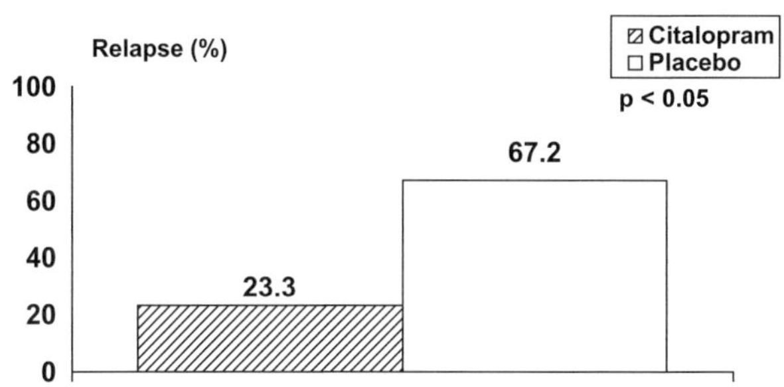

Fig. 9.2 A randomized, double-blind relapse prevention study of citalopram (SSRI) for MDD in the elderly ($n = 121$). [Data extracted from: Klysner, R., Bent-Hansen, J., Hansen, H.L., *et al.* (2002). Efficacy of citalopram in the prevention of recurrent depression in elderly patients: Placebo-controlled study of maintenance therapy. *British Journal of Psychiatry*, 181, 129–135.]

the evidence suggests that continued pharmacotherapy with the antidepressant that brought about clinical response or remission of symptoms does afford greater protection from depressive relapse/recurrence than switching to placebo. A meta-analysis of continued antidepressant treatment for the prevention of depressive relapse reports a 70% reduction in relapse rates (95% CI: 62–78%;

Table 9.4 Double-blind, placebo-substitution and relapse: Studies involving newer antidepressants.

Study	Lead-in AD Duration	Double-blind AD Duration	*N*	Results
Kishimoto *et al.*, 1994	Mianserin minimum 3 months	Mianserin vs Pbo 72 weeks	22	Relapse rate drug < Pbo (44.4% vs 100.0%)
Ferreri *et al.*, 1997	Amineptine 12 weeks	Amineptine vs Pbo 36 weeks	284	Relapse rate drug < Pbo (6.6% vs 18.6%)
Feiger *et al.*, 1999	Nefazodone 16 weeks	Nefazodone vs Pbo 36 weeks	131	Relapse rate drug < Pbo (1.8% vs 18.3%)
Versiani *et al.*, 1999	Reboxetine 6 weeks	Reboxetine vs Pbo 46 weeks	283	Relapse rate drug < Pbo (22% vs 56%)
Rouillon *et al.*, 2001	Milnacipran 22 weeks	Milnacipran vs Pbo 52 weeks	214	Relapse rate drug < Pbo (16.3% vs 23.6%)
Dalery *et al.*, 2001	Tianeptine 6 weeks	Tianeptine vs Pbo 66 weeks	185	Relapse rate drug = Pbo
Thase *et al.*, 2001	Mirtazapine 12 weeks	Mirtazapine vs Pbo 40 weeks	185	Relapse rate drug < Pbo (19.7% vs 43.8%)
Weihs *et al.*, 2002	Bupropion SR 8 weeks	Bupropion SR vs Pbo 44 weeks	423	Relapse rate drug < Pbo
Gelenberg *et al.*, 2003	Nefazodone 28 weeks	Nefazodone vs Pbo 52 weeks	165	Relapse rate drug < Pbo (30.6% vs 47.5%)

(*Continued*)

Table 9.4 (*Continued*)

Study	Lead-in AD Duration	Double-blind AD Duration	*N*	Results
Montgomery *et al.*, 2004	Venlafaxine 24 weeks	Venlafaxine vs Pbo 52 weeks	225	Relapse rate drug < Pbo (22% vs 55%)
Amsterdam *et al.*, 2004	Gepirone IR 6 weeks	Gepirone IR vs Pbo 6 weeks	70	Relapse rate drug < Pbo
Keller *et al.*, 2005	Gepirone ER 12 weeks	Gepirone ER vs Pbo 44 weeks	250	Relapse rate drug < Pbo (23.0% vs 34.7%)
Perahia *et al.*, 2006	Duloxetine 12 weeks	Duloxetine vs Pbo 26 weeks	278	Relapse rate drug < Pbo (17.4% vs 28.5%)
Rickels *et al.*, 2007	Desvenlafaxine 12 weeks	Desvenlafaxine vs Pbo 24 weeks	300	Relapse rate drug < Pbo (24% vs 42%)
Goodwin *et al.*, 2009	Agomelatine 10 weeks	Agomelatine vs Pbo 24 weeks	339	Relapse rate drug 9 < Pbo (21.3% vs 56.1%)
Perahia *et al.*, 2009	Duloxetine 28–34 weeks	Duloxetine vs Pbo 24 weeks	288	Relapse rate drug < Pbo (14.4% vs 33.1%)

Abbreviations: AD = antidepressant, Pbo = placebo, XR, ER = extended release, IR = immediate release.

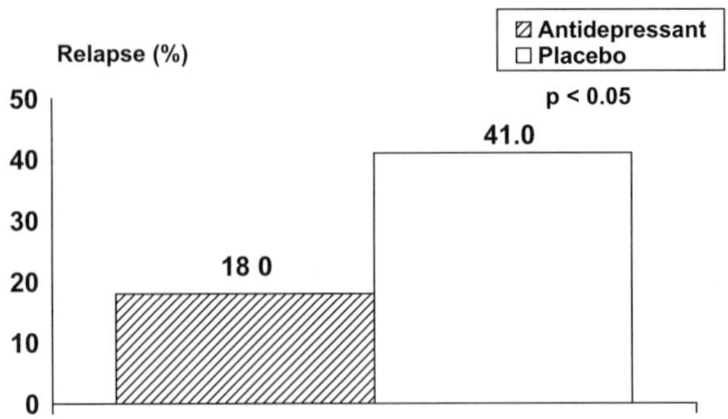

Fig. 9.3 Meta-analysis: Prevention of MDD relapse during continued treatment with antidepressants (31 RCTs, $n = 4410$). [Data extracted from: Geddes, J.R., Carney, S.M., Davies, C., *et al.* (2003). Relapse prevention with antidepressant drug treatment in depressive disorders: A systematic review. *The Lancet*, 361, 653–661.]

$p < 0.00001$) among patients who continue antidepressant treatment that those switched to placebo (Geddes *et al.*, 2003) (Fig. 9.3). In addition to supporting the need for continued pharmacotherapy for depression, these studies raise a number of important questions worth discussing in further detail.

9.2 Special Topics in the Pharmacotherapy of Relapse Prevention

9.2.1 *Long-term efficacy differences among antidepressants*

Eight studies comparing the long-term efficacy of antidepressants have been conducted (Table 9.5). Studies comparing the prophylactic effects of paroxetine and imipramine (Claghorn *et al.*, 1993), moclobemide and fluoxetine (Lonnqvist *et al.*, 1995), sertraline and fluvoxamine (Franchini *et al.*, 1997), mirtazapine and amitriptyline (Montgomery *et al.*, 1998), nefazodone and imipramine (Anton *et al.*, 1994), sertraline and imipramine (Koran *et al.*, 2001), or fluoxetine and venlafaxine XR (Keller *et al.*, 2007a and b, Kocsis *et al.*, 2007) report no difference in long-term prophylaxis between treatment groups.

Table 9.5 Long-term antidepressant comparator studies and relapse.

Study	Lead-in AD Duration	Double-blind AD Duration	*N* Design	Results (relapse rates)
Claghorn *et al.*, 1993	PAX or IMI 6 weeks	PAX or IMI or Pbo 52 weeks	145 DBPS	Imipramine = Paroxetine < Pbo (8% vs 15% vs 25%, resp.)
Anton *et al.*, 1994	NEF, IMI or Pbo 8 weeks	NEF, IMI or Pbo 52 weeks	276 Extension	Nefazodone = Imipramine < Pbo (9% vs 8% vs 25%, resp.)
Lonnqvist *et al.*, 1995	MOCL or FLX 6 weeks	MOCL or FLX 12 weeks	59 Extension	Moclobemide = Fluoxetine (7% vs 3%, resp.)
Stewart *et al.*, 1997	PHEN or IMI 30 weeks	PHEN, IMI or Pbo 24 weeks	60[a] DBPS	Phenelzine < Pbo (23% vs 87%) Imipramine = Pbo (41% vs 47%)
Franchini *et al.*, 1997	TCAs Variable	SERT or FLUV 96 weeks	64 Switch	Sertraline = Fluvoxamine (22% vs 18% resp.)
Montgomery *et al.*, 1998	MIR, AMI or Pbo 6 weeks	MIR, AMI or Pbo 104 weeks	217 Extension	Mirtazapine = Amitriptyline < Pbo (4.1% vs 11.6% vs 28.1%)
Koran *et al.*, 2001	SERT or IMI[b] 12 weeks	SERT or IMI 16 weeks	307 Extension	Sertraline = Imipramine (17% vs 22%, resp.)
Keller *et al.*, 2007a and b	VEN or FLX	VEN or FLX or Pbo	715	Venlafaxine = Fluoxetine < Pbo[a]
Kocsis *et al.*, 2007	10 weeks	2.5 years[c]	DBPS[a]	

[a]Patients (either unipolar or bipolar) with atypical and chronic major depressive episode.
[b]Non-responders following 12 weeks of treatment with either imipramine or sertraline were crossed over to the alternative agent for another 12 weeks of treatment. Patients who were non-responders during the acute phase and crossed-over to the alternative treatment had higher relapse rates than those who responded to the initial agent.
[c]10 week open-label phase compared fluoxetine with venlafaxine. Patients were randomized to c/w their antidepressant vs switch to placebo at the beginning of continuation phase (6 months), then during the first visit of a first maintenance phase (12 months), followed by the first visit of the second maintenance phase (12 months). For each time period, venlafaxine and fluoxetine decreased relapse rates relative to placebo, with no difference between the two active treatments.
Abbreviations: Pbo = placebo; AD = antidepressant, DBPS = double-blind placebo substitution, PAX = paroxetine, IMI = imipramine, NEF = nefazodone, MOCL = moclobemide, FLX = fluoxetine, PHEN = Phenelzine, TCAs = tricyclic antidepressants, MIR = mirtazapine, SERT = sertraline. VEN = venlafaxine XR.

Finally, Stewart *et al.* (1997) randomized patients with atypical major depression (unipolar of bipolar) who had responded following treatment with either the MAOI phenelzine or the TCA imipramine, to continue treatment with the same antidepressant or undergo a switch to placebo. Phenelzine but not imipramine was more effective in preventing a depressive relapse than placebo. This finding further supports the notion that agents that also include a dopaminergic component (i.e., MAOIs) can be more effective in atypical depression than agents which influence serotonin and norepinephrine but not dopamine (i.e., the TCAs) (also see Chap. 4). However, two important limitations should be noted. While the study blind was maintained with regards to whether a patient was on active medication or placebo in these two studies, raters as well as patients were aware whether patients were in the phenelzine or imipramine arm of the study. In addition, the study also involved patients with bipolar disorder that appear to be particularly prone to suffer manic relapses during treatment with TCAs (Nemeroff *et al.*, 2001).

9.2.2 *Optimal duration of long-term therapy*

Perhaps one of the most important questions in the long-term pharmacotherapy of depression is how long must MDD patients who have experienced full symptom remission continue their antidepressant treatment regimen in order to minimize the risk of depressive relapse or recurrence. In the aforementioned meta-analysis by Geddes *et al.*, no relationship was found between the duration of treatment preceding randomization and the treatment effect or the absolute risk of relapse following randomization to either continue with antidepressant treatment or switch to placebo during the continuation and/or maintenance phases. The risk of relapse among patients who continued on antidepressants was 16% for patients treated for 1–2 months prior to randomization versus 18% for patients treated for 4–6 months prior to randomization. Similarly, the risk of relapse among patients who were switched to placebo was 40% for patients treated for 1–2 months prior to randomization versus 35% for patients treated for 4–6 months prior to randomization. However, it is important to note that these analyses involve the duration of treatment during the pre-randomization period rather than the duration of remission which may, in turn, better predict the absolute risk of relapse following randomization to continued pharmacotherapy versus placebo.

In contrast to the meta-analysis by Geddes *et al.*, Reimherr *et al.* (1998) demonstrated that the duration of the continuation phase of treatment did influence the treatment effect. This study involved varying the continuation phase of treatment of MDD by randomizing fluoxetine-(20 mg for 12 weeks) remitters to either continue treatment with fluoxetine (20 mg) for 50 weeks, continue treatment with fluoxetine for 38 weeks followed by switching to placebo for 12 weeks, continue treatment with fluoxetine for 14 weeks followed by switching to placebo for 36 weeks, or continue treatment with placebo for 50 weeks. Relapse rates were lower among the patients who continued to take fluoxetine compared with those transferred to placebo in both the first interval, after 24 total weeks of treatment (fluoxetine, 26.4%; placebo, 48.6%), and the second interval, after 38 total weeks of treatment (fluoxetine, 9.0%; placebo, 23.2%). In the third interval, after 62 total weeks of treatment, rates were not significantly different between the groups (fluoxetine, 10.7%; placebo, 16.2%). The results of this study suggest that patients treated with fluoxetine for 12 weeks whose depressive symptoms remit should continue treatment with fluoxetine for at least an additional 26 weeks in order to minimize their risk of suffering a depressive relapse. However, any benefit of continuing on fluoxetine versus switching to placebo following at least 26 weeks of continuation treatment was not demonstrated in this study. More recently, however, Keller *et al.* (2007a and b; Kocsis *et al.*, 2007) randomized patients who had recovered from MDD (in remission for 1.5 years) on either fluoxetine or venlafaxine to either continue on their antidepressant for an additional year or switch to placebo. Continuing antidepressant was found to result in fewer MDD recurrences than switching to placebo. Finally, in a small study, Kupfer *et al.* (1992; Table 9.1) randomized 20 patients who had maintained remission on a combination of imipramine with or without interpersonal therapy for three years to continue treatment with imipramine versus placebo-substitution for an additional two years. Greater relapse rates among placebo than imipramine-treated patients were reported in that study. This study has yet to be replicated.

9.2.3 *Long-term dosing and risk of relapse*

Another relevant clinical question is whether the dose of antidepressants can be decreased following remission of symptoms without increasing the likelihood of experiencing a depressive relapse. If this were possible, it would also represent a useful treatment strategy for antidepressant remitters who experience intolerable side effects. To date, five studies randomizing patients who responded to a given dose to continued treatment with the same versus a lower dose have been published. These studies involve the use of maprotiline (Rouillon *et al.*, 1991), imipramine (Frank *et al.*, 1993), amineptine (Ferreri *et al.*, 1997), phenelzine (Davidson & Raft, 1984), and paroxetine (Franchini *et al.*, 1998). Continuing the same dose was found to be superior to lowering the dose for maprotiline (from 75–150 mg to 75 mg versus 37.5 mg for 52 weeks), imipramine (full dose that led to remission versus half of that dose for 156 weeks), phenelzine (full dose that led to response versus gradual taper of 15 mg per month), and paroxetine (from 40 mg to 40 mg versus 20 mg for 112 weeks), but not amineptine (from 200 mg to 200 mg versus 100 mg for 36 weeks). More recently, a meta-analysis pooling these five trials confirmed a higher relapse rate among patients randomized to continue on a lower dose of antidepressants than the dose that originally helped bring about symptom improvement (Papakostas *et al.*, 2007a) (Fig. 9.4).

Another question relevant to clinical practice, given that a significant proportion of patients either seek to lower their antidepressant dose or even decide to discontinue antidepressants during long-term treatment due to side effects, is whether decreasing the dose following remission affords any prophylaxis from depressive relapse than discontinuing antidepressant treatment altogether.

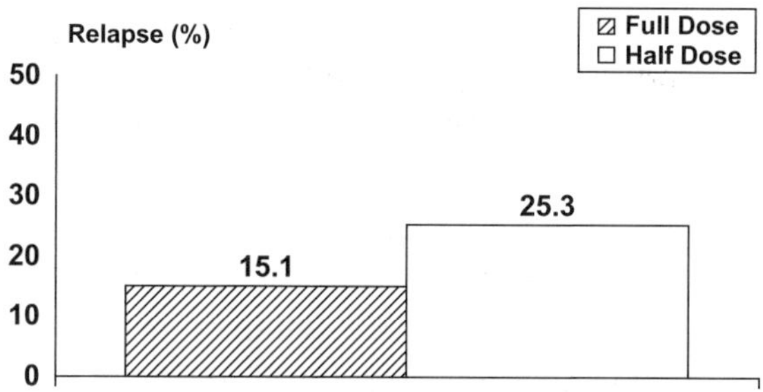

Fig. 9.4 Meta-analysis: Prevention of MDD relapse during continued treatment with antidepressants at their full versus half dose (5 RCTs, $n = 1009$). [Data extracted from: Papakostas, G.I., Perlis, R.H., Seifert, C., & Fava, M. (2007). Antidepressant dose reduction and the risk of relapse in major depressive disorder. *Psychotherapy and Psychosomatics*, 76(5), 266–270.]

Two studies compare decreasing the dose of an antidepressant following remission of symptoms versus placebo-substitution of that antidepressant (Montgomery & Dunbar, 1993; Rouillon *et al.*, 1991 a/b). These studies involve the use of maprotiline (Rouillon *et al.*, 1991 a/b), or paroxetine (Montgomery & Dunbar, 1993), and both demonstrate greater efficacy in preventing depressive relapses following a dose reduction than switching to placebo. Finally, studies examining whether increasing the dose following remission affords greater prophylaxis than maintaining the same dose overall as well as among patients with a history of highly recurrent depression have yet to be conducted.

9.2.4 Continuing adjunctive agents during long-term therapy

The results of post-hoc analyses of uncontrolled (Souza *et al.*, 1990), as well as controlled studies (Reynolds *et al.*, 1996) suggest that discontinuation of adjunctive (to antidepressants) medications (i.e., lithium, perphenazine, or both) results in greater relapse rates than for patients who either remitted without the use of adjunctive treatments (Reynolds *et al.*, 1996) or continued on the adjunctive treatment that brought about remission (Souza *et al.*, 1990).

However, only a handful of trials focus on the long-term efficacy (i.e., relapse prevention) of specific adjunctive treatment strategies for treatment-resistant major depressive disorder (TRD). Three randomized, double-blind, placebo-substitution trials focus on the use of lithium augmentation for TRD. Prien *et al.* (1984/86) randomized 150 patients with unipolar major depression who had remitted following treatment with a combination of imipramine and lithium to either continued treatment with the combination of imipramine and lithium, versus treatment with lithium alone, imipramine alone, or a switch to placebo. The combination of imipramine and lithium was not found to reduce the risk of depressive relapse more so than continued treatment with imipramine monotherapy. Similarly, the results of a small ($n = 12$), double-blind study also do not support the use of continued lithium augmentation versus TCA monotherapy for the long-term prophylaxis of MDD which responded to a TCA-lithium combination (Hardy *et al.*, 1997). Subsequently, however, Bauer *et al.* (2000) conducted a double-blind, placebo-substitution of lithium versus continued treatment with adjunctive lithium among patients who had responded to a combination of antidepressants and lithium, and found greater prophylaxis for lithium- than placebo-treated patients (Fig. 9.5). The results of the latter of these

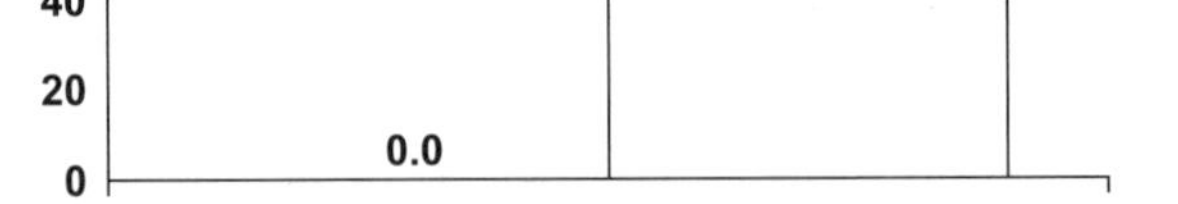

Fig. 9.5 Prevention of MDD relapse with lithium augmentation of antidepressants: A randomized, double-blind study ($n = 30$). [Data extracted from: Bauer, M., Bschor, T., Kunz, D., *et al.* (2000). Double-blind, placebo-controlled trial of the use of lithium to augment antidepressant medication in continuation treatment of unipolar major depression. *American Journal of Psychiatry*, 157, 1429–1435.]

three trials are interesting in light of the evidence that does not conclusively support antidepressant effects for lithium augmentation during the acute-phase of treatment of TRD (also see Chap. 6). Given the proven efficacy of lithium in bipolar depression, one possibility that would account for this discrepancy is the presence of patients with bipolar disorder misclassified as having unipolar depression (i.e., given the proven efficacy of lithium in bipolar but not unipolar depression, one would expect a population of patients diagnosed with unipolar depression, who subsequently remitted following the addition of lithium to their treatment regimen, to be "enriched" with patients with bipolar disorder "misclassified" as unipolar compared to a general population of MDD patients). Interestingly enough, two of these studies report patients diagnosed with "unipolar depression" using standard research screening tools relapsing into mania during the trial (Bauer *et al.*, 2000; Prien *et al.*, 1984/86).

There is a paucity of studies focusing on the long-term efficacy of newer augmentation and combinations strategies. More recently, Rapaport *et al.* (2006) did not report any difference in relapse rates following double-blind, placebo-substitution of risperidone among patients with SSRI-resistant MDD who had improved following risperidone augmentation (Fig. 9.6). Unfortunately, the long-term

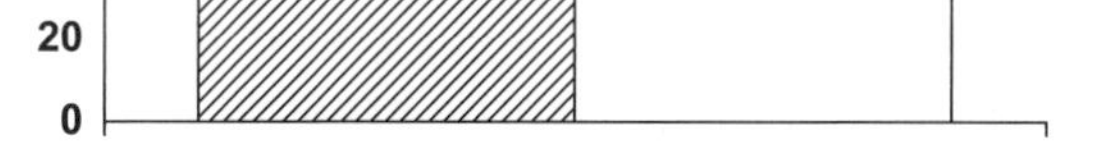

Fig. 9.6 Prevention of MDD relapse during treatment with risperidone augmentation of citalopram (SSRI): A randomized, double-blind study ($n = 241$). [Data extracted from: Rapaport, M.H., Gharabawi, G.M., Canuso, C.M., *et al.* (2006). Effects of risperidone augmentation in patients with treatment-resistant depression: Results of open-label treatment followed by double-blind continuation. *Neuropsychopharmacology*, 31, 2505–2513.]

prophylaxis for other adjunctive strategies discussed in Chaps. 5 or 6 has yet to be studied.

9.2.5 *Instituting antidepressants among non-medicated remitters*

Indirect evidence supporting the notion that un-medicated MDD remitters may benefit from the institution or re-introduction of pharmacotherapy with respect to their long-term prophylaxis comes by way of three studies (Anton *et al.*, 1994; Montgomery *et al.*, 1992/93 and 1998). These three trials compared placebo-remitters who received continuation treatment with placebo with either citalopram-remitters who received continuation treatment with citalopram (Montgomery *et al.*, 1992/93), nefazodone-remitters who received continuation treatment with nefazodone (Anton *et al.*, 1994), TCA-remitters who received continuation treatment with TCAs (Anton *et al.*, 1994; Montgomery *et al.*, 1988), or mirtazapine-remitters who received continuation treatment with mirtazapine (Montgomery *et al.*, 1988). Greater prophylaxis was demonstrated among antidepressant-remitters who continued on antidepressants than placebo-remitters who continued on placebo, suggesting that possibly even placebo-remitters can benefit from prophylaxis with antidepressants. However, it is important to point out that placebo-remitters may differ from un-medicated remitters, the latter group involving patients who either achieved remission following treatment with antidepressants or achieved spontaneous remission of symptoms. In contrast, placebo-remitters achieved symptom improvement following the expectation that they may be receiving active treatment. These data do suggest that the presence of a placebo response does not rule out the possibility of a true benefit from antidepressant treatment in the same subject. This is consistent with the view that patients exposed to antidepressants may respond to placebo effects, true drug effects, or a combination of both.

To date, two studies provide direct evidence suggesting that initiating or re-introducing antidepressant treatment may also benefit unmedicated MDD remitters with respect to their long-term prophylaxis from depressive relapse. Specifically, Bjork *et al.* (1983) and Lepine *et al.* (2004) demonstrated that initiating treatment with zimeldine (Bjork *et al.*, 1983) or sertraline (Lepine *et al.*, 2004) for patients with remitted unipolar major depression who had been unmedicated for at least one (Bjork *et al.*, 1983) or two months (Levine *et al.*, 2004) is more effective than placebo in preventing subsequent relapses.

However, whether patients who have chosen to discontinue treatment for some duration without suffering a depressive relapse benefit from re-instituting the same versus another antidepressant treatment has also not been studied, while the relative benefits of initiating or re-instituting antidepressant treatment for prophylaxis among patients with remitted MDD as a function of either the duration of remission or the time since treatment discontinuation have also not been reported. This information would be especially important in guiding the timing and frequency of follow-up as well as the standard of care for patients with remitted MDD who either decide to discontinue pharmacotherapy or did not receive treatment of their most recent major depressive episode.

9.2.6 *Timing of symptom improvement and risk of relapse*

To date, three studies specifically address whether the timing of clinical response during the acute phase of pharmacotherapy of MDD holds any predictive value with regards to the relative likelihood of experiencing a depressive relapse on continued pharmacotherapy versus placebo-substitution (McGrath *et al.*, 2000; Nierenberg *et al.*, 2004; Stewart *et al.*, 1998). The underlying rationale for these studies is that an early and sustained antidepressant response, defined as improvement which occurs in the first two weeks of treatment that is not followed by subsequent worsening of symptoms, is as likely to occur with placebo as is with antidepressant treatment, while a delayed sustained response (which occurs following at least two weeks of treatment that is not followed by subsequent worsening of symptoms) is more likely to occur with antidepressant than placebo-treatment. According to this hypothesis, patients who experience a delayed onset of clinical response should be more likely to benefit from continued pharmacotherapy than patients who respond within two weeks of initiation of treatment. To date, one of two studies involving the use of fluoxetine (McGrath *et al.*, 2000; Stewart *et al.*, 1998), and one study involving mirtazapine (Nierenberg *et al.*, in 2004) report greater prophylaxis with continued antidepressant treatment than placebo in patients with a delayed sustained response to either fluoxetine or mirtazapine, but not in patients with an early sustained response. However, these studies do not take into account the degree of residual symptomatology during the time of placebo-substitution, which appears to be lower among patients who have had an early sustained response than a late sustained response (Papakostas *et al.*, 2007b). In turn, a lower degree of residual symptoms may explain why there is no difference in drug versus placebo prophylaxis for early responders, since the degree of residual symptoms is known to confer an increased risk of depressive relapse (Faravelli *et al.*, 1986; Kanai *et al.*, 2003; Paykel *et al.*, 1995; Simons *et al.*, 1986). Therefore, the hypothesis that patients who experience a sustained improvement as early as the first two weeks of treatment do not benefit from continued antidepressant treatment needs to be re-tested, stratifying or controlling for depression severity during randomization.

9.2.7 *Treatment-resistance and risk of relapse*

Another question is whether the degree of treatment resistance of a given depressive episode holds any predictive value with regards to subsequent recurrence following clinical improvement that is independent of other possible confounding factors such as residual depression severity. Nierenberg *et al.* (1990) reported a relapse rate as high as 52% over the course of approximately 29 months of follow-up among 66 outpatients with TRD who responded to lithium augmentation of TCAs despite continuation of treatment. Flint and Rifat (2001) report lower relapse rates (67% versus 18%)

among patients who responded to first-line treatment (TCA with or without lithium) and were maintained on that treatment than patients who did not respond to first-line treatment but responded to and were maintained on second-line treatment (MAOI with or without lithium). Similarly, Koran *et al.* (2001) also reported lower relapse rates (51% versus 72%) among patients who responded to and were maintained on a "first-line" treatment (sertraline or imipramine) than patients who did not respond to a first-line treatment but responded to and were maintained on a "second-line" treatment (cross-over between imipramine and sertraline). More recently, using the Sequenced Treatment Alternatives to Relieve Depression (STAR*D) study dataset, Rush *et al.* (2006) also described higher relapse rates among patients who required more treatments to achieve remission of their depressive episode than those who required fewer. That a history of treatment resistance predicts higher chances of relapse during the continuation-maintenance phases of treatment was also confirmed in a large, multi-center study of electroconvulsive therapy (ECT) as continuation-maintenance–phase treatment for MDD (Rasmussen *et al.*, 2009).

Although these studies suggest that treatment resistance confers an increased risk of depressive relapse, it is important to keep in mind that these studies were not designed to answer this specific question. In addition, the treatments used differed, and this may have led to a difference in relapse rates. A prospectively designed study comparing relapse rates among patients with various degrees of treatment resistance who eventually respond to antidepressants of the same class (i.e., switching from one SSRI to another) would be required to control for this confounding factor. In addition, clinician and patient knowledge of the degree of treatment-resistance may also introduce bias. Therefore, both clinician and patient would have to be blinded regarding whether patients responded to the first or second treatment. Switching non-responders to antidepressants of the same class would make such a design more feasible since the risks versus benefits of continuing on one antidepressant versus switching to an equivalent one would be equivalent. Such a study would yield useful knowledge regarding tailoring treatment for MDD patients who achieved remission of symptoms following several treatments (i.e., more frequent follow-up visits, longer follow-up periods, more timely identification and targeting of side effects).

9.3 Treatment of Depressive Relapse/Recurrence

Of the common clinical scenarios that may occur during the natural course of treatment of MDD, perhaps the least is known regarding the pharmacotherapy of depressive relapse. There is anecdotal evidence to suggest increasing the dose to alleviate depressive symptoms in MAOI-(Mann, 1983) and TCA-treated patients (Cohen & Baldessarini, 1985; Zetin *et al.*, 1983) who suffered a depressive relapse. In addition, small open-label trials also report good success following increasing the dose (Fava *et al.*, 1995; Franchini *et al.*, 2000), switching to bupropion (McGrath *et al.*, 2002), or adding bromocriptine (McGrath *et al.*, 1995) for the treatment of depressive relapse in SSRI-treated patients, or switching to SSRIs for the treatment of depressive relapse in TCA-treated patients (Papakostas *et al.*, 2003).

In a larger study ($n = 501$), 57–72% of fluoxetine-remitted patients who subsequently relapsed while on fluoxetine responded following an increase in the dose of fluoxetine (from 20 mg to 40 mg daily or from 90 mg weeks to 90 mg twice a week) (Schmidt *et al.*, 2002), while 62% of fluoxetine-remitters who subsequently relapsed following double-blind, placebo-substitution of fluoxetine responded following re-initiation of fluoxetine (Fava *et al.*, 2002). Very similar results were reported in a similar study involving long-term treatment with duloxetine (Fava *et al.*, 2006). However, double-blind placebo-controlled trials focusing on the efficacy of antidepressants in the treatment of depressive relapse have yet to be published. Similarly, whether it is preferable to treat a depressive relapse with the pharmacologic agent that brought about symptom remission versus switching to a different agent is unknown. In a retrospective chart review, Remillard *et al.* (1994) reported a 57%

response rate when an antidepressant that had successfully been employed in the past was used to treat a given depressive episode, compared to a 65% response rate when a new antidepressant was used. However, double-blind comparator studies on the subject have yet to be conducted.

Chapter 10

Pharmacologic Strategies to Enhance Antidepressant Tolerability

10.1 Adjunctive Therapy

10.1.1 *Sexual dysfunction*

Antidepressant-induced sexual dysfunction is among the most common adverse events reported during treatment with a number of antidepressants (see Chaps. 2–4). A number of agents have been reported to alleviate antidepressant-associated sexual dysfunction in case reports/series or small open-label trials. These agents include antidepressants such as bupropion (Ashton & Rosen, 1998; Chengappa *et al.*, 2001; Gitlin *et al.*, 2002; Labbate & Pollack, 1994; Labbate *et al.*, 1997), mianserin (Dolberg *et al.*, 2002), mirtazapine (Alevizos *et al.*, 2005), trazodone and nefazodone (Michael *et al.*, 1999; Michael & O'Donnell, 2000; Reynolds, 1997; Stryjer *et al.*, 2009), psychostimulants (Bartlik *et al.*, 1995) and other dopaminergic agents such as ropinirole (Worthington *et al.*, 2002), pramipexole (Sporn *et al.*, 2000), amantadine (Balogh *et al.*, 1992; Balon, 1996; Shrivastava *et al.*, 1995), and a host of other drugs including yohimbine (Balon, 1993; Hollander & McCarley, 1992; Jacobson, 1992; Keller Ashton *et al.*, 1997; Price & Grunhaus, 1990), granisetron (Nelson *et al.*, 1997), cyproheptadine (Aizenberg *et al.*, 1995; Arnott & Nutt, 1994; Cohen, 1992; Keller Ashton *et al.*, 1997; Lauerma, 1996; McComick *et al.*, 1990; Sovner, 1984; Steele & Howell, 1986), loratadine (Brubaker, 2002), bethanechol (Gross, 1982), pregabalin (Oulis *et al.*, 2008), and gingko bilboa (Ashton *et al.*, 2000; Cohen & Bartlik, 1998; Ellison and DeLuca, 1998).

A number of case reports (Ashton, 1999; Ashton & Bennett, 1999; Balon, 1998 and 1999; Gupta *et al.*, 1999a and b; Nurnberg *et al.*, 1999a; Rosenberg, 1999; Schaller & Behar, 1999), retrospective chart reviews (Price, 1998), and open-label trials (Damis *et al.*, 1999; Fava *et al.*, 1998; Nurnberg *et al.*, 1999b, c, 2007, and in press; Seidman *et al.*, 2003) also report on the use of adjunct sildenafil for antidepressant-associated sexual dysfunction. These open-label trials report improvements in sexual function in 69–90% of patients following the addition of sildenafil. For verdenafil, there is only a single case report suggesting it may be effective in alleviating SSRI-associated sexual dysfunction (Anghelescu & Urbanek, 2005).

However, only a fraction of these potential treatment strategies have been subject to controlled investigation. The promising, open-label trials involving sildenafil augmentation were soon followed by five double-blind, placebo-controlled trials reporting greater improvement in sexual function among adjunct (to SSRIs, TCAs, venlafaxine) sildenafil- than placebo-treated men with antidepressant-associated sexual dysfunction (Fava *et al.*, 2006a; Nurnberg *et al.*, 2003; Orr *et al.*, 2006; Seidman *et al.*, 2001; Tignol *et al.*, 2004) (Fig. 10.1).

These studies provide strong support suggesting the use of sildenafil augmentation to enhance overall sexual functioning as well as specific-domain functioning (desire, arousal, orgasm) among men with antidepressant-induced sexual dysfunction (Fava *et al.*, 2006a).

More recently, the results of a randomized, double-blind, placebo-controlled trial of sildenafil for the treatment of women with antidepressant-associated sexual dysfunction were also published, and suggested a significantly greater improvement in overall sexual function as well as in some (orgasm, enjoyment) but not other (desire, arousal) specific domains (Nurnberg *et al.*, 2008).

One alternative adjunct strategy to sildenafil for antidepressant-induced sexual dysfunction is bupropion. In fact, adjunct bupropion was found to be the most popular strategy for antidepressant-associated sexual dysfunction in one survey of clinicians (Dording *et al.*, 2003). Initial open-label trials of adjunctive bupropion for antidepressant-associated sexual dysfunction were soon followed

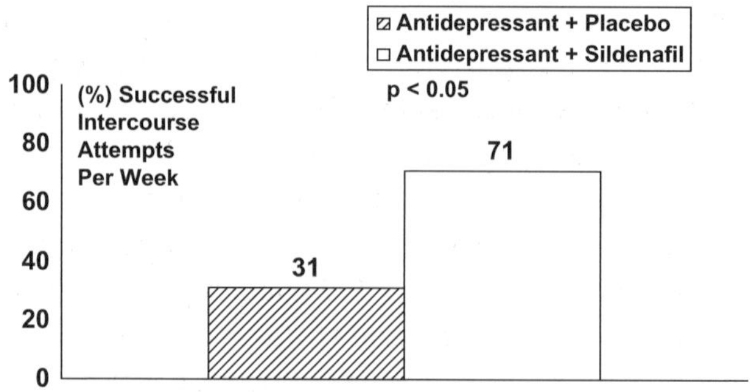

Fig. 10.1 Sildenafil in men with antidepressant-associated erectile dysfunction: A randomized, double-blind study (n = 142). [Data extracted from: Fava, M., Nurnberg, H.G., Seidman, S.N., *et al.* (2006). Efficacy and safety of sildenafil in men with serotonergic antidepressant-associated erectile dysfunction: Results from a randomized, double-blind, placebo-controlled trial. *Journal of Clinical Psychiatry*, 67, 240–246.]

by a negative, probably underpowered and under-dosed double-blind, placebo-controlled trial for bupropion SR (150 mg/day; n = 30; Masand *et al.*, 2001). A subsequent, larger (n = 42; mostly women) double-blind, randomized trial did report bupropion augmentation (300 mg/day) to be more effective than placebo in alleviating some aspects of SSRI-associated sexual dysfunction (desire, but not overall functioning, arousal or orgasm) (Clayton *et al.*, 2004). However, this finding was not replicated by a subsequent study of similar design employing lower doses of bupropion than the study by Clayton *et al.* (Bupropion SR 150 mg, n = 41 — DeBattista *et al.*, 2005a).

The results of a double-blind, randomized trial also suggest significant improvement following the use of 3 gm but not 1.5 gm daily of adjunctive Maca Root (L.Meyenii) for antidepressant-induced sexual dysfunction among women with MDD (Dording *et al.*, 2008). Placebo-controlled trials are pending (clinicaltrials.gov NCT00575328 and 00568126).

There have also been several "negative" double-blind studies on this topic. Michelson *et al.* (2000) randomized 57 women successfully treated with SSRIs but who reported worsening of sexual function during SSRI treatment to receive adjunctive buspirone (15–30 mg), amantadine (50–100 mg) or placebo for eight weeks, and found no difference between the three groups in terms of improvement in sexual functioning. Baldwin *et al.* (2008) randomized men and women who were experiencing SSRI-induced sexual dysfunction to receive adjunctive treatment with either VML-670 (a serotonin 1A-receptor agonist similar to buspirone) or placebo. No difference in the degree of improvement in sexual side effects was noted between the two treatment groups. Similarly, Michelson *et al.* (2002) randomized 118 SSRI-treated women to receive adjunctive mirtazapine (15–30 mg), yohimbine (5.4–10.8 mg), olanzapine (2.5–5 mg) or placebo for six weeks. Again, there was no difference between the four groups in terms of improvement in sexual functioning. Pae *et al.* (2009) reported no difference in sexual functioning among patients with antidepressant-resistant depression who received adjunctive treatment with methylphenidate than placebo. Finally, there are also negative placebo-controlled trials of granisetron (Jespersen *et al.*, 2004; Nelson *et al.*, 2001), ginkgo bilboa (Kang *et al.*, 2002; Wheatley, 2004), and ephedrine (Meston, 2004) for antidepressant-associated sexual dysfunction.

10.1.2 *Fatigue and hypersomnia*

Case reports/series (Berigan, 2001; Even *et al.*, 2004; Holder *et al.*, 2002; Keller-Ashton, 2004; Menza *et al.*, 2000; Nasr, 2004; Schwartz *et al.*, 2002) and small, open-label trials (De Battista *et al.*, 2004; Lundt, 2004; Markovitz & Wagner, 2003; Schwartz *et al.*, 2004a) had initially suggested the potential utility of modafinil augmentation in MDD outpatients with antidepressant-associated or residual fatigue and hypersomnia. Subsequently, two double-blind trials were published. In the first such study, DeBattista *et al.* (2003) examined 136 MDD outpatients with incomplete response to a number of antidepressants who were complaining of fatigue and/or hypersomnia who were then randomized to receive modafinil augmentation (100–400 mg) versus placebo for a total of six weeks. Overall, there was no difference between the two groups at endpoint in terms of improvement in hypersomnia or fatigue. However, a significantly greater improvement in hypersomnia and fatigue scores early on (week 1–2) among modafinil than placebo-treated patients was reported. In the second study, Fava *et al.* (2005) examined 311 MDD outpatients with an incomplete response to an SSRI also complaining of fatigue and hypersomnia who were randomized to receive modafinil augmentation (200 mg) versus placebo for eight weeks. No significant differences in improvement in hypersomnia or fatigue between the two groups were reported. However, a post-hoc analysis recently published on a pooled dataset from the two aforementioned modafinil augmentation studies [Fava *et al.* (2005) and DeBattista *et al.* (2003)] revealed a greater resolution of daytime somnolence but not fatigue among modafinil- than placebo-treated patients (Fava *et al.*, 2007) (Fig. 10.2).

More recently, in a randomized, double-blind, placebo-controlled trial, Dunlop *et al.* (2007) found a greater resolution of lethargic symptoms (hypersomnia symptoms as measured by the Hamilton Depression Rating Scale — HDRS) among MDD patients who received SSRI-modafinil co-therapy than SSRI monotherapy (in contrast to the above-mentioned studies by Fava *et al.* and DeBattista

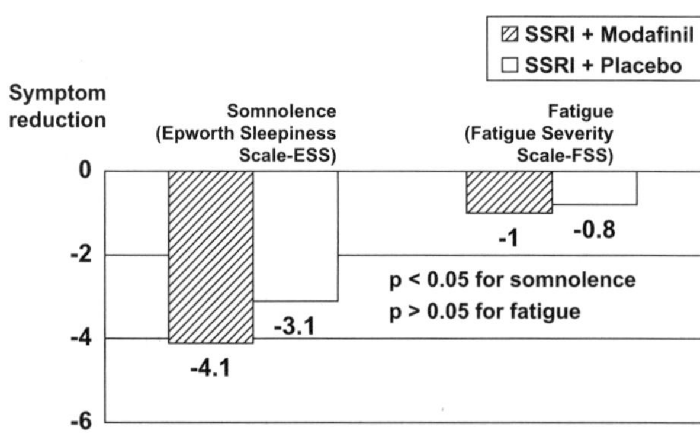

Fig. 10.2 Modafinil augmentation for SSRI-associated somnolence & fatigue: A pooled-analysis of 2 Clinical Trials ($n = 348$). [Data extracted from: Fava, M., Thase, M.E., DeBattista, C., *et al.* (2007). Modafinil augmentation of selective serotonin reuptake inhibitor therapy in MDD partial responders with persistent fatigue and sleepiness. *Annals of Clinical Psychiatry*, 19(3), 153–159.]

et al., modafinil was added at the onset of SSRI treatment rather than at the end of SSRI treatment).

Earlier anecdotal reports (Masand *et al.*, 1998) focusing on the use of psychostimulants for residual or SSRI-associated fatigue were recently confirmed in a randomized, double-blind, placebo-controlled trial. Specifically, Ravindran *et al.* (2008) reported a greater resolution of symptoms of fatigue and apathy among SSRI-treated patients with MDD who received adjunctive methylphenidate than placebo.

Only case reports/series evidence supports the use of adjunct atomoxetine (Papakostas *et al.*, 2006), bupropion (Green, 1997; Schonfeldt-Lecuona *et al.*, 2006) for SSRI-associated fatigue.

10.1.3 *Insomnia, anxiety, and "activation"*

As discussed in Chaps. 2–4, insomnia, anxiety and jitteriness are among the most common adverse events reported during treatment with antidepressants. Amsterdam *et al.* (1994) first reported a significant reduction in jitteriness and anxiety among 54 fluoxetine-treated MDD outpatients who received alprazolam augmentation (0.5–4 mg daily). Subsequently, a double-blind study of clonazepam versus placebo co-initiation with fluoxetine revealed greater improvements in anxiety and insomnia in clonazepam than placebo-treated patients (Londborg *et al.*, 2000), while a double-blind, placebo-controlled trial of eszopiclone and fluoxetine co-initiation revealed a greater resolution of insomnia among eszopiclone- than placebo-treated groups (Fava *et al.*, 2006b) (Fig. 10.3). More recently, co-therapy of MDD with paroxetine and zolpidem (Ji *et al.*, 2007), or escitalopram and zolpidem controlled release (zolpidem CR — Fava *et al.*, 2008) was also found to result in a greater resolution of insomnia than paroxetine or escitalopram monotherapy. In parallel, a double-blind study of zolpidem versus placebo augmentation of SSRIs for patients with SSRI-remitted MDD who continued to experience clinically significant insomnia revealed a greater improvement in quality of sleep among patients treated with adjunctive zolpidem than placebo (Asnis *et al.*, 1999) (Fig. 10.4).

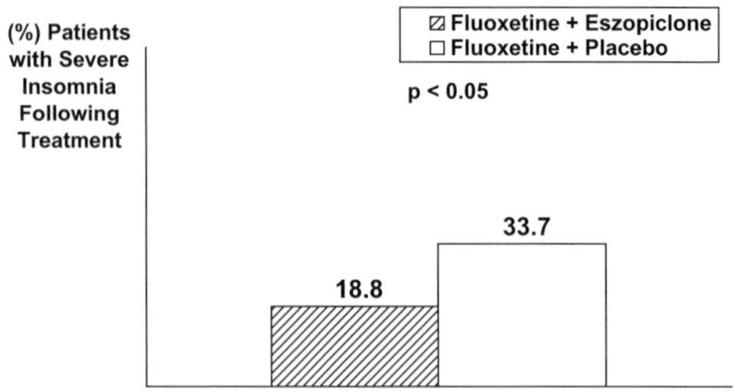

Fig. 10.3 A randomized, double-blind trial of eszopiclone augmentation of fluoxetine: Rates of severe insomnia at the end of treatment ($n = 545$). [Data extracted from: Fava, M., McCall, W.V., Krystal, A., *et al.* (2006). Eszopiclone co-administered with fluoxetine in patients with insomnia coexisting with major depressive disorder. *Biological Psychiatry*, 59, 1052–1060.]

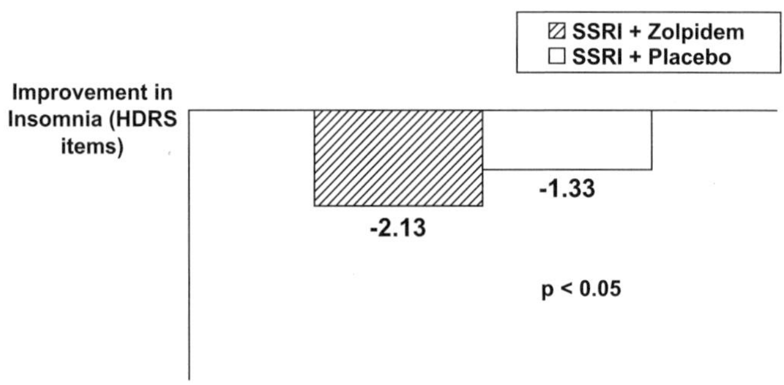

Fig. 10.4 Zolpidem for persistent insomnia in SSRI-treated depressed patients: A randomized, double-blind trial ($n = 190$). HDRS: Hamilton Depression Rating Scale [Data extracted from: Asnis, G.M., Chakraburtty, A., DuBoff, E.A., *et al.* (1999). Zolpidem for persistent insomnia in SSRI-treated depressed patients. *Journal of Clinical Psychiatry*, 60, 668–676.]

The adjunctive use of benzodiazepines for TCA-induced insomnia is supported by several studies including a double-blind, placebo-controlled augmentation study of triazolam with various TCAs for MDD (Cohn, 1983), a double-blind, co-therapy study of alprazolam with desipramine for MDD (Fawcett *et al.*, 1987), and a double-blind co-therapy study of triazolam with imipramine for MDD (Dominguez *et al.*, 1984). Adjunctive treatment with bentazepam was also reported to result in lower anxiety symptoms than placebo in clomipramine-treated MDD patients in one double-blind study (Calcedo Ordonez *et al.*, 1992).

Anecdotal reports supporting the use of melatonin for the treatment of sleep disturbance in depression (Dalton *et al.*, 2000; deVries & Peeters, 1997) were soon followed by a "positive" double-blind, placebo-controlled trial of melatonin (5–10 mg, slow release formulation) as an adjunct to fluoxetine for the treatment of residual sleep disturbance among patients who were fluoxetine-responders or -remitters (Dolberg *et al.*, 1998).

Case reports, and open-label trials (Bertschy *et al.*, 2005; Jacobsen, 1990; Metz & Shader, 1990; Nierenberg & Keck, 1989) also suggest the potential utility of trazodone for antidepressant-associated insomnia, the most popular adjunctive strategy for antidepressant-induced insomnia in one survey of clinicians (Dording *et al.*, 2003). In fact, the results of a double-blind, cross-over study confirmed the utility of this treatment strategy for fluoxetine or bupropion-treated patients experiencing insomnia (Nierenberg *et al.*, 1994).

There is also anecdotal evidence regarding the use of quetiapine, an atypical antipsychotic agent, for the treatment of insomnia associated with phenelzine treatment (Sokolski & Brown, 2006). Gingko bilboa has been reported to increase sleep efficiency and decrease the number of nighttime awakenings in trimipramine-treated patients (Hemmeter *et al.*, 2001). Finally, the results of a randomized clinical trial suggest that co-initiation therapy of escitalopram with cognitive behavioral therapy which specifically targets insomnia in MDD is more effective than escitalopram monotherapy in reducing depressive symptoms overall as well as insomnia specifically (Manber *et al.*, 2008).

To date, only a single open-label study suggesting the potential utility of augmentation of the SSRIs with the atypical neuroleptic aripiprazole for residual anxiety symptoms in MDD has been published (Adson *et al.*, 2005). Similarly, there is an open-label study focusing on the use of adjunctive valproic acid for agitation among SSRI-treated patients with MDD (DeBattista *et al.*, 2005b).

Finally, two double-blind studies suggest greater decreases in symptoms of agitation and hostility among depressed outpatients randomized to receive treatment with a tricyclic antidepressant in addition to a typical neuroleptic than patients treated with a tricyclic antidepressant alone (Rickels *et al.*, 1967 and 1972). These studies have yet to be replicated with the use of newer agents (both antidepressants and atypical antipsychotic agents).

10.1.4 *Akathisia and bruxism*

Akathisia and bruxism are commonly reported during treatment with a number of newer antidepressants (see Chaps. 2–4). A series of reports of adjunctive buspirone for the treatment of bruxism associated with the use of SSRIs or venlafaxine have been published (Bostwick & Jaffee, 1999; Ellison & Stanziani, 1993; Jaffee & Bostwick, 2000; Romanelli *et al.*, 1996; Pavlovic, 2004). In addition, there is anecdotal evidence for the usefulness of the selective β-adrenergic receptor antagonist propranolol for SSRI-induced akathisia (Fleischhacker, 1991; Lipinski *et al.*, 1989). There is also anecdotal evidence to suggest the use of Botulinum toxin type A injections for severe bruxism and dystonia secondary to SSRI use (Chen & Swope, 2005).

10.1.5 *Gastrointestinal symptoms*

Nausea is commonly associated with premature discontinuation of treatment, while the incidence of antidepressant-induced nausea has been reported to range between 20–40% during the course of treatment with newer antidepressants such as the SSRIs, venlafaxine and bupropion (DeVane, 2003). There have been reports of the use of adjunctive 5HT4-selective agonist and cholinergic enhancers cisapride or mosapride in alleviating venlafaxine- (Johnna, 1996) or fluvoxamine-emergent nausea (Ueda *et al.*, 2001). Similarly, there are also reports suggesting the use of the selective 5HT3-receptor antagonist ondasetron for bupropion-emergent nausea (Lara *et al.*, 2001). Finally, there is anecdotal evidence for the use of Gorei-san (TJ-17) (Yamada *et al.*, 1999 and 2003) or mirtazapine (Caldis & Gair, 2004) for the treatment of SSRI-associated nausea.

10.1.6 *Weight gain*

Although the long-term treatment of MDD with a number of antidepressants carries a significant risk of weight gain (see Chaps. 2–4), there is only a single retrospective report (Carpenter *et al.*, 2002), and a small, open-label, short-term study (Van Ameringen *et al.*, 2002) of adjunctive treatment with the anticonvulsant topiramate for SSRI-associated weight gain (Van Ameringen *et al.*, 2002). Similarly, there is only a single case series describing the treatment of SSRI-associated weight gain with the reversible lipase inhibitor orlistat (Schwartz & Beale, 2003).

Ironically, the SSRIs appear to carry a lower risk of weight gain than several other older as well as some newer agents (see Chaps. 2–4). However, only a small ($n = 8$) open-label study of augmentation of TCAs with the opioid-receptor antagonist naltrexone for TCA-induced weight gain has been published to date (Zimmermann *et al.*, 1997), suggesting that naltrexone may attenuate weight loss and decrease food cravings acutely (i.e., eight weeks). Similarly, only a case report focuses on the use of adjunctive orlistat for weight gain in patients treated with the TCAs amitriptyline (Anghelesu *et al.*, 2000) and nortriptyline (Schwartz & Beale, 2003). Finally, a small ($n = 6$) open-label trial examining the potential utility of adjunctive orlistat combined with exercise for antidepressant-associated weight gain has also been published (Schwartz *et al.*, 2004b). Orlistat-treated patients lost an average of 2.5 lb over the course of seven weeks, while an un-blinded control group consisting of five subjects on antidepressants who did not receive orlistat (only exercise) gained an average of 0.5 lb over the course of seven weeks. The difference in weight change between these two groups, however, was not statistically significant. In addition, it is unclear what antidepressant agents these subjects were prescribed.

More recently, the use of the atypical antipsychotic agents has also been expanded for treatment-resistant mood and anxiety disorders (see Chaps. 5 and 6). For the treatment of atypical antipsychotic-induced weight gain, there are case reports/series involving the use of orlistat (Anghelescu *et al.*, 2000; Schwartz & Beale, 2003), the histamine-2 receptor (H-2) antagonist nizatidine (Sacchetti *et al.*, 2000), or the NMDA-receptor antagonist amantadine (Floris *et al.*, 2001; Gracious *et al.*, 2002), as well as open-label trials involving the use of amantadine (Bahk *et al.*, 2004), the norepinephrine-dopamine reuptake inhibitor bupropion (Gadde *et al.*, 2006), the anticonvulsants topiramate (Kim *et al.*, 2006; Levy *et al.*, 2007; Tramontina *et al.*, 2007) and zonisamide (Wang *et al.*, 2008), or the histamine-1 receptor (H-1) agonist/histamine-3-receptor (H-3) antagonist β-histine (Poyurovsky *et al.*, 2005). However, only a fraction of these agents have been subjects of study in randomized, double-blind trials.

Amantadine augmentation of the atypical antipsychotic agent olanzapine was found to be more effective than placebo in attenuating olanzapine-induced weight gain in one double-blind trial (Debert *et al.*, 2004). Three (Baptista *et al.*, 2007; Klein *et al.*, 2006; Wu *et al.*, 2008), but not a fourth (Baptista *et al.*, 2006) double-blind, randomized clinical trials also report adjunctive metformin, an inhibitor of hepatic gluconeogenesis used for the treatment of diabetes mellitus, to be more effective than placebo in preventing olanzapine-induced weight gain. There is also a positive, double-blind study of adjunctive topiramate (anticonvulsant) for olanzapine-related adiposity in women (Nickel *et al.*, 2005). However, neither adjunctive famotidine, nizatadine (H-2 antagonists) (Cavazzoni *et al.*, 2003; Poyurovsky *et al.*, 2004), nor sibutramine (serotonin-norepinephrine-dopamine reuptake inhibitor) (Henderson *et al.*, 2006) were more effective than placebo in limiting olanzapine-induced weight gain. Finally, there is also evidence suggesting a potential role for diet, exercise and/or nutritional education (Alvarez-Jimenez *et al.*, 2006; Kwon *et al.*, 2006; Milano *et al.*, 2007; Scocco *et al.*, 2006) in the prevention of olanzapine-induced weight gain.

10.1.7 *Anticholinergic and other side effects*

A number of case reports or small open-label trials focus on the use of cholinergic agents (i.e., bethanechol, pilocarpine) and cholinesterase inhibitors (i.e., donepezil) in the management of

TCA- or SSRI-related dry mouth and constipation (Jacobsen & Comas-Diaz, 1999), the α-2 adrenergic antagonist yohimbine for TCA-associated xerostomia (Bagheri *et al.*, 1992 and 1994; Rispail *et al.*, 1990) and orthostasis (Hyatt & Messer, 1986; Lacomblez *et al.*, 1989; Lecrubier *et al.*, 1981; Seibyl *et al.*, 1989), and the selective α-adrenergic agonist midodrine for TCA-associated orthostasis (Maskall & Lam, 1993). A small double-blind study comparing yohimbine with the secretagogue anetholtrithione for TCA-induced xerostomia reported greater increases in salivary flow during treatment with yohimbine than anetholtrithione (Bagheri *et al.*, 1997).

For other adverse events, there are case reports of the anticholinergic benztropine for venlafaxine-induced night sweats (Pierre & Guze, 2000), and of selective α-adrenergic receptor antagonists for reboxetine-associated dysuria and urinary hesitancy (Demyttenaire *et al.*, 2001; Demyttenaire & Huygens, 2002; Kasper, 2002; Kasper & Wolf, 2002). There is also a case report of adjunct valproate for the prophylaxis of migraines associated with SSRI use (Delva *et al.*, 1999).

10.1.8 *Cognitive side effects*

Cholinesterase inhibitors such as donepezil have been used anecdotally for the management of antidepressant-related memory loss (Jacobsen & Comes-Diaz, 1999), although the results of a small, randomized, double-blind, placebo-controlled trial focusing on the use of adjunctive galantamine for the improvement of cognition in patients with antidepressant-remitted MDD did not demonstrate greater improvements in cognitive functioning among galantamine- than placebo-treated patients (Elgamal & MacQueen, 2008).

10.2 Switching Antidepressants Due to Intolerance

An alternative strategy to targeting side effects with adjunctive pharmacotherapeutic approaches is to switch to a different agent altogether. This practice, however, is grossly understudied. Specifically, open-label trials focusing on the acute phase of treatment support switching from one SSRI to another (Brown & Harrison, 1995; Calabrese *et al.*, 2003; Schaefer *et al.*, 2004; Thase *et al.*, 1997 and 2002; Zarate *et al.*, 1996). A second SSRI trial appears to be reasonably effective and well tolerated in these cases, with rates of discontinuation due to intolerance ranging from 0% to roughly 10% in these studies. Double-blind studies have yet to be conducted. There is also an open-label study describing switching from an SSRI or venlafaxine to duloxetine due to intolerance, which also reports similarly low rates of discontinuation due to intolerance (Wohlreich *et al.*, 2005). In addition, very few studies have focused on switching from one agent or class of agents to another due to a specific adverse event. To date, there are only two open-label trials focusing on switching to bupropion for SSRI-associated sexual dysfunction (Dobkin *et al.*, 2006; Walker *et al.*, 1993). Both report an improvement in sexual functioning and depressive symptoms following the switch. Finally, even less is known regarding the practice of switching from one agent to another during the continuation and maintenance phase in remitted patients. In a small chart review, Posternak and Zimmerman (2002) reported a 0% relapse rate among nine (mostly SSRI-treated) remitted patients switched to another SSRI or a non-SSRI antidepressant.

Summary and Conclusion of Part III

An ever-growing number of studies reporting on the prophylactic effects of long-term pharmacotherapy for Major Depressive Disorder (MDD) make a compelling argument for the need for long-term pharmacotherapy for MDD. As a result, it is becoming increasingly apparent to clinicians and patients alike that the long-term compliance with treatment is necessary in order to successfully recover from MDD and restore the pre-morbid level of functioning. The sum of the literature focusing on this topic suggests several factors to be highly relevant with regards to therapeutic decisions involving the prevention and treatment of MDD relapse/recurrence.

1. Tolerability is a critical factor in determining the optimal continuation/maintenance dose. A dose reduction appears to be associated with an increase in relapse rate, although it is preferable to decrease the antidepressant dose versus discontinuing the antidepressant altogether.
2. A history of multiple depressive relapse/recurrences, particularly while on an antidepressant therapy, is an important factor in determining the optimal duration of follow-up therapy. The optimal duration of continuation/maintenance therapy is nine months (of sustained remission), although patients with recurrent depression may benefit from longer treatment durations.
3. A history of treatment-resistance or -refractoriness is an important factor in determining the follow-up interval. Patients with resistant depression are at higher risk for MDD relapse/recurrence and, therefore, should be followed more closely (shorter durations of follow-up intervals).
4. Although there is a paucity of data on the topic, it is recommended to continue adjunctive therapy following remission of symptoms for, at least, 6–9 months. Adjunctive therapy may then be withdrawn before the antidepressant is withdrawn.
5. Although there is a paucity of data on the topic, patients who suffer from a depressive relapse/recurrence may benefit from an increase in antidepressant dose.

In light of the overwhelming evidence supporting a critical role for continued pharmacotherapy treatment among MDD remitters in order to prevent a depressive relapse, improving antidepressant tolerability in order to facilitate treatment adherence is of paramount importance when treating MDD. During the course of the past few years, there appears to be a dramatic increase in the number of controlled trials focusing on the use of adjunctive pharmacotherapeutic strategies in order to alleviate a number of side effects of the antidepressants. The majority of these studies focus on the treatment of antidepressant-induced sexual dysfunction, insomnia, anxiety, fatigue, and hypersomnia. Of these, sildenafil augmentation for antidepressant-induced sexual dysfunction in men (desire, arousal, and orgasm dysfunction), adjunctive benzodiazepines or other GABA-ergic agents for antidepressant-induced anxiety and insomnia, and metformin for antipsychotic-induced weight gain appear to be best supported strategies, with several positive, double-blind, placebo-controlled studies each. There is preliminary evidence to support the use of adjunctive sildenafil in women with antidepressant-associated sexual dysfunction (orgasm dysfunction). For bupropion augmentation in sexual dysfunction, there is one positive (300 mg daily dose; greater resolution of decreased desire but not arousal or orgasm dysfunction), and two negative studies (150 mg daily dose). Negative double-blind, placebo-controlled studies have been published on the use of adjunctive buspirone, amantadine, mirtazapine, yohimbine, olanzapine, granisetron, ephedrine, and gingko bilboa for antidepressant-induced sexual dysfunction.

Melatonin and trazodone appear promising for SSRI-associated insomnia, although evidence supporting their use has yet to be replicated. Modafinil augmentation appears to be effective in hypersomnia but not fatigue among patients with depression, while there also appears to be a role for methylphenidate augmentation of SSRIs for fatigue and apathy in MDD.

Despite the dramatic increase in double-blind studies, numerous practices, many of which appear promising, have yet to be subject to controlled comparison. A sustained effort in conducting controlled trials of adjunctive pharmacotherapeutic strategies for antidepressant-associated adverse events and educating clinicians regarding the timely identification, and evidence-based treatment of such adverse events is necessary in order to improve the standard of care for depression. In general, clinicians should take into consideration the following elements when deciding to target antidepressant-associated adverse events:

1. Ensuring that symptoms reported do, indeed, represent side effects rather than a partial recurrence of major depressive disorder, since the management of these two conditions differs. A late emergence of symptoms (with respect to the time an antidepressant agent was prescribed or increased in dose, the intensity of which progressively strengthens in the absence of dose-escalation) may signify a partial depressive relapse/recurrence. In contrast, early emerging symptoms, the intensity of which appears to be dose-related, may represent adverse events.
2. The tolerability profile of the adjunctive agent used to target antidepressant-associated adverse events: it is important to ensure that the side effects of the adjunctive drug employed do now outweight the side effect of the antidepressant.
3. The likelihood of drug–drug interactions when adding a drug to target an adverse event: increased antidepressant levels may further compound side effects, while decreased levels may contribute to a depressive relapse/recurrence.
4. Compliance: in general, it is easier for patients to remember to take fewer pills.

Part IV

Future Directions in Treatment Development

Over the last few decades, the monoamine theory of depression has guided the discovery and development of dozens of new treatments for major depressive disorder (MDD) (Part I of this book). Thus, at the present time, the vast majority of both initial (first-line) as well as subsequent treatment strategies for MDD focus on the use of monoaminergic agents (either alone, in sequence, or in combination), with the addition of a few non-monoaminergic agents as adjuncts; the efficacy, tolerability and safety of which is poorly understood. Due to their established efficacy, tolerability, and long-term safety, psychiatrists will, undoubtedly, continue to largely rely on monoamine–based treatments for MDD in the near future. However, there is emerging evidence suggesting a potential role for non-monoaminergic–based treatments as monotherapies for MDD. These studies offer promise for the development of novel treatments for depression, and are reviewed in the fourth and final section of this book.

Specifically, Chap. 11 focuses on drugs that act on non-monoaminergic neurotransmitter systems (γ-aminobutyric acid, acetylcholine, glutamate, glycine, etc.), Chap. 12 on drugs that act on the various neuroendocrine axes (adrenal, gonadal, thyroid, etc.), and Chap. 13 on drugs that influence human metabolism (one carbon cycle, acetylation, second messenger systems, omega-3 and -6 fatty acids, etc.) as well as drugs with a mechanism of action that is now well understood (modafinil, hypericum perforatum). Finally, Part IV concludes with Chap. 14, which describes studies focusing on a different approach to treatment development: discovering biologic variables (predictors, moderators, or mediators of response) that can help us "decipher" the underlying biological process of illness and symptom recovery in MDD. Such insights may, in turn, lead to the development of more effective antidepressants as well as help us improve our ability to select individual-based treatments for MDD that would result in superior outcome than random selection.

Chapter 11

Agents Operating on Non-monoaminergic Neurotransmitter Systems

11.1 GABA-ergic Treatments

11.1.1 *Benzodiazepines*

11.1.1.1 *Clinical evidence*

Benzodiazepine drugs bind to the γ-aminobutyric acid (GABA)-A receptor (an ionotropic receptor) and, thereby, reversibly inhibit the closing of a chloride channel, resulting in an augmentation of chloride ion cellular efflux (Obata & Yamahura, 1988). Benzodiazepines do not possess any direct monoaminergic activity (i.e., affinity for monoamine receptors or transporters). To date, over 36 double-blind studies comparing the benzodiazepines as monotherapy to placebo for the treatment of depressive disorders have been published. (Feighner *et al.*, 1979, 1983a and b; Laakman *et al.*, 1995; Lipman *et al.*, 1986; Mendels *et al.*, 1986; Raskin *et al.*, 1974; Rickels *et al.*, 1970, 1985, 1987 and 1991; Tyrer *et al.*, 1988; Weissman *et al.*, 1992) and/or standard antidepressants (Ansseau *et al.*, 1984 and 1991; Banerji *et al.*, 1989; Ceskova *et al.*, 1989; Eriksson *et al.*, 1987; Fawcett *et al.*, 1987; Feighner *et al.*, 1979, 1983a and b; Goldberg *et al.*, 1986; Hamouz *et al.*, 1980; Hubain *et al.*, 1990; Imlah *et al.*, 1985; Johnson *et al.*, 1979; Laakman *et al.*, 1995; Lapierre *et al.*, 1994; Laws *et al.*, 1990; Lemoine *et al.*, 1991; Lenox *et al.*, 1984; Lipman *et al.*, 1986; Martins, 1966; Mendels *et al.*, 1986; Montgomery *et al.*, 1970; Overall *et al.*, 1987; Raskin *et al.*, 1974; Remick *et al.*, 1985 and 1988; Richards *et al.*, 1982;Rickels *et al.*, 1970, 1973, 1985, 1987 and 1991; Rush *et al.*, 1985; Russell *et al.*, 1978; Singh *et al.*, 1988; Tiller *et al.*, 1989a/b; Tyrer *et al.*, 1988; Verner, 1969; Weissman *et al.*, 1992). In fact, there are more double-blind studies of benzodiazepines as monotherapy for depression than for any other non-monoaminergic agent as well as for many standard monoaminergic–based treatments.

A number of these studies, however, either include a large proportion of patients with psychotic symptoms (Ceskova *et al.*, 1989; Laakman *et al.*, 1995; Lenox *et al.*, 1984; Raskin *et al.*, 1974; Verner, 1969), or include patients with anxiety but not depressive disorders (Martins, 1966; Montgomery *et al.*, 1970; Rickels *et al.*, 1970; Tyrer *et al.*, 1988) in their study population. Others either do not sufficiently define the depressive disorder studied (Laws *et al.*, 1990), or do not sufficiently measure depressive symptoms (Imlah *et al.*, 1985). The remaining trials are outlined in Tables 11.1 [placebo and tricyclic antidepressant (TCA)-controlled], 11.2 (TCA comparator only), and 11.3 (other antidepressant as comparator).

Of the nine placebo-controlled studies listed in Table 11.1, six involve the use of alprazolam, two involve the use of diazepam and two the use of chlordiazepoxide (Rickels *et al.*, 1987 involves both alprazolam and diazepam). Five studies involving alprazolam, one involving chlordiazepoxide, and one involving diazepam demonstrate a greater reduction of depressive symptom severity among benzodiazepine- than placebo-treated patients. In addition, of 29 TCA-benzodiazepine comparisons (Fig. 11.1), 20 report no difference in the degree of depressive symptom resolution between the two treatment groups at endpoint, while nine report TCAs to be superior in efficacy to the benzodiazepines.

Whether benzodiazepines and TCAs exert similar antidepressant effects on all depressive symptoms or symptom clusters remains unclear. A post-hoc analysis of a double-blind, placebo-controlled trial comparing alprazolam with imipramine reported that alprazolam-treated patients demonstrated the largest effect sizes on symptoms of middle insomnia, late insomnia, psychic and somatic anxiety, and depersonalization, while imipramine-treated

Table 11.1 Double-blind, placebo-controlled studies of benzodiazepine monotherapy for major depression.

Study	N/Duration	Agents	Results[a]
Feighner *et al.*, 1979	279 4 weeks	Chlordiazepoxide 40–60 mg Amitriptyline 100–150 mg Both combined at above doses	B + TCA > B = TCA = Pbo week 1 B + TCA > B = TCA > Pbo week 2, 4
Feighner *et al.*, 1983a	129 6 weeks	Alprazolam 0.5–4.5 mg Imipramine 25–225 mg	Alprazolam > Pbo week 1, 2, 4, 6 Imipramine > Pbo week 2, 4, 6 Alprazolam = TCA throughout
Feighner *et al.*, 1983b	723 6 weeks	Alprazolam 0.5–4.5 mg Imipramine 25–225 mg	Alprazolam > Pbo week 2, 4, 6 Imipramine > Pbo week 2, 4, 6 Alprazolam > TCA week 2 only
Rickels *et al.*, 1985	504 6 weeks	Alprazolam 0.5–4.5 mg Doxepin 25–225 mg Amitriptyline 25–225 mg	Alprazolam > Pbo week 1, 4, 6 Amitriptyline > Pbo week 1, 4, 6 Doxepin > Pbo week 1, 4, 6 B = TCA1 = TCA2 throughout
Lipman *et al.*, 1986	425 8 weeks	Chlordiazepoxide 30–60 mg Imipramine 75–150 mg	Chlordiazepoxide > Pbo wk 1 but not wk 8 Imipramine > Pbo week 8 Chlordiazepoxide > TCA week 1 but TCA > Chlordiazepoxide week 8

(*Continued*)

Table 11.1 *(Continued)*

Study	*N*/Duration	Agents	Results[a]
Mendels *et al.*, 1986	79	Alprazolam1–5 mg	Alprazolam > Pbo week 6
	6 weeks	Imipramine 25–225 mg	Imipramine > Pbo week 6
			Alprazolam = Imipramine weeks 1–6.
Rickels *et al.*, 1987	241	Alprazolam 0.5–4.5 mg	Alprazolam > Pbo week 1, 4 and week 6
	6 weeks	Diazepam 5–45 mg	Diazepam > Pbo week 1 but not week 4, 6
		Imipramine 25–225 mg	TCA > Pbo week 4, 6
			TCA = Alprazolam > Diazepam week 6
Rickels *et al.*, 1991	259	Adinazolam 10–60 mg	Adinazolam > Pbo week 2 but not week 6
	6 weeks	Imipramine 25–150 mg	Diazepam > Pbo week 2 and week 6
		Diazepam 5–30 mg	TCA > Pbo week 6
			TCA > Diazepam = Adinazolam week 6
Weissman *et al.*, 1992	35	Alprazolam 1.5–4.5 mg	Alprazolam > TCA week 2 but B = TCA week 6
	6 weeks	Imipramine 75–225 mg	Alprazolam > Pbo week 1,2 but not week 6
			TCA > Pbo week 2 but not week 6

Abbreviations: B = benzodiazepine, TCA = tricyclic antidepressant, Pbo = placebo.
[a]Difference in change in depression severity during treatment.

Table 11.2 Double-blind studies of benzodiazepine monotherapy in major depression with TCA comparator (no placebo control).

Study	*N*/Duration	Treatments	Results[a]
Rickels *et al.*, 1973	138 4 weeks	Amitriptyline 25–100 mg Diazepam 5–20 mg Phenobarbital 30–120 mg	Diazepam = TCA = Phenobarbital week 4
Johnson *et al.*, 1979	66 4 weeks	Nortriptyline 75–150 mg Diazepam 7.5–15 mg	Diazepam = TCA week 1, 2, 3, 4
Annseau *et al.*, 1984	126 6 weeks	Doxepin 50–225 mg Alprazolam 1–4.5 mg	Alprazolam = TCA week 1, 2, 4, 6
Remick *et al.*, 1985	54 6 weeks	Desipramine 75–225 mg Alprazolam 1.5–4.5 mg	Alprazolam = TCA week 6
Rush *et al.*, 1985	49 6 weeks	Imipramine 25–300 mg Alprazolam 0.5–6 mg	TCA > Alprazolam week 6
Goldberg *et al.*, 1986	60 6 weeks	Imipramine 25–225 mg Alprazolam 0.5–4.5 mg	Alprazolam = TCA week 6
Eriksson *et al.*, 1987	81 6 weeks	Amitrityline 25–225 mg Alprazolam 0.5–4.5 mg	Alprazolam = TCA week 1, 2, 4, 6
Overall *et al.*, 1987	90 6 weeks	Imipramine 75–300 mg Alprazolam 1.5–6 mg	Alprazolam > TCA week 1, 2 but not week 4, 6

(*Continued*)

Table 11.2 *(Continued)*

Study	*N*/Duration	Treatments	Results[a]
Fawcett *et al.*, 1987	79 6 weeks	Alprazolam 1–6 mg Desipramine 50–300 mg Both combined at above doses	B > TCA = B + TCA week 1 B = TCA = B + TCA week 2, 4, 6
Remick *et al.*, 1988	52 6 weeks	Desipramine 25–225 mg Alprazolam 0.5–4.5 mg	Alprazolam > TCA week 2 but not 4, 6
Singh *et al.*, 1988	130 6 weeks	Amitriptyline 25–225 mg Alprazolam 0.5–4.5 mg	Alprazolam > TCA weeks 1, 2, 3 but not weeks 4, 5, 6
Banerji *et al.*, 1989	104 4 weeks	Amitriptyline 50–150 mg Alprazolam 1–3 mg	TCA > Alprazolam week 1, 2 but not week 4
Hubain *et al.*, 1990	30 6 weeks	Amitriptyline 100–125 mg Alprazolam 4–9 mg	TCA > Alprazolam week 3, 4 but not week 6
Annseau *et al.*, 1991	66 4 weeks	Amitriptyline 150–225 mg Diazepam 30–45 mg	TCA > Diazepam week 4
Lemoine *et al.*, 1991	118 6 weeks	Prazepam 20–60 mg Clomipramine 75–150 mg	Prazepam = TCA week 1, 2, 3, 4
Lapierre *et al.*, 1994	43 6 weeks	Alprazolam 20–60 mg Amitriptyline 75–150 mg	Alprazolam < TCA week 6

Abbreviations: B = benzodiazepine, TCA = tricyclic antidepressant.
[a]Difference in change in depression severity during treatment.

Table 11.3 Double-blind studies of benzodiazepine monotherapy in major depression with other active comparators (no placebo control).

Study	*N*/Duration	Treatments	Results[a]
Russell *et al.*, 1978	46 3 weeks	Diazepam 20–40 mg Mianserin 40–80 mg	Mianserin > Diazepam week 3
Hamouz *et al.*, 1980	80 4 weeks	Diazepam 20–40 mg Mianserin 40–80 mg	Mianserin > Diazepam week 2, 3, 4
Richards *et al.*, 1982	93 6 weeks	Diazepam 15–30 mg Mianserin 60–120 mg Trazodone 100–200 mg	Diazepam = Mianserin = Trazodone week 1, 2, 4, 8
Tiller *et al.*, 1989a and b	28 8 weeks	Diazepam 15–45 mg Moclobemide 150–450 mg	Diazepam > MAOI week 1, 4 but not week 8 ($p = 0.058$)

Abbreviation: MAOI = monoamine oxidase inhibitor.
[a]Difference in change in depression severity during treatment.

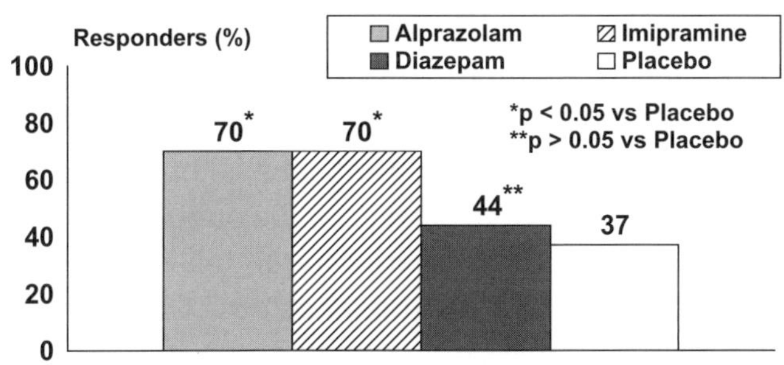

Fig. 11.1 Alprazolam, diazepam, and imipramine (TCA) for major depression: A randomized, double-blind study ($n = 147$). [Data extracted from: Rickels, K., Chung, H.R., Csanalosi, I.B., *et al.* (1987). Alprazolam, diazepam, imipramine, and placebo in outpatients with major depression. *Archives of General Psychiatry*, 44, 862–866.]

patients demonstrated the largest effect sizes for dysphoria, guilt, hopelessness, helplessness, psychic anxiety and somatic anxiety (Leon *et al.*, 1993). However, none of the 11 studies in which benzodiazepines were reported to be as effective as TCAs overall that also employed a specific measure of anxiety [i.e., the Hamilton anxiety rating scale (HARS — Hamilton, 1959) or the Covi anxiety scale (Covi *et al.*, 1979)] demonstrated greater anxiolysis among benzodiazepine than TCA-treated patients (Annseau *et al.*, 1984; Eriksson *et al.*, 1987; Fawcett *et al.*, 1987; Feighner *et al.*, 1983a and b; Goldberg *et al.*, 1986; Johnson *et al.*, 1979; Lemoine *et al.*, 1991; Mendels *et al.*, 1986; Singh *et al.*, 1988; Weissman *et al.*, 1992).

Relatively few studies compare benzodiazepines to antidepressants other than the TCAs (Table 11.3). Specifically, two studies report mianserin to be more effective than diazepam in the treatment of depression (Hamouz *et al.*, 1980; Russel *et al.*, 1978), while a third reports diazepam to be as effective as mianserin and trazodone (Richards *et al.*, 1982). A fourth study suggests earlier improvement in depressive symptoms among patients treatsed with diazepam than moclobemide, with no significant difference in antidepressant efficacy between treatments at endpoint (Tiller *et al.*, 1989a and b). However, in the latter study, seven patients on moclobemide required initiation of adjunctive treatment with the benzodiazepine nitrazepam (5–10 mg) for insomnia during the trial, which may have served to attenuate any difference in efficacy between the two agents at endpoint. Studies comparing benzodiazepines to selective serotonin reuptake inhibitors (SSRIs) or newer antidepressants for depressive disorders have yet to be published. Finally, aside from a small ($n = 5$) open-label trial involving the use of baclofen (Post *et al.*, 1991), the role of the metabotropic GABA-B receptor in depression remains, to date, unexplored.

In summary, the majority of studies report greater efficacy following treatment with benzodiazepines than placebo for unipolar depression, and equivalent efficacy between benzodiazepine and antidepressant comparators. In fact, in a meta-analysis of double-blind clinical trials of benzodiazepines for depression, Petty *et al.* (1995) conclude that alprazolam, the best studied of the benzodiazepines in depression, was superior to placebo and equivalent to the TCAs in efficacy, and may possess a more rapid onset of antidepressant action than the TCAs. However, the authors noted that studies do not support antidepressant effects for diazepam and chlordiazepoxide. One possible explanation for this discrepancy may be due to the relatively smaller number of studies for diazepam and chlordiazepoxide compared to alprazolam. Alternatively, Petty *et al.* (1995) raise the possibility that, given the differences in receptor affinity for these agents, doses of alprazolam, diazepam, and chlordiazepoxide used in their respective studies may not have been equivalent. Specifically, while alprazolam has been assumed to be 10 times more potent than diazepam and 50 times more potent than chlordiazepoxide *in vitro*, placebo-controlled studies of chlordiazepoxide employ dose ranges of 30–60 mg daily while diazepam studies employ maximum doses of 5–45 mg (Johnson *et al.*, 1979; Rickels *et al.*, 1973). However, the usual dosing for alprazolam in placebo-controlled studies was as high as 0.5–4.5 mg daily. Therefore, while this argument would explain why results for chlordiazepoxide were at best modest, the same cannot be said for diazepam. Nevertheless, further studies involving multiple-dose comparisons for the various benzodiazepines would address this issue.

A third possible explanation may be due to the relatively rapid time from ingestion to peak plasma concentration for alprazolam which is just over one hour (Greenblatt & Wright, 1993). Since benzodiazepine administration has been reported to increase dopaminergic transmission as a result of suppression of GABA-ergic inhibitory tone (Dewey *et al.*, 1992 and 1997), a more rapid increase in dopaminergic tone may result in greater euphoric effects in alprazolam than chlordiazepoxide-treated patients, although this would not explain the findings from studies involving diazepam, an agent with an equivalent time to peak plasma concentration as alprazolam (Friedman *et al.*, 1992). Finally, these agents may differ in their relative affinity for various GABA-A receptor subtypes (Sieghart, 1995), the relevance of which will be discussed in the following paragraphs.

11.1.1.2 *Treatment limitations*

Despite the evidence supporting a potential role for benzodiazepine monotherapy for the treatment of depression, several factors prohibit their use as first-, second-, or third-line agents, including the fact that none of these drugs has received a depression indication from the U.S. Food and Drug Administration (FDA). The most obvious is the lack of continuation and maintenance-phase data for the treatment of depression: although it is clear that some of these drugs may help resolve depressive symptoms in the short term, their long-term efficacy, safety and tolerability remains to be established. Other factors include: (1) their abuse potential (Woods *et al.*, 1992), (2) their potential for developing tolerance (Woods *et al.*, 1992) to some of their physiologic (Fujita *et al.*, 1999; Roy-Byrne *et al.*, 1993) and clinical effects (i.e., sedation, alertness, memory function, verbal learning — Fujita *et al.*, 1999; Roy-Byrne *et al.*, 1993) and, thereby the theoretical potential of perhaps developing tolerance to their antidepressant effects, and (3) concerns pertaining to the risks associated with abrupt withdrawal of sub-chronic and chronic treatment such as rebound anxiety, insomnia, upset stomach, tremors and, rarely seizures, particularly following discontinuation of benzodiazepines with relatively shorter half-lives (Chouinard, 2004; Rickels *et al.*, 1990; Schweizer *et al.*, 1990).

Whether or not patients demonstrate tolerance to any antidepressant effects of the benzodiazepines could, potentially, be examined in long-term clinical studies. However, in addition to posing clinical risks, the potential for benzodiazepine withdrawal may also pose obstacles when designing relapse prevention studies for depression (which often employ the double-blind, placebo-substitution study design illustrated in Chap. 10). In light of this, relapse prevention studies specifically designed for benzodiazepine or benzodiazepine-like agents for depression could, alternatively, compare patients randomized to continue on the same benzodiazepine dose versus being randomized to a gradual dose tapering of the benzodiazepine, rather than abrupt placebo-substitution. Finally, yet another limitation of treatment with benzodiazepines is their sedating effect.

In fact, it appears that considerable sedation with the benzodiazepines is achieved at receptor occupancies much lower (i.e., 15–27%; Abadie *et al.*, 1996; Fujita *et al.*, 1999; Innis *et al.*, 1991; Shinotoh *et al.*, 1989; Viebaek *et al.*, 1993) than those required in order for these agents to demonstrate maximal effects on cerebral glucose metabolism, reported to occur at approximately 40% receptor occupancy (Ishizuka *et al.*, 1989).

11.1.1.3 *Neuropharmacology of GABA-A receptors*

GABA-A receptors are composed of a combination of five subunits (Barnard *et al.*, 1998). A large number of different subunit types have been identified to date (i.e., α- 1–5, β- 1–4, γ- 1–3, δ, ε, π, ρ- 1–3), with the subunit composition of various GABA-A receptors in the human brain appearing to vary depending on the brain region within which they are located (Bernard *et al.*, 1998). For example, the α-1 subtype appears to be the most widely distributed in the human brain (Abadie *et al.*, 1996; Maeda *et al.*, 2003) and, primarily, appears to mediate the sedating effects of the benzodiazepines or benzodiazepine-like agents. Other receptor subtypes appear to be distributed in a more region-specific manner.

Classical benzodiazepines including diazepam, clonazepam, triazolam, alprazolam bind with equivalent affinity to the α-1, α-2, α-3, and α-5 subtypes (Sanna *et al.*, 2002; Sieghart, 1995), while agents designed as hypnotics such as zolpidem, zaleplon, and eszopiclone, bind to the α-1 subtype with much greater affinity than the α-2 or α-3 subtype, and have no affinity for the α-5 subtype (Sanna *et al.*, 2002).

Administration of classical benzodiazepines as well as relatively α-1-selective agents has been shown to result in wide-spread binding to benzodiazepine receptors in many cortical, limbic and striatal areas (Fujita *et al.*, 1999; Maeda *et al.*, 2002; McLeod *et al.*, 2002; Shintoh *et al.*, 1996), resulting in a global, non-selective reduction in brain metabolism (de Wit *et al.*, 1991; Gillin *et al.*, 1996; Mintzer *et al.*, 2001; Roy-Byrne *et al.*, 1993; Volkow *et al.*, 1995 and 1998; Wang *et al.*, 2000). In fact, the classical benzodiazepines appear to have their greatest effects in reducing CNS metabolism in the thalamus (Volkow *et al.*, 1995 and 1998), an area implicated in the mediation of the sedative effects of benzodiazepines (Volkow *et al.*, 1995 and 1998; Wang *et al.*, 2000) rather than cortico-limbic areas thought to be principally involved in mood regulation (Phillips *et al.*, 2003a and b).

Of perhaps greatest relevance to the development of treatments for mood as well as substance-use disorders is the α-5 GABA-A receptor subtype. α-5 receptors are found in greatest concentrations in areas involved in the regulation of mood (Phillips *et al.*, 2003a and b) such as the anterior cingulate, the hippocampus, the insular cortex, as well as brain areas involved in the development of drug addiction including the anterior portion of the ventral striatum where the nucleus accumbens, a key structure in the mesolimbic reward system, is located (Lingford-Hughes, 2002; Maeda *et al.*, 2002; McLeod *et al.*, 2002). Animal studies suggest that administration of selective α-5 receptor antagonists may, in fact, antagonize ethanol's neurobehavioral effects (McKay *et al.*, 2004), while selective α-5 receptor inverse agonists have been reported to improve cognition in animals (Chambers *et al.*, 2003). Such effects may be related to the presence of α-5 receptors in the nucleus accumbens and hippocampus, respectively. Therefore, agents which serve as mixed agonists/antagonists for the α-5 receptor subtype might minimize the risk of physiological and psychological dependence or cognitive slowing seen with GABA-receptor agonists as well as serve as potential candidates for the development of new antidepressant agents.

11.1.1.4 *Conclusion*

Despite a number of limitations in relation to standard, monoamine-based antidepressants, benzodiazepines may serve as an option for many patients with resistant or refractory depression (Kishimoto, 1988), and certainly as an augmentation strategy in selected depressed populations (see Chap. 5). In addition, the discovery of GABA-ergic agonists, antagonists or mixed agonists/antagonists which are relatively selective or the α-2, α-3 or α-5 receptor subtypes may represent the next step in the development of GABA-ergic treatments for major depressive disorder (MDD) (Atack, 2003; Mehta & Ticku, 1999), including the treatment of cognitive, memory and attentional impairment in depression (Sternfeld *et al.*, 2004), as well as the treatment of resistant and refractory depression.

11.1.2 *Barbiturates*

Similar to the benzodiazepines, the barbiturates drugs, at lower doses, bind to and reversibly inhibit the closing of the γ-amino-butyric acid (GABA)-A receptor (Mehta & Ticku, 1999). However, at higher doses, barbiturates can open the chloride channel even in the absence of GABA (Mehta & Ticku, 1999). For this reason, it is thought that barbiturates carry a higher risk of abuse (Zawertailo *et al.*, 2003), and can be more lethal following an overdose than benzodiazepines (Johns, 1977; Melander *et al.*, 1991; Mendelson & Rich, 1993). As a result, barbiturates have been largely replaced by benzodiazepines in clinical practice. Randomized, double-blind studies conducted during the late 1960s had suggested amylobarbitone (Hunter *et al.*, 1967), and phenobarbital (Wheatley, 1969) to be as effective as TCA therapy for the treatment of depression. Subsequently, Rickels *et al.* (1973) randomized 138 patients with "non-psychotic depression" to treatment with phenobarbital, diazepam or amitriptyline, and reported equivalent efficacy between the three treatment groups at endpoint. However, to date, placebo-controlled studies for barbiturates in depression have not been published.

11.1.3 *Other GABA-ergic agents*

Fengabine administration has been thought to result in an increase in central nervous system (CNS) GABA-ergic stone, although the exact mechanism by which fengabine influences GABA-ergic function remains unclear (Lloyd *et al.*, 1987). To date, two reports of fengabine for depression have been published. The first involves a description of the results of six randomized, double-blind studies in which 398 in- and out-patients with MDD or a major depressive episode in the setting of bipolar disorder were randomized to treatment with fengabine versus a TCA for a total of four weeks (Magni *et al.*, 1989). The second report describes the results of a small ($n = 16$) double-blind study of four weeks duration in which fengabine was compared to clomipramine for MDD and/or dysthymia (Nielsen *et al.*, 1990). Both reports confirm equivalent antidepressant efficacy between the two treatment groups.

Viqualine is a serotonin-reuptake inhibitor and serotonin-releasing agent with benzodiazepine-like effects (Faravelli *et al.*, 1988). A double-blind, placebo-controlled study involving switching to viqualine in treatment-resistant depression (TRD) has been published, demonstrating greater antidepressant efficacy for viqualine versus placebo (Faravelli *et al.*, 1988). However, it is unlikely that the benzodiazepine-like effects of viqualine contributed to its antidepressant efficacy in that study, since patients randomized to placebo also received treatment with the benzodiazepine drug lorazepam.

A number of anticonvulsants also principally act on the GABA-ergic system. Gabapentin (Bryans & Wustrow, 1999), pregabalin (Bryans & Wustrow, 1999), and vigabatrin (French, 1999), for example, are GABA structural analogues that inhibit the degradation of GABA by the enzyme GABA-transaminase, while tiagabine is a GABA reuptake inhibitor (Czuczwar & Patsalos, 2001). Although the mechanism of action of the anticonvulsant agent levetiracetam has not been fully elucidated, levetiracetam has been shown to promote chloride influx at the GABA-A receptor by inhibiting GABA-A-receptor modulators such as zinc (Rigo *et al.*, 2002). Ganaxolone and retigabine are newer agents currently in the pre-clinical phase of development as anticonvulsants. These agents also possess a GABA-ergic mechanism of action that has not been fully elucidated but appears to differ from the mechanism of other GABA-ergic anticonvulsants (Czuczwar & Patsalos, 2001).

Randomized, double-blind, placebo-controlled trials do not support the use of adjunctive gabapentin in the treatment of manic episodes in patients with bipolar disorder (Pande *et al.*, 2000a), or for bipolar prophylaxis (Vieta *et al.*, 2006). Similarly, a randomized, double-blind, placebo-controlled trial did not demonstrate greater anxiolytic efficacy for gabapentin monotherapy than placebo in patients with panic disorder (Pande *et al.*, 2000b). However, the results of a randomized, double-blind, placebo-controlled trial support the use of gabapentin monotherapy in social anxiety disorder (Pande *et al.*, 1999). Similarly, randomized, double-blind, placebo-controlled studies have been published supporting the use of pregabalin (Bech, 2007; Feltner *et al.*, 2003 and 2008; Montgomery *et al.*, 2006 and 2008; Pande *et al.*, 2003; Pohl *et al.*, 2005; Rickels *et al.*, 2005) for the treatment of generalized anxiety disorder, as well as for pregabalin in the treatment of social anxiety disorder (Pande *et al.*, 2004). In fact, treatment of generalized anxiety disorder with pregabalin has also been shown to be more effective than placebo in reducing depressive symptoms as well as anxiety symptoms (Stein *et al.*, 2008).

However, although the results of one randomized, double-blind, placebo-controlled trial demonstrated greater anxiolytic effects for tiagabine monotherapy in GAD (Pollack *et al.*, 2005), this was not supported by subsequent, placebo-controlled trials (Pollack *et al.*, 2008). Similarly, the results of a randomized, double-blind, placebo-controlled trial do not support the use of tiagabine for the treatment of primary insomnia (Roth *et al.*, 2006), although tiagabine does appear to increase slow-wave sleep (stages 3 and 4) at the expense of stage 1 sleep in patients with primary insomnia or healthy controls (Roth *et al.*, 2006; Walsh *et al.*, 2005 and 2006). Finally, there is evidence to support the use of pregabalin (Arnold *et al.*, 2008; Crofford *et al.*, 2005 and 2008; Mease *et al.*, 2008), and gabapentin (Arnold *et al.*, 2007) for the treatment of fibromyalgia. None of these compounds have been studied as monotherapy for unipolar depressive disorders or for patients with anxious MDD or with comorbid painful symptoms of MDD.

For levetiracetam, there are open-label trials focusing on its use as monotherapy for social anxiety disorder (Simon *et al.*, 2004), or as adjunctive treatment for major depressive episodes in patients with bipolar disorder (Post *et al.*, 2005), refractory anxiety disorders (Kinrys *et al.*, 2007a), or refractory post-traumatic stress disorder (Kinrys *et al.*, 2006). However, the results of a randomized, double-blind, placebo-controlled study do not support the use of levetiracetam in the treatment of social anxiety disorder (Zhang *et al.*, 2005).

Interestingly enough, some case reports suggest that treatment with the anticonvulsant gabapentin may reduce aggression and impulsivity in patients with a variety of disorders including dementia (Goldenberg *et al.*, 1998; Hawkins *et al.*, 2000; Miller, 2001; Regan & Gordon, 1997), stroke (Low & Brandes, 1999), borderline personality disorder (Biancosino *et al.*, 2002), conduct disorder (Gupta *et al.*, 2000; Ryback & Ryback, 1995), post-encephalitic epilepsy (Kaufman *et al.*, 2002), and in elderly patients with a variety of psychiatric diagnoses (Sheldon *et al.*, 1998) although there have also been reports of gabapentin-associated aggression (Lee *et al.*, 1996; Pinninti & Mahajan, 2001; Tallian *et al.*, 1996; Wolf *et al.*, 1995). Studies focusing on the use of gabapentin for MDD with prominent anger and irritability are lacking. Levetiracetam does not appear to be effective in reducing aggression/impulsivity in patients with impulsive aggression (Mattes, 2008).

11.2 Glycine and Glutamate-Based Treatments

11.2.1 *Neuropharmacology*

Glycine and glutamate serve as the primary excitatory neurotransmitters in the human brain where they participate in many functions through activation of several ionotropic receptors, including the α-amino-3-hydroxy-5-methyl-4-isoxazole propionate (AMPA), N-methyl-D-aspartate (NMDA), and kainate receptors, as well as the type I–VIII metabotropic glutamate receptors (Waterhouse *et al.*, 2003). To date, much more is known regarding the function of the NMDA receptor than the AMPA or kainate receptors (Waterhouse *et al.*, 2003). NMDA receptors consist of an NR-1 subunit along with a combination of four distinct NR-2 subunits (2A, 2B, 2C, 2D), with the distribution of NR-2 subunits varying according to each brain region (Lynch & Guttman, 2002). NMDA receptors include distinct binding sites on their exterior for L-glutamate, glycine and d-serine, which serve as co-agonists for the receptor (Scaton, 1993), with glycine and serine binding to the NR-1 subunit and glutamate binding to the NR-2 subunit (Lynch & Guttmann, 2002). The simultaneous binding of glutamate and glycine to the NMDA receptor results in an increase in permeability of the channel to sodium and calcium ions (Parsons *et al.*, 1996).

11.2.2 *NMDA-active agents*

A number of compounds including the hallucinogen phenylcyclidene (PCP), as well as amantadine, memantine, and ketamine, are non-competitive antagonists of the NMDA receptor (Parsons *et al.*, 1996). These compounds bind to a site on the NMDA receptor on the NR-2 subunit, termed the PCP binding site, located within the channel (Waterhouse, 2003). When bound to the receptor, these agents inhibit the neuronal influx of sodium and calcium (Parsons *et al.*, 1996).

Over the course of the past decade, evidence has been accumulating suggesting that, in extreme cases of NMDA receptor over-stimulation, calcium influx-mediated neuronal dysfunction or even neurotoxicity may occur (Sattler & Tymianski, 2001). In fact, such NMDA-mediated excitotoxicity has been proposed to play a central role in the underlying pathophysiology of a number of medical conditions and illnesses (Lipton & Rosenberg, 1994) including ischemia/stroke, hyperglycemia, human immunodeficiency virus (HIV)-related encephalopathy, Huntington's and Parkinson's disease, as well as MDD (Hashimoto *et al.*, 2004; Sapolsky *et al.*, 2000). In addition, it has been hypothesized that NMDA-receptor antagonists may possess neuroprotective properties and, as a result, antidepressant effects (Stahl & Grady, 2003). In parallel, a number of studies also suggest that administration of NMDA antagonists results in an increase in central nervous system (CNS) dopaminergic activity (Breier *et al.*, 1998; Deep, 1999; Kegeles *et al.*, 2000; Smith *et al.*, 1998; Vollenweider *et al.*, 2000), a separate mechanism which would also suggest antidepressant effects for glutamatergic agents.

Despite such promising hypotheses, clinical evidence supporting an antidepressant role for glutamatergic agents remains, disappointingly, limited. Specifically, in addition to augmentation studies involving the use of amantadine or ketamine (described in Chap. 6), there is also evidence, mainly stemming from small open-label trials, suggesting that NMDA antagonists such as amantadine (Dietrich *et al.*, 2000; Ferszt *et al.*, 1999), and memantine (Ferguson *et al.*, 2003; Forest clinical trial MEM-MD-09) may possess antidepressant effects when used as monotherapy for MDD.

Double-blind studies of NMDA-receptor antagonists as monotherapy for depression are limited. In one such study, Vale *et al.* (1971) reported amantadine monotherapy to be superior to placebo for the treatment of depression. Similarly, Berman *et al.* (2000) randomized seven subjects with MDD or major depression in the setting of bipolar disorder to receive intravenous ketamine versus placebo over three days, and reported a robust reduction in depression severity in ketamine but not placebo-treated patients (Fig. 11.2). However, many patients also experienced transient cognitive deficits, perceptual disturbances and other psychotic-like symptoms in that study. More recently, a double-blind, placebo-controlled trial involving the use of memantine (5–20 mg daily for eight weeks) for the treatment of MDD ($n = 32$) did not reveal greater reduction in depressive symptom severity among memantine- than placebo-treated patients (Zarate *et al.*, 2006). A randomized, double-blind, placebo-controlled trial of memantine as monotherapy for MDD is currently under way (NCT00040261).

A major limitation in testing and potential development of NMDA antagonists as antidepressants is that, similar to PCP although to various degrees, these agents can possess hallucinogenic

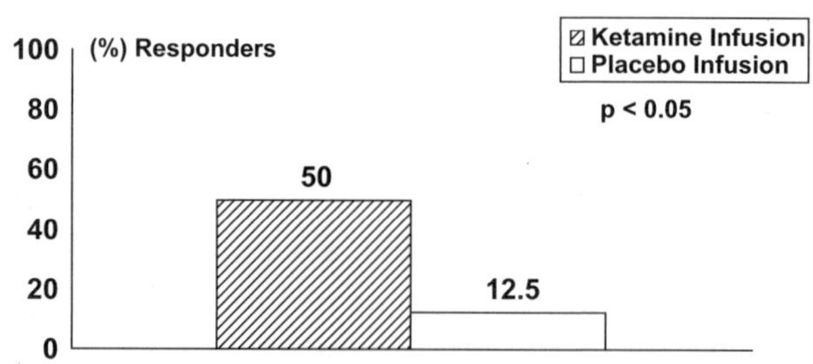

Fig. 11.2 Antidepressant effects 72 hours post-infusion of ketamine for depression: A randomized, double-blind study ($n = 7$). [Data extracted from: Berman, R.M., Cappiello, A., Anand, A., *et al.* (2000). Antidepressant effects of ketamine in depressed patients. *Biological Psychiatry*, 47, 351–354.]

properties and may even induce psychotic-like symptoms in subjects with or without a history of psychosis. Although primarily associated with the use of PCP and ketamine, there are also reports of an induction of hallucinations or psychotic-like symptoms during treatment with amantadine (Armbruster *et al.*, 1974; Borison *et al.*, 1979; Fahn *et al.*, 1971; Guay, 1994; Harper & Knothe, 1973; Macchio *et al.*, 1993; Pimentel & Hughes, 1991; Snoey & Bessen, 1990; Strong *et al.*, 1991; Wilcox, 1985), and memantine (Jarvis & Figgitt, 2003), particularly when used at higher doses and in patients with impaired drug clearance.

The emergence of these psychotic-like symptoms has been correlated to ketamine-induced pro-dopaminergic activities in the striatum (Breier *et al.*, 1998; Vollenweider *et al.*, 2000). However, it has been hypothesized that, unlike the agents PCP, ketamine, and memantine which bind to the NR2A and NR2B subunits with equal preference, treatment with agents that selectively bind to the NR-2B subunit of the NMDA receptor, such as eliprodil and ifenprodil (Avenet *et al.*, 1997), may spare patients of cognitive side effects and psychotic-like symptoms (Avenet *et al.*, 1997; Lynch & Guttmann, 2002).

11.2.3 *Other glutamatergic agents*

The potential role of ionotropic AMPA, kainate, or metabotropic glutamate receptor antagonists in alleviating CNS diseases is, largely, unknown. Bergink and Westenberg (2005) randomized outpatients with panic disorder to receive treatment with LY354740 (100 or 200 mg daily), a potent and selective agonist for metabotropic glutamate receptors 2 and 3 (mGlu 2/3), versus paroxetine or placebo and did not report a difference in anxiolytic efficacy between LY354740 and placebo (paroxetine was found to be more effective than placebo). In a subsequent study, however, Dunayevich *et al.* (2008) randomized patients with GAD to treatment with LY544344 (8 or 16 mg daily), a LY354740 pro-drug that increases LY354740 bioavailability, versus placebo for a total of eight weeks. A greater anxiolytic effect was observed among patients who received 16 mg a day of LY544344 than placebo. Studies focusing on MDD have not been conducted to date.

Riluzole is an agent shown to inhibit the release of glutamic acid as well as non-competitively inhibit the NMDA receptors (Doble, 1996). To date, the results of a small ($n = 19$), open-label trial involving the use of riluzole (100–200 mg, 6 weeks) for MDD resistant to numerous antidepressants has been published (Zarate *et al.*, 2004). Thirty-two percent of patients enrolled in that study experienced a clinical response (50% or greater symptom improvement).

Lamotrigine, an anticonvulsant agent, acts by inhibiting glutamate release (Davies, 1995; Papakostas & Zarate, 2007). There is evidence from randomized, double-blind, placebo-controlled studies to support the use of lamotrigine for the treatment of major depressive episodes (but not manic episodes) in patients with bipolar disorder (see Chap. 5). However, at least three [GlaxoSmithKline protocols SCA 20022; SCAA2011 (105–613); SCA 20025] double-blind, placebo-controlled trials ($n = 900$) focusing on the use of lamotrigine as monotherapy for MDD have been conducted. None of these studies demonstrated any benefit for lamotrigine monotherapy versus placebo (Fig. 11.3).

A small, randomized, double-blind, placebo-controlled trial demonstrated greater efficacy for lamotrigine monotherapy than

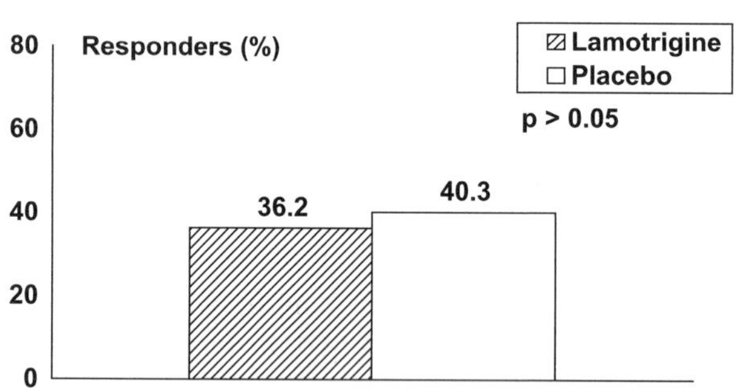

Fig. 11.3 Antidepressant effects of lamotrigine for MDD: A randomized, double-blind study ($n = 300$). [Data extracted from the clinical trial results of GlaxoSmithKline-funded protocol SCA20025.]

placebo in the treatment of post-traumatic stress disorder (PTSD) (Hertzberg *et al.*, 1999). However, studies specifically designed to evaluate the efficacy of lamotrigine for patients with comorbid MDD and PTSD have yet to be conducted.

11.2.4 *Glycinergic agents*

Early studies had also suggested potential antidepressant effects for the glycine site partial agonist d-cycloserine (Crane, 1959 and 1961), an agent that was widely used as an antitubercular agent in the 1950s. Specifically, in a retrospective study, Crane (1959) reported a significant improvement in mood in more than half of 50 patients suffering from tuberculosis as well as chronic depression during treatment with d-cycloserine. Shortly thereafter, Crane (1961) reported a significant reduction in depressive symptoms among 30 patients with tuberculosis and comorbid anxiety and "depressive neuroses" during open-label treatment with d-cycloserine. Subsequent studies of d-cycloserine for depression have not been published.

11.3 Agents with Combined GABA-ergic and Glutamatergic Activity

11.3.1 *Anticonvulsants*

These include certain anticonvulsants such as valproate (Perucca, 2002), topiramate, felbamate, and remacemide (Meldrum, 1996). In addition to their GABA-ergic and glutamatergic effects, these agents also influence the function of several other neuronal structures. Valproate, a short-branched chain fatty acid that is incorporated into neuronal membranes substituting for naturally occurring phospholipids (Siafaka-Kapadai *et al.*, 1998), also blocks voltage-gated sodium channels (Perucca, 2002), and is an inhibitor of histone deacetylase (Harwood & Agam, 2003). Topiramate also appears to act on the sodium channel (Meldrum, 1996). Felbamate blocks the L-type calcium channels, and also may prolong sodium channel inactivation. Finally, the desglycinated metabolite of remacemide also prolongs inactivation of sodium channels (Meldrum, 1996).

Randomized, double-blind, placebo-controlled trials have documented the efficacy of valproic acid as monotherapy in the treatment of manic episodes and major depressive episodes in patients with bipolar disorder, as well as in the prophylaxis of bipolar disorder (see Chap. 5). However, only one open-label study supporting the use of valproate as monotherapy for unipolar depression has been published to date. In that study, Davis *et al.* (1996) treated 33 outpatients with MDD with valproate monotherapy in an open-label fashion for eight weeks, and reported a 54% response rate at endpoint.

In addition, some (Giakas *et al.*, 1990; Herrmann, 1998; Hollander *et al.*, 2003; Horne & Lindley, 1995; Kavoussi & Coccaro, 1998; Kunik *et al.*, 1998; Lott *et al.*, 1995; Mellow *et al.*, 1993; Sival *et al.*, 2004; Stein *et al.*, 1995; Wilcox, 1995) but not other studies (Hollander *et al.*, 2001; Puryear *et al.*, 1995; Sival *et al.*, 2002) suggest the potential utility of valproate monotherapy for the treatment of anger/aggression in patients with a variety of primary diagnoses including seizure disorder (Giakas *et al.*, 1990), axis-I disorders (Kavoussi & Coccaro, 1998), axis-II disorders (Hollander *et al.*, 2003; Kavoussi & Coccaro, 1998; Stein *et al.*, 1995; Wilcox, 1995), dementia (Herrmann, 1998; Kunik *et al.*, 1998; Lott *et al.*, 1995; Mellow *et al.*, 1993; Sival *et al.*, 2002 and 2004), and organic brain syndrome (Horne & Lindley, 1995). Although treatment with the SSRIs has also been shown to reduce anger and aggression in MDD (Coccaro *et al.*, 1997; Fava *et al.*, 1991, 1993, 1996, 1997; Kavoussi *et al.*, 1994; Salzman *et al.*, 1995), as many as one in four SSRI-treated patients do not experience any reduction in anger/aggression following adequate treatment (Coccaro *et al.*, 1997). However, randomized, double-blind, placebo-controlled trials of valproate as monotherapy or augmentation for MDD patients who present with prominent anger/aggression or with residual anger/aggression following treatment with serotonin norepinephrine reuptake inhibitors (SNRIs) or SSRIs have yet to be published.

With respect to topiramate, there are randomized, placebo-controlled trials suggesting it is not more effective than placebo when used either as an adjunct (Roy Chengappa *et al.*, 2006) or as monotherapy (Delbello *et al.*, 2005; Kushner *et al.*, 2006) for the treatment of manic episodes in patients with bipolar disorder, although results of a single-blind study suggest it is as effective as the norepinephrine-dopamine reuptake inhibitor bupropion when used as an adjunct to mood stabilizers for the treatment of major depressive episodes in patients with bipolar disorder (McIntyre *et al.*, 2002).

However, there is emerging evidence to suggest that, similar to other anticonvulsants, topiramate may also reduce anger/aggression in patients with a variety of neuropsychiatric disorders (Fhager *et al.*, 2003; Janowsky *et al.*, 2003; Nickel C *et al.*, 2005a; Nickel MK *et al.*, 2004). In fact, the results of a double-blind, randomized, placebo-controlled trial of topiramate as monotherapy for women with MDD suggest a greater reduction in depressive symptoms and irritability among patients treated with topiramate than placebo (Nickel C *et al.*, 2005a) (Fig. 11.4). This study has yet to be replicated.

In addition, uncontrolled (Woods *et al.*, 2004) as well as controlled reports (Bray *et al.*, 2003; Loew *et al.*, 2006; McElroy *et al.*, 2004; Nickel C *et al.*, 2005a; Nickel MK *et al.*, 2004, 2005; Reife *et al.*, 2000) suggest that some patients may experience weight loss following treatment with topiramate. However, studies of topiramate monotherapy for

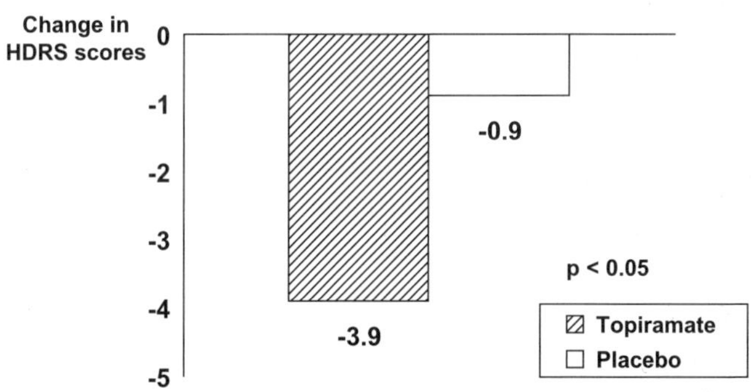

Fig. 11.4 Antidepressant effects of topiramate for women with MDD: A randomized, double-blind study ($n = 64$). [Data extracted from Nickel, C., Lahmann, C., Tritt, K., *et al.* (2005). Topiramate in treatment of depressive and anger symptoms in female depressive patients: A randomized, double-blind, placebo-controlled study. *Journal of Affective Disorders*, 87(2–3), 243–252.]

obese patients with MDD have not been published. Furthermore, randomized, double-blind, placebo-controlled trials support the use of topiramate as monotherapy (McElroy *et al.*, 2003, 2004 and 2007) or adjunctive treatment (Claudino *et al.*, 2007) for binge-eating disorder, as well as monotherapy in bulimia nervosa (Hedges *et al.*, 2003; Hoopes *et al.*, 2003; Nickel C *et al.*, 2005b). However, studies focusing on the use of topiramate for the treatment of MDD with comorbid eating disorders have yet to be published. Randomized, double-blind, placebo-controlled trials do not suggest topiramate as either monotherapy (Tucker *et al.*, 2004) or adjunctive treatment (Lindley *et al.*, 2007) to be particularly effective in the treatment of PTSD.

Studies focusing on the use of felbamate and remacemide for MDD or bipolar disorder have not been published.

11.4 Other Anticonvulsants

Although several anticonvulsants do not appear to directly influence the function of either the GABA-ergic or glutamatergic system, we chose to include their discussion in the same chapter as other anticonvulsants. These agents include the sodium channel–blocking agents carbamazepine, oxcarbazepine (a structural analogue of carbamazepine), phenytoin (Davies, 1995), and mexiletine (Monk & Brogden, 1990), the calcium-channel blocker ethosuximide (Davies, 1995), and the sodium/calcium channel blocker zonisamide (Oommen & Mathews, 1999).

Although the efficacy of carbamazepine in the treatment of manic episodes in patients with bipolar disorder has been well documented in randomized, double-blind, placebo-controlled trials (see Chap. 5), there is only a single report focusing on the use of carbamazepine as monotherapy for MDD. Specifically, Zhang *et al.* (2008) demonstrated a greater reduction in depressive symptoms among patients with MDD randomized under double-blind conditions to treatment with carbamazepine monotherapy than placebo (Fig. 11.5).

Unlike carbamazepine, oxcarbazepine does not appear to be effective in the treatment of mania in patients with bipolar disorder (Wagner *et al.*, 2006).

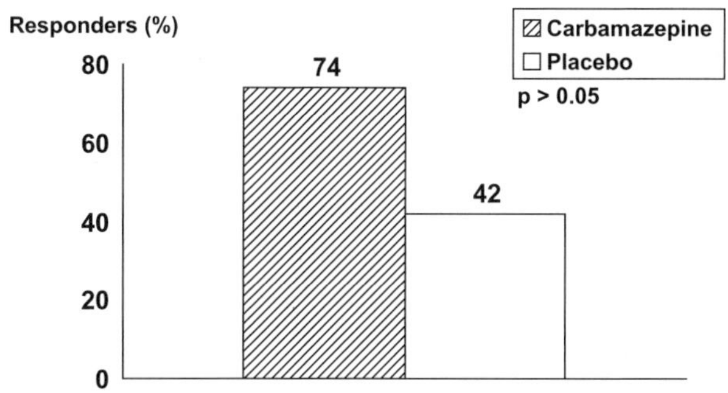

Fig. 11.5 Antidepressant effects of carbamazepine for MDD: A randomized, double-blind study ($n = 89$). [Data extracted from Zhang, Z.J., Tan, Q.R., Tong, Y., *et al.* (2008). The effectiveness of carbamazepine in unipolar depression: A double-blind, randomized, placebo-controlled study. *Journal of Affective Disorders*, 109(1–2), 91–97.]

In addition, similar to several other anticonvulsants, there are reports of anti-aggressive effects for carbamazepine (Cowdry & Gardner, 1988; Foster *et al.*, 1989; Gardner & Chowdry, 1986; Gleason & Schneider, 1990; Luchins, 1983 and 1984; Mattes, 1990; Neppe, 1983), as well as oxcarbazepine (Bellino *et al.*, 2005). However, randomized, double-blind, placebo-controlled trials of carbamazepine or oxcarbazepine or augmentation for MDD patients who present with prominent anger/aggression or with residual anger/aggression following treatment with SSRIs/SNRIs have yet to be published.

Studies focusing on the use of the mexiletine, zonisamide, or phenytoin as monotherapy for unipolar depression have not been published. For mexiletine, there is a randomized, double-blind, placebo-controlled study focusing on its use in manic episodes among patients with bipolar disorder, which did not demonstrate a greater anti-manic effect for mexiletine than placebo (Schaffer & Levitt, 2005). For zonisamide, there is a randomized, double-blind, placebo-controlled trial supporting its use as monotherapy for binge eating disorder (McElroy *et al.*, 2006), as well as open-label trials focusing on its use as an adjunct for treatment-resistant anxiety (Kinrys *et al.*, 2007b), or for the treatment of major depressive episodes in patients with bipolar disorder (Anand *et al.*, 2005; Ghaemi *et al.*, 2006; McElroy *et al.*, 2005). Finally, for phenytoin, there is only one single, open-label trial focusing on its use for the treatment of PTSD (Bremner *et al.*, 2004) as well as one randomized, double-blind, placebo-controlled trial focusing on its use as an adjunct (to the typical antipsychotic agent haloperidol) in the treatment of manic episodes among patients with either bipolar disorder or schizoaffective disorder of bipolar type (Mishory *et al.*, 2000). Greater anti-manic effects were reported for phenytoin- than placebo-treated patients.

11.5 Neurokinin-Receptor Antagonists

11.5.1 *Neuropharmacology*

Neurokinin receptors and their endogenous ligand, substance P, are highly expressed in areas of the brain involved in the regulation of mood and thought to be involved in the pathophysiology of depression including the striatum, nucleus accumbens, amygdala, hippocampus, locus coeruleus, and raphe nuclei (Bergstrom *et al.*, 2004). Of the 3 NK receptor subtypes identified in humans (NK 1, 2, 3), the NK1 receptor appears to be the principal CNS receptor (Hargreaves, 2002).

11.5.2 *Clinical evidence*

Thus far, several double-blind, placebo-controlled studies for neurokinin-1 (NK1) — receptor antagonists have been published. The first study involved randomizing 213 MDD patients to treatment with aprepitant (otherwise known as MK-869 or L-754030) 300 mg versus paroxetine 20 mg versus placebo for a total of six weeks (Kramer *et al.*, 1998). Aprepitant was found to be more effective than placebo at week 1 and throughout week 6, and as effective as paroxetine. However, five subsequent double-blind, placebo-controlled trials of aprepitant failed to show greater efficacy for aprepitant than placebo (Keller *et al.*, 2006), as did two separate randomized, double-blind, placebo-substitution trials of aprepitant for aprepitant-remitted MDD (i.e., relapse prevention trials; Merck aprepitant protocol 65; NCT00048594 and NCT00035048).

A separate double-blind study involving a separate NK1-receptor antagonist termed "compound A" or L-759274 involving 128 MDD patients randomized to treatment with 40 mg daily of L-759274 versus placebo for six weeks revealed greater resolution of depressive symptoms and a similar trend towards statistical significance ($p = 0.07$) for greater response rates for L-759274 that placebo at week 6 (Kramer *et al.*, 2004) (Fig. 11.6). Similarly as with aprepitant, the results of a subsequent double-blind study comparing two doses of L-759274 with paroxetine 20 mg and placebo were also interpreted as inconclusive, since there was no difference in endpoint efficacy between the three treatment groups (Kramer, 2001; Krishnan, 2002). Two separate paroxetine- and placebo-controlled trials (BN16430, BN16568) sponsored by Roche focusing on a different NK1 antagonist also failed to demonstrate greater efficacy for the NK1 antagonist than placebo.

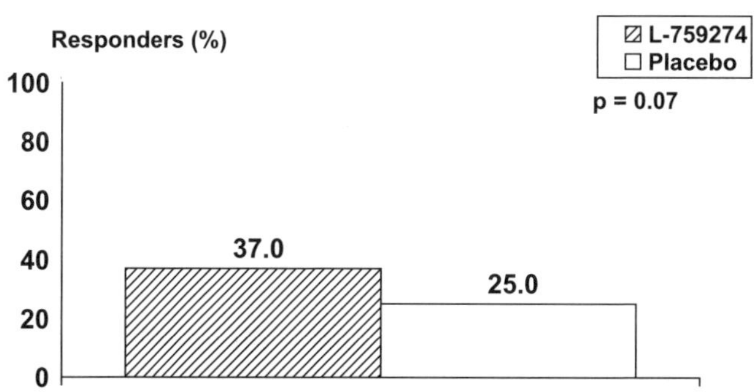

Fig. 11.6 Substance P (NK1) receptor antagonist for MDD: A randomized, double-blind study ($n = 128$). NK1: Neurokinin-1. [Data extracted from: Kramer, M.S., Winokur, A., Kelsey, J., *et al.* (2004). Demonstration of the efficacy and safety of a novel substance P (NK1) receptor antagonist in major depression. *Neuropsychopharmacology*, 29, 385–392.]

There is also a randomized, double-blind, placebo-controlled trial sponsored by GlaxoSmithKline focusing on a different NK1 antagonist (GW679769) as monotherapy for MDD (NCT00413023), the results of which have not yet been published. Finally, randomized, double-blind, placebo-controlled studies involving the use of an NK-2-selective receptor antagonist (saredutant) as monotherapy for MDD are currently under way (www.clinicaltrials.gov: NCT00336713, NCT00415142, NCT00250627, NCT00256113, NCT00250601, NCT00250614).

Little is known regarding the *in-vivo* CNS properties of the NK1 antagonist. Neuroimaging studies suggest that greater than 80% occupancy is obtained with daily doses of aprepitant of approximately 30 mg, while greater than 95% occupancy is obtained with doses of aprepitant of, approximately, 300 mg (Bergstrom *et al.*, 2004). Interestingly enough, at doses of 300 mg of aprepitant, side effects are mild which suggests that, similar to the SSRIs and unlike the benzodiazepines or 5HT1A agonists (see section on benzodiazepines as well as Chap. 5 for further details), significant receptor occupancy can be achieved at initial (and relatively well-tolerated) doses of the drug. In fact, certain side effects including nausea, fatigue and sexual dysfunction appear to occur at lower rates with aprepitant 300 mg than with paroxetine (Kramer *et al.*, 1998). Therefore, should NK1 antagonists prove efficacious for depression, the ability to achieve near-maximum occupancy with starting doses of NK1 antagonists would greatly simplify the clinical use of NK1 antagonists for depression in primary care and specialty-treatment settings, since minimally effective doses could be prescribed during the initial clinic visit.

In summary, due to their novel, non-monoaminergic mechanism, substance P-receptor antagonists would also be of interest as mono- or adjunctive-treatments for TRD. In addition, due to their anti-emetic properties (Olver, 2004), NK-receptor antagonists may prove effective as adjunctive treatment for the prevention and treatment of antidepressant-induced nausea or GI-upset.

11.6 Nicotinic Receptor–Based Treatments

11.6.1 *Neuropharmacology*

The nicotinic receptor is an ionotropic receptor consisting of five subunits (Paterson & Nordberg, 2000). In the human central nervous system, 11 different types of subunits have been identified (α2–9, β2–4), with most nicotinic receptors consisting of a combination of α and β subunits (Paterson & Nordberg, 2000). The most abundant and widespread nicotinic receptors in the mammalian CNS are the $\alpha 4\beta 2$ (i.e., consisting of α4 and β2 subunits), $\alpha 3\beta 4$, $\alpha 3\beta 2$, and α7 (i.e., consisting of five α7 subunits) (Shytle *et al.*, 2002a). Binding of acetylcholine results in an increased permeability to sodium, potassium and calcium ions (Shytle *et al.*, 2002a). The downstream effects of increased ionic permeability depend on whether the receptors are located in a presynaptic, postsynaptic, or axonal distribution. Presynaptic receptors are involved in the release of numerous neurotransmitters including the monoamines, glutamate and GABA, axonal receptors primarily involved in the release of GABA, while postsynaptic receptors provide excitatory input, although the overwhelming component of excitatory input in the CNS is glutamatergic (Dani, 2001).

11.6.2 *Nicotinic-receptor agonists*

Clinical studies supporting the notion that agents with predominantly nicotinic-agonist activity may possess antidepressant properties are limited. A series of small open-label trials suggest that treatment of depression in non-smokers with trans-dermal nicotine often results in a rapid and robust reduction in depressive symptoms in many patients (Haro & Drucker-Colin, 2004a and b; Salin-Pascual *et al.*, 1995, 1996, 1998, 2002). However, all but one (Haro & Drucker-Colin, 2004a and b) of these studies were of very short duration (4–8 days) which is a serious limitation given the propensity for nicotinic cholinergic receptors to desensitize following continued nicotinic agonism (Paterson & Nordberg, 2000), a process which, in turn, could undermine any potential for sustained antidepressant effects. Haro and Drucker-Colin (2004a and b) administered transdermal nicotine (17.5 mg daily) five days a week for six months and reported a significant decrease in Hamilton depression Rating Scale scores (from a mean of 29.7 to a mean of 10.8), baseline to endpoint. However, a subsequent double-blind, placebo-controlled study of transdermal nicotine for depression in non-smokers did not reveal any difference in efficacy at endpoint between treatments (Cox *et al.*, 2003). Unfortunately, the study was probably underpowered ($n = 6$), and of very short duration (8 days) to be informative. More recently, McClernon *et al.* (2006) published the results of a small ($n = 11$), four-week, double-blind, placebo-controlled trial of nicotine (patch) versus placebo for depressive symptoms in non-smokers. Consistent with the desensitization hypothesis, a greater resolution of depressive symptoms was demonstrated among nicotine- than placebo-treated patients early-on (day 1, weeks 1, 2, 3) but not at endpoint.

In addition to the "desensitization" effect, a serious obstacle in testing and, potentially, developing pro-nicotinergic-based treatments for depression is the risk of abuse associated with nicotinic-receptor agonism, which is thought to be secondary to nicotinic receptor–mediated dopamine release in mesolimbic brain areas associated with reward processing (Rice & Cragg, 2004). Nicotine appears to bind to several nicotinic receptor subtypes, including the $\alpha4\beta2$, as well as the $\alpha3\beta4$ and $\alpha3\beta2$ subtypes (Rush *et al.*, 2002). As a result, administration of nicotine results in widespread changes in CNS blood flow and metabolism, simultaneously involving numerous cortical and striatal areas (Domino *et al.*, 2000a and b; Stapleton *et al.*, 2003; Zubieta *et al.*, 2001). However, it appears that craving is linked to nicotine-mediated changes in midbrain and thalamic blood flow (Rose *et al.*, 2003), while the effects of nicotine on cognition and memory appear to be mediated by blood-flow changes in the anterior cingulate and prefrontal cortex (Ernst *et al.*, 2001; Ghatan *et al.*, 1998). In parallel, similar to the GABA-ergic and glutamatergic system, evidence is beginning to emerge suggesting that the various nicotinic-receptor subtypes may be involved in different functions including memory, cognition and behavioral re-enforcement/addiction. For example, both the $\alpha 4\beta 2$ (Chen *et al.*, 2003; Cohen *et al.*, 2003; Sharples *et al.*, 2000) as well as $\alpha 3\beta 4$ and $\alpha 3\beta 2$ (Miller *et al.*, 2002) have been reported to play a key role in acetylcholine-mediated dopamine release in areas involved in behavioral re-enforcement and addiction including the striatum, ventral tegmental area and nucleus accumbens, while some studies suggest that the $\alpha 7$ receptor does not play a predominant role in dopamine release in the striatum (Salimen *et al.*, 2004). In contrast, agonist activity at the $\alpha 7$ receptor has been linked to cognitive functions including learning and memory in pre-clinical studies (Levin *et al.*, 1999; Van Kampen *et al.*, 2004). Therefore, developing specific nicotinic receptor ligands, such as $\alpha 7$ receptor agonists (Levin & Rezvani, 2002), $\alpha 4\beta 2$-receptor partial agonists (similar to varenicline) (Glover & Rath, 2007), or mixed nicotinic-receptor agonists/antagonists may offer opportunities to develop novel treatments for depression as well as treatments which target cognitive dysfunction and inattention in depression. In addition, some studies have linked smoking cessation to an increased risk of depressive relapse or worsening of depressive symptoms in patients with a history of depression who quit smoking while remitted (Glassman *et al.*, 2001). Therefore, the treatment or maintenance of depression with agents selective for certain nicotinic receptors or with mixed nicotinic-receptor agonist/antagonist properties in patients considering smoking cessation may be preferable with respect to minimizing the risk of depressive relapse or worsening of depressive symptoms than the administration of conventional monoaminergic agents alone.

11.6.3 *Cholinesterase inhibitors*

Cholinesterase inhibitors, currently being used for the treatment of Alzheimer's disease (Trinh *et al.*, 2003), possess pro-cholinergic and pro-nicotinergic activity. Specifically, these agents inhibit the enzyme acetyl cholinesterase, involved in the catabolism of acetylcholine. Galantamine, a cholinesterase inhibitor, has also been reported to allosterically potentiate the activity of nicotinic acetylcholine receptors. The results of a double-blind, placebo-controlled trial of galantamine combined with venlafaxine did not demonstrate a greater resolution of depressive or cognitive symptoms among non-demented elderly patients with MDD (see Chap. 5). Similarly, a randomized, double-blind, placebo-controlled trial also did not demonstrate any anti-manic effects for adjunctive donepezil (cholinesterase inhibitor) (Eden Evins *et al.*, 2006).

11.6.4 *Nicotinic-receptor antagonists*

There is little evidence to suggest a potential role for nicotinic-receptor antagonists as monotherapy for depression, although several antidepressants also possess nicotinic-receptor antagonist effects (see Chaps. 2–4 for further details). Shytle *et al.*, (2002b) reported greater improvements in a number of depressive symptoms including irritability, mood swings, attention, restlessness, anxiety, and impulsivity among four children with MDD and comorbid Tourette's disorder randomized to treatment with the nicotinic-receptor antagonist ($\alpha4\beta2$, $\alpha3\beta2$, $\alpha7$) mecamylamine (2.5–7.5 mg for 8 weeks) than placebo. There was also a trend ($p = 0.06$) towards greater improvement in depressed mood among mecamylamine- than placebo-treated patients in that study. No studies for mecamylamine or other selective nicotinic-receptor antagonists as monotherapy for MDD have been published (the results of an augmentation trial are presented in Chap. 6). Finally, the results of a randomized, double-blind, placebo-controlled pilot study suggested antidepressant effects for scopolamine, an antagonist of muscarinic and nicotinic acetylcholine receptors, when used as monotherapy to treat MDD or major depressive episodes in patients with bipolar disorder (Furey & Drevets, 2006).

11.7 Cannabinoids and Endocannabinoids

Clinical studies supporting the notion that cannabinoid-selective treatments may possess antidepressant effects are limited. Specifically, following an encouraging open-label trial (Stockings, 1947) in which 20 of 27 patients with neurotic depression improved following open-label treatment with 60–90 mg of synhexyl, a synthetic tetrahydrocannabinol (THC) analogue, subsequent open-label (Pond, 1948), and double-blind trials (Ablon & Goodwin, 1974; Kotin *et al.*, 1973; Parker & Wrigley, 1950) of either synhexyl or THC for depression have been discouraging, with many patients developing severe adverse reactions including depersonalization, derealization, dysphoria, anxiety, drowsiness, dizziness, paranoid ideation, cognitive slowing, confusion, amotivation, emotional blunting and apathy.

Taken together, these studies do not support a potential antidepressant role for relatively non-selective endocannabinoid-receptor agonists such as THC and synhexyl. In addition, the paucity of more selective cannabinoidergic agents, coupled with our relatively limited understanding of the function of this neurotransmitter system, have until recently proven to be major obstacles in exploring the potential role of cannabinoidergic agents for depression. However, over the course of the past several years, much has been discovered regarding the human cannabinoidergic system. To date, at least two main classes of endocannabinoid receptors (CB1, CB2), metabotropic receptors involved in the inhibition of excitatory and inhibitory neurotransmitter release in the CNS, and at least two major [anandamine (*n*-arachidonylethanolamine) 2-arachidonylgylycerol] as well as three minor endocannabinoid agonists [noladin ether (2-arachidonylglycerol ether), virodhamine (O-arachidoylethanolamine) and *n*-arachidonyldopamine)] have been identified, along with a number of enzymes involved in endocannabinoid-agonist synthesis and reuptake (Porter & Felder, 2001; Van der Stelt & Di Marzo, 2003). A greater understanding of the anatomy and function of the cannabinoidergic system, coupled with the development of pro- or anti-cannabinoidergic agents that specifically target some but not all elements of that neurotransmitter system, may offer new opportunities to test for novel treatments for depression. For example, it has been hypothesized that the endocannabinoidergic system, among other processes, may play a key role in anxiety as well as the perception of pain and nausea (Porter & Felder, 2001; Van der Stelt & Di Marzo, 2003). Therefore, in addition to a possible role in alleviating treatment-resistant depression, as suggested by their novel, non-monoaminergic mechanism, selective cannabinoidergic agonists/antagonists may also be of interest as potential treatments which target painful, anxious or hostile symptoms of depression, as well as antidepressant-induced nausea or weight gain (Porter & Felder, 2001; Van der Stelt & Di Marzo, 2003).

11.8 Opioidergic Therapies

11.8.1 *Opioid-receptor antagonists*

Both an open-label (Cohen *et al.*, 1984) and a double-blind, placebo-controlled, cross-over study (Terenius *et al.*, 1977) report a worsening of depressive symptoms following treatment of depression with the opioid-receptor antagonist naloxone. Subsequent studies have not been conducted. Open-label data suggest modest antidepressant effects of the opioid-receptor antagonist naltrexone in depressed alcoholics (Salloum *et al.*, 1998).

11.8.2 *Opioid-receptor agonists*

The majority of studies involving the use of opioid-receptor agonists are of very short duration (hours), and offer conflicting results. Kline *et al.* (1977), for example, first reported antidepressant effects within hours in two patients with unipolar depression following a single, open-label infusion of β-endorphin. In contrast, Extein *et al.* (1981) reported no significant antidepressant or anxiolytic effects among nine patients with unipolar depression a few hours following a single open-label infusion of morphine. Similar to open-label infusion studies, double-blind, placebo-controlled, cross-over studies of β-endorphin infusion for unipolar depression also report conflicting results, with one study (Gerner *et al.*, 1980), but not another (Extein *et al.*, 1981; Pickar *et al.*, 1981) demonstrating greater improvement in depressive symptoms a few hours following β-endorphin infusion than placebo infusion.

Only two open-label studies of longer duration (days to weeks) report the use of opiate agonists for depression. Lehmann *et al.* (1971) reported an 80% improvement rate among 10 patients with depressive disorders including "neurotic depression" ($n = 5$) or "psychotic bipolar depression" ($n = 5$) treated with a combination of dexedrine and meperidine. In contrast, Varga *et al.* (1982) reported a 0% response rate among 12 depressed outpatients following daily codeine treatment (90–180 mg) for an undisclosed number of weeks. Finally, there is a case report of TRD successfully treated following a switch to tramadol monotherapy (Shapira *et al.*, 2001). Tramadol, structurally similar to venlafaxine (Markowitz & Patrick, 1998) is a μ-opioid receptor agonist with relatively weak serotonin and norepinephrine reuptake inhibitor properties (Raffa *et al.*, 1992).

11.8.3 *Mixed agonists/antagonists*

Fink *et al.* (1970) first reported the use of agents with mixed agonist/antagonist opioidergic activity for depression, when he reported a dramatic improvement in mood among 10 severely depressed patients refractory to treatment with TCAs who were then treated with cyclazocine monotherapy in an open-label fashion for eight weeks. Subsequently, in a double-blind, placebo-controlled, cross-over study, Emrich *et al.* (1982a and b) reported 8 of 13 patients with MDD, who had not responded following treatment with placebo for one week, rapidly improved (within 1 week) when they were switched to buprenorphine, a partial μ-opioid receptor agonist and κ-opioid receptor antagonist (Walsh & Eissenberg, 2003). Since this encouraging study, however, only a case report (Callaway, 1996) and a small open-label trial (Bodkin *et al.*, 1995) focusing on the use of buprenorphine for depression have been published. A 40% response rate following six weeks of buprenorphine monotherapy among 10 outpatients with refractory depression was reported in the latter report.

Overall, it appears that the use of opiate antagonists has an unclear role in the treatment of depressive symptoms, while the treatment of depression with classic opiate agonists, agents which are full agonists at μ-, κ-, as well as δ-opioid receptors, does not appear promising based on studies conducted to date. In addition, the prolonged administration of classic opiate agonists that would be required in order to help depressed patients sustain remission during the continuation and maintenance phases of treatment would carry a significant risk of opiate abuse. For these reasons, opiate antagonists and classical opiate agonists are unlikely as potential candidates for testing as future antidepressants. However, small studies involving the use of mixed opioid agonist/antagonists for depression offer promise. These agents have the advantage of a lower abuse potential than classical opiate agonists (Walsh & Eissenberg, 2003), and may prove useful for the treatment of resistant/refractory depression or when targeting somatic/painful symptoms of depression.

11.9 Other Neurotransmitter Systems

Opipramol is a tricyclic compound with no reuptake-inhibiting properties but with pronounced D2-, 5-HT2-, and H1-antagonist potential as well as high affinity to σ receptors (σ-1 and σ-2) (Möller *et al.*, 2001). The results of a randomized, double-blind, placebo-controlled trial revealed a greater reduction in anxiety among patients with generalized anxiety disorder treated with opipramole than placebo (Möller *et al.*, 2001). The results of an open-label study also report a 60% response rate following monotherapy with the selective σ-1 receptor agonist igmesine (Hayashi & Su, 2004) for depression (Leaderbetter *et al.*, 1999). In fact, a subsequent double-blind study revealed greater efficacy for igmesine- than placebo-treated depressed outpatients (Leaderbetter *et al.*, 1999). However, treatment effect in that study appeared to be confounded by an interaction of treatment by center and hospitalization status and, as a result, the validity of the study findings was questioned (Leaderbetter *et al.*, 1999). A randomized, double-blind, placebo-controlled trial focusing on the use of a new σ-1 receptor agonist (SA4503) as monotherapy for MDD is currently under way (NCT00551109).

Similarly, the results of a double-blind study comparing the 5HT1A-receptor antagonist buspirone, with the antihistaminic agent hydroxyzine and placebo for GAD, reported greater reductions in depressive symptom scores among hydroxyzine than placebo-treated patients, while symptom resolution during treatment with hydroxyzine was equivalent to buspirone (Lader & Scotto, 1998). However, patients with a comorbid mood disorder were excluded from that trial while studies focusing on the use of hydroxyzine or other anti-histaminergic agents for depression have not been published to date.

In parallel, a number of case reports suggest rapid alleviation of depressive symptoms following the administration of the angiotensin-converting enzyme inhibitor captopril (Cohen & Zubenko, 1988; Deicken, 1986; Germain & Chouinard, 1988 and 1989; Vuckovic *et al.*, 1991; Zubenko & Nixon, 1984). The authors of these case reports attributed the observed antidepressant effects on the ability of captopril to inhibit enkephalin metabolism. Subsequent studies have not been published. Finally, studies focusing on the use of agents with selective galanin-, nociceptin-, neuropeptide Y- or cholinergic muscarinic activity as treatments for depression are lacking.

Chapter 12

Neuroendocrine-Based Agents

12.1 Hypothalamic-Pituitary-Gonadal Axis (HPG)

12.1.1 *Estrogen*

A growing body of evidence supports the efficacy of estrogen therapy (ET) as monotherapy for the treatment of depressive disorders in specific sub-populations. Overall, it appears that treatment with estrogen has been successfully used in women suffering from depressive symptoms during periods of intense hormone fluctuations, such as the premenstrual phase (Smith *et al.*, 1995), the postpartum period (Ahokas *et al.*, 2000; Gregoire *et al.*, 1996), and the transition to menopause (Soares *et al.*, 2001). In contrast, studies including sub-populations in which estrogen levels are more constant (e.g., postmenopausal women) have shown less compelling evidence of estrogen's antidepressant efficacy (Cohen *et al.*, 2003; George *et al.*, 1973; Morrison *et al.*, 2004; Saletu *et al.*, 1995). Table 12.1 summarizes the double-blind studies involving estrogen therapy for the treatment of depressive disorders in menopausal women.

The efficacy of transdermal 17β estradiol (E2; 200 µg/day) for the treatment of postpartum depression was demonstrated in a double-blinded, placebo-controlled study (Gregoire *et al.*, 1996). Women ($n = 61$) suffering from treatment-resistant postpartum depression were randomized to receive treatment with either E2 or placebo for three months, followed by E2 plus progesterone (versus placebo arm) for an additional period of three months. After four weeks of treatment, 50% of women receiving E2 had shown significant

Table 12.1 Double-blind estrogen treatment studies (monotherapy) for menopausal depression.

Study	*N*	Population studied	Duration	Study design	Results
Campbell & Whitehead, 1977	64	Severe menopausal MDD	2 months per drug	E (oral CE) vs PL; 2XB, cross-over	E > PL
Schmidt *et al.*, 1997	20	Perimenopausal MDD	6 weeks	E (oral CE) vs PL	E > PL
Thomson, 1977	16	Mixed menopausal	2 months	E (oral CE) vs PL, 2XB	E = PL
Coope, 1981	55	Menopausal MDD	6 months per drug	E (oral CE) vs PL; 2XB, cross-over	Mild improvement E = PL
Schmidt *et al.*, 2000	34	Perimenopausal depression	3 or 6 weeks	E2 (50μg, T), Vs PL; 2XB	Partial/full remission in 80% w/E2; PL = 22%
Soares *et al.*, 2001	50	Perimenopausal depression	3 months	E2 (100μg, T) Vs PL; 2XB	Full remission in 60% w/E2; PL = 20%
Morrison *et al.*, 2004	57	Postmenopausal depression	2 months	E2 (100μg, T) VS PL; 2XB	E2 = PL

Abbreviations: MDD = major depressive disorder; E = estrogen-treated group; E2 = estradiol; T = transdermal use; CE = conjugated estrogens — usually 0.625 mg/day; PL = placebo; 2XB = double-blind; cross-over = cross-over.

response, compared to 26% on placebo. Response to E2 increased progressively during the remaining five months of treatment.

An eight-week, open-label trial utilizing a different route of administration (sub-lingual 17β estradiol) also resulted in a rapid antidepressant response among 23 women with postnatal depression; within two weeks of treatment, clinical recovery was seen in 19 of 23 patients (Ahokas *et al.*, 2001). The same investigators also showed positive results with sublingual E2 for the treatment of postpartum psychosis ($n = 10$ — Ahokas *et al.*, 2000).

Three open-label trials have also focused on the use of estrogen for the treatment of depressive disorders among perimenopausal women; subjects in these trials received treatment for a total of 4–8 weeks, with remission rates ranging from 60% to 70% (Cohen *et al.*, 2003; Rasgon *et al.*, 2001 and 2002). In addition, two double-blind, placebo-controlled trials (with a total of 84 subjects) have also demonstrated the efficacy of transdermal 17β E2 for the treatment of depressive disorders (MDD, dysthymia, or minor depression) among perimenopausal women. In one three-week study ($n = 34$), the treatment of depression among perimenopausal women with patches containing estradiol (50 μg/day) resulted in a greater resolution of depressive symptoms than treatment with placebo (Schmidt *et al.*, 2000). In a larger sample ($n = 50$), 12 weeks of treatment with 100 μg of transdermal E2 promoted a 68% remission of depression in perimenopausal women randomly assigned to receive hormone treatment, compared to 20% in the placebo group (Soares *et al.*, 2001) (Fig. 12.1).

Double-blind, placebo-controlled trials focusing on the use of estrogen for the treatment of depression in populations of women with mixed menopausal status have shown some positive (Campbell *et al.*, 1977; Ditkoff *et al.*, 1991) as well as negative (Coope, 1981; Thompson & Oswald, 1977) results. Interestingly enough, when the population treated was restricted to postmenopausal women (i.e., surgically-induced menopause or women reporting more than 12 months without menses), results of treatment with estrogen were mostly negative. This appears to be true both in double-blind, placebo-controlled studies (Morrison *et al.*, 2004; Saletu *et al.*, 1995)

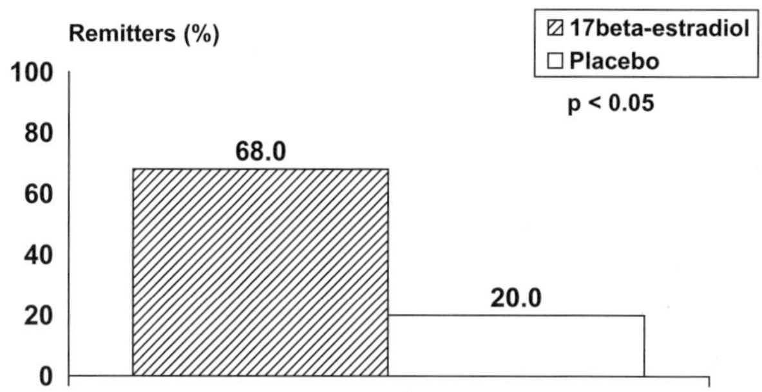

Fig. 12.1 Estradiol for depression in peri-menopausal women: A randomized, double-blind study ($n = 50$). [Data extracted from: Soares, C.N., Almeida, O.P., Joffe, H., & Cohen, L.S. (2001). Efficacy of estradiol for the treatment of depressive disorders in perimenopausal women: A double-blind, randomized, placebo-controlled trial. *Archives of General Psychiatry*, 58, 529–534.]

as well as open-label trials (Cohen *et al.*, 2003; Schneider *et al.*, 1977). In one small study ($n = 12$) including postmenopausal women with depression, significant improvement of depressive symptoms was noted among patients who received oral conjugated estrogens for six months, compared to those who did not receive any treatment (Carranza-Lira & Valentino-Figueroa, 1999). However, the subjects enrolled in the latter study were not randomized, but rather assigned to receive estrogen based on the existence/absence of clinical contraindications to hormone therapy and on their personal decision to receive hormonal treatment. Finally, a randomized, double-blind, placebo-controlled trial focusing on the use of a 17β E2 patch versus placebo for women with perimenopausal major depressive disorder (MDD) as well as insomnia and hot flashes is currently under way (NCT00227942).

Some have hypothesized that the effect of estrogen on depression could be mediated by resolution of vasomotor symptoms (VMS — hot flashes, night sweats) or insomnia. Others suggest that estrogen exerts a direct neuromodulatory effect, and may treat depression independently of its effect on vasomotor symptoms (Rubinow *et al.*, 1998). However, the use of transdermal estradiol has shown superior efficacy compared to placebo even when hot flushes were not present (Schmidt *et al.*, 2000). In addition, women with depression treated with transdermal estradiol were able to sustain an antidepressant benefit obtained with E2 even after a four-week washout period, despite the re-emergence of vasomotor symptoms (Soares *et al.*, 2001). These findings support the notion that estrogens have effects on mood that are independent from the effects mediated through alleviation of VMS.

Differences in the pharmacokinetic aspects of estrogen preparations may contribute to the lack of consistency between studies on the effect of estrogen treatment on mood (Halbreich & Kahn, 2001; Soares, 2003). Transdermal administration of estradiol avoids "first pass" circulation through the liver and gastrointestinal absorption, and provides a rapid rise in the serum concentration of estradiol and nearly constant serum levels over the entire application period (Ramachandran & Fleisher, 2000). Oral estrogen preparations, in contrast, are metabolized through the hepatic portal system, resulting in higher conversion to a less active metabolite (estrone) and consequently lower bioavailability of estradiol (Fraser & Wang, 1998). Perhaps as a consequence, most estrogen metabolites focusing on the use of oral preparations (conjugated equine estrogen or piperazine sulfate estrone) do not support mood-enhancing effects for estrogen (Coope, 1981; Strickler *et al.*, 1977).

12.1.2 *Progesterone*

Progesterone has been more systematically studied as a monotherapy for depressive symptoms associated with premenstrual syndrome (PMS). Specifically, 10 randomized, placebo-controlled studies including more than 600 subjects have utilized either progesterone suppositories administered vaginally or rectally (200–800 mg/day) or oral progesterone (200–600 mg/day) for the treatment of physical and mood symptoms associated with PMS (Andersch & Hahn, 1985; Corney *et al.*, 1990; Dennerstein *et al.*, 1985; Freeman *et al.*, 1990 and 1995; Madocks *et al.*, 1986; Magill, 1995; Rapkin *et al.*, 1987; Van der Meer *et al.*, 1983; Vanselow *et al.*, 1996). Only one study ($n = 20$) revealed some positive effects on irritability and depressive symptoms for progesterone (Van der Meer *et al.*, 1983).

In contrast, a number of studies have attempted to examine the extent to which the administration of depot-medroxiprogesterone acetate (D-MPA), as a contraceptive method, may result in the *worsening* rather than alleviation of mood symptoms. For instance, in one population-based prospective study of 183 D-MPA users and 274 non-users, there was an association between D-MPA use and the occurrence of depressive symptoms (Civic *et al.*, 2000). Similarly, the use of natural progesterone suppositories led to negative mood effects on postmenopausal women in a small, placebo-controlled trial ($n = 36$) (Andreen *et al.*, 2003). In contrast, however, the use of transdermal progesterone for 12 weeks did not significantly change mood characteristics in 80 postmenopausal women randomized to receive active treatment or placebo (Wren *et al.*, 2003). In summary, studies focusing on the role of depot-MPA in worsening mood show the absence of an effect or a minimal increase in negative mood symptoms, and are by no ways definitive (Gupta *et al.*, 2001; Westhoff *et al.*, 1995).

12.1.3 *Androgens*

There is a long history of the use of androgens as antidepressants, with a number of reports published particularly during the pre-monoamine era (Altschule & Tillotson, 1948; Danziger & Blank, 1942; Danziger *et al.*, 1944). In the first double-blind, controlled study of androgen monotherapy ever published, 52 patients suffering from a variety of depressive disorders (i.e., MDD, bipolar depression, psychotic depression, or dysthymic disorder) were randomized to receive androgen therapy (mestrolone, 300–450 mg oral daily) or placebo for a total of six weeks (Itil *et al.*, 1984). There were no differences in the degree of reduction of depressive symptom severity between the two treatment groups. Five subsequent double-blind studies of androgen monotherapy (testosterone or dehydroepiandrosterone-DHEA) for depression have been published to date. Seidman *et al.* (2001 and 2006) randomized 32 hypogonadal men (total testosterone level < 350 ng/dl) with MDD to receive 200 mg of testosterone by intramuscular injection (IM) weekly or placebo for six weeks, and reported no significant differences in the degree of reduction of depressive symptom severity or the degree of improvement in sexual functioning between the two treatment groups. Perry *et al.* (2002) randomized 15 elderly (> 50 years of age) males to receive either 100 mg or 200 mg weekly IM testosterone for six weeks. Five patients remitted, with no differences in the degree of resolution of depressive symptoms between the two groups. Schmidt *et al.* (2005) randomized men (n = 23) and women (n = 23) with midlife-onset (ages 45–65) MDD and minor depression to receive either DHEA (up to 450 mg/day) or placebo for a total of six weeks. A greater resolution of depressive symptoms was reported in DHEA- than placebo-treated patients (Fig. 12.2). Seidman *et al.* (2009) randomized 23 men with dysthymic disorder and low testosterone levels to receive 200 mg testosterone cyprionate in every 10 days or placebo for six weeks. Greater resolution of depressive symptoms was noted among testosterone- than placebo-treated men. Finally, Shores *et al.* (2009) randomized hypogonadol older men with dysthymic disorder or minor depression to receive 7.5 g testosterone gel or placebo for 12 weeks. Greater resolution of depressive symptoms for testosterone- than placebo-treated men was reported.

Studies have also been published focusing on the effects of testosterone monotherapy on depressive symptoms among

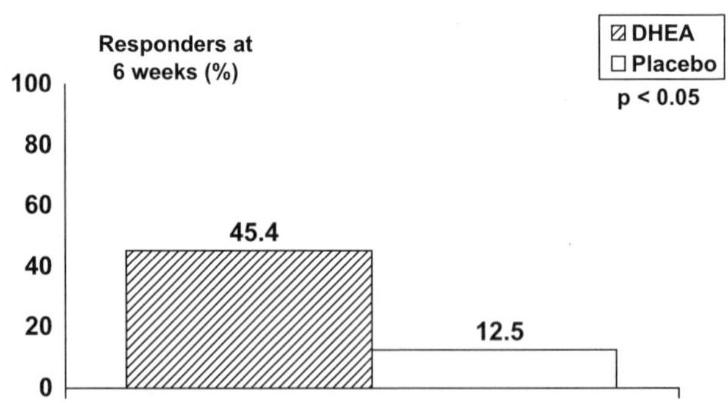

Fig. 12.2 Dehydroepiandrosterone (DHEA) for midlife-onset major and minor depression: A randomized, double-blind study (n = 46). [Data extracted from: Schmidt, P.J., Daly, R.C., Bloch, M., *et al.* (2005). Dehydroepiandrosterone monotherapy in midlife-onset major and minor depression. *Archives of General Psychiatry*, 62, 154–162.]

non-depressed elderly patients. Cavallini *et al.* (2004) randomized 120 elderly men (age 65 y/o and older) to treatment with testosterone undecanoate (160 mg/day), propionyl-L-carnitine/acetyl-L-carnitine 2/2 gm/day, or placebo for six months. Greater improvements in depressed mood, fatigue and sexual functioning were reported in subjects treated with testosterone- or L-carnitine compared to placebo. More recently, however, Haren *et al.* (2005) reported no difference in the resolution of depressive symptoms among elderly subjects following 12 months of treatment with either oral testosterone undecanoate (80 mg twice daily) or placebo.

A number of studies have also examined the use of testosterone for the treatment of depressive symptoms or depression in patients who were tested positive for the human immunodeficiency virus (HIV+). Three open-label studies have been published, including a total of 313 hypogonadal, HIV+ men who received treatment with 400 mg of testosterone IM bi-weekly, for a total of 8–12 weeks (Rabkin & Wagner, 1995; Rabkin *et al.*, 1999; Wagner *et al.*, 1998). These studies report response rates ranging between 64–86% for the subgroup of patients with depressive symptoms or with a formal diagnosis of MDD. In fact, in the study by Rabkin *et al.* (1999), when 84 testosterone-responders were randomized to either switch to placebo or continue treatment with testosterone (in a double-blind fashion) for an additional period of six weeks, a significant increase in depressive symptom scores was found in the placebo-treated patients, but not among the testosterone-treated patients.

Two out of three subsequent double-blind studies also support the use of testosterone for the treatment of depressive symptoms or depression in HIV+ patients. Grinspoon *et al.* (2000) randomized 52 HIV+ hypogonadal men with acquired immunodeficiency syndrome (AIDS) to receive treatment with testosterone (300 mg, IM, every 3 weeks) or placebo for a total of six months. A statistically significant decrease in depressive symptoms in testosterone- but not placebo-treated patients was observed. Rabkin *et al.* (2000) randomized 74 HIV+ men, 26 of who also met criteria for MDD, to receive treatment with testosterone (400 mg IM bi-weekly) or placebo for six weeks. A greater reduction in depressive symptoms among testosterone- than placebo-treated patients was reported.

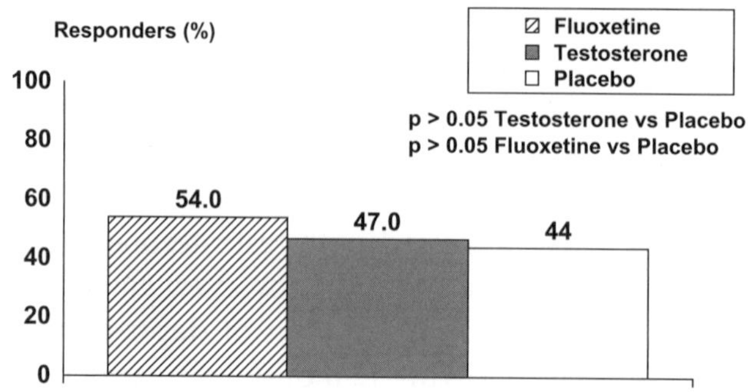

Fig. 12.3 Testosterone versus fluoxetine (SSRI) for depression and fatigue in HIV/AIDS: A randomized, double-blind study ($n = 123$). [Data extracted from: Rabkin, J.G., Wagner, G.J., McElhiney, M.C., *et al.* (2004). Testosterone versus fluoxetine for depression and fatigue in HIV/AIDS: A placebo-controlled trial. *Journal of Clinical Psychopharmacology*, 24, 379–385.]

This finding was also confirmed within the subgroup of patients with a formal diagnosis of MDD. However, when Rabkin *et al.* (2004) randomized 123 HIV+ outpatients who also met criteria for either MDD, dysthymic disorder, or minor depression to treatment with fluoxetine (up to 60 mg), testosterone (400 mg IM every other week), or placebo for a total duration of eight weeks, greater improvement in fatigue but not depression severity was reported among testosterone than fluoxetine- or placebo-treated patients (Fig. 12.3).

However, there is a paucity of studies focusing on the use of androgens for the treatment of depression among patients with other medical conditions commonly associated with hypogonadism. A double-blind, placebo-controlled trial of testosterone replacement (100 mg IM every two weeks) among hypogonadal men with angina revealed greater improvements in self-reported mood among testosterone- than placebo-treated patients (Malkin *et al.*, 2004). In contrast, a small ($n = 10$), double-blind study did not reveal any significant difference in the reduction in depressive symptoms among outpatients with Parkinson's disease who received treatment with testosterone (5 mg/day in gel form) or placebo (Okun *et al.*, 2002). Lastly, anecdotal evidence supports the use of IM testosterone in leuprolide-induced depression (Freeman & Freeman, 2003).

Symptoms of depression, anxiety, as well as decreased libido have also been described in postmenopausal women who present with low testosterone levels, including surgically-induced menopausal women. Shifren *et al.* (2000) conducted a double-blind, placebo-controlled trial involving 75 surgically induced menopausal women (ages 31 to 56) who were randomized to receive treatment with either testosterone (patches containing 150 or 300 μg) or placebo for 12 weeks. All subjects also received concomitant treatment with oral conjugated estrogens. Women treated with testosterone reported greater psychological well-being and a significant improvement in mood, anxiety, and sexual functioning than women who received placebo. Administration of testosterone appeared to be well tolerated, without significant occurrence of acne or hirsutism.

12.1.4 *Dehydroepiandrosterone (DHEA)*

To date, only four studies have examined the role of the natural androgen and estrogen precursor DHEA as monotherapy for depression. Wolkowitz *et al.* (1997) reported a significant decrease in depression symptom severity among six patients with MDD and low basal plasma DHEA levels following treatment with 30–90 mg oral DHEA daily for four weeks. In a subsequent, double-blind study, 22 outpatients suffering from MDD were randomized to receive treatment with either oral DHEA (90 mg/day) or placebo for six weeks (Wolkowitz *et al.*, 1999a). A greater reduction in depression severity scores was reported in DHEA- than placebo-treated patients. Finally, Rabkin *et al.* (2006) reported a greater resolution of depressive symptoms among 145 patients with either minor depression or dysthymic disorder and comorbid HIV/AIDS treated with DHEA than placebo. In addition to these three trials focusing on the treatment of depression, a double-blind study involving 24 women with adrenal insufficiency who received DHEA (50 mg) versus placebo for six weeks revealed a significant decrease in self-reported depressive and anxiety symptoms among DHEA- but not placebo-treated women (Allolio *et al.*, 1999).

12.1.5 *Other gonadotropic agents*

Benkert *et al.* (1975) reported robust but transient (lasting only a few hours) improvement among 6 of 12 women treated with intravenous luteinizing-hormone releasing hormone (LHRH, 500 mcg). Freeman *et al.* (1993) treated seven patients with premenstrual syndrome, two of whom also met criteria for MDD, with open-label IM (depot) gonadotropin-releasing hormone agonist (GnRH) for four weeks. Depressive symptoms were significantly reduced in non-MDD patients from baseline to endpoint, but slightly worsened in MDD patients (Freeman *et al.*, 1993). Finally, a randomized, double-blind, placebo-controlled trial focusing on the use of raloxifene (selective estrogen receptor modulator) versus rimostil (phytoestrogen) versus estradiol as monotherapy for perimenopausal women with MDD is currently under way (NCT00030147).

12.2 Hypothalamic-Pituitary-Adrenal Axis (HPA)

12.2.1 *Corticosteroids*

Only two trials examine the use of the synthetic corticosteroid dexamethasone in the treatment of depression. Arana and Forbes (1991) first reported a 75% response rate among 16 subjects with MDD or a major depressive episode in the setting of bipolar disorder, 10 days after a single, 4–8 mg intravenous (I.V.) injection of dexamethasone. In a subsequent, two-week, double-blind study involving 37 MDD outpatients, Arana *et al.* (1995) reported greater response rates in subjects treated with dexamethasone (monotherapy with oral form, 4 mg for 4 days) than placebo (response rates of 37% versus 6%, respectively). However, there is a paucity of evidence for the use of other forms of corticosteroids as monotherapy for the treatment of depression. Two double-blind studies report acute (within hours) antidepressant effects after intravenous cortisol or hydrocortisone infusion in MDD patients (DeBattista *et al.*, 2000; Goodwin *et al.*, 1992) (Fig. 12.4). However, to date, long-term studies have not been published.

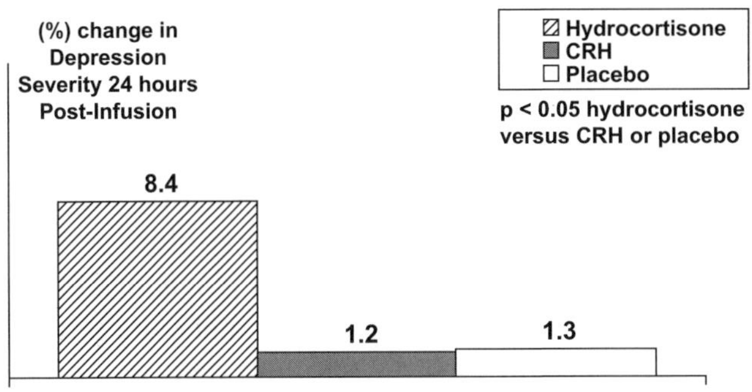

Fig. 12.4 Intravenous hydrocortisone and CRH for depression: A randomized, double-blind study ($n = 22$). [Data extracted from: DeBattista, C., Posener, J.A., Kalehzan, B.M., & Schatzberg, A.F. (2000). Acute antidepressant effects of intravenous hydrocortisone and CRH in depressed patients: A double-blind, placebo-controlled study. *American Journal of Psychiatry*, 157, 1334–1337.]

12.2.2 *Steroid synthesis inhibitors*

A number of reports, mostly published during the 1970s and 1980s, support the use of steroid synthesis inhibitors such as metyrapone, ketoconazole, and aminoglutethimide, for the treatment of depressive symptoms or depression in patients with hypercortisolemia due to medical causes such as Cushing's syndrome or Cushing's disease (Wolkowitz & Reus, 1999). These were followed by numerous case studies (Anand *et al.*, 1995; Bech *et al.*, 1999; Brown *et al.*, 2001; Murphy, 1991; Sovner & Fogelman, 1996), and open-label trials (Ghadirian *et al.*, 1995; Murphy *et al.*, 1991 and 1998; Raven *et al.*, 1996; Thakore & Dinan, 1995; Wolkowitz *et al.*, 1993) focusing on the use of steroid synthesis inhibitors as monotherapy for depression. Some of these reports focused exclusively on MDD patients (Anand *et al.*, 1995; Bech *et al.*, 1999; Murphy, 1991; Raven *et al.*, 1996; Sovner & Fogelman, 1996; Thakore & Dinan, 1995), or a major depressive episode in the setting of bipolar disorder (Brown *et al.*, 2001), while other studies contained both patients with MDD as well as those with a major depressive episode in the setting of bipolar disorder (Wolkowitz *et al.*, 1993), or even patients with MDD, bipolar depression, and psychotic MDD (Ghadirian *et al.*, 1995; Murphy *et al.*, 1991 and 1998). The duration of treatment for the open-label trials ranged from two to eight weeks, with response rates ranging from 55% to 100%.

To date, three controlled trials for steroid synthesis inhibitors as monotherapy for MDD have been published. A small ($n = 8$), single-blind, placebo-controlled, cross-over trial of four weeks' duration revealed a greater decrease in depressive symptom severity among metyrapone-treated patients compared to placebo (O'Dwyer *et al.*, 1995). However, a subsequent double-blind study by Malison *et al.* (1999) involving 16 depressed outpatients who were treated with ketoconazole (up to 1200 mg/day) or placebo did not reveal any difference in efficacy between the two treatment groups. Similarly, a double-blind study conducted by Wolkowitz *et al.* (1999b) involving MDD outpatients ($n = 20$) randomized to receive treatment with ketoconazole (400–800 mg/day) or placebo also did not reveal any difference in efficacy between the two groups. However, in the latter study, a greater decrease in depressive symptom scores during ketoconazole- than placebo-treatment was reported among the subset of patients who were hypercortisolemic at baseline.

12.2.3 Steroid- and CRF-receptor antagonists

R121919 is an antagonist for corticotropin-releasing factor-1 (CRF-1) receptors at central nervous system (CNS) (Heinrichs *et al.*, 2002). To date, there is only a single, open-label trial focusing on the use of R121919 (4–80 mg, 4 weeks) for the treatment of MDD ($n = 24$) (Kunzel *et al.*, 2003). Thirteen patients responded in that study (9 remitted). However, the results of a randomized, double-blind, placebo- and sertraline-controlled trial focusing on the use of a different CRF-1–receptor antagonist for MDD (CP-316,311) did not demonstrate any antidepressant effects for CP-316,311 (Binneman *et al.*, 2008). Several other randomized, double-blind, placebo-controlled trials focusing on the use of various CRF-receptor antagonists (ONO-2333Ms; BMS-562086) are also currently under way (NCT00514865; NCT00135421).

RU486, also known as mifepristone, acts as an antagonist of glucocorticoid and progesterone receptors (Attardi *et al.*, 2004). A case report of mifepristone for the treatment of psychotic depression and

Cushing's syndrome (Chu *et al.*, 2001) was soon followed by an open-label study of mifepristone for psychotic MDD (Belanoff *et al.*, 2002). Thirty patients were enrolled in the latter study, and treated with 50 mg, 600 mg, or 1200 mg of mifepristone daily for a very short duration (7 days). Response rates for depressive symptoms were 18.2%, 50% and 33% for each of the three treatment groups, respectively. Response rates for psychotic symptoms were 36.4%, 70% and 66.7% for each of the three treatment groups, respectively. While a double-blind, cross-over study involving five patients with psychotic MDD who were randomized to receive either 600 mg of mifepristone or placebo for a relatively short duration (4 days) revealed no statistically significant difference in antidepressant or antipsychotic effect between the two treatment groups (Belanoff *et al.*, 2001), a subsequent, larger ($n = 221$) study of longer duration (4 weeks) revealed a significantly greater reduction in the severity of psychotic but not depressive symptoms following treatment with mifepristone than placebo (DeBattista *et al.*, 2006) (Fig. 12.5). Further studies are needed to assess the potential usefulness of this compound in the treatment of psychotic depression.

The results of a small ($n = 4$), open-label study of mifepristone (200 mg/day for up to 8 weeks) for the treatment of non-psychotic

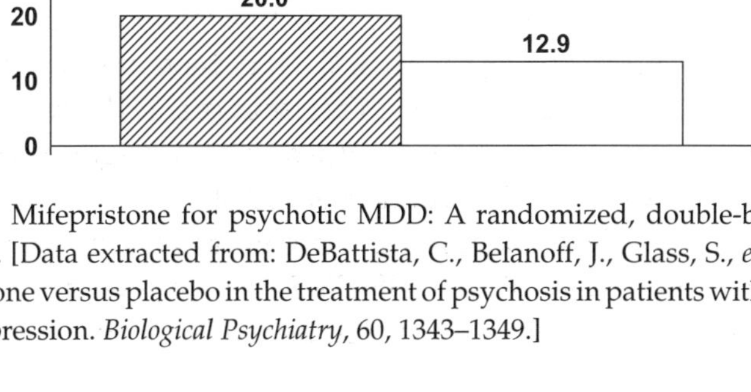

Fig. 12.5 Mifepristone for psychotic MDD: A randomized, double-blind study ($n = 221$). [Data extracted from: DeBattista, C., Belanoff, J., Glass, S., *et al.* (2006). Mifepristone versus placebo in the treatment of psychosis in patients with psychotic major depression. *Biological Psychiatry*, 60, 1343–1349.]

MDD did not reveal a significant reduction in depressive symptom severity during treatment (Murphy *et al.*, 1993). In a recent study, 20 subjects with bipolar depression were treated with 600 mg/day of mifepristone or placebo in a double-blind cross-over fashion. After six weeks of treatment, depressive symptom scores were significantly reduced among patients treated with mifepristone but not among those treated with placebo. Other benefits were also noted among patients in the active treatment group that were not observed among placebo-treated patients, including improvement in spatial working memory performance, spatial recognition memory and verbal fluency (Young *et al.*, 2004).

12.3 Hypothalamic-Pituitary-Thyroid Axis (HPT)

Following the publication of an open-label trial (Kastin *et al.*, 1972) in which four of five depressed patients experienced an improvement in depressive symptoms following the use of parenteral (I.V.) thyrotropin-releasing hormone (TRH), a number of double-blind, placebo-controlled, parallel or cross-over studies have been published reporting robust yet transient (lasting a few hours) improvements in mood following TRH administration as monotherapy (Benkert *et al.*, 1974; Ehrensing *et al.*, 1974; Itil *et al.*, 1974; Prange *et al.*, 1972; Szuba *et al.*, 2005; Van Den Burgh *et al.*, 1976) (Fig. 12.6).

However, not all such studies were able to replicate this finding (Hollister *et al.*, 1974; Takahashi *et al.*, 1973; Vogel *et al.*, 1977). The majority of these studies included mixed unipolar/bipolar patient populations, and employed a wide range of TRH dosages (200–1000 mcg). To date, sustained antidepressant effects (i.e., past 48 hours post-administration) for I.V. TRH have yet to be demonstrated. Controlled trials involving the use of oral TRH (ranging from 80–300 mg) for depression have, uniformly, been negative (Karlberg *et al.*, 1978; Kiely *et al.*, 1976; Turek *et al.*, 1974).

A major obstacle in examining whether treatment with TRH, a tripeptide consisting of pGLU-HIS-PRO-NH2, can lead to sustained improvement is that it is rapidly metabolized in serum (Lloyd *et al.*,

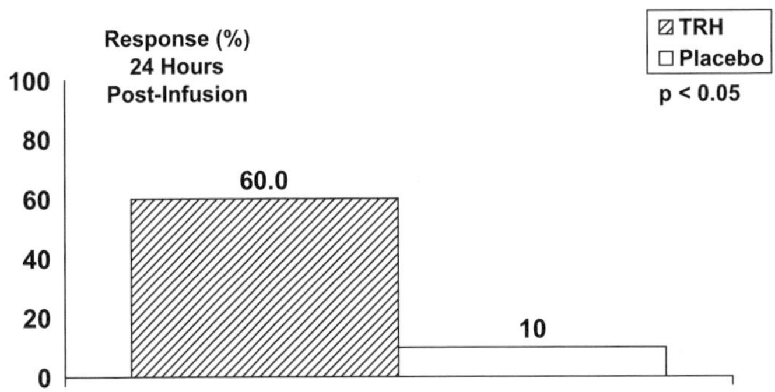

Fig. 12.6 Nocturnal TRH for bipolar major depression: A randomized, double-blind study ($n = 20$). [Data extracted from: Szuba, M.P., Amsterdam, J.D., Fernando, A.T. 3rd., *et al.* (2005). Rapid antidepressant response after nocturnal TRH administration in patients with bipolar type I and bipolar type II major depression. *Journal of Clinical Psychopharmacology*, 25, 325–330.]

2001). Therefore, TRH-analogues not subject to breakdown by TRH metabolizing enzymes including pGLU-GLU-PRO-NH2 (EEP) and pGLU-PHE-PRO-NH2 (EFP) may be better suited for further clinical testing (Lloyd *et al.*, 2001). In addition, the identification and characterization of human TRH-receptor subtypes and, consequently, the development of receptor-specific ligands may present with further opportunities for the development of novel treatments for MDD. In mammals, for example, two receptor subtypes have been identified, termed TRH-R1 and TRH-R2, with the pituitary (involved in TSH release, and, therefore, T3 and T4 release from the thyroid) expressing the former subtype and the cingulated cortex and striatum (involved in mood regulation) expressing the latter subtype (Sun *et al.*, 2003).

12.4 Melatonin and Melatonergic Agents

The results of a small ($n = 6$), double-blind, placebo-controlled cross-over study in patients with MDD did not show any antidepressant effects for melatonin monotherapy (Carman *et al.*, 1976). A subsequent, open-label trial of melatonin for MDD with a seasonal (fall/winter) component also reported very modest response rates (3 out of 17 patients) (Wirz-Justice *et al.*, 1990). However, a double-blind study involving 10 outpatients with MDD or bipolar depression with a winter seasonal component revealed greater reduction in depressive symptoms in the melatonin group (0.25 mg daily) compared to placebo after three weeks of treatment (Lewy *et al.*, 1998). A greater reduction in depression severity was recently reported among peri- and post-menopausal women ($n = 79$) randomized to treatment with melatonin (3 mg) when compared to placebo after six months (Bellipanni *et al.*, 2001). However, melatonin (2 mg for 3 weeks) was not found to be more effective than placebo in the treatment of symptoms of atypical depression among 58 adults with sub-syndromal seasonal affective disorder in one double-blind study (Leppamaki *et al.*, 2003), and did not appear to reduce the risk of relapse more so than placebo among ECT-responders in another double-blind study (Grunhaus *et al.*, 2001). Finally, the results of an open-label trial do not support the use of melatonin for the treatment of depressive symptoms in fibromyalgia patients (Citera *et al.*, 2000).

5-methoxypsoralen (5-MOP) is a melatonin-releasing agent (Souetre *et al.*, 1987). In a double-blind study involving 24 MDD patients randomized to either treatment with the melatonergic agent 5-MOP or placebo for one week, greater decreases in depression severity were reported for the 5-MOP- than the placebo-treated group (Souetre *et al.*, 1988). This study has yet to be replicated.

More recently, treatment with selective M1- and M2-melatonergic-receptor agonists (β-methyl-6-chloromelatonin; Ramelteon) has been reported to result in greater reductions in sleep latency than placebo among outpatients with primary insomnia (Erman *et al.*, 2006; Zemlan *et al.*, 2004). Studies involving these compounds for depression, either as monotherapy or adjunctive treatment, have yet to be published.

The results of one (Ehrensing & Kastin, 1978) but not a second (Ehrensing & Kastin, 1974) double-blind, placebo-controlled trial report greater symptom resolution following five days of treatment of depression with oral melanocyte-stimulating hormone-release inhibiting factor (MIF). Specifically, the former of the two studies demonstrated greater symptom resolution than placebo among patients treated with 75 mg daily but not among those treated with 750 mg daily. In parallel, two double-blind studies also compare oral MIF (60 mg) with imipramine (150 mg daily) for depression (Levy *et al.*, 1982; Van Der Velde, 1983). These studies demonstrated MIF to be either equivalent to imipramine (Levy *et al.*, 1982) or superior to imipramine (Van Der Velde, 1983) following seven days of treatment. In addition, non-responders following seven days of treatment were removed from the study while patients with a partial/full response continued on MIF versus imipramine for an additional three weeks.

A worsening in MIF- but not imipramine-treated patients at endpoint was reported in the former (Levy *et al.*, 1982) but not the later study (Van Der Velde, 1983). Since MIF is a peptide (pPro-Leu-Gly-NH2), questions have been raised regarding the absorption of oral preparations. Greater symptom resolution was reported among MDD patients following five days of treatment with subcutaneous injections of MIF (10 mg/day) versus placebo-treated patients (Ehrensing *et al.*, 1994).

Melanin-concentrating hormone antagonists appear to demonstrate antidepressant, anti-anxiety and anti-obesity effects in animal studies (Doggrell, 2003). Clinical studies for these agents have yet to be published. Finally, melatonergic-receptor antagonists (Dubokovich *et al.*, 2003), although not yet fully characterized, may eventually be of interest for clinical testing as wakefulness-promoting agents, or for the treatment of cognitive symptoms and inattention.

12.5 Other Hormones

Fewer studies examine the role of vasopressin (VP) in depression. A small ($n = 4$) trial published in 1979 reported improvement in cognitive functioning in three patients and in depressive symptoms in four patients with MDD treated with the synthetic VP analog 1-desamo-8-D-arginine vasopressin (DDAVP) (Gold *et al.*, 1979). However, this study was soon followed-up with "negative" double-blind, placebo-controlled trials of lysine vasopressin for the treatment of depression in patients with MDD or bipolar depression ($n = 12$) (Zohar *et al.*, 1985), and DDAVP for the treatment of memory impairment following ECT (Mattes *et al.*, 1989 and 1990). Selective vasopressin VIb-receptor antagonists appear to demonstrate some anti-anxiety and antiobesity effects in animal studies (Griebel *et al.*, 2003). Clinical trials focusing on the use of a vasopressin-receptor antagonist (SSR149415) as monotherapy for MDD are currently under way (NCT00361491; NCT00358631).

Studies for growth hormone (GH) or insulin-like growth factor-1 (IGF-I) in depression have not been published to date. However, greater decreases in depressive symptoms in GH- than placebo-treated patients with GH deficiency have been reported in double-blind studies (Giusti *et al.*, 1998; Soares *et al.*, 1999). Similarly, greater decreases in depressive symptomatology in IGF-I than GH- or placebo-treated obese postmenopausal women have been reported in a different controlled trial (Thompson *et al.*, 1988). More recently, the degree of individual increases in IGF-1 but not GH secretion following the double-blind, placebo-controlled administration of an oral mixture containing glycine, glutamine and niacin (5 g bid) for eight weeks was found to correlate with improved memory and vigor among healthy volunteers (Arwert *et al.*, 2003).

Four double-blind studies involving patients with Alzheimer's disease (Craft *et al.*, 1996 and 1999) or healthy volunteers (Benedict *et al.*, 2004; Kern *et al.*, 2001) suggest that administration of intravenous (Craft *et al.*, 1996 and 1999; Kern *et al.*, 2001) or intranasal (Benedict *et al.*, 2004) insulin, in the absence of hypoglycemia, resulted in improved memory and cognition. One of these trials (Craft *et al.*, 1999) also demonstrated significant improvement in memory and cognition following somatostatin infusion. However, the use of intranasal insulin for the improvement of mood and cognitive function in depression has not yet been studied.

Finally, although studies of cholecystokinin-B (CCK-B), CCK-2 (the principal CNS receptor; Herranz, 2003) receptor antagonists for depression have not been published, double-blind, placebo-controlled trials of CCK-B receptor antagonists for panic disorder (Kramer *et al.*, 1995; Pande *et al.*, 1999; Sramek *et al.*, 1995), and generalized anxiety disorder (Adams *et al.*, 1995) have consistently yielded negative results.

Chapter 13

Metabolic-Based and Other Agents

13.1 Metabolic-Based Agents

13.1.1 *Elements of the "one carbon cycle"*

13.1.1.1 *S-adenosylmethionine* (*SAMe*)

SAMe, folate, vitamin B12, and homocysteine are linked in the "one carbon cycle", as homocysteine and 5-methyltetrahydrofolate (5MTHF), a product of folate, are required for the formation of SAMe.

SAMe is a naturally occurring molecule available commercially in Europe since the late 1970s as a treatment for depression and other conditions but introduced in the U.S. in a stable, enteric-coated oral form only in 1999, where it has become a popular dietary supplement. SAMe is found throughout the human body, with particularly high concentrations in the liver, adrenal glands, and the pineal gland. It appears to be uniformly distributed in the brain where it serves as the major donor of methyl groups required in the synthesis of all three monoamine neurotransmitters, as well as many neuronal second messengers and neuronal membranes (Papakostas *et al.*, 2003; Papakostas, 2009).

SAMe has been marketed for over 25 years in Europe as an antidepressant, but was released in the U.S. as an over-the-counter dietary supplement under the Dietary Health and Supplement Act (DHSEA) in 1999. The antidepressant efficacy of SAMe has been studied in over 45 randomized, controlled trials involving depressed adults in Europe and the United States (Hardy *et al.*, 2003). These studies have used parenteral (IV and IM) and oral preparations of SAMe toluenesulfonate (SAMe tosylate) and, to a lesser extent, SAMe 1,4-butanedisulphonate (Bressa, 1994).

After an initial, serendipitous observation of mood elevation in patients treated with SAMe (Pinzello & Andreoli, 1972), Fazio *et al.* (1973) reported "remission" in 14 of 35 depressed patients in an open trial of parenteral SAMe. In 1975, Agnoli *et al.* (1975) reported marked improvement of depression in 30 of 51 patients given intramuscular SAMe. Following these three reports, a large number of open studies (Andreoli *et al.*, 1977; Barberi & Pusateri, 1978; Carney *et al.*, 1986; Mantero & Pastorino, 1976; Salvadorini *et al.*, 1980) showed that treatment with parenteral SAMe was followed by marked improvement in a substantial proportion of patients. Lipinski *et al.* (1984), using intravenous SAMe in a single-blind study of inpatient depressives, reported improvement or remission in seven of nine subjects. Antidepressant response was rapid and well tolerated.

Several double-blind studies showed that parenteral SAMe, compared with a number of standard TCAs such as clomipramine, amitriptyline, and imipramine, was generally equally or more effective, and tended to produce an earlier response (often within 3–7 days) and fewer side effects (Bell *et al.*, 1988; Dele Chiaie *et al.*, 2002; Janicak *et al.*, 1988). In the two largest double-blind studies, Pancheri *et al.* (2002) and Delle Chiaie *et al.* (2002) found the efficacy of 400 mg daily of intramuscular (IM) SAMe to be equivalent to that of 150 mg daily of oral imipramine in $n = 293$ and $n = 295$ outpatients with major depressive disorder (MDD). Similarly, in two double-blind studies examining the efficacy of IM or intravenous (IV) SAMe compared with placebo, parenteral SAMe was significantly more effective (Caruso *et al.*, 1984; Janicak *et al.*, 1988), but not in a third study (Carney *et al.*, 1986). However, in the latter trial, when Carney *et al.* (1986) examined the efficacy of SAMe versus placebo in the subset of patients with endogenous depression, they did find SAMe to be more effective in treating depression than placebo. Overall, common side effects reported with SAMe include GI distress, jitteriness, insomnia, and possible exacerbation or unmasking of manic symptoms. In addition, some have raised a possible concern regarding potential increases in homocysteine levels in patients administered with SAMe, although studies of SAMe administered in humans do not reveal any impact on homocysteine levels (Loehrer *et al.*, 1997).

Although parenteral SAMe appears to be an effective antidepressant, it is unclear whether similar clinical efficacy can be achieved with its oral preparation. The administration of SAMe orally is associated with a significant rise of cerebrospinal fluid (CSF) SAMe, suggesting that it crosses the blood–brain barrier in humans (Bottiglieri *et al.*, 1990; Castagna *et al.*, 1995). Overall, in controlled clinical trials of oral SAMe, doses have generally been between 800–1600 mg/day although there has been no systematic exploration of dose-response.

In an open trial involving the use of oral SAMe in depressed outpatients (Rosenbaum *et al.*, 1990; Fava *et al.*, 1990), eight (73%) of the original 11 patients were considered to be responders. However, when Fava *et al.* (1992) evaluated the efficacy of oral SAMe in a double-blind, placebo-controlled study in 39 depressed outpatients, there was no significant difference between SAMe and placebo in the degree of improvement of depressive symptoms. In retrospect, this result may have been attributable to lack of stability of the particular oral preparation of SAMe used for that trial. In fact, soon after completion of that study, the U.S. Food and Drug Administration (FDA) forced all of the United States sites of clinical trials on SAMe to stop their studies because of technical issues regarding data on the dissolution of the SAMe tablets (Fava *et al.*, 1992). More recently, Di Rocco *et al.* (2000) reported a 75% response rate among 13 outpatients with Parkinson's disease and comorbid MDD who were treated with SAMe in an open-label fashion. However, the formulation of SAMe used in that study was not reported.

In contrast to the study by Fava *et al.*, double-blind studies by Kagan *et al.* (1990) and Salmaggi *et al.* (1993) both found oral SAMe (1600 mg/day) to be more effective than placebo in treating depressive symptoms among inpatients with MDD ($n = 18$) and depressed postmenopausal women ($n = 60$) (Fig. 13.1).

In addition, in active comparator trials, Bell *et al.* (1990) and De Vanna *et al.* (1992) showed the efficacy of oral SAMe (1600 mg/day) to be comparable to that of desipramine and imipramine in

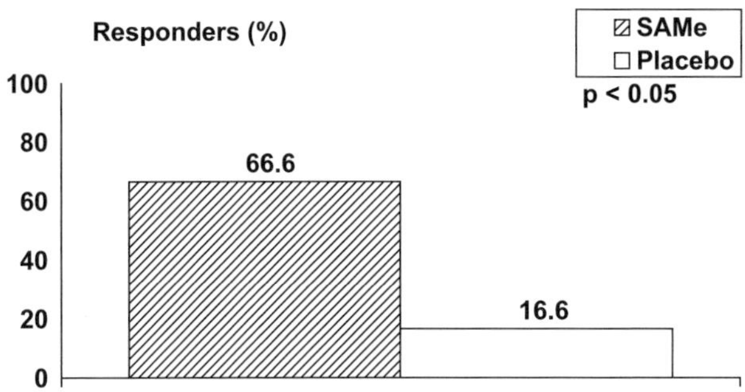

Fig. 13.1 Oral S-adenosylmethionine (SAMe) for depression: A randomized, double-blind study ($n = 18$). [Data extracted from: Kagan, B.L., Sultzer, D.L., Rosenlicht, N., & Gerner, R.H. (1990). Oral S-adenosylmethionine in depression: A randomized, double-blind, placebo-controlled trial. *American Journal of Psychiatry*, 147, 591–595.]

depressed populations ($n = 25$ and 22, respectively). In a recent large study, Delle Chiaie *et al.* (2002) found the efficacy of oral SAMe to be equivalent to that of imipramine in 281 outpatients with MDD. A summary of double-blind studies and their findings is presented in Table 13.1.

In a meta-analysis of prospective, randomized clinical trials comparing SAMe with placebo which was compiled following the publication of the most recent such study (Salmaggi *et al.*, 1993), SAMe demonstrated a superior response rate when compared with placebo, with an average global effect size of 17.0% (Bressa, 1994). Furthermore, when studies comparing SAMe with TCAs were analyzed (Bressa, 1994), a global response of 61% for SAMe and 59% for TCAs was demonstrated. A more recent meta-analysis of depression trials commissioned by the Agency for Healthcare Research and Quality (AHRQ) was similarly concluded. When the data from 47 controlled trials were pooled, SAMe (parenteral or enteral) was associated with an overall effect size of −0.65 (95% CI: −1.05, −0.25) compared with placebo, translating into about a clinically meaningful 5 to 6 point improvement on the Hamilton Depression Rating Scale (Hamilton, 1960). On the other hand, when SAMe was compared with active comparators (tricyclic antidepressants), the effect size

Table 13.1 Selected controlled studies of SAMe in MDD.[a]

Study	Design	SAMe/dose	Comparator	Result
Caruso *et al.*, 1984	3w DB ($n = 25$)	200 mg IM	Placebo ($n = 24$)	SAMe > Pbo
Carney *et al.*, 1986	2w DB ($n = 15$)	200 mg IV	Placebo ($n = 17$)	SAMe = Pbo[b]
Bell *et al.*, 1988	2w DB ($n = 11$)	400 mg IV	Imipramine 150 mg PO ($n = 11$)	SAMe > IMI
Janicak *et al.*, 1988	2w DB ($n = 7$)	400 mg IV	Imipramine 150 mg PO ($n = 3$)	SAMe = IMI
	2w DB ($n = 7$)	400 mg IV	Placebo ($n = 5$)	SAMe > Pbo
Kagan *et al.*, 1990	3w DB ($n = 9$)	1600 mg PO	Placebo ($n = 9$)	SAMe > Pbo
Bell *et al.*, 1990	4w DB ($n = 12$)	1600 mg PO	Desipramine 250 mg PO ($n = 13$)	SAMe = DMI
Fava *et al.*, 1992	6w DB ($n = 24$)	1600 mg PO	Placebo ($n = 31$)	SAMe = Pbo
De Vanna *et al.*, 1992	6w DB ($n = 11$)	1600 mg PO	Imipramine 150 mg PO ($n = 11$)	SAMe = IMI
Salmaggi *et al.*, 1993	30d DB ($n = 30$)	1600 mg PO	Placebo ($n = 30$)	SAMe > Pbo
Pancheri *et al.*, 2002	4w DB ($n = 146$)	400 mg IM	Imipramine 150 mg PO ($n = 147$)	SAMe = IMI
Delle Chiaie *et al.*, 2002	4w DB ($n = 143$)	1600 mg PO	Imipramine 150 mg PO ($n = 138$)	SAMe = IMI
	6w DB ($n = 147$)	400 mg IM	Imipramine 150 mg PO ($n = 148$)	SAMe = IMI

[a]Published in English language peer-reviewed journals between 1980 and 2003. Minimum 2 weeks' duration. HAM-D as primary outcome measure. No data overlap with other publications.
[b]SAMe = PBO overall but SAMe > PBO for endogenous MDD.
Abbreviations: PBO = Placebo, DMI = Desipramine, IMI = Imipramine.

was 0.08 (95% CI: 0.17, 0.32), suggesting equivalent efficacy (Hardy *et al.*, 2003). A randomized, double-blind, placebo-controlled trial focusing on the use of SAMe as monotherapy for MDD is currently under way (NCT00101452).

13.1.1.2 *Folates and other B-vitamins*

To date, two studies focusing on the use of methyltetrahydrofolate (MTHF) as a monotherapy for MDD have been published. In an open-label trial of six-week duration, Guaraldi *et al.* (1993) reported an 81% response rate following treatment with MTHF among elderly depressed patients. However, the results of a double-blind study comparing MTHF versus trazodone among 96 patients aged 65 or older with MDD and comorbid dementia (mini-mental status exam score of 12–23) did not reveal any differences in efficacy between the two treatments (Passeri *et al.*, 1991 and 1993). For vitamin B12 (cyanocobalamin) monotherapy, there is only a single, double-blind trial involving 27 outpatients with seasonal Affective Disorder (SAD) (Oren *et al.*, 1994). In that study, there was no difference in antidepressant efficacy between the two treatment groups following five weeks of treatment. For pyridoxine (vitamin B6), an open-label trial and a double-blind, placebo-controlled, cross-over trial have been published. In the open-label trial (Holsboen *et al.*, 1985), 11/20 women with MDD were reported to have achieved remission following four weeks of combined treatment with pyridoxine (40 mg TiD) and estradiol (10 mg). In the double-blind, cross-over study, pyridoxine (20 mg BiD) was reported to be more effective than placebo in alleviating depressive symptoms among women who had recently started oral contraceptives (Adams *et al.*, 1973). Finally, there is only anecdotal evidence suggesting potential antidepressant effects for tetrahydrobiopterin (BH4) (Curtius *et al.*, 1982 and 1983).

13.1.2 *Agents acting on neuronal "second messenger" systems*

13.1.2.1 *Anatomy of the "second messenger" system*

In the human body, metabotropic receptors are linked via G-proteins, to one of two second messenger systems: (1) adenylate cyclase (AC)/cyclic adenosine monophosphate (cAMP), and (2) phosphatidylinositol (PI)/diacylglycerol (DAG) (Shelton, 2000). G proteins can be either stimulatory (Gs) or inhibitory (Gi).

In the AC/cAMP second messenger system, binding of a ligand to a receptor linked to Gs results in the binding of Gs to the enzyme AC that, in turn, produces cAMP from adenosine triphosphate (ATP). cAMP then activates protein kinase A which, in turn, activates transcription factors (such as cAMP response element (CRE) binding protein — CREB) which subsequently, influence gene expression including the expression of brain-derived neurotrophic factor (BDNF). A number of monoamine and non-monoamine metabotropic neurotransmitter receptors utilize the AC/cAMP second messenger system. Specifically, several glutamatergic metabotropic receptors (II–VIII), the γ-aminobutyric acid-B receptor, the serotonin 1-family of receptors (1A-F), the α-2A adrenergic receptor, as well as the D2–D4 dopaminergic receptors appear to be linked to Gi (leading to decreased cAMP production), while serotonin 4, 6, 7, receptors, the β-1 adrenergic receptor family, and the D1 and D5 dopaminergic receptors appear to be linked to Gs (leading to increased cAMP production).

In the PI/DAG second messenger system, binding of a ligand to a receptor linked to a Gs results in the binding of Gs to the enzyme phospholipase C, which activates calcium influx and converts PI to DAG. DAG then activates phospholipase C which inhibits phospholipase A and also activates transcription factors (such as CREB) which, in turn, influence gene expression (such as BDNF). Receptors which utilize the PI/DAG second messenger system include glutamatergic metabotropic receptors 1 and 5, the serotonin 2 receptor subtypes, as well as the α-1 adrenergic-receptor subtypes. These receptors are linked to Gs (leading to increased conversion of PI to DAG).

13.1.2.2 *Phosphodiesterase inhibitors*

Rolipram is a selective inhibitor of the phosphodiesterase (PDE) IV enzyme, responsible for hydrolysis of the cAMP and cyclic guanosine monophosphate (cGMP), particularly in nerve and immune cells (Renau, 2004; Zhu *et al.*, 2001). Following two open-label trials (Horowski & Sastre-Hernandez, 1985; Zeller *et al.*, 1984) involving the use of the selective phosphodiesterase type IV inhibitor rolipram for the treatment of mixed populations of patients with depression (unipolar and bipolar), several double-blind studies have been published comparing rolipram with tricyclic antidepressants for depression (Bertolino *et al.*, 1988; Bobon *et al.*, 1988; Eckmann *et al.*, 1988; Guiot-Goffioul *et al.*, 1987; Hebenstreit *et al.*, 1989; Scott *et al.*, 1991). Treatment of depression with rolipram (0.75–1 mg TiD) was reported to be equivalent to treatment with tricyclic antidepressants in five studies (Bertolino *et al.*, 1988; Bobon *et al.*, 1988; Eckmann *et al.*, 1988; Guiot-Goffioul *et al.*, 1987; Hebenstreit *et al.*, 1989). However, a sixth study in which 50 inpatients with major depression were randomized to treatment with rolipram (0.5 mg TiD) versus amitriptyline for six weeks reported greater symptom resolution among amitriptyline- than rolipram-treated patients (Scott *et al.*, 1991). Although it was argued that the results of the latter study may have been due to the under-dosing of rolipram, a subsequent dose-finding study suggested that treatment with 0.5 mg TiD was superior to treatment with either 0.25 mg or 0.75 mg TiD, with no difference in efficacy between the latter two doses (Fleischhacker *et al.*, 1992). Placebo-controlled studies for rolipram or other PDE-IV inhibitors as monotherapy for depression have yet to be published.

13.1.2.3 *Inositol*

Inositol is an isomer of glucose that is a key precursor to PI. The results of a small ($n = 28$) double-blind, placebo-controlled study involving the use of inositol monotherapy (12 g/day) for outpatients with either MDD or bipolar depression did not reveal any difference in efficacy between the two groups (Levine *et al.*, 1995). Similarly, a meta-analysis of placebo-controlled monotherapy as well as augmentation studies of inositol for depression did not show any evidence of therapeutic benefit for inositol (Taylor *et al.*, 2004).

13.1.2.4 *Other agents*

Tamoxifen is an inhibitor of protein kinase C. To date, two pilot, randomized, double-blind, placebo-controlled trials suggest greater anti-manic effects for tamoxifen monotherapy when used to treat manic episodes in patients with bipolar disorder (Kulkarni *et al.*, 2006; Zarate *et al.*, 2007). Studies in the treatment of MDD or major depressive episodes in patients with bipolar disorder have yet to be published.

Glycogen synthase kinase-3 (GSK-3) is a serine threonine kinase that is normally highly active in cells, and is deactivated by signals originating from numerous signaling pathways (i.e., protein kinase A, protein kinase C, etc.). Targets of GSK-3 are numerous depending on the signaling pathway that is acting upon it. Although it has been hypothesized that inhibitors of GSK-3, involved in NMDA-mediated apoptosis (Takadera *et al.*, 2004) and also inhibited by lithium (Hongisto *et al.*, 2003; Ryves & Harwood, 2001), may be useful for the treatment of bipolar disorder and depression (Gould *et al.*, 2004), clinical studies have yet to be conducted.

Human phase III trials of recombinant methionyl human brain-derived neurotrophic factor have already been undertaken for amyotrophic lateral sclerosis (but not depression) (Ochs *et al.*, 2000). Unfortunately, side effects encountered at higher doses (including paresthesias, sleep disturbance, agitation) preclude further clinical study.

Finally, GW856553 is a novel compound, currently in development for the treatment of MDD. GW856553 inhibits a protein which is responsible for the production of cytokines (P38a kinase inhibitor). A randomized, double-blind, placebo-controlled trial of GW856553 as monotherapy for MDD is currently under way (NCT00569062).

13.1.3 *Essential fatty acids*

13.1.3.1 *Overview*

Omega-3 (ω-3) and ω-6 fatty acids are naturally occurring essential polyunsaturated fatty acids (PUFA) (Lands, 1992). They are classified according to the position of the first double bond with respect to the methyl (CH3-) end of the molecule (designated as the omega-carbon). For example, the ω-3s have the double (unsaturated) bond at the third carbon, the ω-6s at the 6th carbon, and so forth. Because humans cannot desaturate ω-3 and ω-6 fatty acids, these must be obtained from the diet, and are therefore "essential". The predominant ω-3 fatty acids include the long-chain ω-3 fatty acids docosahexanoic acid (DHA) and eicosapentaenoic acid (EPA), which are found primarily in fish (Stensby, 1969); and the shorter-chain α-linolenic acid (ALA), obtained from land-based plants such as flaxseed (Simopulos *et al.*, 1986 and 1992). ω-6 fatty acids include the 18-carbon linoleic acid (LA), and the 20-carbon arachidonic acid (AA) and are derived primarily from vegetable oils (Leaf & Weber, 1987).

ω-3 fatty acids are incorporated in the neuronal membrane (Lands, 1992) rendering the membrane more fluid, and thereby affecting the conformation and activities of membrane-bound receptors and enzymes that regulate neurotransmitter signaling (Heron *et al.*, 1980). In addition, membrane-bound phospholipids containing ω-3 fatty acids may regulate intracellular signal transduction by inhibiting G-protein and phospholipase C-mediated hydrolysis of PI into the second messenger molecules inositol triphosphate and DAG(Sperling *et al.*, 1993).

13.1.3.2 *Clinical studies*

Although several double-blind studies support the use of adjunctive treatment with ω-3 fatty acids (primarily ethyl-EPA) for treatment-resistant depression (see Chap. 6), to date, a number of trials also focus on the use of ω-3 fatty acids as monotherapy for MDD. Nemets *et al.* (2006) conducted a double-blind, placebo-controlled trial of a DHA-EPA mix (400 and 200 mg, respectively) as monotherapy for childhood depression (Nemets *et al.*, 2006). A greater resolution in depressive symptoms was reported for children treated with ω-3 fatty acids than placebo (Fig. 13.2). Similarly, Su *et al.* (2008) conducted a double-blind, placebo-controlled trial of ω-3 fatty acids (2.2 gram EPA, 1.2 gram DHA) for the treatment of post-partum MDD. A greater resolution of depressive symptoms was reported among women who received ω-3 fatty acids than placebo.

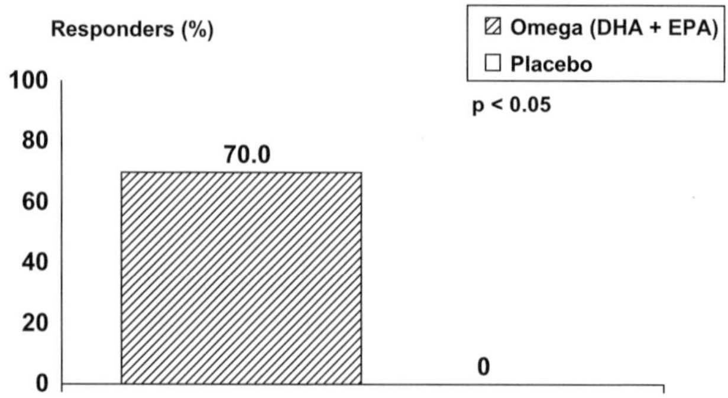

Fig. 13.2 Omega-3 fatty acids for childhood MDD: A randomized, double-blind study ($n = 28$). [Data extracted from: Nemets, H., Nemets, B., Apter, A., *et al.* (2006). Omega-3 treatment of childhood depression: A controlled, double-blind pilot study. *American Journal of Psychiatry*, 163, 1098–1100.]

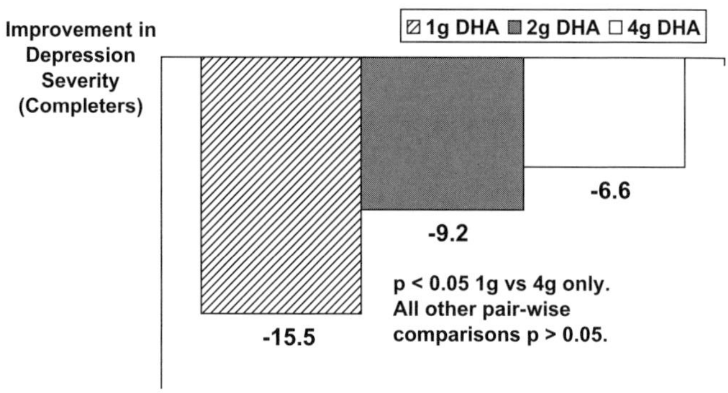

Fig. 13.3 A double-blind, randomized, "dose-finding" study of docosahexanoic acid (DHA) for MDD ($n = 35$). [Data extracted from: Mischoulon, D., Best-Popescu, C., Laposata, M., *et al.* (2008). A double-blind dose-finding pilot study of docosahexaenoic acid (DHA) for major depressive disorder. *European Neuropsychopharmacology*, 18(9), 639–645.]

In addition, the results of a double-blind, dose-finding study of DHA monotherapy for MDD suggested that a 1-g/day total dose may be more effective than a 2-gram or 4-gram daily total dose (Mischoulon *et al.*, 2008) (Fig. 13.3), although a dose–response relationship for combined EPA/DHA could not be established in a second trial focusing on women with post-partum depression (Freeman *et al.*, 2006).

More recently, Jazayeri *et al.* (2008) randomized MDD patients, in a double-blind fashion, to receive treatment with either fluoxetine (20 mg), EPA (1 gram) or the combination of fluoxetine (20 grams) and EPA (1 gram) for a total of eight weeks. There was no difference in the resolution of depressive symptoms among patients treated with either monotherapy. However, patients who received a combination of the two agents demonstrated a greater resolution of depressive symptoms than patients treated with either monotherapy. Mischoulon *et al.* (in press) randomized 57 MDD patients to receive monotherapy with 1 gram of EPA versus placebo. EPA-treated patients but not placebo-treated patients experienced a significant reduction of MDD symptoms. Finally, the results of a double-blind, placebo-controlled trial of eight-weeks duration involving the use of EPA (1 gram daily) for the treatment of aggression and depressive symptoms among outpatients with borderline personality disorder (MDD excluded) reported greater symptom resolution among EPA- than placebo-treated patients (Zanarini & Frankenberg, 2003).

However, not all studies report encouraging results regarding the use of DHA or EPA in depression. Marangell *et al.* (2003) randomized 36 outpatients with MDD to receive DHA (2 grams) versus placebo for six weeks. Rogers *et al.* (2008) randomized 218 subjects with mild-to-moderate symptoms of depression to receive 1.5 g daily of an EPA-DHA mix (650 and 850 mg, respectively) versus placebo. Freeman *et al.* (2008) randomized 59 women with perinatal MDD (including antenatal and post-partum MDD) to receive treatment with ω-3 fatty acids (1.1 gram EPA, 0.8 gram DHA) versus placebo for eight weeks in addition to supportive psychotherapy. Rees *et al.* (2008) randomized 26 women with perinatal MDD (including antenatal and post-partum MDD) to receive treatment with ω-3 fatty acids (1.6 gram DHA, 0.4 gram EPA) versus placebo for six weeks. Grenyer *et al.* (2007) randomized 83 outpatients with MDD to receive treatment with either 3 g DHA-EPA mix (2.2 gram and 0.8 gram, respectively) or placebo. No difference in the degree of symptom reduction between the two treatment groups was reported in any of these five trials. Similarly, the results of a randomized, double-blind, placebo-controlled study ($n = 119$) do not support the use of DHA (220 mg) for the prevention of perinatal MDD (Doornbos *et al.*, 2009). Several randomized, double-blind, placebo-controlled trials focusing on the use of ω-3 fatty acids as monotherapy for adults (NCT00361374; NCT00238758; NCT00096798), or adolescents with MDD (NCT00312897) are currently under way.

13.1.4 *Carnitine*

L-acetylcarnitine (γ-trimethylammonium-β-acetatoxybutyrate), produced in mitochondria from carnitine, is found in various human organs including the central nervous system. L-acetylcarnitine (LAC) contains carnitine and acetyl moieties, both of which have neurobiological properties. Carnitine is important in the β-oxidation of fatty acids and the acetyl moiety can be used to maintain acetyl-CoA levels (major acetyl group donor for transacetylation) (Pettegrew *et al.*, 2000) (Fig. 13.4).

So far, three double-blind, placebo-controlled studies of various carnitines for depressive disorders (mixed unipolar/bipolar populations) or symptoms have been published. In the first such trial, Bella *et al.* (1990) randomized 60 subjects aged 60–80 years old with chronic depressive disorders to receive L-acetylcarnitine (LAC — 3 grams daily) versus placebo for eight weeks, and reported greater symptom resolution in the LAC- than placebo-treated group with respect to depressive symptoms (Fig. 13.5).

Similarly, Garzya *et al.* (1990) reported greater symptom resolution among 28 elderly (70–80 year old) MDD patients following eight weeks of treatment with LAC (1.5 gram daily) versus placebo. Interestingly enough, both studies also reported that greater resolution for self-reported items relating to (1) motivation/apathy/indifference as well as (2) cognition/alertness/memory and orientation was reported in LAC- than placebo-treated patients, effects

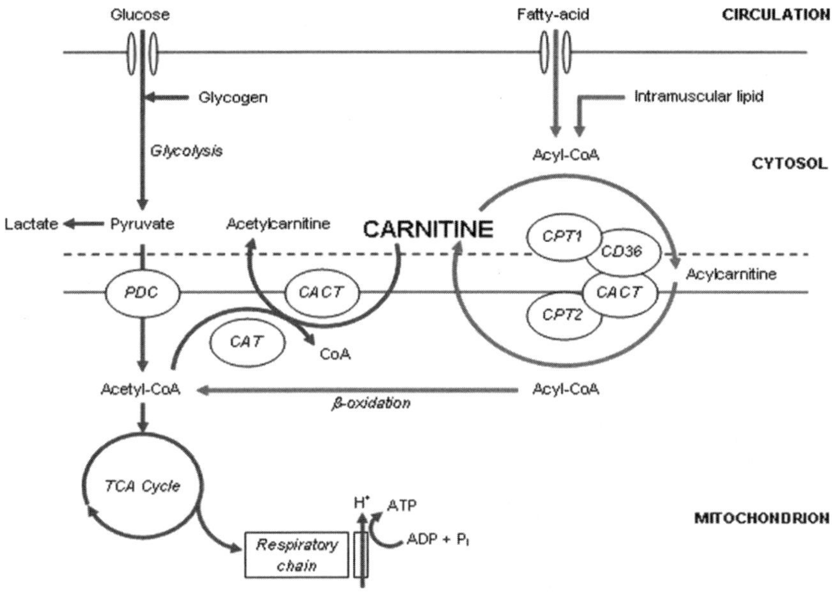

Fig. 13.4 Carnitine and acetylcarnitine metabolism. Carnitine's role in long-chain fatty acid (acyl group) translocation into the mitochondrial matrix, for subsequent β-oxidation is highlighted in red, whereas the role of carnitine as a buffer of excess acetyl-CoA production is highlighted in blue. PDC, pyruvate dehydrogenase complex; TCA, tricarboxylic acid cycle; CAT, carnitine acetyltransferase; CACT, carnitine acylcarnitine translocase; CPT, carnitine palmitoyltransferase; CD36, fatty acid translocase. [Reprinted from Stephens, F.B., Constantin-Teodosiu, D., & Greenhaff, P.L. (2007). New insights concerning the role of carnitine in the regulation of fuel metabolism in skeletal muscle. *Journal of Physiology*, 581(Pt 2), 431–444. with permission from Blackwell Publishing (Copyright 2007).]

which may be related to the procholinergic properties of LAC (Ori *et al.*, 2002; Ricny *et al.*, 1992). More recently, Cavallini *et al.* (2004) reported a significant reduction in depression and fatigue severity among 120 elderly subjects with complaints of depressed mood, fatigue and low libido randomized to treatment with either a combination of LAC (2 g/day) and L-propionyl-carnitine (LPC; 2 g/day) or testosterone undecanoate 160 mg/day than placebo-treated patients. However, subsequent studies focusing on the treatment of depressive disorders with carnitine have yet to be published.

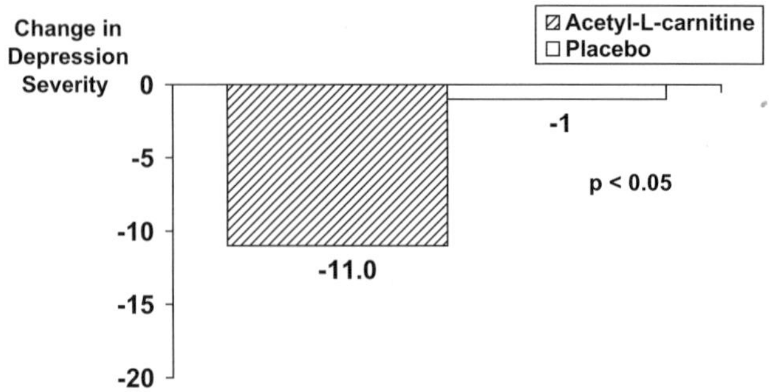

Fig. 13.5 Effect of acetyl-L-carnitine on mood in geriatric patients with dysthymic disorder: A randomized, double-blind study ($n = 60$). [Data extracted from: Bella, R., Biondi, R., Raffaele, R., & Pennisi, G. (1990). Effect of acetyl-L-carnitine on geriatric patients suffering from dysthymic disorders. *International Journal of Clinical Pharmacology Research*, 10, 355–360.]

13.1.5 *Minerals, trace elements, and vitamins (non-B vitamins)*

Chromium is a trace element involved in central nervous system neurotransmission. Following a series of promising case reports of chromium augmentation (McLeod *et al.*, 1999) or monotherapy (McLeod & Golden, 2000) for refractory depression, a small ($n = 15$), double-blind, placebo-controlled study comparing the efficacy of chromium picolinate monotherapy (600 μg daily) versus placebo for the treatment of atypical MDD was conducted (Davidson *et al.*, 2003). A significantly greater response rate for the chromium (7/10) than the placebo (0/5) treated group was reported in that study. However, a subsequent, larger ($n = 115$), double-blind trial of chromium picolinate monotherapy versus placebo for the treatment of atypical MDD revealed no difference in depressive symptom resolution between the two treatment groups (Docherty *et al.*, 2004).

A double-blind, placebo-controlled study of ferrous sulfate (80 mg/day of elemental iron) versus placebo for the treatment of unexplained fatigue among women ($n = 144$, patients with anemia, depression excluded) revealed a greater reduction in complaints of fatigue and anxiety but not depression among iron- than placebo-treated women (Verdon *et al.*, 2003). A double-blind, placebo-controlled study of selenium (100, 200, 300 mcg/day) versus placebo among 501 healthy subjects, however, did not reveal any mood-enhancing benefits of selenium (Rayman *et al.*, 2006). Studies of iron or selenium supplementation for depression have not been published. Finally, there is only anecdotal evidence suggesting potential antidepressant effects for vitamin C (ascorbic acid) (Brody, 2002; Cocchi *et al.*, 1980), and vitamin D (Gloth *et al.*, 1999).

13.2 Agents with Unknown Mechanism of Action

13.2.1 *Herbal remedies*

13.2.1.1 *Hypericum perforatum*

Nearly 2,500 years ago, Hippocrates was among the first to describe psychotropic effects for *Hypericum perforatum*. Although the mechanism of action of *Hypericum perforatum* has yet to be elucidated, the efficacy of *Hypericum perforatum* extracts for the treatment of depression has been widely studied in dozens of randomized, controlled trials, cumulatively containing hundreds of patients, with earlier studies mostly published in German (Kasper, 2001), and more recent studies in English (see Tables 13.2 and 13.3). Controls used in these studies range from placebo, to various tricyclic or tetracyclic agents (amitriptyline, imipramine, maprotiline), to selective serotonin reuptake inhibitors (fluoxetine, sertraline, paroxetine, and citalopram).

One of these trials also examines the use of two preparations of Hypericum containing a different (10-fold) concentration in Hyperforin, one of several compounds contained in Hypericum extracts. These studies are quantitatively summarized in a recent meta-analysis (Werneke *et al.*, 2004). This analysis included all but seven (Bjerkenstedt *et al.*, 2005; Fava *et al.*, 2005; Gastpar *et al.*, 2006; Kasper *et al.*, 2006; Moreno *et al.*, 2006; Randlov *et al.*, 2006; Uebelhack *et al.*, 2004) randomized, double-blind, placebo-controlled trials and

Table 13.2 Selected double-blind, placebo-controlled studies of Hypericum for depression.[a]

Study	*N*, duration	Hypericum	Result[b]
Sommer & Harrer, 1994	105, 4 weeks	LI160 900 mg	H > Pbo
Hubner *et al.*, 1994	39, 4 weeks	LI160 900 mg	H > Pbo
Hansgen *et al.*, 1994	72, 4 weeks	LI160 900 mg	H > Pbo
Laakman *et al.*, 1998	147, 6 weeks	WS5573 900 mg (0.5% hyperforin) or 900 mg (5% hyperforin)	H(5%) > Pbo H(0.5%) = Pbo
Schrader *et al.*, 1998	162, 6 weeks	Ze117 500 mg (0.5% hypericin)	H > Pbo
Philipp *et al.*, 1999	263, 8 weeks	STEI300 (0.2% hypericin) 1050 mg (2% hyperforin)	H = Pbo H = Imipramine
Kalb *et al.*, 2001	72, 6 weeks	WS5572 (1.5% hyperforin)	H > Pbo
Shelton *et al.*, 2001	200, 8 weeks	LI160 1200 mg	H = Pbo
Lecrubier *et al.*, 2002	375, 6 weeks	WS5570 (0.1–0.3% hypericin) 900 mg (3–6% hyperforin)	H > Pbo
HDTSG, 2002	340, 8 weeks	LI160 (0.1–0.3% hypericin) 900–1500 mg	H = Pbo H = Sertraline
Uebelhack *et al.*, 2004	140, 6 weeks	STW 3-VI 900 mg	H > Pbo
Bjerkenstedt *et al.*, 2005	163, 4 weeks	LI160 900 mg	H = Fluoxetine H = Pbo
Fava *et al.*, 2005	135, 12 weeks	LI160 900 mg (0.1–0.3% hypericin)	H > Fluoxetine H = Pbo
Gastpar *et al.*, 2006	388, 6 weeks	STW3-VI	H > Pbo H = Citalopram
Kasper *et al.*, 2006	332, 6 weeks	WS5570 600 or 1200 mg	H > Pbo
Moreno *et al.*, 2006	72, 8 weeks	? 900 mg	H < Pbo H < Fluoxetine
Randlov *et al.*, 2006	150, 6 weeks	PM235 810 mg (0.12–0.18 hypericin)	H = Pbo

[a]Published in English language peer-reviewed journals. No data overlap with other publications.
[b]Difference in change in depression severity.
Abbreviations: HDTSG = Hypericum depression treatment study group, Pbo = Placebo, H = Hypericum, LI160 = Product of Lichtwer Pharma, STEI300 = product of Steiner Arzneimittel, Ze117 = product of Zeller AG, WS5570–3 = products of Willmar Schwabe pharmaceuticals, HDTSG = Hypericum depression trial study group.

reported greater efficacy among Hypericum- than placebo-treated patients (risk ratio 1.97, 95% CI: 1.40–2.14). Of the seven trials not included in the meta-analysis, three found Hypericum to be superior (Gastpar *et al.*, 2006; Kasper *et al.*, 2006; Uebelhack *et al.*, 2004), one

Table 13.3 Selected, double-blind (non-placebo) controlled studies of Hypericum for depression.[a]

Study	N, duration	Hypericum	Comparator	Result
Vorbach *et al.*, 1994	135, 6 weeks	LI160 900 mg	Imipramine 75 mg	H = Imipramine
Harrer *et al.*, 1994	102, 4 weeks	LI160 900 mg	Maprotiline 75 mg	H = Maprotiline
Wheatley, 1997	165, 6 weeks	LI160 900 mg	Amitriptyline 75 mg	H < Amitriptyline
Vorbach *et al.*, 1997	209, 6 weeks	LI160 1800 mg	Imipramine 150 mg	H = Imipramine
Schrader *et al.*, 2000	240, 6 weeks	Ze117 750 mg	Fluoxetine 20 mg	H = Fluoxetine
Woelk *et al.*, 2000	324, 6 weeks	Ze117 500 mg (0.2% hypericin)	Imipramine 150 mg	H = Imipramine
Van Gurp *et al.*, 2002	78, 12 weeks	Hypericum 900–1800 mg (0.3% hypericin)	Sertraline 50–100 mg	H = Sertraline
Szegedi *et al.*, 2005	251, 6 weeks	WS5570 900 mg (0.12–0.28% hypericin) (3–6% hyperforin)	Paroxetine 20 mg	H > Paroxetine

[a]Published in English language peer-reviewed journals. Difference in change in depression severity as primary outcome measure. No data overlap with other publications.
H = Hypericum, LI160 = Product of Lichtwer Pharma, Ze117 = product of Zeller AG, WS5570 = products of Willmar Schwabe pharmaceuticals.

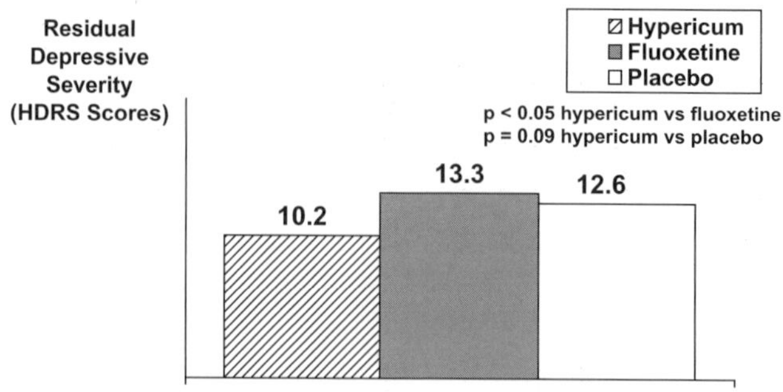

Fig. 13.6 *Hypericum perforatum* (St. John's Wort) versus fluoxetine (SSRI), for MDD: A randomized, double-blind study (n = 135). HDRS: Hamilton Depression Rating Scale. [Data extracted from: Fava, M., Alpert, J., Nierenberg, A.A., *et al.* (2005). A double-blind, randomized trial of St John's wort, fluoxetine, and placebo in major depressive disorder. Journal of Clinical Psychopharmacology, 25, 441–447.]

inferior (Fava *et al.*, 2005) (Fig. 13.6) and three equivalent to placebo in efficacy (Bjerkenstedt *et al.*, 2005; Fava *et al.*, 2005; Randlov *et al.*, 2006) although the study by Fava *et al.* (2005) demonstrated the superiority of Hypericum over the SSRI fluoxetine.

A separate meta-analysis also demonstrated lower rates of premature discontinuation of treatment due to adverse events among Hypericum- than TCA-treated patients (odds ratio 0.25, 95% CI: 0.14–0.45) and comparable rates when compared to SSRI- (odds ration 0.6; 95% CI: 0.31–1.15) or placebo- (odds ration 0.61; 95% CI: 0.28–1.31) treated patients (Knuppel & Linde, 2004). Finally, recent evidence from a randomized, double-blind, placebo-substitution trial of *Hypericum perforatum* among patients with MDD who responded to a six-week, open-label trial of *Hypericum perforatum* (WS5570 900 mg daily) suggest lower relapse rates among patients who receive *Hypericum perforatum* than those who receive placebo during the continuation (26 weeks) but not maintenance phase of therapy (52 weeks) (Kasper *et al.*, 2008).

Despite the cumulative evidence provided by numerous double-blind trials and compiled by recent meta-analyses suggesting antidepressant properties for Hypericum extracts, it remains unclear which of the several components contained in the multitude of commercially available extracts is responsible for the clinical effects of *Hypericum perforatum*. To date, a number of broad groups of compounds contained in *Hypericum perforatum* extracts have been identified as having pharmacological effects. These include naphthodianthrones, phenylpropanes, biflavones, tannins and proanthrocyanidins, flavonol glycosides, xanthones, phloroglucinols, essential oils and amino acids (Nahrstedt & Butterweck, 1997). Although hypericin, a compound with affinity only for the NMDA, neuropeptide Y and σ receptors (Cott, 1997; Gobbi *et al.*, 2001), was originally thought to be responsible for the antidepressant effects of Hypericum (Bladt & Wagner 1994), a subsequent trial suggested the antidepressant effects of Hypericum to be related to the concentration of hyperforin (Laakman *et al.*, 1998), a compound which has been shown to inhibit the vesicular uptake of the monoamines (Chatterjee *et al.*, 1998; Gobbi *et al.*, 2001; Muller *et al.*, 1998; Roz *et al.*, 2002 and 2003) by dissipating the synaptic vesicle membrane, which is the major driving force for vesicular monoamine uptake and storage (Roz & Rehavi, 2003).

Unfortunately, however, only a minority of studies report on the hyperforin (Kalb *et al.*, 2001; Laakman *et al.*, 1998; Lecrubier *et al.*, 2002; Philipp *et al.*, 1999) or hypericin (Fava *et al.*, 2002; HDTSG *et al.*, 2002; Lecrubier *et al.*, 2002; Philipp *et al.*, 1999; Schrader *et al.*, 1998; Woelk *et al.*, 2000; Van Gurp *et al.*, 2002) concentration of the preparation used, making it difficult to explore the relationship between hyperforin/hypericin concentrations and outcome. For example, hyperforin concentrations were not reported among four of five studies that did not demonstrate greater efficacy for Hypericum than placebo (Bjerkenstedt *et al.*, 2005; Fava *et al.*, 2002 HDTSG, 2002; Shelton *et al.*, 2001), nor among any study published prior to 1998. In addition, among studies that did report hyperforin concentrations, concentrations varied twelve-fold from 0.5% (Laakman *et al.*, 1998) to 1.5% (Kalb *et al.*, 2001), to 6% (Lecrubier *et al.*, 2002). To complicate matters further, there also appears to have been great variation in the concentration of hyperforin/hypericin contained in each pill even within studies (i.e., Lecrubier *et al.* report a content of 3–6% for hyperforin). Therefore, to what degree variations in the content of pharmacologically active agents between the various Hypericum preparations used in placebo-controlled trials contribute to the discrepancy in study findings remains unclear. Further clinical trials examining variations in the hyperforin/hypericin and other component concentrations of the extract are necessary in order to clarify the potential role of these pleiotropic molecules. In turn, establishing which compounds are responsible for the antidepressant effects of *Hypericum perforatum* and exploring their neuropharmacologic properties can lead to the development of novel treatments for depression as well as further insights into the mechanisms of what constitutes clinical response in MDD.

13.2.1.2 *Ginseng*

Very little evidence exists supporting the use of other herbal remedies as antidepressants or anxiolytics. The results of an open-label trial of ginseng for depressive symptoms among postmenopausal women with climacteric syndromes (Tode *et al.*, 1999) were soon followed by a positive, double-blind, placebo-controlled trial (Wiklund *et al.*, 1999). In addition, a greater improvement in mood has been reported among a group of middle managers (Ussher *et al.*, 1995) or healthy volunteers (Wiklund *et al.*, 1994) treated with ginseng extracts than placebo. However, the results of other double-blind, placebo-controlled studies do not support the use of ginseng for fatigue (Hartz *et al.*, 2004), or in the rehabilitation of geriatric patients (Thommessen & Laake, 1996).

13.2.1.3 *Kava kava*

An early meta-analysis of seven placebo-controlled trials of kava kava for anxiety symptoms among patients with a variety of disorders reported greater anxiolysis among kava- than placebo-treated patients (Pittler & Ernst, 2000). However, a subsequent, double-blind, placebo-controlled study did not demonstrate greater anxiolysis among kava- than placebo- treated patients with generalized anxiety disorder (Connor & Davidson, 2002). Similarly, a subsequent double-blind study also did not support the use of kava kava for anxiety among patients with either generalized anxiety disorder, agoraphobia or social phobia (Lehrl, 2004) although kava-treated patients did report an overall better quality of sleep as well as feeling more rested in the morning than placebo-treated patients. In parallel, the results of an open-label trial suggest some anxiolytic but no significant antidepressant effects following administration of kava kava to perimenopausal women (Cagnacci *et al.*, 2003). Finally, the results of a more recent, double-blind, 3-weeks cross-over study of kava (250 mg daily) or placebo for "elevated anxiety" demonstrated greater anxiolytic effects for kava- than placebo-treated patients (Sarris *et al.*, 2009). Placebo-controlled trials of kava as monotherapy for MDD have not been published to date, although a randomized, double-blind, placebo-controlled trial of kava–*Hypericum perforatum* combination therapy for MDD suggested some antidepressant effects for combination therapy early-on (i.e., the first 4 weeks) of treatment (Sarris *et al.*, 2009).

13.2.1.4 *Valerian root and Ginkgo bilboa*

For valerian root, there is only a single open-label study evaluating its potential usefulness when used in combination with *Hypericum perforatum* for depression (Muller *et al.*, 2003). Doses for valerian root used in that study were 500 mg and 100 mg daily. For *Ginkgo bilboa* there are two positive placebo-controlled trials of 8- or 14-weeks duration suggesting it may be effective in enhancing memory in cognitively intact middle-aged volunteers (Wesnes *et al.*, 2002 and 2004). However, studies focusing on the use of gingko, valerian root as monotherapy for depression have yet to be published.

13.2.2 *Modafinil*

Modafinil (Provigil) is FDA-approved for the treatment of narcolepsy. It is commercially available in racemic form (Donovan *et al.*, 2003). The exact mechanism of action of modafinil is unknown, although modafinil-induced increases in anterior hypothalamic histamine levels (Ishizuka *et al.*, 2003), posterior hypothalamic glutamate levels (Ferraro *et al.*, 1999), nucleus accumbens dopamine levels (Ferraro *et al.*, 1996a), as well as modafinil-induced decreases in posterior hypothalamic and cortical GABA levels (Ferraro *et al.*, 1996b; Tanganelli *et al.*, 1995) have been suggested as possible mechanisms mediating the wakefulness-promoting effects of modafinil.

Only anecdotal evidence supports the use of modafinil as monotherapy for depression (Berkowitz, 2005; Kaufman *et al.*, 2002; Lundt, 2004; Price, 2005; Rabkin *et al.*, 2004; Sugden & Bourgeois, 2004). Several controlled adjunctive studies of modafinil for depression have been presented or published, and are reviewed in Chaps. 5, 6 and 10.

13.2.3 *Pivagabine*

Similar to modafinil, receptor- or transporter-affinity studies for pivagabine have not been published to date. However, there are reports suggesting an increased concentration of cortical and hypothalamic corticotropin-releasing factor (CRF) following treatment of rats with pivagabine (Follesca *et al.*, 2000), while pivagabine administration has been reported to attenuate stress-induced changes in GABA-A receptor function and CRF concentrations in the rat brain (Serra *et al.*, 1999). In fact, pre-treatment with pivagabine resulted in a greater attenuation of CRF release following experimentally induced psychological stress in humans than placebo (Gerra *et al.*, 2001).

To date, uncontrolled trials focusing on the treatment of climacteric-associated anxiety/depression (Giglotti *et al.*, 1997), or double-depression (Terranova *et al.*, 1997) suggest a potential antidepressant role for pivagabine. In parallel, a double-blind, placebo-controlled trial of pivagabine for "neurasthenia" suggested greater overall improvement among pivagabine- than placebo-treated patients (Pizzolato *et al.*, 1997). Similarly, the results of a double-blind, placebo-controlled study do suggest greater improvements in the quality of sleep among pivagabine- than placebo-treated outpatients with anxiety and comorbid insomnia (Negri, 1997). Studies of pivagabine in MDD have yet to be conducted.

Chapter 14

Biological Predictors, Moderators, and Mediators of Efficacy

14.1 Definition and Significance of Mediators of Outcome

Several goals need to be vigorously and simultaneously pursued in order to further enhance our ability to successfully treat patients with major depressive disorder (MDD).

These include:

1. Improving our knowledge regarding the efficacy, safety and tolerability of contemporary agents for depression (Chaps. 1–4).
2. Developing treatment algorithms which would take into account the presenting demographic and clinical features of patients in order to deliver existing therapies in a safer, better tolerated, and more effective manner (Chaps. 1–4).
3. Testing the combination of existing therapies from the onset of treatment (Chap. 5).
4. Testing pharmacologic and non-pharmacologic strategies for TRD (Chaps. 6–8).
5. Enhancing our ability to maintain wellness among treatment-remitters, and refine the tolerability of antidepressants (Chaps. 9 and 10).
6. Developing novel pharmacological therapies (Chaps. 11–13).

More recently, efforts have also been focused on elucidating biologic markers that may serve as predictors, mediators, or moderators of outcome (efficacy) following the acute-phase of treatment of MDD with *specific* antidepressant agents. In Chap. 1, we defined predictors

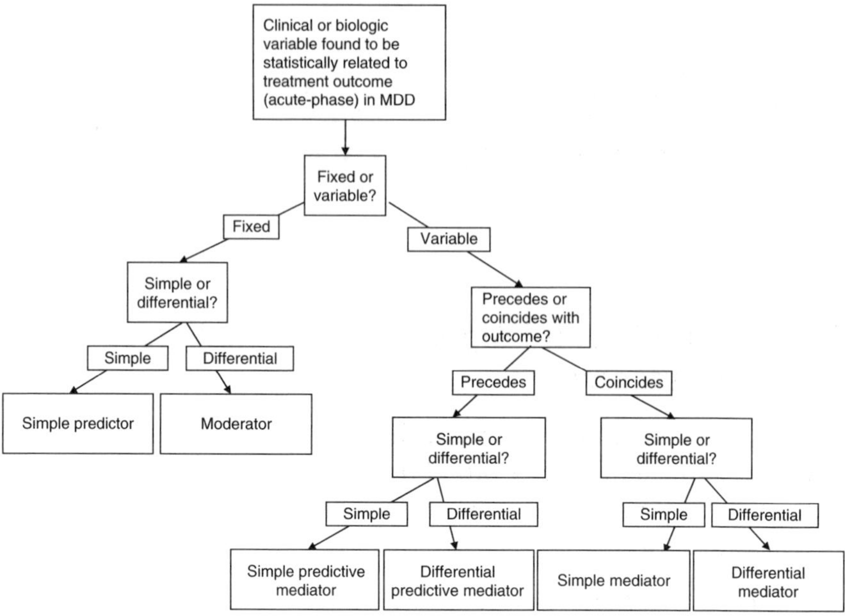

Fig. 14.1 Schematic depiction of definitions.

and moderators of treatment and outlined their potential applications in the treatment of MDD. Mediators of outcome are measurable changes (usually biologic) that occur during treatment and correlate with treatment outcome. These changes can either precede the outcome (in which case they may also predict outcome — "predictive mediators") or temporally coincide with the outcome ("simple mediators"). Differential mediators of outcome are also possible (changes that predict or correlate with an event following treatment with one agent but not another) (see Fig. 14.1).

In addition to their potential utility as treatment predictors or moderators (if they happen to be predictive mediators or differential predictive mediators; see Chap. 1 regarding the utility of treatment predictors and moderators), mediators of efficacy outcome can be very useful for the following reasons:

1. They may provide mechanistic insights into the underlying pathophysiology of depression as well as symptom resolution

in depression. This may result in the identification of new molecular targets for drug development or the definition of distinct MDD subtypes.

2. They may be used in screening for potential new antidepressants (for example, selecting for agents that also result in similar changes in clinical or preclinical settings).
3. They may be used in the formal drug approval process (clinical trials may employ such changes as a proxy for an antidepressant effect, this would be particularly advantageous if these changes occur quickly or are more robust than antidepressant changes, thereby reducing study time and/or sample size).

To date, numerous studies have explored several potential markers of outcome during the acute phase of treatment of MDD. Studies stemming from three separate fields appear to offer the most promise: (i) genetics, (ii) neurophysiology, and (iii) molecular biology. In the following paragraphs, we will review the evidence suggesting the role of biologic markers in predicting antidepressant treatment outcome in MDD (symptom improvement, response, remission).

14.2 Genetic Markers

A number of reports explore various genetic markers as predictors of clinical response to antidepressants in MDD. The vast majority of these focus on genes coding for proteins directly involved in the monoaminergic system, including tryptophan hydroxylase (TPH; the rate-limiting step in serotonin synthesis), tyrosine hydroxylase (TOH), the serotonin transporter (5HTT), the norepinephrine transporter (NET), various norepinephrine (NE-) or serotonin (5HT-) receptors, the monoamine oxidase enzyme (MAO), and the catechol-O-methyltransferase enzyme (COMT; also involved in the catabolism of the monoamines). The overwhelming majority of these studies involve treatment with the selective serotonin reuptake inhibitors (SSRIs) (see Table 14.1).

Table 14.1 State of the evidence for genetic predictors of outcome (efficacy).

Protein	Gene polymorphism	Replicated?	Treatment
5HTT	Insertion/deletion (promoter)	Y	SSRI
		N	Venlafaxine
		N	Mirtazapine
		N	TCA
		N	Atomoxetine[a]
	VTNR intron 2	Y	SSRI
NET	T182C	N	Milnacipran
	G2677T	N	Milnacipran
TPH	A218C	Y	SSRI
5HT2	A1438G	Y	SSRI
	T102C	N	SSRI
	C(1354)T	N	SSRI
5HT1A	C1019G	N	SSRI
alpha-2 AR	C-1297G	N	Milnacipran
MAO-A	Promoter VNTR	N	SSRI
	T941G	N	Mirtazapine
MAO-B	A644G	N	SSRI
COMT	Val158met (rs4680)	Y	SSRI
		N	Mirtazapine
		N	Milnacipran
IL-1 beta	c511T	Y	SSRI
BDNF	val66met	N	SSRI
	C3435T	N	SSRI
	G2677T	Y	SSRI
	C1236T	N	SSRI
GSK-3beta	50T/C	N	Lithium[a]
G-protein beta-3	C825T	N	SSRI
		N	TCA
p75 neurotrophin receptor	missense polymorphism (S250L)	N	SSRI
FKBP5	rs4713916	N	SSRI
ABCB1	G2677T	Y	SSRI
	3437C	N	SSRI
	2677G	N	SSRI
	1236T	N	SSRI
GRIK4	rs1954787	N	SSR

(*Continued*)

Table 14.1 (*Continued*)

Protein	Gene polymorphism	Replicated?	Treatment
TREK1	KCNK2	N	SSRI
SERPINE1	rs2227631-G/rs1799889-4G	N	SSRI
UCN3	rs10904481	N	SSRI/TCA
CD3E	rs2231449	N	SSRI/TCA
	rs2231449	N	SSRI
PSMD9	rs1043307	N	SSRITCA
	rs1043307	N	TCA
PSMD13	rs3817629	N	SSRI
STAT3	rs3809758	N	SSRI/TCA
	rs3744483	N	TCA
PRKCSH	rs34095	N	SSRI/TCA
	rs160841	N	SSRI
CYP3A4	rs2242480	N	SSRI
PSMA7	rs2057169	N	SSRI
	rs2057168	N	SSRI
	rs2281740	N	SSRI
	rs3746651	N	SSRI
CRHR2	rs917195	N	TCA
	rs3809758	N	TCA
DIO1	C785T	N	T3

[a]Augmentation of antidepressants

5HTT = serotonin transporter; NET = norepinephrine transporter; TPH = tryptophan hydroxylase; 5HT2 = serotonin-2 receptor; 5HT1A = seronin 1A receptor; MAO-A PR = monoamine oxidase A isoenzyme; MAO-A = monoamine oxidase A isoenzyme; COMT = catechol-O-methyltransferase; IL-1 beta = interleukin-1 beta; BDNF = brain-derived neurotrophic factor; ABCB1 = p-glycoprotein; GRIK4 = kainate 4 glutamatergic receptor; GSK-3 beta = glycogen synthase kinase 3-beta; G-protein beta-3 = G-protein beta-3; SSRI = selective serotonin reuptake inhibitor; TCA = tricyclic antidepressant; T3 = triiodothyronine; SERPINE1 = plasminogen activator inhibitor type 1; alpha-2 AR = alpha-2 adrenergic-receptor; CD3E = CD3e molecule, epsilon; STAT3 = Signal transducer and activator of transcription 3; PRKCSH = Protein kinase C substrate 80K-H; CYP3A4 = Cytochrome P450, family 3, subfamily A, polypeptide 4; CRHR2 = Corticotropin-releasing hormone receptor 2; PSMD9 = proteasome 26S non-ATPase subunit 9; PSMD13 = proteasome 26S non-ATPase subunit 13; PSMA7 = Proteasome subunit, alpha type 7; UCN3 = Urocortin 3; Dio1 = type 1 deiodinase.

14.2.1 *Studies involving SSRI therapy*

14.2.1.1 *Genes coding for TPH and 5HTT*

Three studies suggest that patients with a specific polymorphism (A218C) in the gene coding for the TPH enzyme are less likely to experience a reduction of depressive symptoms during SSRI therapy than those without such polymorphism (Ham *et al.*, 2007; Serretti *et al.*, 2001a and b), although this was not confirmed in three other studies (Hong *et al.*, 2005; Kato *et al.*, 2007; Peters *et al.*, 2004; Yoshida *et al.*, 2002b).

Early-on, the results of some (Arias *et al.*, 2003; Durham *et al.*, 2004; Bozina *et al.*, 2008; Hong *et al.*, 2006; Kato *et al.*, 2006; Kronenberg *et al.*, 2007; Ng *et al.*, 2006; Rausch *et al.*, 2002; Serreti *et al.*, 2001; Smeraldi *et al.*, 1998; Smits *et al.*, 2008; Wilkie *et al.*, 2009; Yu *et al.*, 2002; Zanardi *et al.*, 2000 and 2001) but not all (Dmitrzak-Weglarz *et al.*, 2007; Kim *et al.*, 2000; Kraft *et al.*, 2005; Minov *et al.*, 2001; Peters *et al.*, 2004; Yoshida *et al.*, 2002a) studies also suggested that depressed patients with a certain (insertion/deletion) polymorphism located in the promoter region of the gene coding for the serotonin transporter (5HTTPR) are less likely to experience an improvement in depressive symptoms during SSRI therapy than those without. Several pooled analyses and meta-analyses have, subsequently, confirmed a predictive role for 5HTTPR genotype with regards to SSRI response in MDD, more so for Caucasian than Asian patients (Serretti *et al.*, 2006 and 2007; Smits *et al.*, 2004). More recently, however, Kraft *et al.* (2007) and, subsequently, Hu *et al.* (2007) did not find an association between response to the SSRI citalopram and 5HTTPR genotype among 1,914 subjects who participated in the first level of the Sequenced Treatment Alternatives to Relieve Depression Trial (STAR*D; see Chap. 1 for further details), although a re-analysis of the data suggested a significant association for white, non-Hispanic patients only (Mrazek *et al.*, 2009). Finally, genotype status for a variable-tandem-repeat-polymorphism (VTRP) in intron 2 of the 5HTT gene was also not found to predict SSRI response in five (Hong *et al.*, 2006; Ito *et al.*, 2002; Kim *et al.*, 2000; Smits *et al.*, 2008; Wilkie *et al.*, 2009) out of six studies [Mrazek *et al.* (2009) did not confirm this association].

14.2.1.2 *Genes coding for 5HT-receptors*

Studies examining the role of 5HT2-receptor genotype as a predictor of SSRI response also present conflicting results. Specifically, two studies have identified a specific single nucleotide polymorphism (SNP) in the promoter region of the 5HT2 receptor (A1438G) that appears to be associated with the likelihood of experiencing symptom improvement during SSRI therapy in MDD (Choi *et al.*, 2005; Kato *et al.*, 2006). However, this finding was not confirmed in a third report (Sato *et al.*, 2002). Similarly, a SNP (T102C) in the gene coding for the 5HT2 receptor was found to predict SSRI response in one (Minov *et al.*, 2001), but not three subsequent studies (Cusin *et al.*, 2002; Dmitrzak-Weglarz *et al.*, 2007; Hong *et al.*, 2006). The results of a small study also demonstrate the presence of a separate polymorphism in the 5HT2 gene [C(1354)T] to predict symptom improvement following treatment with paroxetine (Wilkie *et al.*, 2009). Finally, McMahon *et al.* (2006) conducted an analysis of numerous candidate genes as potential predictors of response to open-label citalopram in MDD utilizing the STAR*D level-1 dataset ($n = 1{,}953$). Of 68 candidate genes investigated, only genetic variation at the locus coding for the 5HT2 receptor gene was found to consistently predict clinical outcome (McMahon *et al.*, 2006), with differences in genotype (comparison of two homozygous groups) accounting for an 18% difference in the absolute risk of having no response to treatment.

There are also reports of poorer response to the SSRIs in patients with specific polymorphisms in genes (178C/C) coding for the 5HT3 receptor protein (Kato *et al.*, 2006), and the 5HT1A receptor protein (C1019G) (Hong *et al.*, 2006; Villafuerte *et al.*, 2009; Yu *et al.*, 2006), although an independent effect of 5HT1A genotype (specifically, C1019G polymorphism status) on SSRI response was not confirmed in a fourth study (Arias *et al.*, 2005).

14.2.1.3 *Genes coding for NET or NE-receptors*

A polymorphism (C-1297G) in the gene coding for the α-2 adrenergic-receptor was not found to predict symptom improvement in MDD following open-label treatment with the SSRI paroxetine (Wakeno *et al.*, 2008). Similarly, the results of one study do not suggest a polymorphism (1287A/G) for the gene coding for the NET to predict response to escitalopram (Szczepankiewicz *et al.*, 2007). STAR*D-based data also show no effect of β-1 adrenergic-receptor polymorphisms on citalopram response (Crowley *et al.*, 2008).

14.2.1.4 *Genes coding for MAO and COMT*

Several reports have also focused on genes coding for enzymes involved in the catabolism of monoamines, including MAO and COMT, as predictors of symptom improvement following SSRI treatment. Specifically, a VNTR polymorphism in the promoter region of the A isoenzyme of the MAO gene (MAO-A PR) was found to predict SSRI response in one (Yu *et al.*, 2005), but not three other studies (Cusin *et al.*, 2002; Peters *et al.*, 2004; Yoshida *et al.*, 2002b). There is also a single report suggesting a relationship between COMT genotype (val158met polymorphism) and outcome following SSRI treatment (Arias *et al.*, 2006). This finding was, subsequently, replicated in two more recent reports, which also demonstrated a more robust effect of COMT genotype on SSRI response (fluoxetine) among men than women with MDD (Benedetti *et al.*, 2009; Tsai *et al.*, 2009). Finally, Tadic *et al.* (2007) reported a link between the A644G polymorphism in intron 13 of the MAO-B isoenzyme and slower response to paroxetine among women but not men with MDD.

14.2.1.5 *Genes coding for other proteins*

Relatively fewer studies have focused on genes coding for proteins not *directly* related to the monoaminergic system. Using a STAR*D-based dataset, Perlis *et al.* (2008) demonstrated a relationship between the presence of a variant (KCNK2) in a gene (TREK1) coding for a potassium channel and the likelihood of experiencing symptom improvement following treatment of MDD with the SSRI citalopram. The results of one (Choi *et al.*, 2006) but not three other reports (Domschke *et al.*, in press; Tsai *et al.*, 2003; Szczepankiewicz *et al.*, 2007) suggest brain-derived neurotrophic factor (BDNF) genotype (val66met polymorphism; rs6265) to influence the likelihood of responding to an SSRI. Similarly, no major association was found between various other polymorphisms for the BDNF gene and SSRI response (rs7103411 and rs7124442) (Domschke *et al.*, in press). The presence of specific SNPs in the gene coding for the methyltetrahydrofolate reductase enzyme (C677T) (Mischoulon *et al.*, 2003), methionine synthase enzyme (A2756G), or nitric oxide synthase enzyme (C276T) (Yu *et al.*, 2003b) also do not appear to predict SSRI response. Finally, variants of the S100A10 (encoding p11, a protein involved in the function of the 5HT1B receptor) or *HDAC5* (encoding a histone deacetylase) genes do not appear to influence SSRI response in MDD (Perlis *et al.*, 2008; Tzang *et al.*, 2008).

In a recent study, Kato *et al.* (2008a) examined the possible association of three functional ABCB1 gene (the gene coding for p-glycoprotein; see Chaps. 2 and 3 for further details) polymorphisms (C3435T, G2677T, and C1236T) with response to paroxetine. There was a significant association of the non-synonymous SNP G2677T with treatment response. Furthermore, wild variant haplotypes (3435C–2677G–1236T) were also associated with relatively poorer response ($p = 0.006$). Findings pertaining to C3435T and G2677T could not be replicated in a subsequent study involving the use of paroxetine (Mihaljevic Peles *et al.*, 2008) although a third study by Nikisch *et al.* (2008) did find a relationship between G2677T and SSRI response.

Paddock *et al.* (2007) reported that genetic variation in a kainic acid–type glutamate receptor (GRIK4) was associated with response to the antidepressant citalopram (marker rs1954787 in the GRIK4 gene, which codes for the kainic acid–type glutamate receptor KA1). The results of a STAR*D-based studies do not suggest polymorphisms coding for the phosphodiesterase (PDE) 11A and 1A-receptor genes (Teranishi *et al.*, 2007), to predict clinical improvement during the treatment of MDD with citalopram. A separate report, however, suggested that a specific polymorphism in the gene coding for the p75 neurotrophin receptor [p75(NTR)] [missense polymorphism (S250L)] was associated with the likelihood of symptom improvement during treatment with the SSRI paroxetine (Gau *et al.*, 2008). There is also a STAR*D-based report suggesting a relationship between the likelihood of achieving remission of symptoms during treatment with the SSRI citalopram and genotype at one of the markers (rs4713916) in the FKBP5 gene, a protein of the hypothalamic-pituitary adrenal (HPA) system modulating the glucocorticoid receptor (Lekman *et al.*, 2008). However, a separate STAR*D-based study did not report a significant association between genotype at various cytochrome genes (CYP2D6, ABCB1, CYP2C19, CYP3A4, and CYP3A5) and symptom improvement in MDD following citalopram treatment (Peters *et al.*, 2008). Tsai *et al.* (2008a) reported polymorphisms for the gene coding for the type 1 plasminogen activator inhibitor (rs2227631-G and rs1799889-4G) to predict treatment response with the SSRI fluoxetine in MDD. Arias *et al.* (2009) did not find several polymorphisms (rs3213207, rs2005976, rs760761 and rs2619522) of the dystrobrevin-binding-protein 1 or dysbindin gene (DTNBP1), to predict SSRI response. DTNBP1 is a protein constituent of the dystrophin-associated protein complex (DPC) of skeletal muscle cells. It is also a part of BLOC-1, or biogenesis of lysosome-related organelles complex 1. Finally, there are reports of poorer response to the SSRIs in patients with specific polymorphisms for the interleukin (IL)-1 β gene (C511T) (Yu *et al.*, 2003a), or the G-protein β3 gene (C825T polymorphism) (Serretti *et al.*, 2003), although separate studies focusing on the C825T polymorphism of the G-protein β3 gene specifically (Hong *et al.*, 2005; Kato *et al.*, 2008b) or other polymorphisms of the G-protein β3 gene [rs334558 (-50 T $>$ C), rs13321783 (IVS7 $+$ 9227 A $>$ G), rs2319398 (IVS7 $+$ 11660 G $>$ T), and rs6808874 (IVS11 $+$ 4251 T $>$ A)] (Tsai *et al.*, 2008b), did not find a link between G-protein β3-genotype and SSRI improvement in MDD.

14.2.2 *Studies involving therapy with other antidepressants*

Studies looking at genetic markers as predictors of response to other non-SSRI antidepressants are much fewer. The results of one study report 5HTTPR genotype to influence the likelihood of responding to the tricyclic antidepressant (TCA) nortriptyline in MDD (Tsapakis *et al.*, 2003), although this could not be replicated in a separate study (Dmitrzak-Weglarz *et al.*, 2007). In parallel, studies do not suggest a relationship between NET genotype (1287A/G polymorphism), BDNF genotype (Val66Met polymorphism) (Szczepankiewicz *et al.*, 2007), or 5HT2A genotype (T102C polymorphism) (Dmitrzak-Weglarz *et al.*, 2007) and antidepressant response to nortriptyline. Similarly, a polymorphism (G2677T) for the ABCB1 gene (see Chaps. 2–4) was not found to predict response to the TCA amitriptyline in one report (Laika *et al.*, 2006).

Two separate studies suggest 5HTTPR genotype to predict response to the serotonin-norepinephrine reuptake inhibitor (SNRI) venlafaxine (Choi *et al.*, 2007), and the 5HT2 α-2 adrenergic receptor inhibitor mirtazapine (Kang *et al.*, 2007a) in MDD. More recently, NET polymorphisms (T-182C and G1287A), but not 5HTT (5HTTPR, 2nd intron VNTR), or 5HT2 receptor (G1438A) genotypes were found to predict symptom improvement following treatment with the SNRI milnacipran (Yoshida *et al.*, 2004). In parallel, COMT (val158met) but not TOH (val81met) genotype was also found to predict response to milnacipran (Yoshida *et al.*, 2008). In a separate study, a polymorphism (C-1297G) in the gene coding for the α-2 adrenergic-receptor was also found to predict symptom improvement in MDD following open-label treatment with milnacipran (Wakeno *et al.*, 2008). However, the presence of a certain polymorphism (C825T polymorphism) for the G-protein β3-gene (Kang *et al.*, 2007b), the MAO-B gene (A644G in intron 13) (Tadic *et al.*, 2007), or the 5HT2 gene (1438A/G polymorphism) (Kang *et al.*, 2007c) was not found to predict response to mirtazapine. Finally, there is also a single study examining the role of MAO-A genotype as a predictor of clinical response to the monoamine-oxidase inhibitor (MAOI) moclobemide (no relationship found; Muller *et al.*, 2001).

Few studies focus on examining the role of genetic polymorphisms in predicting treatment response to augmentation and combination strategies in MDD. In one such study, Michelson *et al.* (2007) reported a greater remission rate (81.8% versus 35.7%) following augmentation of sertraline with atomoxetine than placebo for sertraline-resistant MDD among patients homozygous for the s variant of the 5HTTPR gene. No similar treatment effect for atomoxetine augmentation was observed among patients with other genotypes for the 5HTTPR. In a separate study, Adli *et al.* (2007) reported a significant association between the response to lithium augmentation of antidepressants in antidepressant-resistant depression and the presence of a polymorphism for the glycogen synthase kinase 3-β gene (50T/C single nucleotide polymorphism). More recently, Cooper-Kazaz *et al.* (2009) found a polymorphism for the type 1-deiodiase gene (C785T) to predict symptom improvement following triiodothyronine (T3) augmentation of sertraline. A similar relationship for the DIO1-A1814G polymorphism of the type 1-deiodiase gene or the DIO2-Thr92Ala and DIO2-ORFa-Gly3Asp polymorphisms of the type 2-deiodinase gene was not found (Cooper-Kazaz *et al.*, 2009). Deiodinase is a selenium-dependent enzyme that is involved in synthesizing T3 (from its inactive form thyroxine-T4) or metabolizing T3 (to an inactive form).

14.2.3 *Studies comparing antidepressants*

There are few reports examining genetic predictors of response from randomized, double-blind clinical trials comparing two antidepressants of different classes. Although preliminary, such studies can be useful in genetic markers that may serve as moderators of treatment efficacy. Four such studies focus on 5HTTPR genotype (Dmitrzak-Weglarz *et al.*, in press; Joyce *et al.*, 2003; Murphy *et al.*, 2004; Pollock *et al.*, 2000). In the first such trial, Pollock *et al.* studied 95 elderly (at least 60 years of age) MDD patients treated with either an SSRI (paroxetine) or a TCA (nortriptyline). 5HTTPR genotype was not found to predict treatment response for either medication, or differential treatment response (i.e., the likelihood of responding to one medication versus another). Similarly, in a trial comparing mirtazapine versus paroxetine in elderly patients (at least 65 years of age; $n = 246$), Murphy *et al.* (2004) did not find a statistically significant relationship between 5HTTPR genotype and treatment response for either medication, or differential treatment response. More recently, Dmitrzak-Weglarz *et al.* (in press) did not find 5HTTPR genotype to predict response to the SSRI escitalopram, the TCA nortriptyline, or differential response to either agent in MDD. Finally, Joyce *et al.* (2003) studied 169 MDD patients randomized to treatment with either fluoxetine or nortriptyline, and examined whether 5HTTPR or G-protein β-3-subunit (C825T) genotype influenced symptom improvement following treatment with either of these two agents. For patients younger than 25 years of age, the T allele of the G protein β-3 subunit was associated with a poorer response to nortriptyline. There was no relationship between 5HTTPR genotype and response to treatment with either antidepressant among this age group, nor was there any relationship between G protein β-3 subunit genotype status and response to paroxetine. Among patients 25 years of age or older, however, 5HTTPR genotype predicted response to both fluoxetine and nortriptyline. Findings stemming from this report have yet to be replicated.

Studies comparing escitalopram with nortriptyline for MDD did not demonstrate a link between 5HT2A receptor genotype (T102C polymorphism), NET genotype (1287A/G polymorphism), or BDNF genotype (val66Met polymorphism) and clinical response to either agent or differential response (Dmitrzak-Weglarz *et al.*, in press; Szczepankiewicz *et al.*, 2007). Similarly, Szegedi *et al.* (2005) studied the relationship between the COMT (val158met) polymorphism status and antidepressant response following treatment with paroxetine versus mirtazapine (5HT2 α-2 adrenergic receptor antagonist) in MDD. Patients homozygous for COMT-met showed a poorer response to mirtazapine than patients with other genotypes. A similar finding was not observed during paroxetine treatment. Tadic *et al.* (2007a) studied the relationship between MAO-A (T941G) and polymorphism status and efficacy following treatment of MDD with either mirtazapine or paroxetine. Polymorphism status was found related to treatment outcome for women treated with mirtazapine. A similar relationship was not found for women treated with paroxetine or men treated with either agent. In a separate study, Tadic *et al.* (2007b) examined the relationship between MAO-B polymorphism status (A644G intron 13 polymorphism) and clinical response to paroxetine versus mirtazapine. Genotype status was not predictive of clinical response to either agent among men. Among women, however, genotype status predicted statistically significant slower response to paroxetine but not mirtazapine. Tadic *et al.* (2008) also studied the relationship between (IL)-1 β genotype (C511T) status, and the interleukin-1 receptor antagonist (IL-1Ra) (86 bp)(n) variable number of tandem repeats (VNTR) polymorphism status on response to mirtazapine versus paroxetine. (IL)-1 β genotype (C511T) status was found to predict paroxetine but not mirtazapine response. IL-1Ra genotype status did not predict paroxetine nor mirtazapine response.

Wong *et al.* (2008) conducted a comprehensive genetic analysis focusing on the impact of inflammation-related genes on antidepressant response to the SSRI fluoxetine versus the TCA desipramine among Mexican-American patients with MDD. One-hundred-and-sixty-one (161) single nucleotide polymorphisms (SNPs) of genes coding for proteins involved in steroid pathways or proteasome subunits were analyzed. Four SNPs of three genes were found to predict desipramine responses only (rs917195 of the corticotropin-releasing hormone receptor 2 gene, rs1043307 of the proteasome 26S non-ATPase subunit 9 gene; rs3744483 and rs3809758 of the protein kinase C substrate 80K-H gene), eight SNPs of five genes were found to predict fluoxetine response only (rs2242480 of the cytochrome P450, family 3, subfamily A, polypeptide 4 gene; rs3817629 of the proteasome 26S non-ATPase subunit 13 gene; rs2231449 of the CD3e molecule, epsilon gene; rs160841 of the Protein kinase C substrate 80K-H gene; and rs2057169, rs2057168, rs2281740, rs3746651 of the proteasome subunit, α type 7 gene), while four SNPs of four genes were found to predict both fluoxetine and desipramine responses (rs10904481 of the urocortin 3 gene; rs2231449 of the CD3e molecule, epsilon gene; rs1043307 of the proteasome 26S non-ATPase subunit 9 gene; and rs3809758 of the signal transducer and activator of transcription 3 gene). Finally, in a study comparing mirtazapine with paroxetine for elderly patients with MDD, neither 5HT2 (T102C) nor cytochrome 2D6 (CYP2D6 — presence of duplications — see Chap. 2 for details) genotype status predicted treatment outcome (Murphy *et al.*, 2003).

The major limitation of reports published to date examining the role of genotypes as moderators of response to antidepressants (differential predictors) was that analyses were conducted in a post-hoc fashion. As a result, randomization did not take specific polymorphism status into account. Therefore, it is not possible to directly compare response rates between the two antidepressants among patients with a particular genotype. Nevertheless, these studies are useful in helping to identify potential genetic markers that can serve as moderators of treatment response to various antidepressants, because they control for differences across study (i.e., elements of study design, such as dosing, duration of treatment, and baseline severity of depression, that may confound a significant treatment effect). Therefore, similar exploratory analyses of existing datasets can prove very useful, providing leads for genetic markers that can then be tested as moderators of treatment response using more rigorous methods (prospective studies randomizing MDD patients with specific genotypes to one versus another agent).

14.3 Neurophysiology

14.3.1 *Brain functioning and metabolism*

14.3.1.1 *Positron emission tomography*

A number of studies have examined the potential relationship between functional changes, including changes in regional blood glucose metabolism as measured by positron emission tomography (PET), and clinical response following the treatment of MDD with standard antidepressants (Bench *et al.*, 1995; Brody *et al.*, 1999; Buchsbaum *et al.*, 1997; Kennedy *et al.*, 2001; Little *et al.*, 1996 and 2005; Mayberg *et al.*, 1999 and 2000; Passero *et al.*, 1995). Mayberg *et al.* (2000), for instance, studied the relationship between regional metabolic changes in the central nervous system (CNS) and clinical response following a six-week trial of the SSRI fluoxetine for MDD. The results of her work suggest that metabolism in certain brain areas, as measured by PET, may serve as a mediator of response to the SSRIs. Specifically, she found an increase in brainstem and dorsal cortical metabolism (prefrontal, parietal, anterior cingulate, and posterior cingulate), and a decrease in limbic and striatum metabolism (subgenual cingulate, hippocampus, and insula) from week 1 to week 6 of treatment among fluoxetine responders. Fluoxetine non-responders did not demonstrate changes in these areas during the same treatment period (weeks 1–6).

In a subsequent work, Mayberg *et al.* (2002) reviewed earlier studies examining the relationship between regional metabolic changes and symptom improvement during the treatment of MDD with antidepressants, and concluded that a significant correlation between normalization of frontal hypometabolism and clinical improvement was the best-replicated finding. However, a similar relationship (i.e., between an increase in frontal metabolism and symptom improvement) was also reported during placebo-treatment (Mayberg *et al.*, 2002). The results of the latter study suggest that such changes, at least as detected by the technology available at the time, appear to be related to non-specific (placebo) rather than specific (drug) treatment effects and, therefore, may not serve as robust differential treatment moderators. Little *et al.* (2005), for instance, examined whether there were differences in the relationship between brain metabolism at baseline (predictor or moderator) and symptom improvement between two antidepressants of different classes (the norepinephrine-dopamine reuptake inhibitor (NDRI) bupropion versus the SNRI venlafaxine). For the most part, similar findings predicted symptom improvement for both agents (frontal and left temporal hypometabolism), although some differences emerged [compared with control subjects, bupropion responders ($n = 6$) also had cerebellar hypermetabolism, whereas venlafaxine responders showed bilateral temporal and basal ganglia hypometabolism]. This study has yet to be replicated, either with regards to baseline brain metabolism (i.e., moderator of response), or changes in baseline brain metabolism (i.e., mediator of response).

14.3.1.2 *Functional magnetic resonance imaging*

Functional magnetic resonance imaging (fMRI) is an imaging technology that allows for the precise measurement of brain metabolism. Studies employing the use of fMRI have provided further insight into the relationship between brain functioning following a cognitive task and the likelihood of responding to standard antidepressants in MDD. Specifically, a number of studies have confirmed a relationship between the degree of metabolic activation in the anterior cingulate cortex at baseline following the presentation of a visual (i.e., pictures — Chen *et al.*, 2007; Davidson *et al.*, 2003; Fu *et al.*, 2004, 2007 and 2008), or auditory (i.e., words) stimulus designed to evoke affect (i.e., happiness or sadness) and the likelihood of symptom improvement following open-label treatment with either an SSRI (Chen *et al.*, 2007; Fu *et al.*, 2004 and 2007), an SNRI (Davidson *et al.*, 2003) or CBT (Fu *et al.*, 2008) (predictor of response). These studies provide strong evidence linking the function of the anterior cingulate cortex to treatment response in MDD. Different patterns of activation in various CNS areas (also using fMRI) including the anterior cingulate cortex (Walsh *et al.*, 2007; Langenecker *et al.*, 2007), left middle frontal cortex (Walsh *et al.*, 2007), lateral temporal cortex (Walsh *et al.*, 2007), amygdala (Langenecker *et al.*, 2007), insula (Langenecker *et al.*, 2007) and nucleus accumbens (Langenecker *et al.*, 2007) following cognitive tasks at baseline have also been found to predict SSRI response, findings which have yet to be replicated. Finally, it also appears that the degree of reduction in visual-stimulus–evoked anterior cingulate cortex activation during the course of treatment is correlated to greater symptom improvement in MDD (Fu *et al.*, 2004; Keedwell *et al.*, 2009).

14.3.1.3 *Magnetic resonance spectroscopy*

Magnetic resonance spectroscopy (MRS) is an imaging technology that allows for the chemical characterization of brain tissue. Within the CNS, choline is used in order to synthesize the neurotransmitter acetylcholine and is also used in the synthesis of membrane phospholipids, i.e., sphingomyelin and phosphatidylcholine (Renshaw *et al.*, 1997). The results of one study demonstrated a lower choline to creatinine ratio in the basal ganglia, as measured by MRS, among fluoxetine responders with MDD than non-responders (Renshaw *et al.*, 1997). A separate study reported lower baseline *n*-acetyl aspartate levels (NAA) and choline levels in the hippocampus at baseline to predict symptom improvement following antidepressant (SSRI/TCA) therapy, while an increase in hippocampal NAA and choline levels was found to correlate symptom improvement (mediator) (Block *et al.*, 2009). Finally, with the use of MRS, Iosifescu *et al.* (2008) established a relationship between normalization in measures of brain bioenergetic metabolism (increase in nucleoside triphosphate levels and decrease in phosphocreatine levels) among patients with SSRI-resistant MDD who experienced symptom improvement (clinical response) following T3 augmentation of their SSRI treatment regimen (mediator). This study has yet to be replicated.

14.3.2 *Electroencephalography*

14.3.2.1 *Traditional electroencephalography*

Traditional electroencephalography (EEG) has been studied as a potential biologic predictor, moderator or mediator of treatment response for decades (Bruder *et al.*, 2001; Hunter *et al.*, 2007; Knott *et al.*, 1996 and 2000; Mulert *et al.*, 2007; Rush *et al.*, 1989; Ulrich *et al.*, 1984 and 1988). Most of these studies, however, focused on TCA therapy, and employed a variety of different measures as potential treatment predictors. Knott *et al.* (1996), for example, found lower θ-power from prefrontal leads to predict response following four weeks of treatment of MDD with the TCA imipramine. A greater increase in θ-power from prefrontal leads following 2 weeks of treatment was also found to predict response at four weeks. The same group also published one of the few studies involving traditional EEG that focused on SSRI treatment (paroxetine) (Knott *et al.*, 2000). This study also reported lower prefrontal θ-power at baseline to predict response to treatment (Knott *et al.*, 2000). Other traditional EEG measurements found to predict treatment response include lateralization of baseline α power (Bruder *et al.*, 2001; Ulrich *et al.*, 1984), occipital α power (Bruder *et al.*, 2008), the frequency of non-α epochs (Ulrich *et al.*, 1988), and reduced REM latency at baseline (Rush *et al.*, 1985 and 1989).

14.3.2.2 *Quantitative electroencephalography*

Quantitative electroencephalography (QEEG) involves the use of computer software analysis to deconstruct EEG tracings and quantify parameters including frequency and amplitudes (traditional EEG involves manual readings). A relevant measurement generated by the software traditionally employed by QEEG is referred to as cordance, the calculation of which involves a combination of absolute power (the power of a frequency band) and relative power (the percentage of power in a frequency band compared to the total power across all frequency bands) (Hunter *et al.*, 2007; Leuchter *et al.*, 1994). Cordance of frontal EEG measurements in the θ-band (4–8 Hz) has consistently been found to correlate with antidepressant response in MDD. Specifically, following a number of case reports/series (Cook & Leuchter, 2001; Leuchter *et al.*, 1997), the results of several studies suggest a decrease in θ-cordance from prefrontal EEG leads during the first week of treatment with either an SSRI, an SNRI, or a variety of antidepressants, to predict greater symptom improvement following 4–10 weeks of treatment (Bares *et al.*, 2007 and 2008; Cook *et al.*, 2002 and 2005). In contrast, an increase in prefrontal θ-cordance during the first week of treatment was demonstrated among placebo-responders; suggesting that prefrontal θ-cordance may serve as a differential (predictive) mediator of response to antidepressants versus placebo (Leuchter *et al.*, 2002). Interestingly enough, a report by Hunter *et al.* (2006) suggests that the decrease in prefrontal EEG θ-cordance during the week immediately preceding the initiation of treatment of MDD with antidepressants (fluoxetine, venlafaxine) or placebo (placebo lead-in period) is related to the likelihood of responding to antidepressants but not placebo following nine weeks of treatment (moderator of response).

In conclusion, the sum of the evidence reviewed above suggests a potential role for the change in prefrontal θ-EEG cordance during the first week of treatment in MDD as a mediator and predictor of response to antidepressants but not placebo (differential mediator). Although the exact physiologic relevance of this probable treatment mediator is, at present, unclear, several lines of evidence suggest it may serve as a proxy for changes in underlying prefrontal cortex metabolism (see Hunter *et al.*, 2007 as well as Sec. 14.3.1 of this chapter for further details). The main limitation of this approach (θ-cordance) is that it requires a full EEG for its estimation. As a result, studies have focused on the potential predictive ability of a simplified four-electrode prefrontal EEG (prefrontal θ-band relative power) on antidepressant response. Specifically, two studies have confirmed a decrease in prefrontal θ-band relative power following 1–2 weeks of treatment to predict response to the SSRI in MDD (Iosifescu *et al.*, 2005; Poland *et al.*, 2005). More recently, Iosifescu *et al.* (2005) have computed a composite EEG index (Antidepressant Treatment Response index; ATR) with the intent to result in a more accurate prediction of treatment response.

ATR was recently evaluated in a large trial, termed the rapid identification of treatment effectiveness in major depressive disorder (BRITE-MD) trial (Leuchter *et al.*, 2009). In that study, 220 outpatients with MDD were randomized to receive treatment, under double-blind conditions, with escitalopram 10 mg daily for one week followed by either (1) augmentation with bupropion XL 300 mg/day, (2) switch to bupropion XL 300 mg daily, or (3) continued treatment with escitalopram 10 mg daily for a total of seven weeks. Patients also had QEED measurements at baseline and week 1, and were divided into two groups based on QEEG changes from baseline to week 1: those who had a profile thought to predict symptom improvement following continued treatment with escitalopram 10 mg (ATR+) for an additional seven weeks and those who had a profile thought to be predictive of poor outcome following continued treatment with escitalopram 10 mg (termed ATR−). ATR+ patients were more likely to respond to continued treatment with escitalopram monotherapy than ATR− patients, while ATR− patients were more likely to improve following a switch to bupropion than ATR+ patients. In fact, ATR− patients were more likely to improve following a switch from escitalopram to bupropion monotherapy, while the opposite was true for ATR+ patients (*differential predictive mediator*) (see Fig. 14.2). These results have yet to be replicated. However, if that is confirmed to possess sufficient

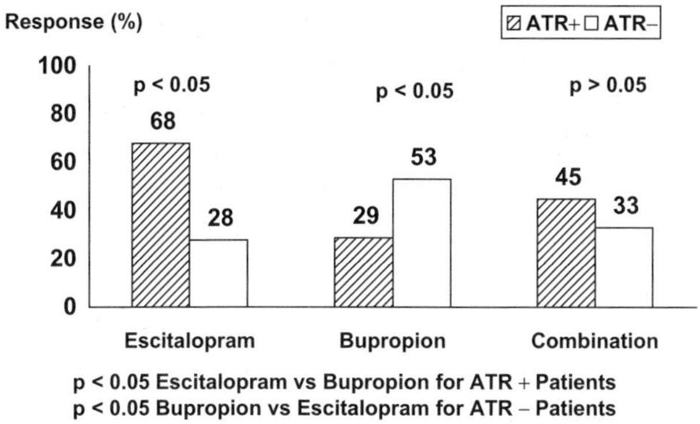

Fig. 14.2 BRITE-MD Trial ($n = 220$). [Data extracted from: Leuchter, A.F., Cook, I.A., Gilmer, W.S., *et al.* (2009). Effectiveness of a quantitative electroencephalographic biomarker for predicting differential response or remission with escitalopram and bupropion in major depressive disorder. *Psychiatry Research*, 169(2), 124–131.]

predictive ability, this or other QEEG indexes based on prefrontal θ-relative power could represent a more cost-effective and user-friendly tool for routine use in the clinic than prefrontal θ-cordance.

14.3.2.3 *Loudness Dependence of Auditory Evoked Potentials (LDAEP)*

Much less is known regarding the potential predictive ability of other EEG-related biomarkers. A number of studies have examined EEG measurements following a stimulus as a predictor of treatment response. Loudness Dependence of Auditory Evoked Potentials (LDAEP) is one such measurement, derived from EEG recordings thought to correspond to the primary auditory cortex following the administration of an auditory stimulus (Hunter *et al.*, 2007). A "strong" LDAEP suggests that the characteristics of evoked potentials following an auditory stimulus are highly dependent on the intensity (loudness) of the auditory stimulus (Hegerl & Juckel, 1993). In contrast, a "weak" LDAEP suggests that evoked potentials following an auditory stimulus do not vary much as a function of how loud the sound is (Hegerl & Juckel, 1993). To date, a variety of clinical studies have demonstrated that patients with "strong" LDAEP at baseline are more likely to respond to treatment with SSRIs than those with "weak" LDEAP (Gallinat *et al.*, 2000; Lee *et al.*, 2005; Linka *et al.*, 2004; Mulert *et al.*, 2002 and 2007; Paige *et al.*, 1994). Changes in LDAEP intensity during SSRI treatment have not been shown to correlate with symptom improvement (Gallinat *et al.*, 2000; Paige *et al.*, 1994). However, the results of a recent report suggest a "strong" LDAEP to predict poor response to the NRI reboxetine in MDD (Linka *et al.*, 2005). This finding was not confirmed in a subsequent report (Mulert *et al.*, 2007). However, in a small ($n = 35$) randomized, open-label trial comparing the SSRI citalopram with the NRI reboxetine for MDD, patients with "strong" LDAEP were more likely to respond to citalopram than reboxetine, while patients with "weak" LDAEP were more likely to response to reboxetine than citalopram (Juckel *et al.*, 2007) (differential predictor or moderator of response). *Double-blind*, randomized clinical trials involving treatment with antidepressants of different class (i.e., SSRI versus NRI) which are specifically designed to examine any potential moderating effects of LDAEP (i.e., randomization based on LDAEP status would also need to occur) have yet to be conducted.

14.3.3 *Brain functional asymmetry* (*dichotic listening*)

Dichotic listening tasks involve auditory stimuli being presented to both the left and the right ears. Potential differences in perception (perceptual asymmetry) are then used as a proxy for brain functional asymmetry. Bruder *et al.* (1990) first studied the relationship between the presence of perceptual asymmetry following dichotic listening tasks at baseline and symptom improvement following treatment with the TCAs. A left-ear advantage (right hemisphere advantage) was significantly more common among non-responders than responders. This was replicated for fluoxetine (SSRI) treatment in two different studies (Bruder *et al.*, 1996 and 2004), and bupropion (NDRI) treatment in a separate study (Bruder *et al.*, 2007) (see Table 14.2).

14.4 Molecular Biology

14.4.1 *Receptor and transporter kinetics*

Numerous studies published to date examine for the relationship between platelet serotonin (5HT) levels, used as a proxy for serotonin transporter (5HTT) kinetics, or direct measures of platelet 5HT kinetics [affinity constant (K_m) and maximal velocity (V_{max})], and the likelihood of responding to antidepressant treatment (Aberg-Wistedt *et al.*, 1981; Bakish *et al.*, 1997; Castrogiovanni *et al.*, 2003; Celada *et al.*, 1992a and b; Figueras *et al.*, 1999; Franke *et al.*, 2003; Gomez-Gil *et al.*, 2004; Gronier *et al.*, 1994; Hrdina *et al.*, 1997; Karege *et al.*, 1994; Kuhs *et al.*, 1992; Lawrence *et al.*, 1994; Lingjaerde *et al.*, 1983; Meltzer *et al.*, 1981; Muck-Seler *et al.*, 2002; Pivac *et al.*, 2003; Spreux-Varoquaux *et al.*, 1996; Victor *et al.*, 1998). Many of these studies suggest that a greater affinity of the 5HTT for 5HT, or greater platelet 5HT levels, predict poorer treatment response. Results of these trials have, however, been inconsistent.

More recently, several studies of rigorous design examining the role of receptor dynamics and kinetics on clinical response have been published. Rausch *et al.* (2001) measured K_m and V_{max} at baseline, 48 hours, 2, 4, and 8 weeks following the initiation of treatment of MDD with the SSRI fluvoxamine. Treatment with fluvoxamine was found to result in an increase in K_m and V_{max} values (K_m is defined as the extra-cellular concentration of serotonin at which transport is half maximal, a proxy for the affinity of the transporter for serotonin — hence a high or increased K_m reflects inhibition or poorer affinity of 5HTT for 5HT). Higher baseline K_m values were associated with a greater resolution of depressive symptoms during treatment (predictor). Earlier increases in K_m and V_{max} were associated with a greater resolution of *anxious* but not depressive symptoms (mediator). In a subsequent study, Rausch *et al.* (2002) measured K_m and V_{max} at baseline and 1, 6, 12, and 24 weeks following the initiation of treatment with fluoxetine. Analyses also controlled for 5HTTPR genotype (see Sec. 14.2.1 of this chapter). Higher baseline K_m values were predictive of response, controlling for 5HTTPR genotype. Fluoxetine significantly increased K_m and

V_{max}. In addition, changes in K_m during treatment were significantly different between responders (greater) and non-responders (mediator), controlling for baseline K_m, dose and 5HTTPR genotype. More recently, Axelson *et al.* (2005) confirmed the latter finding (mediator) when they also reported a significant relationship between the decrease in serotonin reuptake and antidepressant response in MDD. Finally, in a third study by Rausch group, a higher K_m at baseline was also found to result in greater chances of clinical response to the TCA nortriptyline. In fact, there were differences in the changes in K_m values (greater) during treatment among nortriptyline responders (greater) than non-responders, controlling for baseline K_m and nortriptyline plasma level. These findings are intriguing, given that nortriptyline has minimal affinity for the 5HTT (Rausch *et al.*, 2003). If confirmed, changes in 5HTT K_m during treatment may serve as a non-specific treatment moderator of response to antidepressants, a finding that could have several applications in drug development (i.e., selecting agents regardless of mechanism of action which increase K_m in pre-clinical models).

Finally, although much less is known regarding the relationship between monoamine receptor kinetics and symptom improvement in MDD, several studies suggest a potential role for monoamine receptor kinetics as predictors of response. Specifically, some studies report a direct link between the degree of α-2 desensitization during pharmacologic treatment and clinical response. Gurguis *et al.* (1999a), for instance, reported that imipramine led to decreased platelet α-2 receptor coupling and density in responders only. Gurguis *et al.* (1999b) also found that chronic imipramine decreased neutrophil α-2 adrenoreceptor density and coupling to G(s) in imipramine responders only. These studies have yet to be replicated.

14.4.2 *Intracellular signal transduction*

Little information is currently available, although there is potential for significant growth in this area. The results of an, as of yet, unreplicated study reported greater protein kinase A (PKA) activity from human skin cultured fibroblasts at baseline to predict a greater resolution of depressive symptoms following the treatment of MDD with an SSRI antidepressant (Shelton *et al.*, 2004). Antidepressant treatment also appears to reduce cAMP-response element binding protein (CREB) mRNA levels (Iga *et al.*, 2007; Lai *et al.*, 2003), as well as increase in phosphorylated CREB in lymphocytes of MDD patients (Koch *et al.*, 2002). Changes in phosphorylated CREB concentrations (Koch *et al.*, 2002) but not CREB mRNA levels (Iga *et al.*, 2007; Lai *et al.*, 2003) were found to correlate with symptom improvement in MDD.

At least four separate studies have reported a normalization (increase) of low serum BDNF levels among MDD patients following treatment with first-line antidepressants including the SSRIs and venlafaxine (Gervasoni *et al.*, 2005; Huang *et al.*, 2008; Matrisciano *et al.*, 2009; Yoshimura *et al.*, 2007). In fact, one of these studies reported higher post-treatment BDNF levels among MDD patients who responded to treatment with the SSRI paroxetine or the SNRI milnacipran ($n = 26$) than treatment non-responders ($n = 16$) (Yoshimura *et al.*, 2007), while two of these studies reported a positive correlation between symptom improvement and the degree of increase of BDNF levels in MDD (Gervasoni *et al.*, 2005; Matrisciano *et al.*, 2009). However, the results of two subsequent studies did not report a significant correlation between BDNF levels at baseline or the change in BDNF levels during antidepressant treatment with symptom improvement (Hellweg *et al.*, 2008; Huang *et al.*, 2008). More recently, the results of a meta-analysis of studies focusing on the role of BDNF in MDD suggest that BDNF does, indeed, increase during antidepressant therapy (Sen *et al.*, 2008). Further information regarding the molecules described above can be found in Chap. 13.

S100B is a calcium-binding protein produced by astroglial cells that, at nanomolar concentrations, appears to promote neuronal growth while, at larger concentrations (micromolar), may promote apoptosis (Schroeter *et al.*, 2002). S100B has been found to be elevated among MDD patients when compared to healthy control subjects (Schroeter *et al.*, 2008). Higher S100B levels immediately before treatment were found to predict a greater likelihood of clinical improvement following the treatment of MDD inpatients with either an SSRI or a TCA in one small study (Arolt *et al.*, 2003). Finally, a meta-analysis (Schroeter *et al.*, 2008) of three studies (Hetzel *et al.*, 2004; Schroeter *et al.*, 2002 and 2008) demonstrated a significant correlation between a reduction in S100B levels and a reduction in depressive symptoms among MDD patients during antidepressant therapy.

14.4.3 *Inflammatory markers*

Considerably more data are available in this field. Baseline levels or the change in levels of interferon-γ (Kim *et al.*, 2007; Myint *et al.*, 2005), interleukin-4 (Kim *et al.*, 2007; Myint *et al.*, 2005), interleukin-6 (Maes *et al.*, 1995 and 1997; Mikova *et al.*, 2001), interleukin-8 (Eller *et al.*, 2008; Mikova *et al.*, 2001), or interleukin-12 (Lee & Kim, 2006) do not appear to correlate with symptom improvement in MDD following antidepressant treatment, although the results of two subsequent studies do suggest that lower interleukin-6 levels predict a greater probability of symptom resolution in MDD (Lanquillon *et al.*, 2000; Yoshimura *et al.*, 2009). In addition, the results of two studies have identified a correlation between reductions in tumor-necrosis-α levels and symptom improvement in MDD following antidepressant treatment (Eller *et al.*, 2008; Lanquillon *et al.*, 2000). These findings have yet to be replicated on a larger scale.

Table 14.2 State of the evidence for predictors, moderators and mediators.

Genetic markers

- Several genotypes have been found to *predict* response to antidepressants

EEG and QEEG

REM latency at baseline or lateralization of alpha waves at baseline (EEG)

- *Predict* response to antidepressants

Various indexes of change in prefrontal θ-cordance during the first week of treatment (QEEG)

- *Predict* response to antidepressants (predictive *mediator*)
- Possible *mediator* of symptom improvement during antidepressant but not placebo treatment (*predictive differential mediator*) — unreplicated.
- Possible *mediator* of symptom improvement during treatment with one versus a different antidepressant-treatment strategy (*predictive differential mediator*) — unreplicated.

Loudness Dependence of Auditory Evoked Potentials (strong versus weak)

- *Predicts* response to antidepressants
- Possible moderator of response to SSRI versus NRI agents — unreplicated

PET

Normalization of frontal hypometabolism during treatment

- Is a *mediator* of symptom improvement during antidepressant treatment (but not a predictor since the measurement does not precede treatment)

(Continued)

Table 14.2 *(Continued)*

fMRI
Greater degree of metabolic activation of anterior cingulate following an emotional probe (i.e., patient shown pictures or words).
• *Predicts* response to antidepressants and CBT
Greater reduction of the degree of metabolic activation of anterior cingulate following an emotional probe during treatment
• Is a *mediator* of symptom improvement during antidepressant treatment
MRS
Choline to creatinine ratio in the basal ganglia
• *Predicts* response to antidepressants
N-acetylaspartate levels and choline levels in hippocampus
• Predict response and their change during treatment — is also a mediator of response
Increase in nucleoside triphosphate and decrease in phosphocreatine levels — is a mediator of response to T3 augmentation of SSRIs
Others
Dichotic listening (left hemispheric preference), 5HTT K_m at baseline, PKA activity at baseline, interleukin-6 levels at baseline
• *Predict* response to antidepressants
Reduction in tumor-necrosis factor levels, increase in phosphorylated CREB levels, reduction in S100B levels, and increase in BDNF levels
• Possible mediators of symptom improvement in MDD following antidepressant treatment

Summary and Conclusion of Part IV

Several leads are being simultaneously pursued in order to develop novel treatment strategies for MDD. A number of drugs with a non-monoaminergic immediate mechanism of action have or are in the process of being investigated as monotherapy for MDD, including agents acting on various neurotransmitter systems (γ-aminobutyric acid, glutamate, glycine, acetylcholine, neurokinin, σ, etc.), agents acting on various neuroendocrine axes (gonadal, adrenal, thyroid, etc.), or agents which influence human metabolism (fatty acid metabolism, second messenger systems, one carbon metabolism, etc.). Although the sum of the evidence supporting the role of any specific agent or class of agents as monotherapy for MDD is, at best, preliminary, several interesting leads have been presented. For the most part, such leads have suggested that any potential, novel non-monoaminergic agents would have, overall, comparable efficacy and safety when compared to contemporary monoaminergic agents. However, due to their distinct mechanism of action compared to contemporary antidepressants, it is quite possible that robust treatment differences may emerge with respect to the resolution of specific depressive symptoms, symptom clusters, or depressive subtypes. Future studies that (1) confirm antidepressant effects for these agents, and (2) compare their efficacy in treating specific depressive symptoms, symptom clusters, or subtypes of MDD to standard (monoaminergic) pharmacotherapies could help improve the standard of care for MDD.

Finally, preliminary studies have identified a number of putative "biomarkers", relating to genetic, neurophysiologic [particularly quantitative EEG (QEEG)-based measurements as well as measures of prefrontal cortical metabolism], or receptor/transporter kinetic factors (serotonin transporter kinetics), which appear to correlate with symptom improvement during the treatment of MDD with standard antidepressants. Conducting further studies designed to establish reliable, replicable, and robust biological factors which function as predictors, mediators or moderators of clinical improvement in MDD could benefit the field in several ways, from enhancing our ability to develop more effective treatments to improving our ability to chose an individualized pharmacotherapeutic regimen for patients with MDD which would result in a more rapid and robust resolution of depressive symptoms.

Appendix A

Common cytochrome p450 isoenzyme substrates, inhibitors and inducers.

P450 2D6	
Substrates	Tricyclic antidepressants, fluoxetine, atomoxetine, duloxetine, aripiprazole, mirtazapine, mianserin, mCPP β-blockers, antiarrhythmics (mexiletine, flecainide, propafenone, encainide) diltiazem, nifedipine, nisoldipine, codeine, hydroxycodone, oxycodon, tramadol, odansetron, phenothiazines, risperidone, dextromethorphan
Inhibitors	Fluoxetine, paroxetine, sertraline, bupropion, phenothiazines, cocaine, methadone, yohimbine, quinidine, protease inhibitors, antimalarials, cimetidine, lansoprazole, antifungal (terbinafine)
Inducers	Unknown
P450 3A	
Substrates	Sertraline, gepirone, venlafaxine, desvenlafaxine, nefazodone, mirtazapine, trazodone, reboxetine, aripiprazole, pimozide, alprazolam, midazolam, clonazepam, eszopiclone, selegiline, zolpidem, zaleplon, buspirone, carbamazepine, tertiary TCAs, quetiapine, clozapine, ziprasidone, haloperidol, cisapride, ergotamines, alfentanil, fentanyl, methadone, sildenafil, H1 blockers, sibutramine, montelukast, OCPs, testosterone, CA++ channel blockers, cyclosporine, tacrolimus, HMG-CoA reductase inhibitors, amiodarone, propafenone, quinidine, antiretrovirals
Inhibitors	Nefazodone, fluvoxamine, fluoxetine, paroxetine, sertraline, antifungals, macrolide antibiotics, antiretrovirals, quinupristin/dalfopristin, calcium channel blockers, grapefruit juice, cimetidine
Inducers	Carbamazepine, pheytoin, oxcarbazepine, phenobarbital, ritonavir (chronic), efavirenz (also inhibitor), rifampin, *Hypericum perforatum*, modafinil

(*Continued*)

Appendix A (*Continued*)

P450 1A2	
Substrates	Clozapine, duloxetine, mirtazapine, olanzapine, haloperidol, tertiary TCAs, selegiline, tacrine, theophylline, aminophylline, caffeine, R-warfarin, cyclobenzaprine, propafenone, acetaminophen, phenacetin, pro-carcinogens
Inhibitors	Fluvoxamine, fluorquinolones (ciprofloxacin, norfloxacin and others), cimetidine, antiarrhythmics (mexiletine, propafenone), zafirlukast
Inducers	Omeprazole, cigarette smoking, charred meats (arylhydrocarbons), cruciferous vegetables (e.g., brussel sprouts), modafinil
CYP 2C Sub-family	
Substrates	Diazepam, tertiary TCAs, pheytoin, tetrahydrocanabinol (THC), S-warfarin, NSAIDs, celecoxib, piroxicam, dapsone, propranolol, mephenytoin, THC, tolbutamide, glyburide, glipizide, rosiglitazone, tamoxifen, angiotensin II blockers (losartan, valsartan)
Inhibitors	Fluoxetine, fluvoxamine, sertraline, modafinil, tranylcypromine, omeprazole, valproate, isoniazid, ketoconazole, fluconazole, ritonavir, sulfaphenazole, ticlopidine, zafirlukast, fluvstatin, cimetidine
Inducers	Rifampin, phenobarbital, carbamazepine

Appendix B

"State of the evidence": The use of antidepressants in depressive disorders.

	MDD (Adults)	MDD (Elderly)	MDD (Children & Adolescents)	MDD (Post-Partum)	MDD (Alcohol use Dis.)	MDD (Drug use Dis.)	BPD	DD	SAD	MiDD	Psy. MDD
SSRI	+	+	+	+	+	–	–	+	+	+	+
Tianeptine	+										
Venlafaxine	+	–	–								
Desvenlafaxine	+										
Duloxetine	+	+									
Milnacipran	+										
Bupropion	+	–							+		
Reboxetine	+										
Mirtazapine	+	+	–								
Trazodone	+	+									

(Continued)

Appendix B (*Continued*)

	MDD (Adults)	MDD (Elderly)	MDD (Children & Adolescents)	MDD (Post-Partum)	MDD (Alcohol use Dis.)	MDD (Drug use Dis.)	BPD	DD	SAD	MiDD	Psy. MDD
Nefazodone	+				+						
Agomelatine	+										
Selegiline	+										
Moclobemide	+	+						+	−		

- Limited to newer antidepressants [selective serotonin reuptake inhibitors (SSRIs) and more recently-developed agents].
- "+" indicates at least one double-blind, randomized, placebo-controlled trial demonstrating a greater reduction in depressive symptoms during treatment of a depressive disorder with an antidepressant agent than placebo.
- "−" indicates only "negative" double-blind, randomized, placebo-controlled trials (i.e., trials which fail to demonstrate a greater antidepressant effect for a given drug than placebo in a specific population".
- A blank entry indicates no randomized, double-blind, placebo-controlled trials published to date.

Abbreviations

MDD = major depressive disorder; BPD = bipolar disorder — major depressive episode; DD = dysthymic disorder; SAD = seasonal affective disorder; MiDD = minor depressive disorder; Psy. MDD = Psychotic MDD.

Appendix C

"State of the evidence": The use of antidepressants in disorders often comorbid with MDD.

	GAD	PD	SAD	OCD	PTSD	Anorexia Nervosa	Bulimia Nervosa	BED	AD(H)D	FM
SSRI	+	+	+	+	+	+	+	+		+
Tianeptine										
Venlafaxine	+	+	+		+					
Desvenlafaxine										
Duloxetine	+									+
Milnacipran										+
Bupropion									+	
Reboxetine		+								
Mirtazapine			+		+					
Trazodone	+						+			

(*Continued*)

Appendix C *(Continued)*

	GAD	PD	SAD	OCD	PTSD	Anorexia Nervosa	Bulimia Nervosa	BED	AD(H)D	FM
Nefazodone					+					
Agomelatine	+									
Selegiline										
Moclobemide			+							

- Limited to newer antidepressants [selective serotonin reuptake inhibitors (SSRIs) and more recently-developed agents].
- "+" indicates at least one double-blind, randomized, placebo-controlled trial demonstrating a greater reduction in depressive symptoms during treatment of a depressive disorder with an antidepressant agent than placebo.
- A blank entry indicates no "+" randomized, double-blind, placebo-controlled trials published to date.

Abbreviations

GAD = generalized anxiety disorder; PD = panic disorder; SAD = social anxiety disorder; OCD = obsessive compulsive disorder; PTSD = post-traumatic stress disorder; BED = binge-eating disorder; AD(H)D = attention deficit (hyperactivity) disorder; FM = fibromyalgia.

Appendix D

"State of the evidence": The use of antidepressants for the treatment of MDD in patients with comorbid medical disorders.

	Diabetes	MI	Asthma	Post Stroke	Alzheimers	Hemodialysis	IFN-α	HIV	Cancer
SSRI	+	+	+	+	+	+	+	+	+
Tianeptine									
Venlafaxine									
Desvenlafaxine									
Duloxetine									
Milnacipran									
Bupropion									
Reboxetine									
Mirtazapine		+		+					
Trazodone									
Nefazodone									
Agomelatine									
Selegiline									
Moclobemide			+						

- Limited to newer antidepressants [selective serotonin reuptake inhibitors (SSRIs) and more recently-developed agents].
- "+" indicates at least one double-blind, randomized, placebo-controlled trial demonstrating a greater reduction in depressive symptoms during treatment of a depressive disorder with an antidepressant agent than placebo.
- A blank entry indicates no "+" randomized, double-blind, placebo-controlled trials published to date.

Abbreviations

MI = myocardial infarction; IFN-α = interferon-alpha induced depression; HIV = human immunodeficiency virus.

Bibliography

Chapter 1

Alexopoulos, G.S., Kiosses, D.N., Heo, M., *et al.* (2005). Executive dysfunction and the course of geriatric depression. *Biological Psychiatry*, 58(3), 204–210.

Alexopoulos, G.S., Murphy, C.F., Gunning-Dixon, F.M., *et al.* (2008). Microstructural white matter abnormalities and remission of geriatric depression. *American Journal of Psychiatry*, 165(2), 238–244.

Alpert, J.E., Maddocks, A., Nierenberg, A.A., *et al.* (1996). Attention deficit hyperactivity disorder in childhood among adults with major depression. *Psychiatry Research*, 62(3), 213–219.

American Psychiatric Association. (1994). DSM-IV: Diagnostic and statistical manual of mental disorders. 4th ed. Washington, DC: APA.

Angst, J., Scheidegger, P. and Stabl, M. (1993). Efficacy of moclobemide in different patient groups. Results of new subscales of the Hamilton Depression Rating Scale. *Clinical Neuropharmacology*, 16(Suppl 2), S55–62.

Arnold, L.M., Meyers, A.L., Sunderajan, P., *et al.* (2008). The effect of pain on outcomes in a trial of duloxetine treatment of major depressive disorder. *Annals of Clinical Psychiatry*, 20(4), 187–193.

Blazer, D., George, L.K., Landerman, R., *et al.* (1985). Psychiatric disorders. A rural/urban comparison. *Archives of General Psychiatry*, 42(7), 651–660.

Blazer, D.G., Kessler, R.C., McGonagle, K.A. and Swartz, M.S. (1994). The prevalence and distribution of major depression in a national community sample: The National Comorbidity Survey. *American Journal of Psychiatry*, 151(7), 979–986.

Bostwick, J.M. and Pankratz, V.S. (2000). Affective disorders and suicide risk: A reexamination. *American Journal of Psychiatry*, 157(12), 1925–1932.

Breslau, N., Davis, G.C., Peterson, E.L. and Schultz, L. (1997). Psychiatric sequelae of posttraumatic stress disorder in women. *Archives of General Psychiatry*, 54(1), 81–87.

Broadhead, W.E., Blazer, D.G., George, L.K. and Tse, C.K. (1990). Depression, disability days, and days lost from work in a prospective epidemiological survey. *Journal of the American Medical Association*, 264, 2524–2528.

Bruce, M.L., Leaf, P.J., Rozal, G.P., *et al.* (1994). Psychiatric status and 9-year mortality data in the New Haven Epidemiologic Catchment Area Study. *American Journal of Psychiatry*, 151(5), 716–721.

Burns, R.A., Lock, T., Edwards, D.R., *et al.* (1995). Predictors of response to amine-specific antidepressants. *Journal of Affective Disorders*, 35(3), 97–106.

Caligiuri, M.P., Gentili, V., Eberson, S., *et al.* (2003). A quantitative neuromotor predictor of antidepressant non-response in patients with major depression. *Journal of Affective Disorders*, 77(2), 135–141.

Carta, M.G., Carpiniello, B., Kovess, V., *et al.* (1995). Lifetime prevalence of major depression and dysthymia: Results of a community survey in Sardinia. *European Neuropsychopharmacology*, 5 Suppl, 103–107.

Cleary, P. and Guy, W. (1977). Factor analysis of the Hamilton Depression Scale. *Drugs Under Experimental and Clinical Research*, 1, 115–120.

Corey-Lisle, P.K., Nash, R., Stang, P. and Swindle, R. (2004). Response, partial response, and nonresponse in primary care treatment of depression. *Archives of Internal Medicine*, 164(11), 1197–1204.

Davidson, J.R., Meoni, P., Haudiquet, V., *et al.* (2002). Achieving remission with venlafaxine and fluoxetine in major depression: Its relationship to anxiety symptoms. *Depression and Anxiety*, 16(1), 4–13.

De Lisio, G., Maremmani, I., Perugi, G., *et al.* (1986). Impairment of work and leisure in depressed outpatients: A preliminary communication. *Journal of Affective Disorders*, 10, 79–84.

Delini-Stula, A., Mikkelsen, H. and Angst, J. (1995). Therapeutic efficacy of antidepressants in agitated anxious depression — a meta-analysis of moclobemide studies. *Journal of Affective Disorders*, 35(1–2), 21–30.

Demopulos, C., Fava, M., McLean, N.E., *et al.* (1996). Hypochondriacal concerns in depressed outpatients. *Psychosomatic Medicine*, 58(4), 314–320.

Denninger, J.W., Papakostas, G.I., Mahal, Y., *et al.* (2006). Somatic symptoms in outpatients with major depressive disorder treated with fluoxetine. *Psychosomatics*, 47(4), 348–352.

Eaton, W.W., Regier, D.A., Locke, B.Z. and Taube, C.A. (1981). The Epidemiologic Catchment Area Program of the National Institute of Mental Health. *Public Health Reports*, 96(4), 319–325.

Farabaugh, A., Mischoulon, D., Fava, M., *et al.* (2005). The relationship between early changes in the HAMD-17 anxiety/somatization factor items and treatment outcome among depressed outpatients. *International Clinical Psychopharmacology*, 20(2), 87–91.

Farabaugh, A., Sonawalla, S., Johnson, D.P., *et al.* (in press) Early improvements in anxiety, depression, and anger/hostility symptoms and response to antidepressant treatment. *Annals of Clinical Psychiatry*.

Fava, M. (2003). Diagnosis and definition of treatment-resistant depression. *Biological Psychiatry*, 53(8), 649–659.

Fava, M., Bless, E., Otto, M.W., *et al.* (1994b). Dysfunctional attitudes in major depression. Changes with pharmacotherapy. *Journal of Nervous and Mental Disease*, 182(1), 45–49.

Fava, M., Borus, J.S., Alpert, J.E., *et al.* (1997b). Folate, vitamin B12, and homocysteine in major depressive disorder. *American Journal of Psychiatry*, 154(3), 426–428.

Fava, M., Bouffides, E., Pava, J.A., *et al.* (1994a). Personality disorder comorbidity with major depression and response to fluoxetine treatment. *Psychotherapy and Psychosomatics*, 62(3–4), 160–167.

Fava, M., Graves, L.M., Benazzi, F., *et al.* (2006). A cross-sectional study of the prevalence of cognitive and physical symptoms during long-term antidepressant treatment. *Journal of Clinical Psychiatry*, 67(11), 1754–1759.

Fava, M., Hoog, S.L., Judge, R.A., *et al.* (2002). Acute efficacy of fluoxetine versus sertraline and paroxetine in major depressive disorder including effects of baseline insomnia. *Journal of Clinical Psychopharmacology*, 22(2), 137–147.

Fava, M., Labbate, L.A., Abraham, M.E. and Rosenbaum, J.F. (1995). Hypothyroidism and hyperthyroidism in major depression revisited. *Journal of Clinical Psychiatry*, 56(5), 186–192.

Fava, M., Martinez, J.M., Greist, J., *et al.* (2007). The efficacy and tolerability of duloxetine in the treatment of anxious versus non-anxious depression: A post-hoc analysis of an open-label outpatient study. *Annals of Clinical Psychiatry*, 19(3), 187–195.

Fava, M., Rush, A.J., Alpert, J.E., *et al.* (2008). Do outpatients with anxious vs. non-anxious major depressive disorder have different treatment outcomes? A STAR*D report. *American Journal of Psychiatry*, 165, 342–351.

Fava, M., Uebelacker, L.A., Alpert, J.E., *et al.* (1997a). Major depressive subtypes and treatment response. *Biological Psychiatry*, 42(7), 568–576.

Feiger, A.D., Flament, M.F., Boyer, P. and Gillespie, J.A. (2003). Sertraline versus fluoxetine in the treatment of major depression: A combined analysis of five double-blind comparator studies. *International Clinical Psychopharmacology*, 18(4), 203–210.

Flint, A.J. and Rifat, S.L. (1997). Anxious depression in elderly patients. Response to antidepressant treatment. *American Journal of Geriatric Psychiatry*, 5(2), 107–115.

Foley, D., Ancoli-Israel, S., Britz, P. and Walsh, J. (2004). Sleep disturbances and chronic disease in older adults: Results of the 2003 National Sleep Foundation Sleep in America Survey. *Journal of Psychosomatic Research*, 56(5), 497–502.

Frank, E., Rucci, P., Katon, W., *et al.* (2002). Correlates of remission in primary care patients treated for minor depression. *General Hospital Psychiatry*, 24(1), 12–19.

Fredman, L., Weissman, M.M., Leaf, P.J. and Bruce, M.L. (1988). Social functioning in community residents with depression and other psychiatric disorders: Results of the Newhaven Epidemiologic Catchment Area Study. *Journal of Affective Disorders*, 15, 103–112.

Friedman, R.A., Parides, M., Baff, R., *et al.* (1995). Predictors of response to desipramine in dysthymia. *Journal of Clinical Psychopharmacology*, 15(4), 280–283.

Gilmer, W.S., Gollan, J.K., Wisniewski, S.R., *et al.* (2008). Does the duration of index episode affect the treatment outcome of major depressive disorder? A STAR*D report. *Journal of Clinical Psychiatry*, 69(8), 1246–1256.

Grant, B.F. (1995). Comorbidity between DSM-IV drug use disorders and major depression: Results of a national survey of adults. *Journal of Substance Abuse*, 7(4), 481–497.

Grant, B.F. and Harford, T.C. (1995). Comorbidity between DSM-IV alcohol use disorders and major depression: Results of a national survey. *Drug and Alcohol Dependence*, 39(3), 197–206.

Grunhaus, L., Harel, Y., Krugler, T., *et al.* (1988). Major depressive disorder and panic disorder. Effects of comorbidity on treatment outcome with antidepressant medications. *Clinical Neuropharmacology*, 11(5), 454–461.

Grunhaus, L., Rabin, D. and Greden, J.F. (1986). Simultaneous panic and depressive disorder: Response to antidepressant treatments. *Journal of Clinical Psychiatry*. 1986, 47(1), 4–7.

Hamilton, M. (1960). A rating scale for depression. *Journal of Neurology, Neurosurgery and Psychiatry*, 23, 56–62.

Hays, R.D., Wells, K.B., Sherbourne, C.D., *et al.* (1995). Functioning and well-being outcomes of patients with depression compared with chronic general medical illnesses. *Archives of General Psychiatry*, 52(1), 11–19.

Heiligenstein, J.H., Tollefson, G.D. and Faries, D.E. (1994). Response patterns of depressed outpatients with and without melancholia: A double-blind, placebo-controlled trial of fluoxetine versus placebo. *Journal of Affective Disorders*, 30(3), 163–173.

Hirschfeld, R.M., Russell, J.M., Delgado, P.L., *et al.* (1998). Predictors of response to acute treatment of chronic and double depression with sertraline or imipramine. *Journal of Clinical Psychiatry*, 59(12), 669–675.

Howland, R.H., John Rush, A., Wisniewski, S.R., *et al.* (2009). Concurrent anxiety and substance use disorders among outpatients with major depression: Clinical features and effect on treatment outcome. *Drug and Alcohol Dependence*, 99(1–3), 248–260.

Howland, R.H., Wilson, M.G., Kornstein, S.G., *et al.* (2008). Factors predicting reduced antidepressant response: Experience with the SNRI duloxetine in patients with major depression. *Annals of Clinical Psychiatry*, 20(4), 209–218.

Husain, M.M., Rush, J.A., Wisniewski, S., *et al.* (2009). Family history of depression and therapeutic outcome: Findings from STAR*D. *Journal of Clinical Psychiatry*, 70(2), 185–195.

Iosifescu, D.V., Clementi-Craven, N., Fraguas, R., *et al.* (2005). Cardiovascular risk factors may moderate pharmacological treatment effects in major depressive disorder. *Psychosomatic Medicine*, 67(5), 703–706.

Iosifescu, D.V., Howarth, S., Alpert, J.E., *et al.* (2001). T3 blood levels and treatment outcome in depression. *International Journal of Psychiatry in Medicine*, 31(4), 367–373.

Iosifescu, D.V., Nierenberg, A.A., Alpert, J.E., *et al.* (2003). The impact of medical comorbidity on acute treatment in major depressive disorder. *American Journal of Psychiatry*, 160(12), 2122–2127.

Iosifescu, D.V., Renshaw, P.F., Lyoo, I.K., *et al.* (2006). Brain MRI white matter hyperintensities, cardiovascular risk factors, and treatment outcome in major depressive disorder. *British Journal of Psychiatry*, 188, 180–185.

Joffe, R.T. and Regan, J.J. (1989). Personality and response to tricyclic antidepressants in depressed patients. *Journal of Nervous and Mental Disease*, 177(12), 745–749.

Johnson, J., Weissman, M.M. and Klerman, G.L. (1992). Service utilization and social morbidity associated with depressive symptoms in the community. *Journal of the American Medical Association*, 267(11), 478–483.

Joyce, P.R., Mulder, R.T. and Cloninger, C.R. (1994). Temperament predicts clomipramine and desipramine response in major depression. *Journal of Affective Disorders*, 30(1), 35–46.

Judd, L.L., Paulus, M.P., Wells, K.B. and Rapaport, M.H. (1996). Socioeconomic burden of subsyndromal depressive symptoms and major depression in a sample of the general population. *American Journal of Psychiatry*, 153(11), 1411–1417.

Kendler, K.S., Davis, C.G. and Kessler, R.C. (1997). The familial aggregation of common psychiatric and substance use disorders in the National

Comorbidity Survey: A family history study. *British Journal of Psychiatry*, 170, 541–548.

Kessler, R.C., Berglund, P.A., Foster, C.L., *et al.* (1997). Social consequences of psychiatric disorders, II: Teenage parenthood. *American Journal of Psychiatry*, 154(10), 1405–1411.

Kessler, R.C., Foster, C.L., Saunders, W.B. and Stang, P.E. (1995). Social consequences of psychiatric disorders, I: Educational attainment. *American Journal of Psychiatry*, 152(7), 1026–1032.

Kessler, R.C., McGonagle, K.A., Zhao, S., *et al.* (1994). Lifetime and 12-month prevalence of DSM-III-R psychiatric disorders in the United States: Results from the National Comorbidity Survey. *Archives of General Psychiatry*, 51, 8–19.

Kessler, R.C., Nelson, C.B., McGonagle, K.A., *et al.* (1996). Comorbidity of DSM-III-R major depressive disorder in the general population: Results from the US National Comorbidity Survey. *British Journal of Psychiatry Supplement*, (30), 17–30.

Kessler, R.C., Walters, E.E. and Forthofer, M.S. (1998). The social consequences of psychiatric disorders, III: Probability of marital stability. *American Journal of Psychiatry*, 155(8), 1092–1096.

Kocsis, J.H., Leon, A.C., Markowitz, J.C., *et al.* (2009). Patient preference as a moderator of outcome for chronic forms of major depressive disorder with nefazodone, cognitive behavioral analysis system of psychotherapy, or their combination. *Journal of Clinical Psychiatry*, 70(3), 354–361.

Kocsis, J.H., Mason, B.J., Frances, A.J., *et al.* (1989). Prediction of response of chronic depression to imipramine. *Journal of Affective Disorders*, 17(3), 255–260.

Kornstein, S.G., Wohlreich, M.M., Mallinckrodt, C.H., *et al.* (2006). Duloxetine efficacy for major depressive disorder in male vs. female patients: Data from 7 randomized, double-blind, placebo-controlled trials. *Journal of Clinical Psychiatry*, 67(5), 761–770.

Kozel, F.A., Trivedi, M.H., Wisniewski, S.R., *et al.* (2008). Treatment outcomes for older depressed patients with earlier versus late onset of first depressive episode: A sequenced treatment alternatives to relieve depression (STAR*D) report. *American Journal of Geriatric Psychiatry*, 16(1), 58–64.

Lenze, E.J., Mulsant, B.H., Dew, M.A., *et al.* (2003). Good treatment outcomes in late-life depression with comorbid anxiety. *Journal of Affective Disorders*, 77(3), 247–254.

Lepine, J.P., Gastpar, M., Mendlewicz, J. and Tylee, A. (1997). Depression in the community: The first pan-European study DEPRES [Depression Research in European Society]. *International Clinical Psychopharmacology*, 12(1), 19–29.

Lesser, I.M., Castro, D.B., Gaynes, B.N., *et al.* (2007). Ethnicity/race and outcome in the treatment of depression: Results from STAR*D. *Medical Care*, 45(11), 1043–1051.

Lesser, I., Rosales, A., Zisook, S., *et al.* (2008). Depression outcomes of Spanish- and English-speaking Hispanic outpatients in STAR*D. *Psychiatric Services*, 59(11), 1273–1284.

Liebowitz, M.R., Quitkin, F.M., Stewart, J.W., *et al.* (1988). Antidepressant specificity in atypical depression. *Archives of General Psychiatry*, 45(2), 129–137.

Maciejewski, P.K., Prigerson, H.G. and Mazure, C.M. (2000). Self-efficacy as a mediator between stressful life events and depressive symptoms: Differences based on history of prior depression. *British Journal of Psychiatry*, 176, 373–378.

Maddux, R.E., Riso, L.P., Klein, D.N., *et al.* (2009). Select comorbid personality disorders and the treatment of chronic depression with nefazodone, targeted psychotherapy, or their combination. *Journal of Affective Disorders*, 117, 174–179.

Mallinckrodt, C.H., Watkin, J.G., Liu, C., *et al.* (2005). Duloxetine in the treatment of Major Depressive Disorder: A comparison of efficacy in patients with and without melancholic features. *BioMed Central Psychiatry*, 5, 1.

Marcus, R.N. and Mendels, J. (1996). Nefazodone in the treatment of severe, melancholic, and recurrent depression. *Journal of Clinical Psychiatry*, 57(Suppl 2), 19–23.

Marzuk, P.M., Tardiff, K. and Hirsch, C.S. (1992). The epidemiology of murder-suicide. *Journal of the American Medical Association*, 267(23), 3179–3183.

McGrath, P.J., Khan, A.Y., Trivedi, M.H., *et al.* (2008). Response to a selective serotonin reuptake inhibitor (citalopram) in major depressive disorder with melancholic features: A STAR*D report. *Journal of Clinical Psychiatry*, 69(12), 1847–1855.

Mischoulon, D., Burger, J.K., Spillmann, M.K., *et al.* (2000). Anemia and macrocytosis in the prediction of serum folate and vitamin B12 status, and treatment outcome in major depression. *Journal of Psychosomatic Research*, 49(3), 183–187.

Murray, C.J.L. and Lopez, A.D. (1997a). Alternative projections of mortality and disability by cause. 1990–2020: Global burden of disease study. *The Lancet*, 349, 1498–1504.

Murray, C.J.L. and Lopez, A.D. (1997b). Global mortality, disability, and the contribution of risk factors: Global burden of disease study. *The Lancet*, 349, 1436–1442.

Mynors-Wallis, L. and Gath, D. (1997). Predictors of treatment outcome for major depression in primary care. *Psychological Medicine*, 27(3), 731–736.

Nelson, E. and Cloninger, C.R. (1997). Exploring the TPQ as a possible predictor of antidepressant response to nefazodone in a large multi-site study. *Journal of Affective Disorders*, 44(2–3), 197–200.

Nelson, E.C. and Cloninger, C.R. (1995). The tridimensional personality questionnaire as a predictor of response to nefazodone treatment of depression. *Journal of Affective Disorders*, 35(1–2), 51–57.

Newman, J.R., Ewing, S.E., McColl, R.D., *et al.* (2000). Tridimensional personality questionnaire and treatment response in major depressive disorder: A negative study. *Journal of Affective Disorders*, 57(1–3), 241–247.

Newman, S.C. and Bland, R.C. (1991). Suicide risk varies by subtype of depressive disorder. *Acta Psychiatrica Scandinavica*, 83, 420–426.

Nierenberg, A.A. and Amsterdam, J.D. (1990). Treatment-resistant depression: Definition and treatment approaches. *Journal of Clinical Psychiatry*, 51 Suppl, 39–47.

Nierenberg, A.A. and DeCecco, L.M. (2001). Definitions of antidepressant treatment response, remission, nonresponse, partial response, and other relevant outcomes: A focus on treatment-resistant depression. *Journal of Clinical Psychiatry*, 62(Suppl 16), 5–9.

Nierenberg, A.A., Farabaugh, A.H., Alpert, J.E., *et al.* (2000). Timing of onset of antidepressant response with fluoxetine treatment. *American Journal of Psychiatry*, 157(9), 1423–1428.

Nierenberg, A.A., Keefe, B.R., Leslie, V.C., *et al.* (1999). Residual symptoms in depressed patients who respond acutely to fluoxetine. *Journal of Clinical Psychiatry*, 60(4), 221–225.

Nierenberg, A.A., McLean, N.E., Alpert, J.E., *et al.* (1995). Early nonresponse to fluoxetine as a predictor of poor 8-week outcome. *American Journal of Psychiatry*, 152(10), 1500–1503.

Nunes, E.V., Deliyannides, D., Donovan, S. and McGrath, P.J. (1996). The management of treatment resistance in depressed patients with substance use disorders. *Psychiatric Clinics of North America*, 19(2), 311–327.

Ormel, J., Von Korff, M., Oldehinkel, A.J., *et al.* (1999). Onset of disability in depressed and non-depressed primary care patients. *Psychological Medicine*, 29, 847–853.

Ormel, J., Von Korff, M., Ustun, T.B., *et al.* (1994). Common mental disorders and disability across cultures. Results from the WHO collaborative study on psychological problems in general health care. *Journal of the American Medical Association*, 272(22), 1741–1748.

Pampallona, S., Bollini, P., Tibaldi, G., *et al.* (2004). Combined pharmacotherapy and psychological treatment for depression: A systematic review. *Archives of General Psychiatry*, 61(7), 714–719.

Papakostas, G.I. and Fava, M. (2009). Does the probability of receiving placebo influence clinical trial outcome? A meta-regression of double-blind, randomized clinical trials in MDD. *European Neuropsychopharmacology*, 19(1), 34–40.

Papakostas, G.I., Crawford, C.M., Scalia, M.J. and Fava, M. (2007c) Timing of clinical improvement and symptom resolution in the treatment of major depressive disorder. A replication of findings with the use of a double-blind, placebo-controlled trial of *Hypericum perforatum* versus fluoxetine. *Neuropsychobiology*, 56(2–3), 132–137.

Papakostas, G.I., Iosifescu, D.V., Renshaw, P.F., *et al.* (2005b). Brain MRI white matter hyperintensities, cardiovascular risk factors, and one-carbon cycle metabolism in non-geriatric outpatients with major depressive disorder (Part II). *Psychiatry Research: Neuroimaging*, 140(3), 301–307.

Papakostas, G.I., McGrath, P.J., Stewart, J., *et al.* (2008). Psychic and somatic anxiety symptoms as predictors of response to fluoxetine in major depressive disorder. *Psychiatry Research*, 161(1), 116–120.

Papakostas, G.I., Petersen, T., Denninger, J., *et al.* (2003b). Somatic symptoms in treatment-resistant depression. *Psychiatry Research*, 118, 39–45.

Papakostas, G.I., Petersen, T., Denninger, J.W., *et al.* (2004b). Psychosocial functioning during the treatment of major depressive disorder with fluoxetine. *Journal of Clinical Psychopharmacology*, 24(5), 507–511.

Papakostas, G.I., Petersen, T., Farabaugh, A., *et al.* (2003a). Psychiatric comorbidity among responders and nonresponders to nortriptyline in treatment-resistant major depressive disorder. *Journal of Clinical Psychiatry*, 64, 1357–1361.

Papakostas, G.I., Petersen, T., Hughes, M.E., *et al.* (2003b). Functioning and interpersonal relationships as predictors of response in treatment resistant depression. *Comprehensive Psychiatry*, 44, 44–50.

Papakostas, G.I., Petersen, T., Iosifescu, D.V., *et al.* (2004b). Somatic symptoms as predictors of time to onset of response to fluoxetine in major depressive disorder. *Journal of Clinical Psychiatry*, 65, 543–546.

Papakostas, G.I., Petersen, T., Iosifescu, D.V., *et al.* (2004c). Obesity among outpatients with major depressive disorder. *International Journal of Neuropsychopharmacology*, 7, 1–5.

Papakostas, G.I., Petersen, T., Iosifescu, D.V., *et al.* (2003f). Axis III comorbidity in treatment-resistant depression. *Psychiatry Research*, 118, 183–188.

Papakostas, G.I., Petersen, T., Lebowitz, B.D., *et al.* (2005a). The relationship between serum folate, vitamin B12 and homocysteine levels in major depressive disorder and the timing of clinical improvement to fluoxetine. *International Journal of Neuropsychopharmacology*, 8(4), 523–528.

Papakostas, G.I., Petersen, T., Mahal, Y., *et al.* (2004a). Quality of life assessments in major depressive disorder: A review of the literature. *General Hospital Psychiatry*, 26, 13–17.

Papakostas, G.I., Petersen, T., Pava, J., *et al.* (2007a). Hopelessness as a predictor of non-response to fluoxetine in major depressive disorder. *Annals of Clinical Psychiatry*, 19(1), 5–8.

Papakostas, G.I., Petersen, T., Pava, J., *et al.* (2003c). Hopelessness and suicide in treatment-resistant depression: Prevalence and impact on treatment outcome. *Journal of Nervous and Mental Disease*, 191, 444–449.

Papakostas, G.I., Petersen, T., Sklarsky, K.G., *et al.* (2007b). Timing of clinical improvement and symptom resolution in the treatment of major depressive disorder. *Psychiatry Research*, 149(1–3), 195–200.

Papakostas, G.I., Petersen, T., Sonawalla, S., *et al.* (2003e). Serum cholesterol in treatment-resistant depression. *Neuropsychobiology*, 47, 146–151.

Patience, D.A., McGuire, R.J., Scott, A.I. and Freeman, C.P. (1995). The Edinburgh Primary Care Depression Study: Personality disorder and outcome. *British Journal of Psychiatry*, 167(3), 324–330.

Patten, S.B. (1999). Long-term medical conditions and major depression in the Canadian population. *Canadian Journal of Psychiatry*, 44(2), 151–157.

Paykel, E.S., Ramana, R., Cooper, Z., *et al.* (1995). Residual symptoms after partial remission: An important outcome in depression. *Psychological Medicine*, 25(6), 1171–1180.

Pedrelli, P., Feldman, G.C., Vorono, S., *et al.* (2008). Dysfunctional attitudes and perceived stress predict depressive symptoms severity following antidepressant treatment in patients with chronic depression. *Psychiatry Research*, 161(3), 302–308.

Penninx, B.W., Geerlings, S.W., Deeg, D.J., *et al.* (1999). Minor and major depression and the risk of death in older persons. *Archives of General Psychiatry*, 56(10), 889–895.

Peselow, E.D., Fieve, R.R. and DiFiglia, C. (1992). Personality traits and response to desipramine. *Journal of Affective Disorders*, 24(4), 209–216.

Petersen, T., Papakostas, G.I., Bottonari, K., *et al.* (2002). NEO-FFI factor scores as predictors of response to fluoxetine treatment in depressed outpatients. *Psychiatry Research*, 109, 9–16.

Petersen, T., Papakostas, G.I., Posternak, M.A., *et al.* (2005). Empirical testing of two models for staging antidepressant treatment resistance. *Journal of Clinical Psychopharmacology*, 25(4), 336–341.

Posternak, M.A. and Miller, I. (2001). Untreated short-term course of major depression: A meta-analysis of outcomes from studies using wait-list control groups. *Journal of Affective Disorders*, 66(2–3), 139–146.

Posternak, M.A. and Zimmerman, M. (2000). Short-term spontaneous improvement rates in depressed outpatients. *Journal of Nervous and Mental Disease*, 188(12), 799–804.

Quitkin, F.M., McGrath, P.J., Stewart, J.W., *et al.* (1990). Atypical depression, panic attacks, and response to imipramine and phenelzine. A replication. *Archives of General Psychiatry*, 47(10), 935–941.

Quitkin, F.M., Petkova, E., McGrath, P.J., *et al.* (2003). When should a trial of fluoxetine for major depression be declared failed? *American Journal of Psychiatry*, 160(4), 734–740.

Quitkin, F.M., Stewart, J.W., McGrath, P.J., *et al.* (1988). Phenelzine versus imipramine in the treatment of probable atypical depression: Defining syndrome boundaries of selective MAOI responders. *American Journal of Psychiatry*, 145(3), 306–311.

Reich, J.H. (1990). Effect of DSM-III personality disorders on outcome of tricyclic antidepressant-treated nonpsychotic outpatients with major or minor depressive disorder. *Psychiatry Research*, 32(2), 175–181.

Robinson, D.S., Kayser, A., Corcella, J., *et al.* (1985). Panic attacks in outpatients with depression: Response to antidepressant treatment. *Psychopharmacology Bulletin*, 21(3), 562–567.

Rounsaville, B.J., Weissman, M.M., Prusoff, B.A. and Herceg-Baron, R.L. (1979). Marital disputes and treatment outcome in depressed women. *Comprehensive Psychiatry*, 20(5), 483–490.

Rush, A.J., Batey, S.R., Donahue, R.M.J., *et al.* (2001b). Does pretreatment anxiety predict response to either bupropion SR or sertraline? *Journal of Affective Disorders*, 64, 81–87.

Rush, A.J., Carmody, T.J., Haight, B.R., *et al.* (2005). Does pretreatment insomnia or anxiety predict acute response to bupropion SR? *Annals of Clinical Psychiatry*, 17(1), 1–9.

Rush, A.J., Trivedi, M., Carmody, T.J., *et al.* (2004). One-year clinical outcomes of depressed public sector outpatients: A benchmark for subsequent studies. *Biological Psychiatry*, 56(1), 46–53.

Rush, A.J., Trivedi, M.H., Carmody, T.J., *et al.* (2001a). Response in relation to baseline anxiety levels in major depressive disorder treated with bupropion sustained release or sertraline. *Neuropsychopharmacology*, 25(1), 131–138.

Rush, A.J., Wisniewski, S.R., Warden, D., *et al.* (2008). Selecting among second-step antidepressant medication monotherapies: Predictive value of clinical, demographic, or first-step treatment features. *Archives of General Psychiatry*, 65(8), 870–880.

Russell, J.M., Koran, L.M., Rush, J., *et al.* (2001). Effect of concurrent anxiety on response to sertraline and imipramine in patients with chronic depression. *Depression and Anxiety*, 13(1), 18–27.

Sato, T., Hirano, S., Narita, T., *et al.* (1999). Temperament and character inventory dimensions as a predictor of response to antidepressant treatment in major depression. *Journal of Affective Disorders*, 56(2–3), 153–161.

Shea, M.T., Pilkonis, P.A., Beckham, E., *et al.* (1990). Personality disorders and treatment outcome in the NIMH Treatment of Depression Collaborative Research Program. *American Journal of Psychiatry*, 147(6), 711–718.

Silverstone, P.H. and Salinas, E. (2001). Efficacy of venlafaxine extended release in patients with major depressive disorder and comorbid generalized anxiety disorder. *Journal of Clinical Psychiatry*, 62(7), 523–529.

Simon, G.E., Heiligenstein, J.H., Grothaus, L., *et al.* (1998). Should anxiety and insomnia influence antidepressant selection: A randomized comparison of fluoxetine and imipramine. *Journal of Clinical Psychiatry*, 59(2), 49–55.

Sir, A., D'Souza, R.F., Uguz, S., *et al.* (2005). Randomized trial of sertraline versus venlafaxine XR in major depression: Efficacy and discontinuation symptoms. *Journal of Clinical Psychiatry*, 66(10), 1312–1320.

Sonawalla, S., Papakostas, G.I., Petersen, T., *et al.* (2002). Elevated cholesterol levels in major depressive disorder associated with non-response to fluoxetine treatment. *Psychosomatics*, 43, 310–316.

Stewart, A.L., Greenfield, S., Hays, R.D., *et al.* (1989). Functional status and well-being of patients with chronic conditions. Results from the Medical Outcomes Study. *Journal of the American Medical Association*, 262(7), 907–913.

Talati, A., Wickramaratne, P.J., Pilowsky, D.J., *et al.* (2007). Remission of maternal depression and child symptoms among single mothers: A STAR*D-Child report. *Social psychiatry and psychiatric epidemiology*, 42(12), 962–971.

Taylor, B.P., Bruder, G.E., Stewart, J.W., *et al.* (2006). Psychomotor slowing as a predictor of fluoxetine nonresponse in depressed outpatients. *American Journal of Psychiatry*, 163(1), 73–78.

Thase, M.E., Greenhouse, J.B., Frank, E., *et al.* (1997). Treatment of major depression with psychotherapy or psychotherapy-pharmacotherapy combinations. *Archives of General Psychiatry*, 54(11), 1009–1015.

Thase, M.E. and Rush, A.J. (1997). When at first you don't succeed: Sequential strategies for antidepressant nonresponders. *Journal of Clinical Psychiatry*, 58(Suppl 13), 23–29.

Tollefson, G.D., Holman, S.L., Sayler, M.E. and Potvin, J.H. (1994). Fluoxetine, placebo, and tricyclic antidepressants in major depression with and without anxious features. *Journal of Clinical Psychiatry*, 55(2), 50–59.

Trivedi, M.H., Morris, D.W., Pan, J.Y., *et al.* (2005). What moderator characteristics are associated with better prognosis for depression? *Neuropsychiatric Disease and Treatment*, 1(1), 51–57.

Trivedi, M.H., Rush, A.J., Wisniewski, S.R., *et al.* (2006). Evaluation of outcomes with citalopram for depression using measurement-based care in STAR*D: Implications for clinical practice. *American Journal of Psychiatry*, 163(1), 28–40.

Vallejo, J., Gasto, C., Catalan, R., *et al.* (1991). Predictors of antidepressant treatment outcome in melancholia: Psychosocial, clinical and biological indicators. *Journal of Affective Disorders*, 21(3), 151–162.

Weissman, M.M., Leaf, P.J., Holzer, C.E. 3rd., *et al.* (1984). The epidemiology of depression. An update on sex differences in rates. *Journal of Affective Disorders*, 7(3–4), 179–188.

Weissman, M.M., Prusoff, B.A., Thompson, W.D., *et al.* (1978). Social adjustment by self-report in a community sample and in psychiatric outpatients. *Journal of Nervous and Mental Disease*, 166, 317–326.

Wells, K.B., Stewart, A., Hays, R.D., *et al.* (1989). Greenfield, S. and Ware, J.: The functioning and well-being of depressed patients. Results from the Medical Outcomes Study. *Journal of the American Medical Association*, 262(7), 914–919.

Wells, K.B., Strom, R., Sherbourne, C.D. and Meredith, L.S. (1996). Caring for depression: A RAND study. Cambridge: Harvard University Press.

Whisman, M.A. (1999). Marital dissatisfaction and psychiatric disorders: Results from the National Comorbidity Survey. *Journal of Abnormal Psychology*, 108(4), 701–706.

Worthington, J., Fava, M., Agustin, C., *et al.* (1996). Consumption of alcohol, nicotine, and caffeine among depressed outpatients. Relationship with response to treatment. *Psychosomatics*, 37(6), 518–522.

Young, E.A., Kornstein, S.G., Marcus, S.M., *et al.* (2009). Sex differences in response to citalopram: A STAR *D report. *Journal of Psychiatric Research*, 43(5), 503–511.

Zheng, D., Macera, C.A., Croft, J.B., *et al.* (1997). Major depression and all-cause mortality among white adults in the United States. *Annals of Epidemiology*, 7(3), 213–218.

Zlotnick, C., Kohn, R., Keitner, G. and Sella Grotta, S.A. (2000). The relationship between quality of interpersonal relationships and major depressive disorder: Findings from the National Comorbidity Survey. *Journal of Affective Disorders*, 59(3), 205–215.

Zuckerman, D.M., Prusoff, B.A., Weissman, M.M. and Padian, N.S. (1980). Personality as a predictor of psychotherapy and pharmacotherapy outcome for depressed outpatients. *Journal of Consulting and Clinical Psychology*, 48(6), 730–735.

Chapter 2

Abdelmalik, N., Ruhé, H.G., Barwari, K., *et al.* (2008). Effect of the selective serotonin reuptake inhibitor paroxetine on platelet function is modified by a SLC6A4 serotonin transporter polymorphism. *Journal of Thrombosis and Haemostaesis*, 6(12), 2168–2174.

Abdelrahman, N., Kleinman, Y., Rund, D. and Da'as, N. (2003). Hyponatremia associated with the initiation of reboxetine therapy. *European Journal of Clinical Pharmacology*, 59(2), 177.

Adler, L.A. and Angrist, B.M. (1995). Paroxetine and akathisia. *Biological Psychiatry*, 37(5), 336–337.

Addis, A. and Koren, G. (2000). Safety of fluoxetine during the first trimester of pregnancy: A meta-analytical review of epidemiological studies. *Psychological Medicine*, 30(1), 89–94.

Agrawal, N.K., Rastogi, A., Goyal, R. and Singh, S.K. (2007). Sertraline-induced hyponatremia in the elderly. *Canadian Journal of Emergency Medical Care*, 9(6), 415.

Ahmed, R. and Eagleton, C. (2008). Toxic epidermal necrolysis after paroxetine treatment. *New Zealand Medical Journal*, 121(1274), 86–89.

Alderman, C.P., Seshadri, P. and Ben-Tovim, D.I. (1996). Effects of serotonin reuptake inhibitors on hemostasis. *Annals of Pharmacotherapy*, 30(11), 1232–1234.

Alevizos, B., Christodoulou, G.N., Ioannidis, C., *et al.* (1989). The efficacy of amineptine in the treatment of depressive patients with irritable bowel syndrome. *Clinical Neuropharmacology*, 12(Suppl 2), S66–76.

Allgulander, C., Florea, I. and Huusom, A.K. (2006). Prevention of relapse in generalized anxiety disorder by escitalopram treatment.*International Journal of Neuropsychopharmacology*, 9(5), 495–505.

Alper, K., Schwartz, K.A., Kolts, R.L. and Khan, A. (2007). Seizure incidence in psychopharmacological clinical trials: An analysis of Food and Drug Administration (FDA) summary basis of approval reports. *Biological Psychiatry*, 62(4), 345–354.

Alpert, J.E., Franznick, D.A., Hollander, S.B. and Fava, M. (2004). Gepirone extended-release treatment of anxious depression: Evidence from a retrospective subgroup analysis in patients with major depressive disorder. *Journal of Clinical Psychiatry*, 65(8), 1069–1075.

Almeida, O.P., Waterreus, A. and Hankey, G.J. (2006). Preventing depression after Stroke: Results from a randomized placebo-controlled trial. *Journal of Clinical Psychiatry*, 67(7), 1104–1109.

Altshuler, L.L., Pierre, J.M., Wirshing, W.C. and Ames, D. (1994). Sertraline and akathisia. *Journal of Clinical Psychopharmacology*, 14(4), 278–279.

Alwan, S., Reefhuis, J., Rasmussen, S.A., *et al.* (2007). National Birth Defects Prevention Study. Use of selective serotonin-reuptake inhibitors in pregnancy and the risk of birth defects. *New England Journal of Medicine*, 356(26), 2684–2792.

Amore, M., Jori, M.C. and AMISERT Investigators. (2001). Faster response on amisulpride 50 mg versus sertraline 50–100 mg in patients with dysthymia or double depression: A randomized, double-blind, parallel group study. *International Clinical Psychopharmacology*, 16(6), 317–324.

Amsterdam, J.D., Brunswick, D.J. and Hundert, M. (2002). A single-site, double-blind, placebo-controlled, dose-ranging study of YKP10A — a putative, new antidepressant. *Prog Neuropsychopharmacol Biological Psychiatry*, 26(7–8), 1333–1338.

Amsterdam, J.D., Garcia-Espana, F., Goodman, D., *et al.* (1997). Breast enlargement during chronic antidepressant therapy. *Journal of Affective Disorders*, 46(2), 151–156.

Amsterdam, J.D. and Shults, J. (2005). Comparison of fluoxetine, olanzapine, and combined fluoxetine plus olanzapine initial therapy of bipolar type I and type II major depression — lack of manic induction. *Journal of Affective Disorders*, 87(1), 121–130.

Anbu, A.T. and Theodore, A. (2006). Fluoxetine withdrawal syndrome in the newborn. *Indian Pediatrics*, 43(1), 66–69.

Andersen, G., Vestergaard, K. and Lauritzen, L. (1994). Effective treatment of post*Stroke* depression with the selective serotonin reuptake inhibitor citalopram. *Stroke*, 25(6), 1099–1104.

Anderson, I.M. (2001). Meta-analytical studies on new antidepressants. *British Medical Bulletin*, 57, 161–178.

Andrade, S.E., McPhillips, H., Loren, D., *et al.* (2009). Antidepressant medication use and risk of persistent pulmonary hypertension of the newborn. *Pharmacoepidemiology and Drug Safety*, 18(3), 246–252.

Andree, B., Thorberg, S.O., Halldin, C. and Farde, L. (1999). Pindolol binding to 5-HT1A receptors in the human brain confirmed with positron emission tomography. *Psychopharmacology*, 144(3), 303–305.

Andreoli, V., Caillard, V., Deo, R.S., *et al.* (2002). Reboxetine, a new noradrenaline selective antidepressant, is at least as effective as fluoxetine in the treatment of depression. *Journal of Clinical Psychopharmacology*, 22(4), 393–399.

Anisman, H., Ravindran, A.V., Griffiths, J. and Merali, Z. (1999). Interleukin-1 beta production in dysthymia before and after Pharmacotherapy. *Biological Psychiatry*, 46(12), 1649–1655.

Appleby, L., Warner, R., Whitton, A. and Faragher, B. (1997). A controlled study of fluoxetine and cognitive-behavioural counselling in the treatment of postnatal depression. *British Medical Journal*, 314(7085), 932–936.

Apseloff, G., Wilner, K.D., Gerber, N. and Tremaine, L.M. (1997). Effect of sertraline on protein binding of warfarin. *Clinical Pharmacokinetics*, 32(Suppl 1), 37–42.

Apter, A., Lipschitz, A., Fong, R., *et al.* (2006). Evaluation of suicidal thoughts and behaviors in children and adolescents taking paroxetine. *Journal of Child and Adolescent Psychopharmacology*, 16(1–2), 77–90.

Argelyan, M., Szabo, Z., Keri, S., *et al.* (2006). The activity of dopamine transporter in depression and the effects of sertraline. *European Neuropsychopharmacology*, 16(s4), 313.

Arinzon, Z.H., Lehman, Y.A., Fidelman, Z.G. and Krasnyansky, I.I. (2002). Delayed recurrent SIADH associated with SSRIs. *Annals of Pharmacotherapy*, 36(7–8), 1175–1177.

Armitage, R. (2000). The effects of antidepressants on sleep in patients with depression. *Canadian Journal of Psychiatry*, 45(9), 803–809.

Arnold, L.M., Hess, E.V., Hudson, J.I., *et al.* (2002). A randomized, placebo-controlled, double-blind, flexible-dose study of fluoxetine in the treatment of women with fibromyalgia. *American Journal of Medicine*, 112(3), 191–197.

Arnold, L.M., McElroy, S.L., Hudson, J.I., *et al.* (2002). A placebo-controlled, randomized trial of fluoxetine in the treatment of binge-eating disorder. *Journal of Clinical Psychiatry*, 63(11), 1028–1033.

Aronson, M.D. and Hafez, H. (1986). A case of trazodone-induced ventricular tachycardia. *Journal of Clinical Psychiatry*, 47(7), 388–399.

Arya, D.K. and Taylor, W.S. (1995). Lactation associated with fluoxetine treatment. *Australian and New Zealand Journal of Psychiatry*, 29(4), 697.

Askinazi, C., Weintraub, R.J. and Karamouz, N. (1986). Elderly depressed females as a possible subgroup of patients responsive to methylphenidate. *Journal of Clinical Psychiatry*, 47(9), 467–469.

Astier, B., Lambas Senas, L., Souliere, F., *et al.* (2003). *In vivo* comparison of two 5-HT1A receptors agonists alnespirone (S-20499) and buspirone on locus coeruleus neuronal activity. *European Journal of Pharmacology*, 459(1), 17–26.

Aström-Lilja, C., Odeberg, J.M., Ekman, E. and Hägg, S. (2008). Drug-induced torsades de pointes: A review of the Swedish pharmacovigilance database. *Pharmacoepidemiology and Drug Safety*, 17(6), 587–592.

Atar, D., Malinin, A., Pokov, A., *et al.* (2007). Antiplatelet properties of escitalopram in patients with the metabolic syndrome: A dose-ranging *in vitro* study. *Neuropsychopharmacology*, 32(11), 2369–2374.

Atar, D., Malinin, A., Takserman, A., *et al.* (2006). Escitalopram, but not its major metabolites, exhibits antiplatelet activity in humans. *Journal of Clinical Psychopharmacology*, 26(2), 172–177.

Avila, A., Cardona, X., Martin-Baranera, M., *et al.* (2003). Does nefazodone improve both depression and Parkinson disease? A pilot randomized trial. *Journal of Clinical Psychopharmacology*, 23(5), 509–513.

Ayonrinde, O.T., Reutens, S.G. and Sanfilippo, F.M. (1995). Paroxetine-induced SIADH. *Medical Journal of Australia*, 163(7), 390.

Bahl, S., Cotterchio, M., Kreiger, N. and Klar, N. (2004). Antidepressant medication use and non-Hodgkin's lymphoma risk: No association. *American Journal of Epidemiology*, 160(6), 566–575.

Bailey, D.L. and Le Melledo, J.M. (2003). Effects of selective serotonin reuptake inhibitors on cholesterol levels in patients with panic disorder. *Journal of Clinical Psychopharmacology*, 23(3), 317–319.

Bak, S., Tsiropoulos, I., Kjaersgaard, J.O., *et al.* (2002). Selective serotonin reuptake inhibitors and the risk of stroke: A population-based case-control study. *Stroke*, 33(6), 1465–1473.

Baker, G.B. and Prior, T.I. (2002). Stereochemistry and drug efficacy and development: Relevance of chirality to antidepressant and antipsychotic drugs. *Annals of Medicine*, 34(7–8), 537–543.

Bakish, D., Ravindran, A., Hooper, C. and Lapierre, Y. (1994). Psychopharmacological treatment response of patients with a DSM-III diagnosis of dysthymic disorder. *Psychopharmacology Bulletin*, 30(1), 53–59.

Bakker, A., van Balkom, A.J. and van Dyck, R. (2000). Selective serotonin reuptake inhibitors in the treatment of panic disorder and agoraphobia. *International Clinical Psychopharmacology*, 15(Suppl 2), S25–30.

Baldwin, D.S., Cooper, J.A., Huusom, A.K. and Hindmarch, I. (2006). A double-blind, randomized, parallel-group, flexible-dose study to evaluate the tolerability, efficacy and effects of treatment discontinuation with escitalopram and paroxetine in patients with major depressive disorder. *International Clinical Psychopharmacology*, 21(3), 159–169.

Balestrieri, G., Cerudelli, B., Ciaccio, S. and Rizzoni, D. (1992). Hyponatraemia and seizure due to overdose of trazodone. *British Medical Journal*, 304(6828), 686.

Baliga, R.R. and McHardy, K.C. (1993). Syndrome of inappropriate antidiuretic hormone secretion due to fluvoxamine therapy. *British Journal of Clinical Practice*, 47(2), 62–63.

Ball, C.J. (1993). Fluvoxamine and SIADH. *British Journal of Clinical Practice*, 47(4), 227.

Bandelow, B., Andersen, H.F. and Dolberg, O.T. (2007). Escitalopram in the treatment of anxiety symptoms associated with depression. *Depression and Anxiety*, 24(1), 53–61.

Bangs, M.E., Emslie, G.J., Spencer, T.J., *et al.* (2007). Efficacy and safety of atomoxetine in adolescents with attention-deficit/hyperactivity disorder and major depression. *Journal of Child and Adolescent Psychopharmacology*, 17(4), 407–420.

Barclay, T.S. and Lee, A.J. (2002). Citalopram-associated SIADH. *Annals of Pharmacotherapy*, 36(10), 1558–1563.

Bardin, E.D. and Krieger, J.N. (1990). Pharmacological priapism: Comparison of trazodone- and papaverine-associated cases. *International Urology and Nephrology*, 22(2), 147–152.

Bauer, M., Hellweg, R. and Baumgartner, A. (1996). Fluoxetine-induced akathisia does not reappear after switch to paroxetine. *Journal of Clinical Psychiatry*, 57(12), 593–594.

Beasley, C.M. Jr., Ball, S.G., Nilsson, M.E., *et al.* (2007). Fluoxetine and adult suicidality revisited: An updated meta-analysis using expanded data sources from placebo-controlled trials. *Journal of Clinical Psychopharmacology*, 27(6), 682–686.

Beasley, C.M. Jr., Dornseif, B.E., Bosomworth, J.C., *et al.* (1991a). Fluoxetine and suicide: A meta-analysis of controlled trials of treatment for depression. *British Medical Journal*, 303(6804), 685–692.

Beasley, C.M. Jr., Dornseif, B.E., Pultz, J.A., *et al.* (1991b). Fluoxetine versus trazodone: Efficacy and activating-sedating effects. *Journal of Clinical Psychiatry*, 52(7), 294–299.

Beasley, C.M. Jr., Masica, D.N., Heiligenstein, J.H., *et al.* (1993). Possible monoamine oxidase inhibitor-serotonin uptake inhibitor interaction: Fluoxetine clinical data and preclinical findings. *Journal of Clinical Psychopharmacology*, 13(5), 312–320.

Beckmann, H., Athen, D., Olteanu, M. and Zimmer, R. (1979). DL-phenylalanine versus imipramine: A double-blind controlled study. *Archiv für Psychiatrie und Nervenkrankheiten*, 227, 49–58.

Benazzi, F. (1998). Nefazodone withdrawal symptoms. *Canadian Journal of Psychiatry*, 43(2), 194–195.

Bengtsson, B.O., Wiholm, B.E., Myrhed, M. and Walinder, J. (1994). Adverse experiences during treatment with zimeldine on special licence in Sweden. *International Clinical Psychopharmacology*, 9(1), 55–61.

Berard, A., Ramos, E., Rey, E., *et al.* (2007). First trimester exposure to paroxetine and risk of cardiac malformations in infants: The importance of dosage. Birth Defects Research Part B. *Developmental and Reproductive Toxicology*, 80(1), 18–27.

Berk, M., Jacobson, B.F. and Hurly, E. (1995). Fluoxetine and hemostatic function: A pilot study. *Journal of Clinical Psychiatry*, 56(1), 14–16.

Berle, J.O., Steen, V.M., Aamo, T.O., *et al.* (2004). Breastfeeding during maternal antidepressant treatment with serotonin reuptake inhibitors: Infant exposure, clinical symptoms, and cytochrome p450 genotypes. *Journal of Clinical Psychiatry*, 65(9), 1228–1234.

Berry, R.B., Yamaura, E.M., Gill, K. and Reist, C. (1999). Acute effects of paroxetine on genioglossus activity in obstructive sleep apnea. *Sleep*, 22(8), 1087–1092.

Bersani, G., Pozzi, F., Marini, S., *et al.* (1991). 5-HT2 receptor antagonism in dysthymic disorder: A double-blind placebo-controlled study with ritanserin. *Acta Psychiatrica Scandinavica*, 83(4), 244–248.

Bertschy, G. and Vandel, S. (1993). Fluoxetine-related indifference and akathisia. A case report. *Therapie*, 48(2), 158–159.

Bhagwagar, Z., Wylezinska, M., Taylor, M., *et al.* (2004). Increased brain GABA concentrations following acute administration of a selective serotonin reuptake inhibitor. *American Journal of Psychiatry*, 161(2), 368–370.

Bhakta, S.G. and Andrade, C. (in press). Melatonin treatment of shoulder and-neck dyskinesia possibly related to fluoxetine treatment. *World Journal of Biological Psychiatry.*

Bielski, R.J., Cunningham, L., Horrigan, J.P., *et al.* (2008). Gepirone extended-release in the treatment of adult outpatients with major depressive disorder: A double-blind, randomized, placebo-controlled, parallel-group study. *Journal of Clinical Psychiatry*, 69(4), 571–577.

Birdsall, T.C. (1998). 5-Hydroxytryptophan: A clinically-effective serotonin precursor. *Alternative Medicine Review*, 3(4), 271–280.

Black, B. and Uhde, T.W. (1992). Acute dystonia and fluoxetine. *Journal of Clinical Psychiatry*, 53(9), 327.

Blanco, C., Schneier, F.R., Schmidt, A., *et al.* (2003). Pharmacological treatment of social anxiety disorder: A meta-analysis. *Depression and Anxiety*, 18(1), 29–40.

Blier, P. and Ward, N.M. (2003). Is there a role for 5-HT1A agonists in the treatment of depression? *Biological Psychiatry*, 53(3), 193–203.

Blouin, A.G., Blouin, J.H., Perez, E.L., *et al.* (1988). Treatment of bulimia with fenfluramine and desipramine. *Journal of Clinical Psychopharmacology*, 8(4), 261–269.

Blumenfield, M., Levy, N.B., Spinowitz, B., *et al.* (1997). Fluoxetine in depressed patients on dialysis. *International Journal of Psychiatry in Medicine*, 27(1), 71–80.

Boffa, E. and Lofchy, J. (2000). Paroxetine and tardive akathisia. *Canadian Journal of Psychiatry*, 45(4), 398.

Bogetto, F., Bellino, S., Revello, R.B. and Patria, L. (2002). Discontinuation syndrome in dysthymic patients treated with selective serotonin reuptake inhibitors: A clinical investigation. *CNS Drugs*, 16(4), 273–283.

Bolden-Watson, C. and Richelson, E. (1993). Blockade by newly-developed antidepressants of biogenic amine uptake into rat brain synaptosomes. *Life Sciences*, 52(12), 1023–1029.

Bolo, N.R., Hode, Y., Nedelec, J.F., *et al.* (2000). Brain pharmacokinetics and tissue distribution *in vivo* of fluvoxamine and fluoxetine by fluorine magnetic resonance spectroscopy. *Neuropsychopharmacology*, 23(4), 428–438.

Bondi, M., Menozzi, M., Bertolini, M.G., *et al.* (2000). Metabolic effects of fluoxetine in obese menopausal women. *Journal of Endocrinological Investigation*, 23, 280–286.

Bonierbale, M., Lancon, C. and Tignol, J. (2003). The ELIXIR study: Evaluation of sexual dysfunction in 4557 depressed patients in France. *Current Medical Research and Opinion*, 19(2), 114–124.

Bonin, B., Vandel, P., Sechter, D. and Bizouard, P. (1997). Paroxetine and galactorrhea. *Pharmacopsychiatry*, 30(4), 133–134.

Bonin, B., Vandel, P. and Vandel, S. (1994). Fluvoxamine and galactorrhea. A case report. *Therapie*, 49(2), 149–151.

Boral, G.C. and Shah, L.P. (1989). The beneficial effects of amineptine (Survector 100) in the treatment of depression: Preliminary results of an Indian multicenter trial. *Clinical Neuropharmacology*, 12(Suppl 2), S51–57.

Bornstein, S. (1979). Cross-over trial comparing the antidepressant effects of amineptine and maprotiline. *Current Medical Research and Opinion*, 6(2), 107–110.

Bosch, X. and Vera, M. (1998). Aplastic anaemia during treatment with fluoxetine. *The Lancet*, 351(9108), 1031.

Bostwick, J.M. and Jaffee, M.S. (1999). Buspirone as an antidote to SSRI-induced bruxism in 4 cases. *Journal of Clinical Psychiatry*, 60(12), 857–860.

Boucher, N., Bairam, A. and Beaulac-Baillargeon, L. (2008). A new look at the neonate's clinical presentation after in utero exposure to antidepressants in late pregnancy. *Journal of Clinical Psychopharmacology*, 28(3), 334–339.

Bouras, N. and Bridges, P. (1982). Bromocriptine in depression. *Current Medical Research and Opinion* 1982; 8, 150–153.

Bouman, W.P., Pinner, G. and Johnson, H. (1998). Incidence of selective serotonin reuptake inhibitor (SSRI) induced hyponatraemia due to the syndrome of inappropriate antidiuretic hormone (SIADH) secretion in the elderly. *International Journal of Geriatric Psychiatry*, 13(1), 12–15.

Bourgeois, J.A., Babine, S.E. and Bahadur, N. (2002). A case of SIADH and hyponatremia associated with citalopram. *Psychosomatics*, 43(3), 241–242.

Boyer, P., Lecrubier, Y., Stalla-Bourdillon, A. and Fleurot, O. (1999). Amisulpride versus amineptine and placebo for the treatment of dysthymia. *Neuropsychobiology*, 39(1), 25–32.

Braitberg, G. and Curry, S.C. (1995). Seizure after isolated fluoxetine overdose. *Annals of Emergency Medicine*, 26(2), 234–237.

Breitbart, W., Rosenfeld, B., Kaim, M. and Funesti-Esch, J. (2001). A randomized, double-blind, placebo-controlled trial of psychostimulants for the treatment of fatigue in ambulatory patients with human immunodeficiency virus disease. *Archives of Internal Medicine*, 161(3), 411–420.

Brennan, D., MacManus, M., Howe, J. and McLoughlin. (1988). Neuroleptic malignant syndrome' without neuroleptics. *British Journal of Psychiatry*, 152, 578–579.

Brewster, U.C., Ciampi, M.A., Abu-Alfa, A.K. and Perazella, M.A. (2003). Addition of sertraline to other therapies to reduce dialysis-associated hypotension. *Nephrology (Carlton)*, 8(6), 296–301.

Bridge, J.A., Iyengar, S., Salary, C.B., *et al.* (2007). Clinical response and risk for reported suicidal ideation and suicide attempts in pediatric antidepressant treatment: A meta-analysis of randomized controlled trials. *Journal of the American Medical Association*, 297(15), 1683–1696.

Brodie-Meijer, C.C., Diemont, W.L. and Buijs, P.J. (1999). Nefazodone-induced clitoral priapism. *International Clinical Psychopharmacology*, 14(4), 257–258.

Bronzo, M.R. and Stahl, S.M. (1993). Galactorrhea induced by sertraline. *American Journal of Psychiatry*, 150(8), 1269–1270.

Bross, R. and Hoffer, L.J. (1995). Fluoxetine increases resting energy expenditure and basal body temperature in humans. *American Journal of Clinical Nutrition*, 61(5), 1020–1025.

Brown, E.S., Vigil, L., Khan, D.A., *et al.* (2005). A randomized trial of citalopram versus placebo in outpatients with asthma and major depressive disorder: A proof of concept study. *Biological Psychiatry*, 58(11), 865–870.

Brunswick, D.J., Amsterdam, J.D., Fawcett, J., *et al.* (2000). Fluoxetine and norfluoxetine plasma concentrations during relapse prevention treatment. Presented at the 40th Annual Meeting of the New Clinical Drug Evaluation Unit of the National Institute of Mental Health, Boca Raton, Florida.

Brzezinski, A.A., Wurtman, J.J., Wurtman, R.J., *et al.* (1990). d-Fenfluramine suppresses the increased calorie and carbohydrate intakes and improves the mood of women with premenstrual depression. *Obstetrics and Gynecology*, 76(2), 296–301.

Bull, S.A., Hunkeler, E.M., Lee, J.Y., *et al.* (2002). Discontinuing or switching selective serotonin-reuptake inhibitors. *Annals of Pharmacotherapy*, 36(4), 578–584.

Burke, D. and Fanker, S. (1996a). Fluoxetine and the syndrome of inappropriate secretion of antidiuretic hormone (SIADH) *Australian and New Zealand Journal of Psychiatry*, 30(2), 295–298.

Burke, D. and Franker, S. (1996b). Fluoxetine-induced SIADH: Most likely in the elderly? *Australian and New Zealand Journal of Psychiatry*, 30(2), 299–301.

Calabrese, J.R., Guelfi, J.D., Perdrizet-Chevallier, C. and Agomelatine Bipolar Study Group. (2007). Agomelatine adjunctive therapy for acute bipolar depression: Preliminary open data. *Bipolar Disorder*, 9(6), 628–535.

Calhoun, J.W. and Calhoun, D.D. (1996). Prolonged bleeding time in a patient treated with sertraline. *American Journal of Psychiatry*, 153(3), 443.

Capuron, L., Gumnick, J.F., Musselman, D.L., *et al.* (2002). Neurobehavioral effects of interferon-alpha in cancer patients: Phenomenology and paroxetine responsiveness of symptom dimensions. *Neuropsychopharmacology*, 26(5), 643–652.

Capuron, L., Neurauter, G., Musselman, D.L., *et al.* (2003). Interferon-alpha-induced changes in tryptophan metabolism: Relationship to depression and paroxetine treatment. *Biological Psychiatry*, 54(9), 906–914.

Caracci, G. and Decina, P. (1991). Fluoxetine and Prolonged Seizure. *Convulsive Therapy*, 7(2), 145–147.

Cardenas, L., Houle, S., Kapur, S. and Busto, U.E. (2004). Oral D-amphetamine causes prolonged displacement of [11C]raclopride as measured by PET. *Synapse*, 51(1), 27–31.

Carvajal, G.P., Garcia, D., Sanchez, S.A., *et al.* (2002). Hepatotoxicity associated with the new antidepressants. *Journal of Clinical Psychiatry*, 63(2), 135–137.

Carvalhal, A.S., de Abreu, P.B., Spode, A., *et al.* (2003). An open trial of reboxetine in HIV-seropositive outpatients with major depressive disorder. *Journal of Clinical Psychiatry*, 64(4), 421–424.

Casis, O. and Sanchez-Chapula, J.A. (1998). Mechanism of block of cardiac transient outward K+ current (I(to)) by antidepressant drugs. *Journal of Cardiovascular Pharmacology*, 32(4), 527–534.

Cassano, G.B., Jori, M.C. and AMIMAJOR Group. (2002). Efficacy and safety of amisulpride 50 mg versus paroxetine 20 mg in major depression: A randomized, double-blind, parallel group study. *International Clinical Psychopharmacology*, 17(1), 27–32.

Catalano, G., Catalano, M.C., Epstein, M.A. and Tsambiras, P.E. (2001). QTc interval prolongation associated with citalopram overdose: A case report and literature review. *Clinical Neuropharmacology*, 24(3), 158–162.

Cavanagh, J., Patterson, J., Pimlott, S., *et al.* (2006). Serotonin transporter residual availability during long-term antidepressant therapy does not differentiate responder and nonresponder unipolar patients. *Biological Psychiatry*, 59(4), 301–308.

Cazzullo, C.L., Bessone, E., Bertrando, P., *et al.* (1998). Treatment of depression in HIV-infected patients. *Journal of Psychiatry and Neuroscience*, 23(5), 293–297.

Ceravolo, R., Nuti, A., Piccinni, A., *et al.* (2000). Paroxetine in Parkinsons disease: Effects on motor and depressive symptoms. *Neurology*, 55(8), 1216–1218.

Chambers, C.D., Anderson, P.O., Thomas, R.G., *et al.* (1999). Weight gain in infants breastfed by mothers who take fluoxetine. *Pediatrics*, 104(5), e61.

Chambers, C.D., Hernandez-Diaz, S., Van Marter, L.J., *et al.* (2006). Selective serotonin-reuptake inhibitors and risk of persistent pulmonary hypertension of the newborn. *New England Journal of Medicine*, 354(6), 579–587.

Chambers, C.D., Johnson, K.A., Dick, L.M., *et al.* (1996). Birth outcomes in pregnant women taking fluoxetine. *New England Journal of Medicine*, 335(14), 1010–1015.

Charbonnier, J.F., Reboul, P., Rougier, M., *et al.* (1987). Citalopram. An open study of a highly selective serotonin-uptake inhibitor administered by infusion to depressive patients. *Encephale*, 13(4), 249–254.

Charlier, C., Broly, F., Lhermitte, M., *et al.* (2003) Polymorphisms in the CYP 2D6 Gene: Association with plasma concentrations of fluoxetine and paroxetine.*Therapeutic Drug Monitoring*, 25(6), 738–742.

Chelben, J., Strous, R.D., Lustig, M. and Baruch, Y. (2001). Remission of SSRI-induced akathisia after switch to nefazodone. *Journal of Clinical Psychiatry*, 62(7), 570–571.

Chiasson, L., Law, D.C.W., Leiter, L.A., *et al.* (1989). Fluoxetine has potential in obese NIDDM-multicentre Canadian trial. *Diabetes*, 38, 154A.

Chien, C., Li, C.I., Heckbert, S.R., *et al.* (2006). Antidepressant use and breast cancer risk. *Breast Cancer Research and Treatment*, 95(2), 131–140.

Childs, P.A., Rodin, I., Martin, N.J., *et al.* (1995). Effect of fluoxetine on melatonin in patients with seasonal affective disorder and matched controls. *British Journal of Psychiatry*, 166(2), 196–198.

Chin, C.K., Roe, C.J. and Thomas, G.W. (1996). Fluoxetine: A treatment option for severe symptomatic postural hypotension in a diabetic haemodialysis patient. *Australian and New Zealand Journal of Medicine*, 26(5), 714.

Choi, B.H., Choi, J.S., Yoon, S.H., *et al.* (2001). Effects of norfluoxetine, the major metabolite of fluoxetine, on the cloned neuronal potassium channel Kv3.1. *Neuropharmacology*, 41(4), 443–453.

Choi, J.S., Hahn, S.J., Rhie, D.J., *et al.* (1999). Mechanism of fluoxetine block of cloned voltage-activated potassium channel Kv1.3. *Journal of Pharmacology and Experimental Therapeutics*, 291(1), 1–6.

Choi-Kwon, S., Han, S.W., Kwon, S.U., *et al.* (2006). Fluoxetine treatment in poststroke depression, emotional incontinence, and anger proneness: A double-blind, placebo-controlled study. *Stroke*, 37(1), 156–161.

Chong, S.A. (1995). Fluvoxamine and mandibular dystonia. *Canadian Journal of Psychiatry*, 40(7), 430–431.

Chong, S.A. and Tan, C.H. (1996). Fluvoxamine and akathisia. *Journal of Clinical Psychopharmacology*, 16(4), 334–335.

Chouinard, G., Annable, L. and Bradwejn, J. (1984). An early phase II clinical trial of tomoxetine (LY139603) in the treatment of newly admitted depressed patients. *Psychopharmacology*, 83(1), 126–128.

Chung, K.J., Wang, Y.C., Liu, B.M. and Supernaw, R.B. (2008). Management of ventricular dysrhythmia secondary to trazodone overdose. *Journal of Emergency Medicine*, 35(2), 171–174.

Claire, R.J., Servis, M.E. and Cram, D.L. Jr. (1991). Potential interaction between warfarin sodium and fluoxetine. *American Journal of Psychiatry*, 148(11), 1604.

Clayton, A.H., Pradko, J.F., Croft, H.A., *et al.* (2002). Prevalence of sexual dysfunction among newer antidepressants. *Journal of Clinical Psychiatry*, 63(4), 357–366.

Clayton, A.H., Zajecka, J., Ferguson, J.M., *et al.* (2003). Lack of sexual dysfunction with the selective noradrenaline reuptake inhibitor reboxetine during treatment for major depressive disorder. *International Clinical Psychopharmacology*, 18(3), 151–156.

Cohn, J.B., Collins, G., Ashbrook, E. and Wernicke, J.F. (1989). A comparison of fluoxetine imipramine and placebo in patients with bipolar depressive disorder. *International Clinical Psychopharmacology*, 4(4), 313–322.

Cole, J.A., Ephross, S.A., Cosmatos, I.S. and Walker, A.M. (2007). Paroxetine in the first trimester and the prevalence of congenital malformations. *Pharmacoepidemiology and Drug Safety*, 16(10),1075–1085.

Condon, J. (2003). Serotonergic symptoms in neonates exposed to SSRIs during pregnancy. *Australian and New Zealand Journal of Psychiatry*, 37(6), 777–778.

Connor, D.F., Fletcher, K.E. and Swanson, J.M. (1999). A meta-analysis of clonidine for symptoms of attention-deficit hyperactivity disorder. *Journal of the American Academy of Child and Adolescent Psychiatry*, 38(12), 1551–1559.

Coogan, P.F., Palmer, J.R., Strom, B.L. and Rosenberg, L. (2005). Use of selective serotonin reuptake inhibitors and the risk of breast cancer. *American Journal of Epidemiology*, 162(9), 835–838.

Coogan, P.F., Rosenberg, L., Palmer, J.R., *et al.* (2000). Risk of ovarian cancer according to use of antidepressants, phenothiazines, and benzodiazepines (United States). *Cancer Causes & Control*, 11(9), 839–845.

Coogan, P.F., Strom, B.L. and Rosenberg, L. (2009). SSRI use and breast cancer risk by hormone receptor status. *Breast Cancer Research and Treatment* 23(3), 216–128.

Cornelius, J.R., Salloum, I.M., Ehler, J.G., *et al.* (1997). Fluoxetine in depressed alcoholics. A double-blind, placebo-controlled trial. *Archives of General Psychiatry*, 4(8), 700–705.

Corrigan, M.H., Denahan, A.Q., Wright, C.E., *et al.* (2000). Comparison of pramipexole, fluoxetine, and placebo in patients with major depression. *Depression and Anxiety*, 11(2), 58–65.

Costa e Silva, J.A., Ruschel, S.I., Caetano, D., *et al.* (1997). Placebo-controlled study of tianeptine in major depressive episodes. *Neuropsychobiology*, 35(1), 24–29.

Costei, A.M., Kozer, E., Ho, T., *et al.* (2002). Perinatal outcome following third trimester exposure to paroxetine. *Archives of Pediatric and Adolescent Medicine*, 156(11), 1129–1132.

Cotterchio, M., Kreiger, N., Darlington, G. and Steingart, A. (2000). Antidepressant medication use and breast cancer risk. *American Journal of Epidemiology*, 151(10), 951–957.

Cowen, P.J. and Sargent, P.A. (1997). Changes in plasma prolactin during SSRI treatment: Evidence for a delayed increase in 5-HT neurotransmission. *Journal of Psychopharmacology*, 11(4), 345–348.

Currier, M.B., Molina, G. and Kato, M. (2004). Citalopram treatment of major depressive disorder in hispanic HIV and AIDS patients: A prospective study. *Psychosomatics*, 45(3), 210–216.

Cyr, M. and Brown, C.S. (1996). Nefazodone: Its place among antidepressants. *Annals of Pharmacotherapy*, 30(9), 1006–1012.

Czlonkowska, A.I., Zienowicz, M., Bidzinski, A., *et al.* (2003). The role of neurosteroids in the anxiolytic, antidepressive and anticonvulsive effects of selective serotonin reuptake inhibitors. *Medical Science Monitor*, 9(11), RA270–275.

Dahl, M.L., Olhager, E. and Ahlner, J. (1997). Paroxetine withdrawal syndrome in a neonate. *British Journal of Psychiatry*, 171, 391–392.

Dalery, J., Rochat, C., Peyron, E. and Bernard, G. (1997). The efficacy and acceptability of amineptine versus fluoxetine in major depression. *International Clinical Psychopharmacology*, 12(Suppl 3), S35–38.

Dalton, S.O., Johansen, C., Mellemkjaer, L., *et al.* (2003). Use of selective serotonin reuptake inhibitors and risk of upper gastrointestinal tract bleeding: A population-based cohort study. *Archives of Internal Medicine*, 163(1), 59–64.

Dattilo, P.B. and Nordin, C. (2007). Prolonged QT associated with an overdose of trazodone. *Journal of Clinical Psychiatry*, 68(8), 1309–1310.

Dave, M. (1994). Fluoxetine-associated dystonia. *American Journal of Psychiatry*, 151(1), 149.

Davenport, E. and Velamoor, R. (2002). A case of paroxetine-induced galactorrhea. *Canadian Journal of Psychiatry*, 47(9), 890–891.

Davidson, J., Pearlstein, T., Londborg, P., *et al.* (2001). Efficacy of sertraline in preventing relapse of posttraumatic stress disorder: Results of a 28-week double-blind, placebo-controlled study. *American Journal of Psychiatry*, 158(12), 1974–1981.

Davidson, J.R., Connor, K.M., Hertzberg, M.A., *et al.* (2005). Maintenance therapy with fluoxetine in posttraumatic stress disorder: A placebo-controlled discontinuation study. *Journal of Clinical Psychopharmacology*, 25(2), 166–169.

Davis, L.L., Nugent, A.L., Murray, J., *et al.* (2000). Nefazodone treatment for chronic posttraumatic stress disorder: An open trial. *Journal of Clinical Psychopharmacology*, 20(2), 159–164.

Davis, R.L., Rubanowice, D., McPhillips, H., *et al.* (2007). Risks of congenital malformations and perinatal events among infants exposed to antidepressant medications during pregnancy. *Pharmacoepidemiology and Drug Safety*, 16(10), 1086–1094.

de Abajo., F.J., Garcia-Rodriguez., L.A. (2008). Risk of upper gastrointestinal bleeding associated with selective serotonin reuptake inhibitors and venlafaxine therapy. *Archives of General Psychiatry*, 65(7), 795–803.

de Abajo, F.J., Jick, H., Derby, L., *et al.* (2000). Intracranial haemorrhage and use of selective serotonin reuptake inhibitors. *British Journal of Clinical Pharmacology*, 50(1), 43–47.

De Bellis, M.D., Gold, P.W., Geracioti, T.D. Jr., *et al.* (1993). Association of fluoxetine treatment with reductions in CSF concentrations of corticotropin-releasing hormone and arginine vasopressin in patients with major depression. *American Journal of Psychiatry*, 150(4), 656–657.

de Jong, J.C., van den Berg, P.B., Tobi, H. and de Jong-van den Berg, L.T. (2003). Combined use of SSRIs and NSAIDs increases the risk of gastrointestinal adverse effects. *British Journal of Clinical Pharmacology*, 55(6), 591–595.

De Jonghe, F., Ravinelli, D.P. and Tuynman-Qua, H. (1991). A randomized, double-blind study of Fluoxetine and maprotiline in the treatment of major depression. *Pharmacopsychiatry*, 24, 62–67.

de Maistre, E., Allart, C., Lecompte, T. and Bollaert, P.E. (2002). Severe bleeding associated with use of low molecular weight heparin and selective serotonin reuptake inhibitors. *American Journal of Medicine*, 113(6), 530–532.

de Meester, A., Carbutti, G., Gabriel, L. and Jacques, J.M. (2001). Fatal overdose with trazodone: Case report and literature review. *Acta Clinica Belgica*, 56(4), 258–261.

De Simoni, M.G., De Luigi, A., Clavenna, A. and Manfridi, A. (1992). *In vivo* studies on the enhancement of serotonin reuptake by tianeptine. *Brain Research*, 574(1–2), 93–97.

De Wit, S., Cremers, L., Hirsch, D., *et al.* (1999). Efficacy and safety of trazodone versus clorazepate in the treatment of HIV-positive subjects with adjustment disorders: A pilot study. *Journal of International Medical Research*, 27(5), 223–232.

Dean, A.J., Bell, J., Mascord, D.J., *et al.* (2002). A randomised, controlled trial of fluoxetine in methadone maintenance patients with depressive symptoms. *Journal of Affective Disorders*, 72(1), 85–90.

Deeg, M.A. and Lipkin, E.W. (1996). Hypoglycemia associated with the use of fluoxetine. *Western Journal of Medicine*, 164(3), 262.

Delalleau, B., Dulcire, C., Le Moine, P. and Kamoun, A. (1988). Analysis of the side effects of tianeptine. *Clinical Neuropharmacology*, 11(Suppl 2), S83–89.

Dell'Agnello, G., Ceravolo, R., Nuti, A., *et al.* (2001). SSRIs do not worsen Parkinson's disease: Evidence from an open-label, prospective study. *Clinical Neuropharmacology*, 24(4), 221–227.

Den Boer, J.A. and Westenberg, H.G. (1990). Serotonin function in panic disorder: A double blind placebo controlled study with fluvoxamine and ritanserin. *Psychopharmacology*, 102(1), 85–94.

Dent, L.A. and Orrock, M.W. (1997). Warfarin-fluoxetine and diazepam-fluoxetine interaction. *Pharmacotherapy*, 17(1), 170–172.

DeSanty, K.P. and Amabile, C.M. (2007). Antidepressant-induced liver injury. *Annals of Pharmacotherapy*, 41(7), 1201–1211.

DeSilva, K.E., Le Flore, D.B., Marston, B.J. and Rimland, D. (2001). Serotonin syndrome in HIV-infected individuals receiving antiretroviral therapy and fluoxetine. *AIDS*, 15(10), 1281–1285.

DeVane, C.L., Donovan, J.L., Liston, H.L., *et al.* (2004). Comparative CYP3A4 inhibitory effects of venlafaxine, fluoxetine, sertraline, and nefazodone in healthy volunteers. *Journal of Clinical Psychopharmacology*, 24(1), 4–10.

Devos, D., Dujardin, K., Poirot, I., *et al.* (2008). Comparison of desipramine and citalopram treatments for depression in Parkinson's disease: A double-blind, randomized, placebo-controlled study. *Movement Disorders*, 23(6), 850–857.

Dheenan, S., Venkatesan, J., Grubb, B.P. and Henrich, W.L. (1998). Effect of sertraline hydrochloride on dialysis hypotension. *American Journal of Kidney Diseases*, 31(4), 624–630.

Diav-Citrin, O., Shechtman, S., Weinbaum, D., *et al.* (2008). Paroxetine and fluoxetine in pregnancy: A prospective, multicentre, controlled, observational study. *British Journal of Clinical Pharmacology*, 66(5), 695–705.

Diem, S.J., Blackwell, T.L., Stone, K.L., *et al.* (2007). Use of antidepressants and rates of hip bone loss in older women: The study of osteoporotic fractures. *Archives of Internal Medicine*, 167(12), 1240–1245.

Dominguez-Moran, J.A., Callejo, J.M., Fernandez-Ruiz, L.C. and Martinez-Castrillo, J.C. (2001). Acute paroxysmal dystonia induced by fluoxetine. *Movement Disorders*, 16(4), 767–769.

Doogan, D.P. and Caillard, V. (1992). Sertraline in the prevention of depression. *British Journal of Psychiatry*, 160, 217–222.

Dording, C.M., Mischoulon, D., Petersen, T.J., *et al*. (2002). The pharmacologic management of SSRI-induced side effects: A survey of psychiatrists. *Annals of Clinical Psychiatry*, 14(3), 143–147.

Druckenbrod, R. and Mulsant, B.H. (1994). Fluoxetine-induced syndrome of inappropriate antidiuretic hormone secretion: A geriatric case report and a review of the literature. *Journal of Geriatric Psychiatry and Neurology*, 7(4), 254–256.

Dubini, A., Bosc, M. and Polin, V. (1997). Noradrenaline-selective versus serotonin-selective antidepressant therapy: Differential effects on social functioning. *Journal of Psychopharmacology*, 11(Suppl 4), S17–23.

Dublin, S., Rossing, M.A., Heckbert, S.R., *et al*. (2002). Risk of epithelial ovarian cancer in relation to use of antidepressants, benzodiazepines, and other centrally acting medications. *Cancer Causes & Control*, 13(1), 35–45.

Dumortier, G., Cabaret, W., Stamatiadis, L., *et al*. (2002). Hepatic tolerance of atypical antipsychotic drugs. *Encephale*, 28(6 Pt 1), 542–551.

Duncan, D., Sayal, K., McConnell, H. and Taylor, D. (1998). Antidepressant interactions with warfarin. *International Clinical Psychopharmacology*, 13(2), 87–94.

Dykens, J.A., Jamieson, J.D., Marroquin, L.D., *et al*. (2008). *In vitro* assessment of mitochondrial dysfunction and cytotoxicity of nefazodone, trazodone and buspirone. *Toxicological Science*, 103(2), 335–345.

Edwards, J.G., Goldie, A. and Papayanni-Papasthatis, S. (1989). Effect of paroxetine on the electrocardiogram. *Psychopharmacology*, 97(1), 96–98.

Ehde, D.M., Kraft, G.H., Chwastiak, L., *et al*. (2008). Efficacy of paroxetine in treating major depressive disorder in persons with multiple sclerosis. *General Hospital Psychiatry*, 30(1), 40–48.

Ehrentraut, S., Rothenhausler, H.B., Gerbes, A.L., *et al*. (2002). Acute liver failure in nefazodone therapy? A case report. *Der Nervenarzt*, 73(7), 686–689.

Einarson, A., Bonari, L., Voyer-Lavigne, S., *et al*. (2003). A multicentre prospective controlled study to determine the safety of trazodone and nefazodone use during pregnancy. *Canadian Journal of Psychiatry*, 48(2), 106–110.

Einarson, T.R. and Einarson, A. (2005). Newer antidepressants in pregnancy and rates of major malformations: A meta-analysis of prospective comparative studies. *Pharmacoepidemiology and Drug Safety*, 14(12), 823–827.

Einarson, A., Pistelli, A., Desantis, M., *et al*. (2008). Evaluation of the risk of congenital cardiovascular defects associated with use of paroxetine during pregnancy. *American Journal of Psychiatry*, 165(6), 749–752.

Elizur, A., Wintner, I. and Davidson, S. (1979). The clinical and psychological effects of pemoline in depressed patients — a controlled study. *International Pharmacopsychiatry*, 14(3), 127–134.

Elliott, A.J., Russo, J., Bergam, K., *et al.* (1999). Antidepressant efficacy in HIV-seropositive outpatients with major depressive disorder: An open trial of nefazodone. *Journal of Clinical Psychiatry*, 60(4), 226–231.

Elliott, A.J., Uldall, K.K., Bergam, K., *et al.* (1998). Randomized, placebo-controlled trial of paroxetine versus imipramine in depressed HIV-positive outpatients. *American Journal of Psychiatry*, 155(3), 367–372.

Ellison, J.M. and Stanziani, P. (1993). SSRI-associated nocturnal bruxism in four patients. *Journal of Clinical Psychiatry*, 54(11), 432–434.

El-Mallakh, R.S. (2000). An open study of methylphenidate in bipolar depression. *Bipolar Disorders*, 2(1), 56–59.

Emslie, G.J., Heiligenstein, J.H., Hoog, S.L., *et al.* (2004). Fluoxetine treatment for prevention of relapse of depression in children and adolescents: A double-blind, placebo-controlled study. *Journal of the American Academy of Child and Adolescent Psychiatry*, 43(11), 1397–1405.

Emslie, G.J., Heiligenstein, J.H., Wagner, K.D., *et al.* (2002). Fluoxetine for acute treatment of depression in children and adolescents: A placebo-controlled, randomized clinical trial. *Journal of the American Academy of Child and Adolescent Psychiatry*, 41(10), 1205–1215.

Emslie, G.J., Rush, A.J., Weinberg, W.A., *et al.* (1997). A double-blind, randomized, placebo-controlled trial of fluoxetine in children and adolescents with depression. *Archives of General Psychiatry*, 54(11), 1031–1037.

Emslie, G.J., Ventura, D., Korotzer, A. and Tourkodimitris, S. (2009). Escitalopram in the treatment of adolescent depression: A randomized placebo-controlled multisite trial. *Journal of the American Academy of Child and Adolescent Psychiatry*, 48(7), 721–729.

Engebretsen, K.M., Harris, C.R. and Wood, J.E. (2003). Cardiotoxicity and late onset seizures with citalopram overdose. *Journal of Emergency Medicine*, 25(2), 163–166.

Eralp Bellibas, S. (1999). Ritonavir-fluoxetine interaction. *Antimicrobial Agents and Chemotherapy*, 43(7), 1815.

Fabian, T.J., Amico, J.A., Kroboth, P.D., *et al.* (2004). Paroxetine-induced hyponatremia in older adults: A 12-week prospective study. *Archives of Internal Medicine*, 164(3), 327–332.

Fabre, L.F. (1990). Buspirone in the management of major depression: A placebo-controlled comparison. *Journal of Clinical Psychiatry*, 51 Suppl, 55–61.

Fagius, J., Osterman, P.O., Siden, A. and Wiholm, B.E. (1985). Guillain-Barre syndrome following zimeldine treatment. *Journal of Neurology, Neurosurgery and Psychiatry*, 48(1), 65–69.

Farah, A. (2002). Interferon-induced depression treated with citalopram. *Journal of Clinical Psychiatry*, 63(2), 166–167.

Faull, C.M., Rooke, P. and Baylis, P.H. (1991). The effect of a highly specific serotonin agonist on osmoregulated vasopressin secretion in healthy man. *Clinical Endocrinology (Oxf)*, 35(5), 423–430.

Fava, M., Amsterdam, J.D., Deltito, J.A., *et al.* (1998). A double-blind study of paroxetine, fluoxetine, and placebo in outpatients with major depression. *Annals of Clinical Psychiatry*, 10(4), 145–150.

Fava, M., Graves, L.M., Benazzi, F., *et al.* (2006). A cross-sectional study of the prevalence of cognitive and physical symptoms during long-term antidepressant treatment. *Journal of Clinical Psychiatry*, 67(11), 1754–1759.

Fava, M., Hoog, S.L., Judge, R.A., *et al.* (2002). Acute efficacy of fluoxetine versus sertraline and paroxetine in major depressive disorder including effects of baseline insomnia. *Journal of Clinical Psychopharmacology*, 22(2), 137–147.

Fava, M., Judge, R., Hoog, S.L., *et al.* (2000). Fluoxetine versus sertraline and paroxetine in major depressive disorder: Changes in weight with long-term treatment. *Journal of Clinical Psychiatry*, 61(11), 863–867.

Fava, M. and Rosenbaum, J.F. (1991). Suicidality and fluoxetine: Is there a relationship? *Journal of Clinical Psychiatry*, 52(3), 108–111.

Fava, M., Rosenbaum, J.F., Pava, J.A., *et al.* (1993). Anger attacks in unipolar depression, Part 1: Clinical correlates and response to fluoxetine treatment. *American Journal of Psychiatry*, 150(8), 1158–1163.

Favale, E., Audenino, D., Cocito, L. and Albano, C. (2003). The anticonvulsant effect of citalopram as an indirect evidence of serotonergic impairment in human epileptogenesis. *Seizure*, 12(5), 316–318.

Favale, E., Rubino, V., Mainardi, P., *et al.* (1995). Anticonvulsant effect of fluoxetine in humans. *Neurology*, 45(10), 1926–1927.

Feiger, A.D. (1996). A double-blind comparison of gepirone extended release, imipramine, and placebo in the treatment of outpatient major depression. *Psychopharmacology Bulletin*, 32(4), 659–665.

Feiger, A.D., Heiser, J.F., Shrivastava, R.K., *et al.* (2003). Gepirone extended-release: New evidence for efficacy in the treatment of major depressive disorder. *Journal of Clinical Psychiatry*, 64(3), 243–249.

Feighner, J.P., Boyer, W.F., Tyler, D.L. and Neborsky, R.J. (1990). Adverse consequences of fluoxetine-MAOI combination therapy. *Journal of Clinical Psychiatry*, 51(6), 222–225.

Ferguson, J.M. and Feighner, J.P. (1987). Fluoxetine-induced weight loss in overweight non-depressed humans. *International Journal of Obesity*, 11(Suppl 3), 163–170.

Ferguson, J.M., Mendels, J. and Schwartz, G.E. (2002). Effects of reboxetine on Hamilton Depression Rating Scale factors from randomized, placebo-controlled trials in major depression. *International Clinical Psychopharmacology*, 17(2), 45–51.

Ferguson, J.M., Shrivastava, R.K., Stahl, S.M., *et al.* (2001). Reemergence of sexual dysfunction in patients with major depressive disorder: Double-blind comparison of nefazodone and sertraline. *Journal of Clinical Psychiatry*, 62(1), 24–29.

Ferguson, J.M., Wesnes, K.A. and Schwartz, G.E. (2003). Reboxetine versus paroxetine versus placebo: Effects on cognitive functioning in depressed patients. *International Clinical Psychopharmacology*, 18(1), 9–14.

Fernandes, N.F., Martin, R.R. and Schenker, S. (2000). Trazodone-induced hepatotoxicity: A case report with comments on drug-induced hepatotoxicity. *American Journal of Gastroenterology*, 95(2), 532–535.

Fernandez, F., Levy, J.K., Samley, H.R., *et al.* (1995). Effects of methylphenidate in HIV-related depression: A comparative trial with desipramine. *International Journal of Psychiatry in Medicine*, 25(1), 53–67.

Ferrando, S.J., Goldman, J.D. and Charness, W.E. (1997). Selective serotonin reuptake inhibitor treatment of depression in symptomatic HIV infection and AIDS. Improvements in affective and somatic symptoms. *General Hospital Psychiatry*, 19(2), 89–97.

Ferrando, S.J., Rabkin, J.G., de Moore, G.M. and Rabkin, R. (1999). Antidepressant treatment of depression in HIV-seropositive women. *Journal of Clinical Psychiatry*, 60(11), 741–746.

Ferrari, M.D., Goadsby, P.J., Roon, K.I. and Lipton, R.B. (2002). Triptans (serotonin, 5-HT1B/1D agonists) in migraine: Detailed results and methods of a meta-analysis of 53 trials. *Cephalalgia*, 22(8), 633–658.

Fineberg, N.A., Tonnoir, B., Lemming, O. and Stein, D.J. (2007). Escitalopram prevents relapse of obsessive-compulsive disorder. *European Neuropsychopharmacology*, 17(6–7), 430–439.

Finkel, M.S., Laghrissi-Thode, F., Pollock, B.G. and Rong, J. (1996). Paroxetine is a novel nitric oxide synthase inhibitor. *Psychopharmacology Bulletin*, 32(4), 653–658.

Finkel, S.I., Richter, E.M. and Clary, C.M. (1999). Comparative efficacy and safety of sertraline versus nortriptyline in major depression in patients 70 and older. *International Psychogeriatrics*, 11(1), 85–99.

Fisch, M.J., Loehrer, P.J., Kristeller, J., *et al.* (2003). Fluoxetine versus placebo in advanced cancer outpatients: A double-blinded trial of the Hoosier Oncology Group. *Journal of Clinical Oncology*, 21(10), 1937–1943.

Fisher, A., Davis, M., Croft-Baker, J., *et al.* (2002). Citalopram-induced severe hyponatraemia with coma and seizure. Case report with literature and spontaneous reports review. *Adverse Drug Reactions and Toxicological Reviews*, 21(4), 179–187.

Fleischhacker, W.W. (1991). Propanolol for fluoxetine-induced akathisia. *Biological Psychiatry*, 30(5), 531–532.

Fleishaker, J.C., Francom, S.F., Herman, B.D., *et al.* (2001). Lack of effect of reboxetine on cardiac repolarization. *Clinical Pharmacology and Therapeutics*, 70(3), 261–269.

Flores, G., Perez-Patrigeon, S., Cobos-Ayala, C. and Vergara, J. (2004). Severe symptomatic hyponatremia during citalopram therapy. *BioMed Central Nephrology*, 5(1), 2.

Fluoxetine Bulimia Nervosa Collaborative Study Group. (1992). Fluoxetine in the treatment of bulimia nervosa. A multicenter, placebo-controlled, double-blind trial. Fluoxetine Bulimia Nervosa Collaborative Study Group. *Archives of General Psychiatry*, 49(2), 139–147.

Ford, M.A., Anderson, M.L., Rindone, J.P. and Jaskar, D.W. (1997). Lack of effect of fluoxetine on the hypoprothrombinemic response of warfarin. *Journal of Clinical Psychopharmacology*, 17(2), 110–112.

Fountoulakis, K.N., Samolis, S., Iacovides, A. and Kaprinis, G. (2007). Ecchymoses as an adverse effect of fluoxetine treatment. *Psychiatry Research*, 152(1):91–92.

Freeman, A.M. 3rd., Westphal, J.R., Norris, G.T., *et al.* (1997). Efficacy of ondansetron in the treatment of generalized anxiety disorder. *Depression and Anxiety*, 5(3), 140–141.

Frey, J. and Darbonne, C. (1994). Fluoxetine suppresses human cataplexy: A pilot study. *Neurology*, 44(4), 707–709.

Friedman, E.H. (1990). Fluoxetine-induced akathisia in male OCD patients. *Journal of Clinical Psychiatry*, 51(5), 212.

Fruehwald, S., Gatterbauer, E., Rehak, P. and Baumhackl, U. (2003). Early fluoxetine treatment of post-stroke depression — a three-month double-blind placebo-controlled study with an open-label long-term follow up. *Journal of Neurology*, 250(3), 347–351.

Fryer, J.D. and Lukas, R.J. (1999). Noncompetitive functional inhibition at diverse, human nicotinic acetylcholine receptor subtypes by bupropion, phencyclidine, and ibogaine. *Journal of Pharmacology and Experimental Therapeutics*, 288(1), 88–92.

Fugh-Berman, A. and Cott, J.M. (1999). Dietary supplements and natural products as psychotherapeutic agents. *Psychosomatic Medicine*, 61(5), 712–728.

Fulton-Kehoe, D., Rossing, M.A., Rutter, C., *et al.* (2006). Use of antidepressant medications in relation to the incidence of breast cancer. *British Journal of Cancer*, 94(7), 1071–1078.

Galletly, C., Clark, A. and Tomlinson, L. (1996). Evaluation of dexfenfluramine in a weight loss program for obese infertile women. *International Journal of Eating Disorders*, 19(2), 209–212.

Garattini, S. (1997). Pharmacology of amineptine, an antidepressant agent acting on the dopaminergic system: A review. *International Clinical Psychopharmacology*, 12(Suppl 3), S15–19.

Garattini, S. and Mennini, T. (1989). Pharmacology of amineptine: Synthesis and updating. *Clinical Neuropharmacology*, 12(Suppl 2), S13–18.

Garland, E.J. and Baerg, E.A. (2001). Amotivational syndrome associated with selective serotonin reuptake inhibitors in children and adolescents. *Journal of Child and Adolescent Psychopharmacology*, 11(2), 181–186.

Ghanizadeh, A. (2008). Sertraline-associated hair loss. *Journal of Drugs in Dermatology*, 7(7), 693–694.

Gelenberg, A.J., Wojcik, J.D., Falk, W.E., *et al.* (1990). Tyrosine for depression: A double-blind trial. *Journal of Affective Disorders*, 19(2), 125–132.

Gelenberg, A.J., Wojcik, J.D., Growdon, J.H., *et al.* (1980). Tyrosine for the treatment of depression. *American Journal of Psychiatry*, 137, 622–623.

George, M.S. and Trimble, M.R. (1993). Dystonic reaction associated with fluvoxamine. *Journal of Clinical Psychopharmacology*, 13(3), 220–221.

George, T.P. and Godleski, L.S. (1996). Possible serotonin syndrome with trazodone addition to fluoxetine. *Biological Psychiatry*, 39(5), 384–385.

Gerber, P.E. and Lynd, L.D. (1998). Selective serotonin-reuptake inhibitor-induced movement disorders. *Annals of Pharmacotherapy*, 32(6), 692–698.

Gerlach, M., Double, K., Arzberger, T., *et al.* (2003). Dopamine receptor agonists in current clinical use: Comparative dopamine receptor binding profiles defined in the human striatum. *Journal of Neural Transmission*, 110(10), 1119–1127.

Gerner, R., Estabrook, W., Steuer, J. and Jarvik, L. (1980). Treatment of geriatric depression with trazodone, imipramine, and placebo: A double-blind study. *Journal of Clinical Psychiatry*, 41(6), 216–220.

Gerstenberg, G., Aoshima, T., Fukasawa, T., *et al.* (2003a). Relationship between clinical effects of fluvoxamine and the steady-state plasma concentrations of fluvoxamine and its major metabolite fluvoxamino acid in Japanese depressed patients. *Psychopharmacology*, 167(4), 443–448.

Gerstenberg, G., Aoshima, T., Fukasawa, T., *et al.* (2003b). Effects of the CYP 2D6 genotype and cigarette smoking on the steady-state plasma concentrations of fluvoxamine and its major metabolite fluvoxamino acid in Japanese depressed patients. *Therapeutic Drug Monitoring*, 25(4), 463–468.

Gilaberte, I., Montejo, A.L., de la Gandara, J., *et al.* (2001). Fluoxetine in the prevention of depressive recurrences: A double-blind study. *Journal of Clinical Psychopharmacology*, 21(4), 417–424.

Gill, H.S., DeVane, C.L. and Risch, S.C. (1997). Extrapyramidal symptoms associated with cyclic antidepressant treatment: A review of the literature and consolidating hypotheses. *Journal of Clinical Psychopharmacology*, 17(5), 377–389.

Ginzburg, R. and Rosero, E. (2009). Risk of fractures with selective serotonin-reuptake inhibitors or tricyclic antidepressants. *Annals of Pharmacotherapy*, 66(22), 2037–2041.

Girault, C., Richard, J.C., Chevron, V., *et al.* (1997). Syndrome of inappropriate secretion of antidiuretic hormone in two elderly women with elevated serum fluoxetine. *Journal of Toxicology. Clinical Toxicology*, 35(1), 93–95.

Glassman, A.H., O'Connor, C.M., Califf, R.M., *et al.* (2002). Sertraline treatment of major depression in patients with acute MI or unstable angina. *Journal of the American Medical Association*, 288(6), 701–709.

Gleason, O.C., Yates, W.R., Isbell, M.D. and Philipsen, M.A. (2002). An open-label trial of citalopram for major depression in patients with hepatitis C. *Journal of Clinical Psychiatry*, 63(3), 194–198.

Gleason, O.C., Yates, W.R. and Philipsen, M.A. (2005). Major depressive disorder in hepatitis C: An open-label trial of escitalopram. *Primary Care Companion of the Journal of Clinical Psychiatry*, 7(5), 225–230.

Gleason, O.C., Yates, W.R., Philipsen, M.A., *et al.* (2004). Plasma levels of citalopram in depressed patients with hepatitis C. *Psychosomatics*, 45(1), 29–33.

Gobert, A., Rivet, J.M., Cistarelli, L., *et al.* (1999). Buspirone modulates basal and fluoxetine-stimulated dialysate levels of dopamine, noradrenaline and serotonin in the frontal cortex of freely moving rats: Activation of serotonin1A receptors and blockade of alpha2-adrenergic receptors underlie its actions. *Neuroscience*, 93(4), 1251–1262.

Goldberg, I.K. (1980). L-tyrosine in depression. *The Lancet*, 2, 364–365.

Goldberg, R.J. and Huk, M. (1992). Serotonin syndrome from trazodone and buspirone. *Psychosomatics*, 33(2), 235–236.

Golden, R.N., Nemeroff, C.B., McSorley, P., *et al.* (2002). Efficacy and tolerability of controlled-release and immediate-release paroxetine in the treatment of depression. *Journal of Clinical Psychiatry*, 63(7), 577–584.

Goldstein, D.J., Corbin, L.A. and Sundell, K.L. (1997). Effects of first-trimester fluoxetine exposure on the newborn. *Obstetrics and Gynecology*, 89(5 Pt 1), 713–718.

Goldstein, L., Barker, M., Segall, F., *et al.* (1996). Seizure and transient SIADH associated with sertraline. *American Journal of Psychiatry*, 153(5), 732.

Gonzalez, E., Minguez, L. and Sanguino, R.M. (2000). Galactorrhea after paroxetine treatment. *Pharmacopsychiatry*, 33(3), 118.

González-Pérez, A. and García Rodríguez, L.A. (2005). Breast cancer risk among users of antidepressant medications.*Epidemiology*, 16(1), 101–105.

Goodnick, P.J. (2001). Use of antidepressants in treatment of comorbid diabetes mellitus and depression as well as in diabetic neuropathy. *Annals of Clinical Psychiatry*, 13(1), 31–41.

Gordon, C., Whale, R. and Cowen, P.J. (1998). Sertraline treatment does not increase plasma prolactin levels in healthy subjects. *Psychopharmacology*, 137(2), 201–202.

Gorwood, P., Weiller, E., Lemming, O. and Katona, C. (2007). Escitalopram prevents relapse in older patients with major depressive disorder. *American Journal of Geriatric Psychiatry*, 15(7), 581–593.

Grassi, B., Gambini, O., Garghentini, G., *et al.* (1997). Efficacy of paroxetine for the treatment of depression in the context of HIV infection. *Pharmacopsychiatry*, 30(2), 70–71.

Grassi, L., Biancosino, B., Marmai, L. and Righi, R. (2004). Effect of reboxetine on major depressive disorder in breast cancer patients: An open-label study. *Journal of Clinical Psychiatry*, 65(4), 515–520.

Graudins, A., Vossler, C. and Wang, R. (1997). Fluoxetine-induced cardiotoxicity with response to bicarbonate therapy. *American Journal of Emergency Medicine*, 15(5), 501–503.

Gray, D.S., Fujiyoka, K., Dewine, W. and Bray, G.A. (1992). Fluoxetine treatment of the obese diabetic. *International Journal of Obesity*, 16, 193–198.

Greeno, C.G. and Wing, R.R. (1996). A double-blind placebo controlled trial of the effect of fluoxetine on daily intake in overweight women with and without binge-eating disorders. *American Journal of Clinical Nutrition*, 64, 267–273.

Grof, P., Joffe, R., Kennedy, S., *et al.* (1993). An open study of oral flesinoxan, a 5-HT1A receptor agonist, in treatment-resistant depression. *International Clinical Psychopharmacology*, 8(3), 167–172.

Gross, R., Dannon, P.N., Lepkifker, E., *et al.* (1998). Generalized seizures caused by fluoxetine overdose. *American Journal of Emergency Medicine*, 16(3), 328–329.

Grosbois, B., Milon, D., Dauriac, C., *et al.* (1985). Hematologic disorders (acute agranulocytosis) during treatment with indalpine. *La Presse Medicale*, 14(3), 163–164.

Grubb, B.P., Samoil, D., Kosinski, D., *et al.* (1994). The use of serotonin reuptake inhibitors for the treatment of recurrent syncope due to carotid sinus hypersensitivity unresponsive to dual chamber cardiac pacing. *Pacing and Clinical Electrophysiology*, 17(8), 1434–1436.

Gupta, S., Lentz, B. and Frank, B.L. (2002). A case report of drug-induced dermatitis with weekly fluoxetine. *Prim Care Companion Journal of Clinical Psychiatry*, 4(2), 78–79.

Guzey, C. and Spigset, O. (2006). Low serum concentrations of paroxetine in CYP2D6 ultrarapid metabolizers. *Journal of Clinical Psychopharmacology*, 26(2), 211–212.

Haffmans, P.M. and Vos, M.S. (1999). The effects of trazodone on sleep disturbances induced by brofaromine. *European Psychiatry*, 14(3), 167–171.

Hajdu, P., Ulens, C., Panyi, G. and Tytgat, J. (2003). Drug- and mutagenesis-induced changes in the selectivity filter of a cardiac two-pore background K+ channel. *Cardiovascular Research*, 58(1), 46–54.

Hall, M.J. (1994). Breast tenderness and enlargement induced by sertraline. *American Journal of Psychiatry*, 151(9), 1395–1396.

Hammad, T.A., Laughren, T.P. and Racoosin, J.A. (2006). Suicide rates in short-term randomized controlled trials of newer antidepressants. *Journal of Clinical Psychopharmacology*, 26(2), 203–207.

Haney, E.M., Chan, B.K., Diem, S.J., *et al.* (2007). Association of low bone mineral density with selective serotonin reuptake inhibitor use by older men. *Archives of Internal Medicine*, 167(12), 1246–1251.

Hansen, L. (2003). Fluoxetine dose-increment related akathisia in depression: Implications for clinical care, recognition and management of selective serotonin reuptake inhibitor-induced akathisia. *Journal of Psychopharmacology*, 17(4), 451–452.

Hanzel, D.A., Proia, N.G. and Hudgel, D.W. (1991). Response of obstructive sleep apnea to fluoxetine and protriptyline. *Chest*, 100(2), 416–421.

Haque, R., Enger, S.M., Chen, W. and Petitti, D.B. (2005). Breast cancer risk in a large cohort of female antidepressant medication users. *Cancer Letters*, 221(1), 61–65.

Harel, Z., Biro, F.M. and Tedford, W.L. (1995). Effects of long term treatment with sertraline (Zoloft) simulating hypothyroidism in an adolescent. *Journal of Adolescent Health*, 16(3), 232–234.

Hargrave, R., Martinez, D. and Bernstein, A.J. (1992). Fluoxetine-induced seizures. *Psychosomatics*, 33(2), 236–239.

Haria, M., Fitton, A. and McTavish, D. (1994). Trazodone. A review of its pharmacology, therapeutic use in depression and therapeutic potential in other disorders. *Drugs and Aging*, 4(4), 331–355.

Hartter, S., Wang, X., Weigmann, H., *et al.* (2001). Differential effects of fluvoxamine and other antidepressants on the biotransformation of melatonin. *Journal of Clinical Psychopharmacology*, 21(2), 167–174.

Hauser, P., Khosla, J., Aurora, H., *et al.* (2002). A prospective study of the incidence and open-label treatment of interferon-induced major depressive disorder in patients with hepatitis C. *Molecular Psychiatry*, 7(9), 942–947.

Hauser, P., Soler, R., Reed, S., *et al.* (2000). Prophylactic treatment of depression induced by interferon-alpha. *Psychosomatics*, 41(5), 439–441.

Hauser, R.A. and Zesiewicz, T.A. (1997). Sertraline for the treatment of depression in Parkinson's disease. *Movement Disorders*, 12(5), 756–759.

Hayes, D. (2004). Recent developments in antidepressant therapy in special populations. *American Journal of Managed Care*, 10(6 Suppl), S179–185.

Hellerstein, D.J., Yanowitch, P., Rosenthal, J., *et al.* (1993). A randomized double-blind study of fluoxetine versus placebo in the treatment of dysthymia. *American Journal of Psychiatry*, 150(8), 1169–1175.

Hemels, M.E., Einarson, A., Koren, G., *et al.* (2005). Antidepressant use during pregnancy and the rates of spontaneous abortions: A meta-analysis. *Annals of Pharmacotherapy*, 39(5), 803–809.

Hemrick-Luecke, S.K., Snoddy, H.D. and Fuller, R.W. (1994). Evaluation of nefazodone as a serotonin uptake inhibitor and a serotonin antagonist *in vivo*. *Life Sciences*, 55(7), 479–483.

Hemeryck, A. and Belpaire, F.M. (2002). Selective serotonin reuptake inhibitors and cytochrome P-450 mediated drug-drug interactions: An update. *Current Drug Metabolism*, 3(1), 13–37.

Hendrick, V., Smith, L.M., Suri, R., *et al.* (2003). Birth outcomes after prenatal exposure to antidepressant medication.*American Journal of Obstetrics and Gynecology*, 188(3), 812–815.

Henry, J.A., Alexander, C.A. and Sener, E.K. (1995). Relative mortality from overdose of antidepressants. *British Medical Journal*, 310(6974), 221–224.

Henry, M.E., Moore, C.M., Kaufman, M.J., *et al.* (2000). Brain kinetics of paroxetine and fluoxetine on the third day of placebo substitution: A fluorine MRS study. *American Journal of Psychiatry*, 157(9), 1506–1508.

Hergovich, N., Aigner, M., Eichler, H.G., *et al.* (2000). Paroxetine decreases platelet serotonin storage and platelet function in human beings. *Clinical Pharmacology and Therapeutics*, 68(4), 435–442.

Hertzman, P.A., Blevins, W.L., Mayer, J., *et al.* (1990). Association of the eosinophilia-myalgia syndrome with the ingestion of tryptophan. *New England Journal of Medicine*, 322(13), 869–873.

Hewer, W., Rost, W. and Gattaz, W.F. (1995). Cardiovascular effects of fluvoxamine and maprotiline in depressed patients. *European Archives of Psychiatry and Clinical Neuroscience*, 246(1), 1–6.

Hewlett, W.A., Schmid, S.P. and Salomon, R.M. (2003). Pilot Trial of Ondansetron in the Treatment of 8 Patients with Obsessive-Compulsive Disorder. *Journal of Clinical Psychiatry*, 64(9), 1025–1030.

Himmelhoch, J.M., Schechtman, K. and Auchenbach R. (1984). The role of trazodone in the treatment of depressed cardiac patients. *Psychopathology*, 17(Suppl 2), 51–63.

Hindmarch, I., Kimber, S. and Cockle, S.M. (2000). Abrupt and brief discontinuation of antidepressant treatment: Effects on cognitive function and psychomotor performance. *International Clinical Psychopharmacology*, 15(6), 305–318.

Hinze-Selch, D., Schuld, A., Kraus, T., *et al.* (2000). Effects of antidepressants on weight and on the plasma levels of leptin, TNF-alpha and soluble TNF receptors: A longitudinal study in patients treated with amitriptyline or paroxetine. *Neuropsychopharmacology*, 23(1), 13–19.

Hochstrasser, B., Isaksen, P.M., Koponen, H., *et al.* (2001). Prophylactic effect of citalopram in unipolar, recurrent depression: Placebo-controlled study of maintenance therapy. *British Journal of Psychiatry*, 178, 304–310.

Hoehn-Saric, R., Harris, G.J., Pearlson, G.D., *et al.* (1991). A fluoxetine-induced frontal lobe syndrome in an obsessive-compulsive patient. *Journal of Clinical Psychiatry*, 52(3), 131–133.

Hoehn-Saric, R., Lipsey, J.R. and McLeod, D.R. (1990). Apathy and indifference in patients on fluvoxamine and fluoxetine. *Journal of Clinical Psychopharmacology*, 10(5), 343–345.

Hoehn-Saric, R., Ninan, P., Black, D.W., *et al.* (2000). Multicenter double-blind comparison of sertraline and desipramine for concurrent obsessive-compulsive and major depressive disorders. *Archives of General Psychiatry*, 57(1), 76–82.

Holland, J.C., Romano, S.J., Heiligenstein, J.H., *et al.* (1998). A controlled trial of fluoxetine and desipramine in depressed women with advanced cancer. *Psychooncology*, 7(4), 291–300.

Hollander, E., Allen, A., Steiner, M., *et al.* (2003). Acute and long-term treatment and prevention of relapse of obsessive-compulsive disorder with paroxetine. *Journal of Clinical Psychiatry*, 64(9), 1113–1121.

Hovorka, J., Herman, E. and Nemcova, I. (2000). Treatment of Interictal Depression with Citalopram in Patients with Epilepsy. *Epilepsy and Behavior*, 1(6), 444–447.

Humphries, J.E., Wheby, M.S. and VandenBerg, S.R. (1990). Fluoxetine and the bleeding time. *Archives of Pathology and Laboratory Medicine*, 114(7), 727–728.

Hull, M., Kottlors, M. and Braune, S. (2002). Prolonged coma caused by low sodium and hypo-osmolarity during treatment with citalopram. *Journal of Clinical Psychopharmacology*, 22(3), 337–338.

Hu, X.H., Bull, S.A., Hunkeler, E.M., *et al.* (2004). Incidence and duration of side effects and those rated as bothersome with selective serotonin reuptake inhibitor treatment for depression: Patient report versus physician estimate. *Journal of Clinical Psychiatry*, 65(7), 959–965.

Inder, W.J., Prickett, T.C., Mulder, R.T., *et al.* (2001). Reduction in basal afternoon plasma ACTH during early treatment of depression with fluoxetine. *Psychopharmacology*, 156(1), 73–78.

Invernizzi, G., Aguglia, E., Bertolino, A., *et al.* (1994). The efficacy and safety of tianeptine in the treatment of depressive disorder: Results of a controlled double-blind multi-centre study vs. amitriptyline. *Neuropsychobiology*, 30(2–3), 85–93.

Iraqi, A. and Baickle, E. (2004). A case report of hyponatremia with citalopram use. *Journal of the American Medical Directors Association*, 5(1), 64–65.

Irwin, M. and Spar, J.E. (1983). Reversible cardiac conduction abnormality associated with trazodone administration. *American Journal of Psychiatry*, 140(7), 945–946.

Isbister, G.K., Prior, F.H. and Foy, A. (2001). Citalopram-induced bradycardia and presyncope. *Annals of Pharmacotherapy*, 35(12), 1552–1555.

Ishikawa, M., Ishiwata, K., Ishii, K., *et al.* (2007). High occupancy of sigma-1 receptors in the human brain after single oral administration of fluvoxamine: A positron emission tomography study using [(11)C]SA4503. *Biological Psychiatry*, 62(8), 878–883.

Jan, M.W., ZumBrunnen, T.L., Kazmi, Y.R., *et al.* (2002). Pharmacokinetics of fluvoxamine in relation to CYP2C19 phenotype and genotype. *Drug Metabolism and Drug Interactions*, 19(1), 1–11.

Janowsky, D., Curtis, G., Zisook, S., *et al.* (1983a). Ventricular arrhythmias possibly aggravated by trazodone. *American Journal of Psychiatry*, 140(6), 796–797.

Janowsky, D., Curtis, G., Zisook, S., *et al.* (1983b). Trazodone-aggravated ventricular arrhythmias. *Journal of Clinical Psychopharmacology*, 3(6), 372–376.

Jenkins, S.W., Robinson, D.S., Fabre, L.F. Jr., *et al.* (1990). Gepirone in the treatment of major depression. *Journal of Clinical Psychopharmacology*, 10(Suppl 3), 77S-85S.

Jezova, D. and Duncko, R. (2002). Enhancement of stress-induced pituitary hormone release and cardiovascular activation by antidepressant treatment in healthy men. *Journal of Psychopharmacology*, 16(3), 235–240.

Jiang, G.X., Cheng, Q., Ehrnst, A., *et al.* (1997). Guillain-Barre syndrome in Stockholm County, 1973–1991. *European Journal of Epidemiology*, 13(1), 25–32.

John, L., Perreault, M.M., Tao, T. and Blew, P.G. (1997). Serotonin syndrome associated with nefazodone and paroxetine. *Annals of Emergency Medicine*, 29(2), 287–289.

Jorge, R.E., Robinson, R.G., Arndt, S. and Starkstein, S. (2003). Mortality and post*Stroke* depression: A placebo-controlled trial of antidepressants. *American Journal of Psychiatry*, 160(10), 1823–1829.

Jouvent, R., Abensour, P., Bonnet, A.M., *et al.* (1983). Antiparkinsonian and antidepressant effects of high doses of bromocriptine. An independent comparison. *Journal of Affective Disorders*, 5(2), 141–145.

Judd, F.K., Mijch, A.M. and Cockram, A. (1995). Fluoxetine treatment of depressed patients with HIV infection. *Australian and New Zealand Journal of Psychiatry*, 29(3), 433–436.

Judd, L.L., Rapaport, M.H., Yonkers, K.A., *et al.* (2004). Randomized, placebo-controlled trial of fluoxetine for acute treatment of minor depressive disorder. *American Journal of Psychiatry*, 161(10), 1864–1871.

Judge, R., Parry, M.G., Quail, D. and Jacobson, J.G. (2002). Discontinuation symptoms: Comparison of brief interruption in fluoxetine and paroxetine treatment. *International Clinical Psychopharmacology*, 17(5), 217–225.

Judge, R., Plewes, J.M., Kumar, V., *et al.* (2000). Changes in energy during treatment of depression: An analysis of fluoxetine in double-blind, placebo-controlled trials. *Journal of Clinical Psychopharmacology*, 20(6), 666–672.

Kallen, B.A. and Otterblad Olausson, P. (2007). Maternal use of selective serotonin re-uptake inhibitors in early pregnancy and infant congenital malformations. *Birth Defects Research Part A, Clinical and Molecular Teratology*, 79(4), 301–308.

Kalender, B., Ozdemir, A.C., Yalug, I. and Dervisoglu, E. (2007). Antidepressant treatment increases quality of life in patients with chronic renal failure.*Renal Failure*, 29(7), 817–822.

Kamijima, K., Burt, T., Cohen, G., *et al.* (2006). A placebo-controlled, randomized withdrawal study of sertraline for major depressive disorder in Japan. *International Clinical Psychopharmacology*, 21(1), 1–9.

Kamo, T., Horikawa, N., Tsuruta, Y., *et al.* (2004). Efficacy and pharmacokinetics of fluvoxamine maleate in patients with mild depression undergoing hemodialysis. *Psychiatry and Clinical Neurosciences*, 58(2), 133–137.

Kanner, A.M., Kozak, A.M. and Frey, M. (2000). The use of sertraline in patients with epilepsy: Is it safe? *Epilepsy and Behavior*, 1(2), 100–105.

Kanjanauthai, S., Kanluen, T. and Chareonthaitawee, P. (2008). Citalopram induced torsade de pointes, a rare life threatening side effect. *International Journal of Cardiology*, 131(1), e33–34.

Kasper, S., Laigle, L. and Bayle, F. (2008). Superior antidepressant efficacy og agomelatine versus sertraline: A randomized, double-blind study. *European Neuropsychopharmacology*, 18(s4), s336.

Karson, C.N., Newton, J.E., Livingston, R., *et al.* (1993). Human brain fluoxetine concentrations. *Journal of Psychiatry and Clinical Neurosciences*, 5(3), 322–329.

Kasper, S. and Olie, J.P. (2002). A meta-analysis of randomized controlled trials of tianeptine versus SSRI in the short-term treatment of depression. *European Psychiatry*, 17(Suppl 3), 331–340.

Kaufmann, M.W., Cassem, N.H., Murray, G.B. and Jenike, M. (1984). Use of psychostimulants in medically ill patients with neurological disease and major depression. *Canadian Journal of Psychiatry*, 29(1), 46–49.

Kaye, W.H., Nagata, T., Weltzin, T.E., *et al.* (2001). Double-blind placebo-controlled administration of fluoxetine in restricting- and restricting-purging-type anorexia nervosa. *Biological Psychiatry*, 49(7), 644–652.

Kazal, L.A. Jr., Hall, D.L., Miller, L.G. and Noel, M.L. (1993). Fluoxetine-induced SIADH: A geriatric occurrence? *Journal of Family Practice*, 36(3), 341–343.

Keegan, D., Bowen, R.C., Blackshaw, S., *et al.* (1991). A comparison of fluoxetine and amitriptyline in the treatment of major depression. *International Clinical Psychopharmacology*, 6(2), 117–124.

Keller, M.B., Kocsis, J.H., Thase, M.E., *et al.* (1998). Maintenance phase efficacy of sertraline for chronic depression: A randomized controlled trial. *Journal of the American Medical Association*, 280(19), 1665–1672.

Kelly, J.P., Rosenberg, L., Palmer, J.R., *et al.* (1999). Risk of breast cancer according to use of antidepressants, phenothiazines, and antihistamines. *American Journal of Epidemiology*, 150(8), 861–868.

Kennedy, S.H., Andersen, H.F. and Thase, M.E. (2009). Escitalopram in the treatment of major depressive disorder: A meta-analysis. *Current Medical and Research Opinion*, 25(1), 161–175.

Kennedy, S.H. and Emsley, R. (2006). Placebo-controlled trial of agomelatine in the treatment of major depressive disorder. *European Neuropsychopharmacology*, 16(2), 93–100.

Kennedy, S.H., Rizvi, S., Fulton, K. and Rasmussen, J. (2008). A double-blind comparison of sexual functioning, antidepressant efficacy, and tolerability between agomelatine and venlafaxine XR. *Journal of Clinical Psychopharmacology*, 28(3), 329–333.

Kent, J.M., Coplan, J.D., Lombardo, I., *et al.* (2002). Occupancy of brain serotonin transporters during treatment with paroxetine in patients with social phobia: A positron emission tomography study with 11C McN 5652. *Psychopharmacology*, 164(4), 341–348.

Khan, A., Khan, S., Kolts, R. and Brown, W.A. (2003). Suicide rates in clinical trials of SSRIs, other antidepressants, and placebo: Analysis of FDA reports. *American Journal of Psychiatry*, 160(4), 790–792.

Kharofa, J., Sekar, P., Haverbusch, M., *et al.* (2007). Selective serotonin reuptake inhibitors and risk of hemorrhagic stroke. *Stroke*, 38(11), 3049–3051.

Khouzam, H.R., Monteiro, A.J. and Gerken, M.E. (1998). Remission of cancer chemotherapy-induced emesis during antidepressant therapy with nefazodone. *Psychosomatic Medicine*, 60(1), 89–91.

Kim, K.Y., Craig, J.M. and Hawley, J.M. (2000). Seizure possibly associated with fluvoxamine. *Annals of Pharmacotherapy*, 34(11), 1276–1278.

Kinzie, J.D. and Leung, P. (1989). Clonidine in Cambodian patients with posttraumatic stress disorder. *Journal of Nervous and Mental Disease*, 177(9), 546–550.

Kirby, D., Harrigan, S. and Ames, D. (2002). Hyponatraemia in elderly psychiatric patients treated with Selective Serotonin Reuptake Inhibitors and venlafaxine: A retrospective controlled study in an inpatient unit. *International Journal of Geriatric Psychiatry*, 17(3), 231–237.

Klee, B. and Kronig, M.H. (1993). Case report of probable sertraline-induced akathisia. *American Journal of Psychiatry*, 150(6), 986–987.

Knoppert, D.C., Nimkar, R., Principi, T. and Yuen, D. (2006). Paroxetine toxicity in a newborn after in utero exposure: Clinical symptoms correlate with serum levels. *Therapeutic Drug Monitoring*, 28(1), 5–7.

Koch, S., Perry, K.W., Nelson, D.L., *et al.* (2002). R-fluoxetine increases extracellular DA, NE, as well as 5-HT in rat prefrontal cortex and hypothalamus: An *in vivo* microdialysis and receptor binding study. *Neuropsychopharmacology*, 27(6), 949–959.

Koelkebeck, K., Domschke, K., Zwanzger, P., *et al.* (in press). A case of non-SIADH-induced hyponatremia in depression after treatment with reboxetine. *World Journal of Biological Psychiatry.*

Kole, M.H., Swan, L. and Fuchs, E. (2002). The antidepressant tianeptine persistently modulates glutamate receptor currents of the hippocampal CA3 commissural associational synapse in chronically stressed rats. *European Journal of Neuroscience*, 16(5), 807–816.

Konig, F., Hauger, B., von Hippel, C., *et al.* (2000). Effect of paroxetine on thyroid hormone levels in severely depressed patients. *Neuropsychobiology*, 42(3), 135–138.

Kopelman, P.G., Elliott, M.W., Simonds, A., *et al.* (1992). Short-term use of fluoxetine in asymptomatic obese subjects with sleep-related hypoventilation. *International Journal of Obesity and Related Metabolic Disorders*, 16(10), 825–830.

Koran, L.M., Chuong, H.W., Bullock, K.D. and Smith, S.C. (2003). Citalopram for compulsive shopping disorder: An open-label study followed by double-blind discontinuation. *Journal of Clinical Psychiatry*, 64(7), 793–798.

Koran, L.M., Hackett, E., Rubin, A., *et al.* (2002). Efficacy of sertraline in the long-term treatment of obsessive-compulsive disorder. *American Journal of Psychiatry*, 159(1), 88–95.

Koren, G. and Boucher, N. (2009). Adverse effects in neonates exposed to SSRIs and SNRI in late gestation — Motherisk Update 2008. *Canadian Journal of Clinical Pharmacology*, 16(1), e66–67.

Kornstein, S.G., Bose, A., Li, D., *et al.* (2006). Escitalopram maintenance treatment for prevention of recurrent depression: A randomized, placebo-controlled trial. *Journal of Clinical Psychiatry*, 67(11), 1767–1775.

Kotlyar, M., Golding, M., Brewer E.R. and Carson, S.W. (1999). Possible nefazodone withdrawal syndrome. *American Journal of Psychiatry*, 156(7), 1117.

Kraiczi, H., Hedner, J., Dahlof, P., *et al.* (1999). Effect of serotonin uptake inhibition on breathing during sleep and daytime symptoms in obstructive sleep apnea. *Sleep*, 22(1), 61–67.

Kraus, M.R., Schäfer, A., Faller, H., *et al.* (2002). Paroxetine for the treatment of interferon-alpha-induced depression in chronic hepatitis C. *Alimentary Pharmacology and Therapeutics*, 16(6), 1091–1099.

Kraus, M.R., Schäfer, A., Schöttker, K., *et al.* (2008). Therapy of interferon-induced depression in chronic hepatitis C with citalopram: A randomized, double-blind, placebo-controlled study. *Gut*, 57(4), 531–536.

Kreider, M.S., Bushnell, W.D., Oakes, R. and Wheadon, D.E. (1995). A double-blind, randomized study to provide safety information on switching fluoxetine-treated patients to paroxetine without an intervening washout period. *Journal of Clinical Psychiatry*, 56(4), 142–145.

Kristensen, J.H., Hackett, L.P., Kohan, R., *et al.* (2002). The amount of fluvoxamine in milk is unlikely to be a cause of adverse effects in breastfed infants. *Journal of Human Lactation*, 18(2), 139–143.

Kubera, M., Lin, A.H., Kenis, G., *et al.* (2001). Anti-Inflammatory effects of antidepressants through suppression of the interferon-gamma/interleukin-10 production ratio. *Journal of Clinical Psychopharmacology*, 21(2), 199–206.

Kuhn, K.U., Quednow, B.B., Thiel, M., *et al.* (2003). Antidepressive treatment in patients with temporal lobe epilepsy and major depression: A prospective study with three different antidepressants. *Epilepsy and Behavior*, 4(6), 674–679.

Kulin, N.A., Pastuszak, A., Sage, S.R., *et al.* (1998). Pregnancy outcome following maternal use of the new selective serotonin reuptake inhibitors: A prospective controlled multicenter study. *Journal of the American Medical Association*, 279(8), 609–610.

Kutnowski, M., Daubresse, J.C., Friedman, H., *et al.* (1992). Fluoxetine therapy in obese diabetic and glucose intolerant patients. *International Journal of Obesity*, 16(Suppl 4), S63–S66.

Klysner, R., Bent-Hansen, J., Hansen, H.L., *et al.* (2002). Efficacy of citalopram in the prevention of recurrent depression in elderly patients: Placebo-controlled study of maintenance therapy. *British Journal of Psychiatry*, 181, 29–35.

Lader, M., Andersen, H.F. and Baekdal, T. (2005). The effect of escitalopram on sleep problems in depressed patients. *Human Psychopharmacology*, 20(5), 349–354.

Laine, K., Anttila, M., Heinonen, E., *et al.* (1997). Lack of adverse interactions between concomitantly administered selegiline and citalopram. *Clinical Neuropharmacology*, 20(5), 419–433.

Laine, K., Kytola, J. and Bertilsson, L. (2004). Severe adverse effects in a newborn with two defective CYP2D6 alleles after exposure to paroxetine during late pregnancy. *Therapeutic Drug Monitoring*, 26(6), 685–687.

Lake, M.B., Birmaher, B., Wassick, S., *et al.* (2000). Bleeding and selective serotonin reuptake inhibitors in childhood and adolescence. *Journal of Child and Adolescent Psychopharmacology*, 10(1), 35–38.

Lam, R.W., Gorman, C.P., Michalon, M., *et al.* (1995). Multicenter, placebo-controlled study of fluoxetine in seasonal affective disorder. *American Journal of Psychiatry*, 152(12), 1765–1770.

Lam, Y.W., Alfaro, C.L., Ereshefsky, L. and Miller, M. (2003). Pharmacokinetic and pharmacodynamic interactions of oral midazolam with ketoconazole, fluoxetine, fluvoxamine, and nefazodone. *Journal of Clinical Pharmacology*, 43(11), 1274–1282.

Lambert, M.T., Trutia, C. and Petty, F. (1998). Extrapyramidal adverse effects associated with sertraline. *Progress in Neuropsychopharmacology and Biological Psychiatry*, 22(5), 741–748.

Lane, R. and Baldwin, D. (1997). Selective serotonin reuptake inhibitor-induced serotonin syndrome: Review. *Journal of Clinical Psychopharmacology*, 17(3), 208–221.

Lapierre, Y.D., Silverstone, P., Reesal, R.T., *et al.* (1998). A Canadian multicenter study of three fixed doses of controlled-release ipsapirone in outpatients with moderate to severe major depression. *Journal of Clinical Psychopharmacology*, 18(4), 268–273.

Lara, N., Archer, S.L., Baker, G.B. and Le Melledo, J.M. (2003a). Paroxetine-induced increase in metabolic end products of nitric oxide. *Journal of Clinical Psychopharmacology*, 23(4), 408–412.

Lara, N., Baker, G., Archer, S.L. and Le Melledo, J.M. (2003b). Increased cholesterol levels during paroxetine administration in healthy men. *Journal of Clinical Psychiatry*, 64(12), 1455–1459.

Lash, T.L., Pedersen, L., Cronin-Fenton, D., *et al.* (2008). Tamoxifen's protection against breast cancer recurrence is not reduced by concurrent use of the SSRI citalopram. *British Journal of Cancer*, 99(4), 616–621.

Lauber, C. (1999). Nefazodone withdrawal syndrome. *Canadian Journal of Psychiatry* 44(3), 285–286.

Layton, D., Clark, D.W., Pearce, G.L. and Shakir, S.A. (2001). Is there an association between selective serotonin reuptake inhibitors and risk of abnormal bleeding? Results from a cohort study based on prescription event monitoring in England. *European Journal of Clinical Pharmacology*, 57(2), 167–176.

Lazarus, L.W., Moberg, P.J., Langsley, P.R. and Lingam, V.R. (1994). Methylphenidate and nortriptyline in the treatment of poststroke depression: A retrospective comparison. *Archives of Physical Medicine and Rehabilitation*, 75(4), 403–406.

Lazarus, L.W., Winemiller, D.R., Lingam, V.R., *et al.* (1992). Efficacy and side effects of methylphenidate for post-stroke depression. *Journal of Clinical Psychiatry*, 53(12), 447–449.

Leander, J.D. (1992). Fluoxetine, a selective serotonin-uptake inhibitor, enhances the anticonvulsant effects of phenytoin, carbamazepine, and ameltolide (LY201116). *Epilepsia*, 33(3), 573–576.

Lechin, F., van der Dijs, B., Jara, H., *et al.* (1998). Effects of buspirone on plasma neurotransmitters in healthy subjects. *Journal of Neural Transmission*, 105(6–7), 561–573.

Lecrubier, Y., Boyer, P., Turjanski, S. and Rein, W. (1997). Amisulpride versus imipramine and placebo in dysthymia and major depression. Amisulpride Study Group. *Journal of Affective Disorders*, 43(2), 95–103.

Lecrubier, Y., Puech, A.J., Aubin, F., *et al.* (1988). Improvement by amisulpride of the negative syndrome in non-psychotic subjects: A preliminary study. *Psychiatry and Psychobiology*, 3, 329–333.

Lee, A., Woo, J. and Ito, S. (2004). Frequency of infant adverse events that are associated with citalopram use during breast-feeding. *American Journal of Obstetrics and Gynecology*, 190(1), 218–221.

Lee, M.S. and Nam, J.W. (2000). A case of paroxetine-induced dyskinetic movements. *Journal of Clinical Psychopharmacology*, 20(6), 712–713.

Lekakis, J., Ikonomidis, I., Papoutsi, Z., *et al.* (in press). Selective serotonin re-uptake inhibitors decrease the cytokine-induced endothelial adhesion molecule expression, the endothelial adhesiveness to monocytes and the circulating levels of vascular adhesion molecules. *International Journal of Cardiology.*

Lemke, M.R. (2002). Effect of reboxetine on depression in Parkinson's disease patients. *Journal of Clinical Psychiatry*, 63(4), 300–304.

Lemke, M.R., Brecht, M., Koester, J., *et al.* (2002). Depression and anhedonia in Parkinson's disease. *European Neuropsychopharmacology*, 12(3), S109.

Lemke, M.R. and Wendorff, T. (2000). Differential effects of tricyclic antidepressants and paroxetine on gait performance in depression. *European Neuropsychopharmacology*, 10(3), S254.

Lemoine, P., Achaintre, A., Balvay, G., *et al.* (1981). Double-blind trial of amineptine and clomipramine in the treatment of depression. *Current Medical Research and Opinion*, 7(4), 234–240.

Lemoine, P., Guilleminault, C. and Alvarez, E. (2007). Improvement in subjective sleep in major depressive disorder with a novel antidepressant, agomelatine: Randomized, double-blind comparison with venlafaxine.*Journal of Clinical Psychiatry*, 68(11), 1723–1732.

Leo, R.J. (1996). Movement disorders associated with the serotonin selective reuptake inhibitors. *Journal of Clinical Psychiatry*, 57(10), 449–454.

Leo, R.J., Lichter, D.G. and Hershey, L.A. (1995). Parkinsonism associated with fluoxetine and cimetidine: A case report. *Journal of Geriatric Psychiatry and Neurology*, 8(4), 231–233.

Lepine, J.P., Altamura, C., Ansseau, M., *et al.* (2001). Tianeptine and paroxetine in major depressive disorder, with a special focus on the anxious component in depression: An international, 6-week double-blind study dagger. *Human Psychopharmacology*, 16(3), 219–227.

Lepine, J.P., Caillard, V., Bisserbe, J.C., *et al.* (2004). A randomized, placebo-controlled trial of sertraline for prophylactic treatment of highly recurrent major depressive disorder. *American Journal of Psychiatry*, 161(5), 836–842.

Lesaca, T.G. (1996). Sertraline and galactorrhea. *Journal of Clinical Psychopharmacology*, 16(4), 333–334.

Lesperance, F., Frasure-Smith, N., Koszycki, D., *et al.* (2007). Effects of citalopram and interpersonal psychotherapy on depression in patients with coronary artery disease: The Canadian Cardiac Randomized Evaluation of Antidepressant and Psychotherapy Efficacy (CREATE) trial. *Journal of the American Medical Association*, 297(4), 367–379.

Lesperance, F., Frasure-Smith, N., Laliberte, M.A., *et al.* (2003). An open-label study of nefazodone treatment of major depression in patients with congestive heart failure. *Canadian Journal of Psychiatry*, 48(10), 695–701.

Letizia, C., Kapik, B. and Flanders, W.D. (1996). Suicidal risk during controlled clinical investigations of fluvoxamine. *Journal of Clinical Psychiatry*, 57(9), 415–21.

Levenson, J.L. (1999). Prolonged QT interval after trazodone overdose. *American Journal of Psychiatry*, 156(6), 969–970.

Levenson, J.L. and Fallon, H.J. (1993). Fluoxetine treatment of depression caused by interferon-alpha. *American Journal of Gastroenterology*, 88(5), 760–761.

Levin, O.S. (2007). Coaxil (tianeptine) in the treatment of depression in Parkinson's disease. *Neuroscience and Behavioral Physiology*, 37(4), 419–424.

Levine, L.R., Enas, G.G., Thompson, W.L., *et al.* (1989). Use of fluoxetine: A selective serotonin reuptake inhibitor, in the treatment of obesity. *International Journal of Obesity*, 13, 635–645.

Levine, L.R., Rosenblatt, S. and Bosomworth, J. (1987). Use of a serotonin re-uptake inhibitor, fluoxtine, in the treatment of obesity. *International Journal of Obesity*, 11(Suppl 3), 163–170.

Levinson-Castiel, R., Merlob, P., Linder, N., *et al.* (2006). Neonatal abstinence syndrome after in utero exposure to selective serotonin reuptake inhibitors in term infants. *Archives of Pediatric and Adolescent Medicine*, 160(2), 173–176.

Levkovitz, Y., Caftori, R., Avital, A. and Richter-Levin, G. (2002). The SSRIs drug Fluoxetine, but not the noradrenergic tricyclic drug Desipramine, improves memory performance during acute major depression. *Brain Research Bulletin*, 58(4), 345–350.

Levsky, M.E. and Schwartz, J.B. (1998). Sertraline-induced hyponatremia in an older patient. *Journal of the American Geriatric Society*, 46(12), 1582–1583.

Levy, N.B., Blumenfield, M., Beasley, C.M. Jr., *et al.* (1996). Fluoxetine in depressed patients with renal failure and in depressed patients with normal kidney function. *General Hospital Psychiatry*, 18(1), 8–13.

Limke, K.K., Shelton, A.R. and Elliott, E.S. (2002). Fluvoxamine interaction with warfarin. *Annals of Pharmacotherapy*, 36(12), 1890–1892.

Lingam, V.R., Lazarus, L.W., Groves, L. and Oh, S.H. (1988). Methylphenidate in treating post*Stroke* depression. *Journal of Clinical Psychiatry*, 49(4), 151–153.

Lipinski, J.F. Jr., Mallya, G., Zimmerman, P. and Pope, H.G. Jr. (1989). Fluoxetine-induced akathisia: Clinical and theoretical implications. *Journal of Clinical Psychiatry*, 50(9), 339–342.

Lippmann, S., Bedford, P., Manshadi, M. and Mather, S. (1983). Trazodone cardiotoxicity. *American Journal of Psychiatry*, 140(10), 1383.

Little, K.Y. (1993). d-Amphetamine versus methylphenidate effects in depressed inpatients. *Journal of Clinical Psychiatry*, 54(9), 349–355.

Liu, B.A., Mittmann, N., Knowles, S.R. and Shear, N.H. (1996). Hyponatremia and the syndrome of inappropriate secretion of antidiuretic hormone associated with the use of selective serotonin reuptake inhibitors: A review of spontaneous reports. *Canadian Medical Association Journal*, 155(5), 519–527.

Liu, Z.Q., Cheng, Z.N., Huang, S.L., *et al.* (2001). Effect of the CYP2C19 oxidation polymorphism on fluoxetine metabolism in Chinese healthy subjects. *British Journal of Clinical Pharmacology*, 52(1), 96–99.

Llerena, A., Dorado, P., Berecz, R., *et al.* (2004). Effect of CYP2D6 and CYP2C9 genotypes on fluoxetine and norfluoxetine plasma concentrations during steady-state conditions. *European Journal of Clinical Pharmacology*, 59(12), 869–873.

Lobbezoo, F., van Denderen, R.J., Verheij, J.G. and Naeije, M. (2001). Reports of SSRI-associated bruxism in the family physician's office. *Journal of Orofacial Pain*, 15(4), 340–346.

Loebstein, R. and Koren, G. (1997). Pregnancy outcome and neurodevelopment of children exposed in utero to psychoactive drugs: The Motherisk experience. *Journal of Psychiatry and Neuroscience*, 22(3), 192–196.

Longstreth, G.F. and Hershman, J. (1985). Trazodone-induced hepatotoxicity and leukonychia. *Journal of the American Academy of Dermatology*, 13(1), 149–150.

Loo, H., Hale, A. and D'haenen, H. (2002). Determination of the dose of agomelatine, a melatoninergic agonist and selective 5-HT(2C) antagonist, in the treatment of major depressive disorder: A placebo-controlled dose range study. *International Clinical Psychopharmacology*, 17(5), 239–247.

Loo, H., Saiz-Ruiz, J., Costa E Silva, J.A., *et al.* (2001). Efficacy and safety of tianeptine in the treatment of depressive disorders in comparison with fluoxetine. *Human Psychopharmacology*, 16(S1), S31–S38.

Loo, H., Saiz-Ruiz, J., Costa e Silva, J.A., *et al.* (1999). Efficacy and safety of tianeptine in the treatment of depressive disorders in comparison with fluoxetine. *Journal of Affective Disorders*, 56(2–3), 109–118.

Louik, C., Lin, A.E., Werler, M.M., *et al.* (2007). First-trimester use of selective serotonin-reuptake inhibitors and the risk of birth defects. *New England Journal of Medicine*, 356(26), 2675–2683.

Lowenthal, M.N. (1999). Sertraline-induced hyponatremia in an older patient. *Journal of the American Geriatric Society*, 47(10), 1274.

Lustman, P.J., Clouse, R.E., Nix, B.D., *et al.* (2006). Sertraline for prevention of depression recurrence in diabetes mellitus: A randomized, double-blind, placebo-controlled trial. *Archives of General Psychiatry*, 63(5), 521–529.

Lustman, P.J., Freedland, K.E., Griffith, L.S. and Clouse, R.E. (2000). Fluoxetine for depression in diabetes: A randomized double-blind placebo-controlled trial. *Diabetes Care*, 23(5), 618–623.

Lydiatt, W.M., Denman, D., McNeilly, D.P., *et al.* (2008). A randomized, placebo-controlled trial of citalopram for the prevention of major depression during treatment for head and neck cancer. *Archives of Otolaryngology — Head and Neck Surgergy*, 134(5), 528–535.

Lyketsos, C.G., DelCampo, L., Steinberg, M., *et al.* (2003). Treating depression in Alzheimer disease: Efficacy and safety of sertraline therapy, and the benefits of depression reduction: The DIADS. *Archives of General Psychiatry*, 60(7), 737–746.

Lyliard, R.B., Stahl, S.M., Hertzman, M. and Harrison, W.M. (1997). A double-blind, placebo-controlled study comparing the effects of sertraline versus amitriptyline in the treatment of major depression. *Journal of Clinical Psychiatry*, 58(11), 484–491.

Maany, I. and Dhopesh, V. (1990). Akathisia and fluoxetine. *Journal of Clinical Psychiatry*, 51(5), 210–212.

Macher, J.P. and Mirabaud, C. (1992). A double-blind comparison of moclobemide and amineptine in the treatment of depressed outpatients. *Psychopharmacology*, 106 Suppl, S116–117.

Maes, M., Song, C., Lin, A.H., *et al.* (1999). Negative immunoregulatory effects of antidepressants: Inhibition of interferon-gamma and stimulation of interleukin-10 secretion. *Neuropsychopharmacology*, 20(4), 370–379.

Maes, M., Van de Vyvere, J., Vandoolaeghe, E., *et al.* (1996). Alterations in iron metabolism and the erythron in major depression: Further evidence for a chronic inflammatory process. *Journal of Affective Disorders*, 40(1–2), 23–33.

Magai, C., Kennedy, G., Cohen, C.I. and Gomberg, D. (2000). A controlled clinical trial of sertraline in the treatment of depression in nursing home patients with late-stage Alzheimer's disease. *American Journal of Geriatric Psychiatry*, 8(1), 66–74.

Maggi, L., Palma, E., Miledi, R. and Eusebi, F. (1998). Effects of fluoxetine on wild and mutant neuronal alpha 7 nicotinic receptors. *Molecular Psychiatry*, 3(4), 350–355.

Maggio, R., Scarselli, M., Novi, F., *et al.* (2003). Potent activation of dopamine D3/D2 heterodimers by the antiparkinsonian agents, S32504, pramipexole and ropinirole. *Journal of Neurochemistry*, 87(3), 631–641.

Maheaux, P., Ducros, F., Bourque, J., *et al.* (1997). Fluoxetine improves insulin sensitivity in obese patients with non-insulin-dependant diabetes mellitus independently of weight loss. *International Journal of Obesity and Related Metabolic Disorders*, 21(2), 97–102.

Mander, A., McCausland, M., Workman, B., *et al.* (1994). Fluoxetine induced dyskinesia. *Australian and New Zealand Journal of Psychiatry*, 28(2), 328–330.

Marar, I.E., Towers, A.L., Mulsant, B.H., *et al.* (2000). Effect of paroxetine on plasma vasopressin and water load testing in elderly individuals. *Journal of Geriatric Psychiatry and Neurology*, 13(4), 212–216.

Marchesi, C., Caccherininelli, A., Rossi, A. and Maggini, C. (1998). Is anxious-agitated major depresion responsive to fluoxetine? A double-blind, comparison with amitriptyline. *Pharmacopsychiatry*, 31, 216–221.

Marcoli, M., Maura, G., Tortarolo, M. and Raiteri, M. (1998). Trazodone is a potent agonist at 5-HT2C receptors mediating inhibition of the N-methyl-D-aspartate/nitric oxide/cyclic GMP pathway in rat cerebellum. *Journal of Pharmacology and Experimental Therapeutics*, 285(3), 983–986.

Margolese, H.C. and Chouinard, G. (2000). Serotonin syndrome from addition of low-dose trazodone to nefazodone. *American Journal of Psychiatry*, 157(6), 1022.

Marik, P.E., van Heerden, W. and Steenkamp, V. (1990). Fluoxetine-induced syndrome of inappropriate antidiuretic hormone excretion. *South African Medical Journal*, 78(12), 760–761.

Marino, S., Sessa, E., Di Lorenzo, G., *et al.* (2008). Sertraline in the treatment of depressive disorders in patients with Parkinson's disease. *Neurological Sciences*, 29(6), 391–395.

Markowitz, J.S., DeVane, C.L., Liston, H.L. and Montgomery, S.A. (2000). An assessment of selective serotonin reuptake inhibitor discontinuation symptoms with citalopram. *International Clinical Psychopharmacology*, 15(6), 329–333.

Marnata, J.B., Lamblin, G. and Gineston, J.L. (1991). Fulminant hepatitis probably induced by medifoxamine (Cledial). *Gastroenterol Clinical Biology*, 15(8–9), 659–660.

Martenyi, F., Brown, E.B., Zhang, H., *et al.* (2002). Fluoxetine v. placebo in prevention of relapse in post-traumatic stress disorder.*British Journal of Psychiatry*, 181, 315–320.

Martenyi, F. and Soldatenkova, V. (2006). Fluoxetine in the acute treatment and relapse prevention of combat-related post-traumatic stress disorder: Analysis of the veteran group of a placebo-controlled, randomized clinical trial. *European Neuropsychopharmacology*, 16(5), 340–349.

Martin, K.A., Krahn, L.E., Balan, V. and Rosati, M.J. (2007). Selective serotonin reuptake inhibitors in the context of hepatitis C infection: Reexamining the risks of bleeding.*Journal of Clinical Psychiatry*, 68(7), 1024–1026.

Masand, P.S. and Gupta, S. (1999). Selective serotonin-reuptake inhibitors: An update. *Harvard Review of Psychiatry*, 7(2), 69–84.

Masand, P., Gupta, S. and Dewan, M. (1991a). Suicidal ideation related to fluoxetine treatment. *New England Journal of Medicine*, 324(6), 420.

Masand, P., Murray, G.B. and Pickett, P. (1991b). Psychostimulants in post-stroke depression. *Journal of Neuropsychiatry and Clinical Neurosciences*, 3(1), 23–27.

Masand, P., Pickett, P. and Murray, G.B. (1991c). Psychostimulants for secondary depression in medical illness. *Psychosomatics*, 32(2), 203–208.

Massana, J. (1998). Reboxetine versus fluoxetine: An overview of efficacy and tolerability. *Journal of Clinical Psychiatry*, 59(Suppl 14), 8–10.

Massana, J., Moller, H.J., Burrows, G.D. and Montenegro, R.M. (1999). Reboxetine: A double-blind comparison with fluoxetine in major depressive disorder. *International Clinical Psychopharmacology*, 14(2), 73–80.

Mattox, J.H., Buckman, M.T., Bernstein, J., *et al.* (1986). Dopamine agonists for reducing depression associated with hyperprolactinemia. *Journal of Reproductive Medicine*, 31(8), 694–698.

Maura, G., Marcoli, M., Pepicelli, O., *et al.* (2000). Serotonin inhibition of the NMDA receptor/nitric oxide/cyclic GMP pathway in human neocortex slices: Involvement of 5-HT(2C) and 5-HT(1A) receptors. *British Journal of Pharmacology*, 130(8), 1853–1858.

Mauri, M.C., Laini, V., Cerveri, G., *et al.* (2002). Clinical outcome and tolerability of sertraline in major depression: A study with plasma levels. *Progress in Neuropsychopharmacology and Biological Psychiatry*, 26(3), 597–601.

McCowen, K.C., Garber, J.R. and Spark, R. (1997). Elevated serum thyrotropin in thyroxine-treated patients with hypothyroidism given sertraline. *New England Journal of Medicine*, 337(14), 1010–1011.

McCracken, J. and Kosanin, R. (1984). Trazodone administration during ECT associated with cardiac conduction abnormality. *American Journal of Psychiatry*, 141(11), 1488–1489.

McCue, R.E. and Joseph, M. (2001). Venlafaxine- and trazodone-induced serotonin syndrome. *American Journal of Psychiatry*, 158(12), 2088–2089.

McElroy, S., Young, A.H., Carlsson, A., *et al.* (2008). A double-blind, placebo-controlled study with acute and continuation phase of quetiapine and paroxetine in adults with bipolar depression (Embolden II). Annual Meeting of the Association of European Psychiatrists (AEP).

McFarlane, A., Kamath, M.V., Fallen, E.L., *et al.* (2001). Effect of sertraline on the recovery rate of cardiac autonomic function in depressed patients after acute myocardial infarction. *American Heart Journal*, 142(4), 617–623.

McGrath, P.J., Stewart, J.W., Quitkin, F.M., *et al.* (2006). Predictors of relapse in a prospective study of fluoxetine treatment of major depression. *American Journal of Psychiatry*, 163(9), 1542–1548.

McGrath, P.J., Stewart, J.W., Quitkin, F.M., *et al.* (1994). Gepirone treatment of atypical depression: Preliminary evidence of serotonergic involvement. *Journal of Clinical Psychopharmacology*, 14(5), 347–352.

Meltzer, H.Y., Young, M., Metz, J., *et al.* (1979). Extrapyramidal side effects and increased serum prolactin following fluoxetine, a new antidepressant. *Journal of Neural Transmission*, 45(2), 165–175.

Mendis, N., Hanwella, D.R., Weerasinghe, C., *et al.* (1989). A double-blind comparative study: Amineptine (Survector 100) versus imipramine. *Clinical Neuropharmacology*, 12(Suppl 2), S58–65.

Menza, M.A. (1986). Withdrawal syndrome in a depressed patient treated with trazodone. *American Journal of Psychiatry*, 143(9), 1195.

Menza, M., Defronzo Dobkin, R., Marin, H., *et al.* (2009). A controlled trial of antidepressants in patients with Parkinson disease and depression. *Neurology*, 72(10), 886–892.

Mercke, Y., Sheng, H., Khan, T. and Lippmann, S. (2000). Hair loss in psychopharmacology. *Annals of Clinical Psychiatry*, 12(1), 35–42.

Merlob, P., Stahl, B. and Sulkes, J. (2004). Paroxetine during breast-feeding: Infant weight gain and maternal adherence to counsel. *European Journal of Pediatry*, 163(3), 135–139.

Meyer, J.H., Cho, R., Kennedy, S. and Kapur, S. (1999). The effects of single dose nefazodone and paroxetine upon 5-HT2A binding potential in humans using [18F]-setoperone PET. *Psychopharmacology*, 144(3), 279–281.

Meyer, J.H., Wilson, A.A., Ginovart, N., *et al.* (2001). Occupancy of serotonin transporters by paroxetine and citalopram during treatment of depression: A [(11)C]DASB PET imaging study. *American Journal of Psychiatry*, 158(11), 1843–1849.

Meyer, J.H., Wilson, A.A., Sagrati, S., *et al.* (2004). Serotonin transporter occupancy of five selective serotonin reuptake inhibitors at different doses: An [11C]DASB positron emission tomography study. *American Journal of Psychiatry*, 161(5), 826–835.

Meyers, B.S., Flint, A.J., Rothschild, A.J., *et al.* (2009). A double-blind randomized controlled trial of olanzapine plus sertraline vs olanzapine plus placebo for psychotic depression: The study of pharmacotherapy of psychotic depression (STOP-PD). *Archives of General Psychiatry*, 66(8), 838–847.

Meyers, S. (2000). Use of neurotransmitter precursors for treatment of depression. *Alternative Medicine Review*, 5(1), 64–71.

Michalets, E.L. and Williams, C.R. (2000). Drug interactions with cisapride: Clinical implications. *Clinical Pharmacokinetics*, 39(1), 49–75.

Michelson, D., Amsterdam, J.D., Quitkin, F.M., *et al.* (1999). Changes in weight during a 1-year trial of fluoxetine. *American Journal of Psychiatry*, 156(8), 1170–1176.

Michelson, D., Fava, M., Amsterdam, J., *et al.* (2000a). Interruption of selective serotonin reuptake inhibitor treatment. Double-blind, placebo-controlled trial. *British Journal of Psychiatry*, 176, 363–368.

Michelson, D., Amsterdam, J., Apter, J., *et al.* (2000b). Hormonal markers of stress response following interruption of selective serotonin reuptake inhibitor treatment. *Psychoneuroendocrinology*, 25(2), 169–177.

Michelson, D., Page, S.W., Casey, R., *et al.* (1994). An eosinophilia-myalgia syndrome related disorder associated with exposure to L-5-hydroxytryptophan. *Journal of Rheumatology*, 21(12), 2261– 2265.

Michelson, D., Pollack, M., Lydiard, R.B., *et al.* (1999). Continuing treatment of panic disorder after acute response: Randomised, placebo-controlled trial with fluoxetine. The Fluoxetine Panic Disorder Study Group. *British Journal of Psychiatry*, 174, 213–218.

Mihara, K., Kondo, T., Suzuki, A., *et al.* (2001). Effects of genetic polymorphism of CYP1A2 inducibility on the steady-state plasma concentrations of trazodone and its active metabolite m-chlorophenylpiperazine in depressed Japanese patients. *Pharmacology and Toxicology*, 88(5), 267–270.

Mihara, K., Otani, K., Suzuki, A., *et al.* (1997). Relationship between the CYP2D6 genotype and the steady-state plasma concentrations of trazodone and its active metabolite m-chlorophenylpiperazine. *Psychopharmacology*, 133(1), 95–98.

Millan, M.J., Gobert, A., Lejeune, F., *et al.* (2003). The novel melatonin agonist agomelatine (S20098) is an antagonist at 5-hydroxytryptamine2c receptors, blockade of which enhances the activity of frontocortical dopaminergic and adrenergic pathways. *Journal of Pharmacology and Experimental Therapeutics*, 306(3), 954–964.

Miller, D.K., Wong, E.H., Chesnut, M.D. and Dwoskin, L.P. (2002). Reboxetine: Functional inhibition of monoamine transporters and nicotinic acetylcholine receptors. *Journal of Pharmacology and Experimental Therapeutics*, 302(2), 687–695.

Miller, M. (2002). Depression after cardiac transplant treated with interpersonal psychotherapy and paroxetine. *American Journal of Psychotherapy*, 56(4), 555–561.

Milnes, J.T., Crociani, O., Arcangeli, A., *et al.* (2003). Blockade of HERG potassium currents by fluvoxamine: Incomplete attenuation by S6 mutations at F656 or Y652. *British Journal of Pharmacology*, 139(5), 887–898.

Miranda, H., Ortiz, G., Figueroa, S., *et al.* (2001). Depression scores following migraine treatment in patients attending a specialized center for headache and neurology. *Headache*, 41(7), 680–684.

Misra, M., Papakostas, G.I. and Klibanski, A. (2004). Effects of psychiatric disorders and psychotropic medications on prolactin and bone metabolism. *Journal of Clinical Psychiatry*, 65(12), 1607–1618.

Misri, S., Kim, J., Riggs, K.W. and Kostaras, X. (2000). Paroxetine levels in postpartum depressed women, breast milk, and infant serum. *Journal of Clinical Psychiatry*, 61(11), 828–832.

Mischoulon, D., Dougherty, D.D., Bottonari, K.A., *et al.* (2002). An open pilot study of nefazodone in depression with anger attacks: Relationship between clinical response and receptor binding. *Psychiatry Research*, 116(3), 151–161.

Mockenhaupt, M., Viboud, C., Dunant, A., *et al.* (2008). Stevens–Johnson syndrome and toxic epidermal necrolysis: Assessment of medication risks with emphasis on recently marketed drugs. The EuroSCAR-Study.*Journal of Investigative Dermatology*, 128(1), 35–44.

Mohr, D.C., Boudewyn, A.C., Goodkin, D.E., *et al.* (2001a). Comparative outcomes for individual cognitive-behavior therapy, supportive-expressive group psychotherapy, and sertraline for the treatment of depression in multiple sclerosis. *Journal of Consulting and Clinical Psychology*, 69(6), 942–949.

Mohr, D.C., Goodkin, D.E., Islar, J., *et al.* (2001b). Treatment of depression is associated with suppression of nonspecific and antigen-specific T(H)1 responses in multiple sclerosis. *Archives of Neurology*, 58(7), 1081–1086.

Mohr, D.C., Hart, S.L. and Goldberg, A. (2003). Effects of treatment for depression on fatigue in multiple sclerosis. *Psychosomatic Medicine*, 65(4), 542–547.

Montalbetti, D.J. and Zis, A.P. (1988). Cholinergic rebound following trazodone withdrawal? *Journal of Clinical Psychopharmacology*, 8(1), 73.

Montejo, A.L., Llorca, G., Izquierdo, J.A. and Rico-Villademoros, F. (2001). Incidence of sexual dysfunction associated with antidepressant agents: A prospective multicenter study of 1022 outpatients. Spanish Working Group for the Study of Psychotropic-Related Sexual Dysfunction. *Journal of Clinical Psychiatry*, 62(Suppl 3), 10–21.

Montastruc, J.L., Pelat, M., Verwaerde, P., *et al.* (1998). Fluoxetine in orthostatic hypotension of Parkinson's disease: A clinical and experimental pilot study. *Fundamental and Clinical Pharmacology*, 12(4), 398–402.

Monteleone, P., Catapano, F., Tortorella, A., *et al.* (1995). Plasma melatonin and cortisol circadian patterns in patients with obsessive-compulsive disorder before and after fluoxetine treatment. *Psychoneuroendocrinology*, 20(7), 763–770.

Montgomery, S.A., Dufour, H., Brion, S., *et al.* (1988). The prophylactic efficacy of fluoxetine in unipolar depression. *British Journal of Psychiatry Supplement*, (3), 69–76.

Montgomery, S.A. and Dunbar, G. (1993). Paroxetine is better than placebo in relapse prevention and the prophylaxis of recurrent depression. *International Clinical Psychopharmacology*, 8(3), 189–195.

Montgomery, S.A., Dunner, D.L. and Dunbar, G.C. (1995). Reduction of suicidal thoughts with paroxetine in comparison with reference antidepressants and placebo. *European Neuropsychopharmacology*, 5(1), 5–13.

Montgomery, S., Ferguson, J.M. and Schwartz, G.E. (2003). The antidepressant efficacy of reboxetine in patients with severe depression. *Journal of Clinical Psychopharmacology*, 23(1), 45–50.

Montgomery, S.A., Kennedy, S.H., Burrows, G.D., *et al.* (2004). Absence of discontinuation symptoms with agomelatine and occurrence of discontinuation symptoms with paroxetine: A randomized, double-blind, placebo-controlled discontinuation study. *International Clinical Psychopharmacology*, 19(5), 271–380.

Montgomery, S.A., Nil, R., Durr-Pal, N., *et al.* (2005). A 24-week randomized, double-blind, placebo-controlled study of escitalopram for the prevention of generalized social anxiety disorder. *Journal of Clinical Psychiatry*, 66(10), 1270–1278.

Montgomery, S.A., Olie, J.P., Ahokas, A. and Kennedy, S.H. (2006). Antidepressant efficacy of agomelatine in MDD: Meta-analysis of three pivotal studies. *International Journal of Neuropsychopharmacology*, 9(s1), s1–s309.

Montgomery, S.A., Rasmussen, J.G. and Tanghoj, P. (1993). A 24-week study of 20 mg citalopram, 40 mg citalopram, and placebo in the prevention of relapse of major depression. *International Clinical Psychopharmacology*, 8(3), 181–188.

Moon, C.A.L., Jago, L.W., Wood, K. and Doogan, D.P. (1994). A double-blind comparison of sertraline and clomipramine in the treatment of major depressive disorder and associated anxiety in general practice. *Journal of Psychopharmacology*, 8(3), 171–176.

Moorman, P.G., Berchuck, A., Calingaert, B., *et al.* (2005). Antidepressant medication use [corrected] and risk of ovarian cancer. *Obstetrics and Gynecology*, 105(4), 725–730.

Moorman, P.G., Grubber, J.M., Millikan, R.C. and Newman, B. (2003). Antidepressant medications and their association with invasive breast cancer and carcinoma *in situ* of the breast. *Epidemiology*, 14(3), 307–314.

Moosa, M.Y., Panz, V.R., Jeenah, F.Y. and Joffe, B.I. (2003). African women with depression: The effect of imipramine and fluoxetine on body mass index and leptin secretion. *Journal of Clinical Psychopharmacology*, 23(6), 549–552.

Moreau, X., Azorin, J.M., Lejeune, P.J. and Jeanningros, R. (2000). Red blood cell triiodothyronine uptake in unipolar major depression: Effect of a chronic antidepressant treatment. *Progress in Neuropsychopharmacology and Biological Psychiatry*, 24(1), 23–35.

Morrison, J., Remick, R.A., Leung, M., *et al.* (2001). Galactorrhea induced by paroxetine. *Canadian Journal of Psychiatry*, 46(1), 88–89.

Morrow, G.R., Hickok, J.T., Roscoe, J.A., *et al.* (2003). Differential effects of paroxetine on fatigue and depression: A randomized, double-blind trial from the university of Rochester cancer center community clinical oncology program. *Journal of Clinical Oncology*, 21(24), 4635–4641.

Morrow, G.R., Hickok, J.T. and Rosenthal, S.N. (1995). Progress in reducing nausea and emesis. Comparisons of ondansetron (Zofran), granisetron (Kytril), and tropisetron (Navoban). *Cancer*, 76(3), 343–357.

Moses-Kolko, E.L., Bogen, D., Perel, J., *et al.* (2005). Neonatal signs after late in utero exposure to serotonin reuptake inhibitors: Literature review and implications for clinical applications. *Journal of the American Medical Association*, 293(19), 2372–2383.

Mosholder, A.D. and Willy, M. (2006). Suicidal adverse events in pediatric randomized, controlled clinical trials of antidepressant drugs are associated with active drug treatment: A meta-analysis. *Journal of Child and Adolescent Psychopharmacology*, 16(1–2), 25–32.

Mostert, J.P., Admiraal-Behloul, F., Hoogduin, J.M., *et al.* (2008). Effects of fluoxetine on disease activity in relapsing multiple sclerosis: A double-blind, placebo-controlled, exploratory study. *Journal of Neurology, Neurosurgery, and Psychiatry*, 79(9), 1027–1031.

Movig, K.L., Janssen, M.W., de Waal Malefijt, J., *et al.* (2003). Relationship of serotonergic antidepressants and need for blood transfusion in orthopedic surgical patients. *Archives of Internal Medicine*, 163(19), 2354–2358.

Muck-Seler, D., Pivac, N., Sagud, M., *et al.* (2002). The effects of paroxetine and tianeptine on peripheral biochemical markers in major depression. *Progress in Neuropsychopharmacology and Biological Psychiatry*, 26(7–8), 1235–1243.

Muller, J.C., Pryer, W.W., Gibbons, J.E. and Orgain, E.S. (1955). Depression and anxiety occurring during Rauwolfia therapy. *Journal of the American Medical Association*, 159, 836–839.

Murray, V., von Arbin, M., Bartfai, A., *et al.* (2005). Double-blind comparison of sertraline and placebo in *Stroke* patients with minor depression and less severe major depression. *Journal of Clinical Psychiatry*, 66(6), 708–716.

Musselman, D.L., Lawson, D.H., Gumnick, J.F., *et al.* (2001). Paroxetine for the prevention of depression induced by high-dose interferon alfa. *New England Journal of Medicine*, 344(13), 961–966.

Musselman, D.L., Somerset, W.I., Guo, Y., *et al.* (2006). A double-blind, multicenter, parallel-group study of paroxetine, desipramine, or placebo in breast cancer patients (stages I, II, III, and IV) with major depression. *Journal of Clinical Psychiatry*, 67(2), 288–396.

Muzykewicz, D.A., Newberry, P., Danforth, N., *et al.* (2007). Psychiatric comorbid conditions in a clinic population of 241 patients with tuberous sclerosis complex.*Epilepsy and Behavior*, 11(4), 506–513.

Nakayama, T., Suhara, T., Okubo, Y., *et al.* (2002). *In vivo* drug action of tandospirone at 5-HT1A receptor examined using positron emission tomography and neuroendocrine response. *Psychopharmacology*, 165(1), 37–42.

Nappi, G., Sandrini, G., Granella, F., *et al.* (1990). A new 5-HT2 antagonist (ritanserin) in the treatment of chronic headache with depression. A double-blind study vs amitriptyline. *Headache*, 30(7), 439–444.

Naranjo, C.A., Lane, D., Ho-Asjoe, M. and Lanctot, K.L. (1990). A Bayesian assessment of idiosyncratic adverse reactions to new drugs: Guillain–Barre syndrome and zimeldine. *Journal of Clinical Pharmacology*, 30(2), 174–180.

Narushima, K., Kosier, J.T. and Robinson, R.G. (2002). Preventing post-stroke depression: A 12-week double-blind randomized treatment trial and 21-month follow-up. *Journal of Nervous and Mental Disease*, 190(5), 296–303.

Navari, R.M., Brenner, M.C. and Wilson, M.N. (2008). Treatment of depressive symptoms in patients with early stage breast cancer undergoing adjuvant therapy. *Breast Cancer Research and Treatment*, 112(1), 197–201.

Neely, J.L. (1998). Tonic clonic seizures and tachycardia induced by fluoxetine (Prozac) overdose. *West Virginia Medical Journal*, 94(5), 283–285.

Nemeroff, C.B., Evans, D.L., Gyulai, L., *et al.* (2001). Double-blind, placebo-controlled comparison of imipramine and paroxetine in the treatment of bipolar depression. *American Journal of Psychiatry*, 158(6), 906–912.

Newton, R.E., Marunycz, J.D., Alderdice, M.T. and Napoliello, M.J. (1986). Review of the side-effect profile of buspirone. *American Journal of Medicine*, 80(3B), 17–21.

Nierenberg, A.A. and Keck, P.E. Jr. (1989). Management of monoamine oxidase inhibitor-associated insomnia with trazodone. *Journal of Clinical Psychopharmacology*, 9(1), 42–45.

Nikisch, G., Mathe, A.A., Czernik, A., *et al.* (2004). Stereoselective metabolism of citalopram in plasma and cerebrospinal fluid of depressive patients: Relationship with 5-HIAA in CSF and clinical response. *Journal of Clinical Psychopharmacology*, 24(3), 283–290.

Nisijima, K., Shimizu, M., Abe, T. and Ishiguro, T. (1996). A case of serotonin syndrome induced by concomitant treatment with low-dose trazodone and amitriptyline and lithium. *International Clinical Psychopharmacology*, 11(4), 289–290.

Nonacs, R. and Cohen, L.S. (2003). Assessment and treatment of depression during pregnancy: An update. *Psychiatric Clinics of North America*, 26(3), 547–562.

Nordin, C., Siwers, B. and Bertilsson, L. (1981). Bromocriptine treatment of depressive disorders. Clinical and biochemical effects. *Acta Psychiatrica Scandinavica*, 64(1), 25–33.

Nordeng, H., Lindemann, R., Perminov, K.V. and Reikvam, A. (2001). Neonatal withdrawal syndrome after in utero exposure to selective serotonin reuptake inhibitors. *Acta Paediatrica*, 90(3), 288–291.

Novotny, V. and Faltus, F. (2002). Tianeptine and fluoxetine in major depression: A 6-week randomised double-blind study. *Human Psychopharmacology*, 17(6), 299–303.

Nyth, A.L., Gottfries, C.G., Lyby, K., *et al.* (1992). A controlled multicenter clinical study of citalopram and placebo in elderly depressed patients with and without concomitant dementia. *Acta Psychiatrica Scandinavica*, 86(2), 138–145.

Oberlander, T.F., Misri, S., Fitzgerald, C.E., *et al.* (2004). Pharmacologic factors associated with transient neonatal symptoms following prenatal psychotropic medication exposure. *Journal of Clinical Psychiatry*, 65(2), 230–237.

O'Kane, M., Wiles, P.G. and Wales, J.K. (1994). Fluoxetine in the treatment of obese type 2 diabetic patients.*Diabetic Medicine*, 11, 105–110.

O'Rourke, D., Wurtman, J.J., Wurtman, R.J., *et al.* (1989). Treatment of seasonal depression with d-fenfluramine. *Journal of Clinical Psychiatry*, 50(9), 343–347.

Odeh, M., Beny, A. and Oliven, A. (2001). Severe symptomatic hyponatremia during citalopram therapy. *American Journal of the Medical Sciences*, 321(2), 159–160.

Ohara, K., Tanabu, S., Ishibashi, K., *et al.* (2003). CYP2D6*10 alleles do not determine plasma fluvoxamine concentration/dose ratio in Japanese subjects. *European Journal of Clinical Pharmacology*, 58(10), 659–661.

Oke, A., Adhiyaman, V., Aziz, K. and Ross, A. (2001). Dose-dependent seizure activity associated with fluoxetine therapy. *QJM: Monthly Journal of the Association of Physicians*, 94(2), 113–114.

Olie, P.J. and Kasper, S. (2007). Efficacy of agomelatine, a MT1/MT2 receptor agonist with 5-HT2C antagonistic properties, in major depressive disorder. *International Journal of Neuropsychopharmacology*, 10(5), 661–673.

Olin, J. and Masand, P. (1996). Psychostimulants for depression in hospitalized cancer patients. *Psychosomatics*, 37(1), 57–62.

Olivera, A.A. (1996). A case of paroxetine-induced akathisia. *Biological Psychiatry*, 39(10), 910.

Olivera, A.O. (1997). Sertraline and akathisia: Spontaneous resolution. *Biological Psychiatry*, 41(2), 241–242.

Ono, K., Iwanaga, Y., Mannami, T., *et al.* (2003). Epidemiological evidence of an association between SLC6A2 gene polymorphism and hypertension. *Hypertension Research*, 26(9), 685–689.

Opbroek, A., Delgado, P.L., Laukes, C., *et al.* (2002). Emotional blunting associated with SSRI-induced sexual dysfunction. Do SSRIs inhibit emotional responses? *International Journal of Neuropsychopharmacology*, 5(2), 147–151.

Opler, L.A. (1994). Sertraline and akathisia. *American Journal of Psychiatry*, 151(4), 620–621.

Oral, E.T., Taneli, B., Tunca, Z., *et al.* (2001). Efficacy and acceptability of tianeptine versus sertraline: A multicenter, double-blind, controlled study. *European Neuropsychopharmacology*, 11(3), S206.

Oren, D.A., Moul, D.E., Schwartz, P.J., *et al.* (1994). A controlled trial of levodopa plus carbidopa in the treatment of winter seasonal affective disorder: A test of the dopamine hypothesis. *Journal of Clinical Psychopharmacology*, 14(3), 196–200.

Oswald, P., Souery, D. and Mendlewicz, J. (2003). Fluvoxamine-induced hyperglycaemia in a diabetic patient with comorbid depression. *International Journal of Neuropsychopharmacology*, 6(1), 85–87.

Ota, H., Yamaguchi, Y., Yamaguchi, K., *et al.* (2008). Paroxetine-induced hyponatremia in an elderly man due to the syndrome of inappropriate secretion of antidiuretic hormone. *Nippon Ronen Igakkai Zasshi*, 45(1), 90–94.

Otani, K., Yasui, N., Kaneko, S., *et al.* (1995). Trazodone treatment increases plasma prolactin concentrations in depressed patients. *International Clinical Psychopharmacology*, 10(2), 115–117.

Ouellet, D., Hsu, A., Qian, J., *et al.* (1998). Effect of fluoxetine on pharmacokinetics of ritonavir. *Antimicrobial Agents and Chemotherapy*, 42(12), 3107–3112.

Owens, M.J., Knight, D.L. and Nemeroff, C.B. (2001). Second-generation SSRIs: Human monoamine transporter binding profile of escitalopram and R-fluoxetine. *Biological Psychiatry*, 50(5), 345–350.

Pace-Schott, E.F., Gersh, T., Silvestri, R., *et al.* (2001). SSRI treatment suppresses dream recall frequency but increases subjective dream intensity in normal subjects. *Journal of Sleep Research*, 10(2), 129–142.

Pae, C.U., Kim, Y.J., Won, W.Y., *et al.* (2004). Paroxetine in the treatment of depressed patients with haematological malignancy: An open-label study. *Human Psychopharmacology*, 19(1), 25–29.

Paes de Sousa, M. and Tropa, J. (1989). Evaluation of the efficacy of amineptine in a population of 1,229 depressed patients: Results of a multicenter study carried out by 135 general practitioners. *Clinical Neuropharmacology*, 12(Suppl 2), S77–86.

Page, R.L., Ruscin, J.M., Bainbridge, J.L. and Brieke, A.A. (2008). Restless legs syndrome induced by escitalopram: Case report and review of the literature. *Pharmacotherapy*, 28(2), 271–280.

Pai, V.B. and Kelly, M.W. (1996). Bruising associated with the use of fluoxetine. *Annals of Pharmacotherapy*, 30(7–8), 786–788.

Paile-Hyvärinen, M., Wahlbeck, K. and Eriksson, J.G. (2007). Quality of life and metabolic status in mildly depressed patients with type 2 diabetes treated with paroxetine: A double-blind randomised placebo controlled 6-month trial. *BioMedCentral Family Practice*, 8, 34.

Pancrazio, J.J., Kamatchi, G.L., Roscoe, A.K. and Lynch, C. 3rd. (1998). Inhibition of neuronal Na^+ channels by antidepressant drugs. *Journal of Pharmacology and Experimental Therapeutics*, 284(1), 208–214.

Pande, A.C., Birkett, M., Fechner-Bates, S., *et al.* (1996). Fluoxetine versus phenelzine in atypical depression. *Biological Psychiatry*, 40(10), 1017–1020.

Papakostas, G.I. (2007). Current limitations of antidepressant monotherapy: Tolerability.*Journal of Clinical Psychiatry*, 68(Suppl 10), 11–17.

Papakostas, G.I., Charles, D. and Fava, M. (in press). Are typical starting doses of the selective serotonin reuptake inhibitors sub-optimal? A meta-analysis of randomized, double-blind, placebo-controlled, dose-finding studies in major depressive disorder. *World Journal of Biological Psychiatry*.

Papakostas, G.I. and Fava, M. (2006a). A meta-analysis of clinical trials comparing moclobemide with selective serotonin reuptake inhibitors for the treatment of major depressive disorder. *Canadian Journal of Psychiatry*, 51(12), 783–790.

Papakostas, G.I. and Fava, M. (2006b). Does the probability of receiving placebo influence the likelihood of responding to placebo or clinical trial outcome? A meta-regression of double-blind, randomized clinical trials in MDD. *Neuropsychopharmacology*, 31(s1), s158.

Papakostas, G.I. and Fava, M. (2007). A meta-analysis of clinical trials comparing the serotonin (5HT)-2 receptor antagonists trazodone and nefazodone with a selective serotonin reuptake inhibitor for the treatment of major depressive disorder. *European Psychiatry*, 22(7), 444–447.

Papakostas, G.I., Nelson, J.C., Kasper, S. and Moller, H.J. (2008). A Meta-analysis of clinical trials comparing reboxetine, a norepinephrine reuptake inhibitor, with selective serotonin reuptake inhibitors for the treatment of major depressive disorder. *European Neuropsychopharmacology*, 18(2), 122–127.

Papakostas, G.I., Nutt, D.J., Hallett, L.A, *et al.* (2006a). Resolution of sleepiness and fatigue in the treatment of major depressive disorder: A comparison of bupropion and the selective serotonin reuptake inhibitors. *Biological Psychiatry*, 16(12), 1350–1355.

Papakostas, G.I., Miller, K.K., Petersen, T., *et al.* (2006b). Serum prolactin among outpatients with major depressive disorder during the acute phase of treatment with fluoxetine. *Journal of Clinical Psychiatry*, 67(6), 952–958.

Papakostas, G.I., Petersen, T., Montoya, H., *et al.* (2003). Treatment-related adverse events and outcome in a clinical trial of fluoxetine for depression. *Annals of Clinical Psychiatry*, 15(3–4), 187–192.

Papakostas, Y.G., Markianos, M., Zervas, I.M., *et al.* (2000). Administration of citalopram before ECT: Seizure duration and hormone responses. *Journal of Electroconvulsive Therapy*, 16(4), 356–360.

Papp, L.A. and Gorman, J.M. (1990). Suicidal preoccupation during fluoxetine treatment. *American Journal of Psychiatry*, 147(10), 1380–1381.

Pasini, A., Tortorella, A. and Gale, K. (1992). Anticonvulsant effect of intranigral fluoxetine. *Brain Research*, 593(2), 287–290.

Pastuszak, A., Schick-Boschetto, B., Zuber, C., *et al.* (1993). Pregnancy outcome following first-trimester exposure to fluoxetine (Prozac). *Journal of the American Medical Association*, 269(17), 2246–2248.

Patkar, A.A., Masand, P.S., Krulewicz, S., *et al.* (2007). A randomized, controlled, trial of controlled release paroxetine in fibromyalgia. *American Journal of Medicine*, 120(5), 448–454.

Pazzagli, M., Giovannini, M.G. and Pepeu, G. (1999). Trazodone increases extracellular serotonin levels in the frontal cortex of rats. *European Journal of Pharmacology*, 383(3), 249–257.

Pearson, K.H., Nonacs, R.M., Viguera, A.C., *et al.* (2007). Birth outcomes following prenatal exposure to antidepressants. *Journal of Clinical Psychiatry*, 68(8), 1284–1289.

Pedersen, A.G. (2006). Citalopram and suicidality in adult major depression and anxiety disorders. *Nordic Journal of Psychiatry*, 60(5), 392–399.

Pedersen, A.G. (2005). Escitalopram and suicidality in adult depression and anxiety. *International Clinical Psychopharmacology*, 20(3), 139–143.

Perazella, M.A. (2001). Pharmacologic options available to treat symptomatic intradialytic hypotension. *American Journal of Kidney Diseases*, 38(4 Suppl 4), S26–36.

Peabody, C.A. (1987). Trazodone withdrawal and formication. *Journal of Clinical Psychiatry*, 48(9), 385.

Perucca, E., Marchioni, E., Soragna, D. and Savoldi, F. (1997). Fluoxetine-induced movement disorders and deficient CYP2D6 enzyme activity. *Movement Disorders*, 12(4), 624–625.

Perugi, G., Toni, C., Ruffolo, G., *et al.* (2001). Adjunctive dopamine agonists in treatment-resistant bipolar II depression: An open case series. *Pharmacopsychiatry*, 34(4), 137–141.

Peter, H., Tabrizian, S. and Hand, I. (2000). Serum cholesterol in patients with obsessive-compulsive disorder during treatment with behavior therapy and SSRI or placebo. *International Journal of Psychiatry in Medicine*, 30(1), 27–39.

Peterson, M.C. (2001). Reversible galactorrhea and prolactin elevation related to fluoxetine use. *Mayo Clinic Proceedings*, 76(2), 215–216.

Petersen, T., Dording, C., Neault, N.B., *et al.* (2002). A survey of prescribing practices in the treatment of depression. *Progress in Neuropsychopharmacology Biological Psychiatry*, 26(1), 177–187.

Petracca, G.M., Chemerinski, E. and Starkstein, S.E. (2001). A double-blind, placebo-controlled study of fluoxetine in depressed patients with Alzheimer's disease. *International Psychogeriatrics*, 13(2), 233–240.

Petrakis, I., Carroll, K.M., Nich, C., *et al.* (1998). Fluoxetine treatment of depressive disorders in methadone-maintained opioid addicts. *Drug and Alcohol Dependence*, 50(3), 221–226.

Petty, K.J. (1996). Hyperglycemia associated with paroxetine. *Ann Intern Med*, 125(9), 782.

Pezzella, G., Moslinger-Gehmayr, R. and Contu, A. (2001). Treatment of depression in patients with breast cancer: A comparison between paroxetine and amitriptyline. *Breast Cancer Research and Treatment*, 70(1), 1–10.

Pickett, P., Masand, P. and Murray, G.B. (1990). Psychostimulant treatment of geriatric depressive disorders secondary to medical illness. *Journal of Geriatric Psychiatry and Neurology*, 3(3), 146–151.

Piercey, M.F. (1998). Pharmacology of pramipexole, a dopamine D3-preferring agonist useful in treating Parkinson's disease. *Clinical Neuropharmacology*, 21(3), 141–151.

Piercey, M.F., Smith, M.W. and Lum-Ragan, J.T. (1994). Excitation of noradrenergic cell firing by 5-hydroxytryptamine1A agonists correlates with dopamine antagonist properties. *Journal of Pharmacology and Experimental Therapeutics*, 268(3), 1297–1303.

Pigott, T.A., Prakash, A., Arnold, L.M., *et al.* (2007). Duloxetine versus escitalopram and placebo: An 8-month, double-blind trial in patients with major depressive disorder. *Current Medical and Research Opinion*, 23(6), 1303–1318.

Pigott, T.A., Seay, S.M. (1999). A review of the efficacy of selective serotonin reuptake inhibitors in obsessive-compulsive disorder. *Journal of Clinical Psychiatry*, 60(2), 101–106.

Piontek, C.M., Wisner, K.L., Perel, J.M. and Peindl, K.S. (2001). Serum fluvoxamine levels in breastfed infants. *Journal of Clinical Psychiatry*, 62(2), 111–113.

Pisani, F., Oteri, G., Costa, C., *et al.* (2002). Effects of psychotropic drugs on seizure threshold. *Drug Safety*, 25(2), 91–110.

Pjrek, E., Winkler, D., Konstantinidis, A., *et al.* (2007). Agomelatine in the treatment of seasonal affective disorder. *Psychopharmacology*, 190(4), 575–579.

Plaisant, F., Dommergues, M.A., Spedding, M., *et al.* (2003). Neuroprotective properties of tianeptine: Interactions with cytokines. *Neuropharmacology*, 44(6), 801–809.

Pohl, R., Balon, R., Jayaraman, A., *et al.* (2003). Effect of fluoxetine, pemoline and placebo on heart period and QT variability in normal humans. *Journal of Psychosomatic Research*, 55(3), 247–251.

Portilla-Botelho, M., Ortega-Carnicer, J., Gómez-Grande, M.L. and Martín-Rodríguez, C. (2008). Paroxetine-induced severe hyponatremic rhabdomyolisis. *Medicina Intensiva*, 32(7), 365–366.

Pollock, B.G., Bose, A., Li, D. and Gandhi, C. (2006). Escitalopram in the treatment of diabetic patients with MDD. *Neuropsychopharmacology*, 31(s1), s98.

Pollak, P.T., Mukherjee, S.D. and Fraser, A.D. (2001). Sertraline-induced hypoglycemia. *Annals of Pharmacotherapy*, 35(11), 1371–1374.

Pope, H.G. Jr., Keck, P.E. Jr., McElroy, S.L. and Hudson, J.I. (1989). A placebo-controlled study of trazodone in bulimia nervosa. *Journal of Clinical Psychopharmacology*, 9(4), 254–259.

Post, R.M., Altshuler, L.L., Leverich, G.S., *et al.* (2006). Mood switch in bipolar depression: Comparison of adjunctive venlafaxine, bupropion and sertraline. *British Journal of Psychiatry*, 189, 124–131.

Post, R.M., Gerner, R.H., Carman, J.S., *et al.* (1978). Effects of a dopamine agonist piribedil in depressed patients: Relationship of pretreatment homovanillic acid to antidepressant response. *Archives of General Psychiatry*, 35(5), 609–615.

Potter Van Loon, B.J. (1992). Fluoxetine increases insulin action in obese nondiabetic and in obese non-insulin-dependant diabetic individuals. *International Journal of Obesity*, 16, 79–85.

Prakash, O. and Dhar, V. (2008) Emergence of electric shock-like sensations on escitalopram discontinuation. *Journal Clinial Psychopharmacology*, 28(3), 359–360.

Prasher, V.P. (1993). Seizures associated with fluoxetine therapy. *Seizure*, 2(4), 315–317.

Prendiville, S. and Gale, K. (1993). Anticonvulsant effect of fluoxetine on focally evoked limbic motor seizures in rats. *Epilepsia*, 34(2), 381–384.

Preti, A. (2002). Tomoxetine (Eli Lilly & Co). *Current Opinion on Investigational Drugs*, 3(2), 272–277.

Price, L.H., Charney, D.S., Delgado, P.L. and Heninger, G.R. (1990). Fenfluramine augmentation in tricyclic-refractory depression. *Journal of Clinical Psychopharmacology*, 10(5), 312–317.

Priskorn, M., Sidhu, J.S., Larsen, F., *et al.* (1997). Investigation of multiple dose citalopram on the pharmacokinetics and pharmacodynamics of racemic warfarin. *British Journal of Clinical Pharmacology*, 44(2), 199–202.

Rabkin, J.G, Wagner, G.J. and Rabkin, R. (1999). Fluoxetine treatment for depression in patients with HIV and AIDS: A randomized, placebo-controlled trial. *American Journal of Psychiatry*, 156(1), 101–107.

Raeder, M.B., Bjelland, I., Emil Vollset, S. and Steen, V.M. (2006). Obesity, dyslipidemia, and diabetes with selective serotonin reuptake inhibitors: The Hordaland Health Study. *Journal of Clinical Psychiatry*, 67(12), 1974–1982.

Raison, C.L., Woolwine, B.J., Demetrashvili, M.F., *et al.* (2007). Paroxetine for prevention of depressive symptoms induced by interferon-alpha and ribavirin for hepatitis C. *Alimentary Pharmacology and Therapeutics*, 25(10), 1163–1174.

Rajagopalan, M. and Little, J. (1999). Discontinuation symptoms with nefazodone. *Australian and New Zealand Journal of Psychiatry*, 33(4), 594–597.

Raju, G.V., Kumar, T.C. and Khanna, S. (2000). Seizures associated with sertraline. *Canadian Journal of Psychiatry*, 45(5), 491.

Ramasubbu, R. (1999). Switching to moclobemide to reverse fluoxetine-induced sexual dysfunction in patients with depression. *Journal of Psychiatry and Neuroscience*, 24(1), 45–50.

Rampello, L., Chiechio, S., Raffaele, R., *et al.* (2002). The SSRI, citalopram, improves bradykinesia in patients with Parkinson's disease treated with L-dopa. *Clinical Neuropharmacology*, 25(1), 21–24.

Rampello, L., Nicoletti, G., Raffaele, R. and Drago, F. (1995). Comparative effects of amitriptyline and amineptine in patients affected by anxious depression. *Neuropsychobiology*, 31(3), 130–134.

Rampono, J., Kristensen, J.H., Hackett, L.P., *et al.* (2000). Citalopram and demethylcitalopram in human milk; distribution, excretion and effects in breast fed infants. *British Journal of Clinical Pharmacology*, 50(3), 263–268.

Ranieri, P., Franzoni, S. and Trabucchi, M. (2000). Reboxetine and hyponatremia. *New England Journal of Medicine*, 342(3), 215–216.

Rao, R. (1998). Serotonergic syndrome with trazodone. *Hosp Med*, 59(1), 79.

Rapaport, M.H., Bose, A. and Zheng, H. (2004). Escitalopram continuation treatment prevents relapse of depressive episodes. *Journal of Clinical Psychiatry*, 65(1), 44–49.

Rapaport, M.H., Endicott, J. and Clary, C.M. (2002). Posttraumatic stress disorder and quality of life: Results across 64 weeks of sertraline treatment. *Journal of Clinical Psychiatry*, 63(1), 59–65.

Rapaport, M.H., Lydiard, R.B., Pitts, C.D., *et al.* (2009). Low doses of controlled-release paroxetine in the treatment of late-life depression:

A randomized, placebo-controlled trial. *Journal of Clinical Psychiatry*, 70(1), 46–57.

Rapaport, M.H., Schneider, L.S., Dunner, D.L., *et al.* (2003). Efficacy of controlled-release paroxetine in the treatment of late-life depression. *Journal of Clinical Psychiatry*, 64(9), 1065–1074.

Rapaport, M.H., Wolkow, R., Rubin, A., *et al.* (2001). Sertraline treatment of panic disorder: Results of a long-term study. *Acta Psychiatrica Scandinavica*, 104(4), 289–298.

Rapoport, M.J., Chan, F., Lanctot, K., *et al.* (2008). An open-label study of citalopram for major depression following traumatic brain injury. *Journal of Psychopharmacology*, 22(8), 860–864.

Rasmussen, A., Lunde, M., Poulsen, D.L., *et al.* (2003). A double-blind, placebo-controlled study of sertraline in the prevention of depression in *Stroke* patients. *Psychosomatics*, 44(3), 216–221.

Rasmussen, J., Fulton, K. and Kennedy, S.H. (2006). "SexFx" differentiates depressed and non-depressed populations and demonstrates a favorable sexual side effect profile for agomelatine in the treatment of depression. *International Journal of Neuropsychopharmacology*, 9(s1), 309.

Rasmussen, S.L., Overo, K.F. and Tanghoj, P. (1999). Cardiac safety of citalopram: Prospective trials and retrospective analyses. *Journal of Clinical Psychopharmacology*, 19(5), 407–415.

Rausch, J.L., Pavlinac, D.M. and Newman, P.E. (1984). Complete heart block following a single dose of trazodone. *American Journal of Psychiatry*, 141(11), 1472–1473.

Ravindran, A.V., Guelfi, J.D., Lane, R.M. and Cassano, G.B. (2000). Treatment of dysthymia with sertraline: A double-blind, placebo-controlled trial in dysthymic patients without major depression. *Journal of Clinical Psychiatry*, 61(11), 821–827.

Razavi, D., Kormoss, N., Collard, A., *et al.* (1999). Comparative study of the efficacy and safety of trazodone versus clorazepate in the treatment of adjustment disorders in cancer patients: A pilot study. *Journal of International Medical Research*, 27(6), 264–272.

Reccoppa, L., Welch, W.A. and Ware, M.R. (1990). Acute dystonia and fluoxetine. *Journal of Clinical Psychiatry*, 51(11), 487.

Reeves, R.R. and Bullen, J.A. (1995). Serotonin syndrome produced by paroxetine and low-dose trazodone. *Psychosomatics*, 36(2), 159–160.

Reichmann, H., Brecht, M.H., Koster, J., *et al.* (2003). Pramipexole in routine clinical practice: A prospective observational trial in Parkinson's disease.*CNS Drugs*, 17(13), 965–973.

Rektorova, I., Rektor, I., Bares, M., *et al.* (2005). Cognitive performance in people with Parkinson's disease and mild or moderate depression:

Effects of dopamine agonists in an add-on to L-dopa therapy. *European Journal of Neurology*, 12(1), 9–15.

Rektorova, I., Rektor, I., Bares, M., *et al.* (2003). Pramipexole and pergolide in the treatment of depression in Parkinson's disease: A national multicentre prospective randomized study. *European Journal of Neurology*, 10(4), 399–406.

Renshaw, P.F., Guimaraes, A.R., Fava, M., *et al.* (1992). Accumulation of fluoxetine and norfluoxetine in human brain during therapeutic administration. *American Journal of Psychiatry*, 149(11), 1592–1594.

Rettman, K.S. and McClintock, C. (2001). Hepatotoxicity after short-term trazodone therapy. *Annals of Pharmacotherapy*, 35(12), 1559–1561.

Richards, J.B., Papaioannou, A., Adachi, J.D., *et al.* (2007). Effect of selective serotonin reuptake inhibitors on the risk of fracture. *Archives of Internal Medicine*, 167(2), 188–294.

Richelson, E. and Nelson, A. (1984). Antagonism by antidepressants of neurotransmitter receptors of normal human brain *in vitro*. *Journal of Pharmacology and Experimental Therapeutics*, 230(1), 94–102.

Richman, A., Heinrichs, S.C. (2007). Seizure prophylaxis in an animal model of epilepsy by dietary fluoxetine supplementation. *Epilepsy Research*, 74(1), 19–27.

Rickels, K., Amsterdam, J., Clary, C., *et al.* (1990). Buspirone in depressed outpatients: A controlled study. *Psychopharmacology Bulletin*, 26(2), 163–167.

Rickels, K., Amsterdam, J.D., Clary, C., *et al.* (1991). Buspirone in major depression: A controlled study. *Journal of Clinical Psychiatry*, 52(1), 34–38.

Rickels, K., Downing, R., Schweizer, E. and Hassman, H. (1993). Antidepressants for the treatment of generalized anxiety disorder. A placebo-controlled comparison of imipramine, trazodone, and diazepam. *Archives of General Psychiatry*, 50(11), 884–895.

Rickels, K., Derivan, A., Kunz, N., *et al.* (1996). Zalospirone in major depression: A placebo-controlled multicenter study. *Journal of Clinical Psychopharmacology*, 16(3), 212–217.

Rickels, K., Rynn, M., Iyengar, M. and Duff, D. (2006). Remission of generalized anxiety disorder: A review of the paroxetine clinical trials database. *Journal of Clinical Psychiatry*, 67(1), 41–47.

Riddle, M.A., Brown, N., Dzubinski, D., *et al.* (1989). Fluoxetine overdose in an adolescent. *Journal of the American Academy of Child and Adolescent Psychiatry*, 28(4), 587–588.

Rimele, T.J., Henry, D.E., Lee, D.K., *et al.* (1987). Tissue-dependent alpha adrenoceptor activity of buspirone and related compounds. *Journal of Pharmacology and Experimental Therapeutics*, 241(3), 771–778.

Robert, P. and Montgomery, S.A. (1995). Citalopram in doses of 20–60 mg is effective in depression relapse prevention: A placebo-controlled 6-month study. *International Clinical Psychopharmacology*, 10(Suppl 1), 29–35.

Roberts, R.L., Mulder, R.T., Joyce, P.R., *et al.* (2004). No evidence of increased adverse drug reactions in cytochrome P450 CYP2D6 poor metabolizers treated with fluoxetine or nortriptyline. *Human Psychopharmacology*, 19(1), 17–23.

Robinson, D.S., Rickels, K., Feighner, J., *et al.* (1990). Clinical effects of the 5-HT1A partial agonists in depression: A composite analysis of buspirone in the treatment of depression. *Journal of Clinical Psychopharmacology*, 10(3 Suppl), 67S–76S.

Robinson, R.G., Jorge, R.E., Moser, D.J., *et al.* (2008). Escitalopram and problem-solving therapy for prevention of poststroke depression: A randomized controlled trial. *Journal of the American Medical Association*, 299(20), 2391–2400.

Robinson, R.G., Schultz, S.K., Castillo, C., *et al.* (2000). Nortriptyline versus fluoxetine in the treatment of depression and in short-term recovery after stroke: A placebo-controlled, double-blind study. *American Journal of Psychiatry*, 157(3), 351–359.

Rocca, P., Fonzo, V., Ravizza, L., *et al.* (2002). A comparison of paroxetine and amisulpride in the treatment of dysthymic disorder. *Journal of Affective Disorders*, 70(3), 313–317.

Roccatagliata, G., Murialdo, G., Albano, C., *et al.* (1982). Neuroendocrinological and clinical data upon trazodone treatment in depressed patients. *Neuropsychobiology*, 8(5), 259–268.

Romanelli, F., Adler, D.A. and Bungay, K.M. (1996). Possible paroxetine-induced bruxism. *Annals of Pharmacotherapy*, 30(11), 1246–1248.

Romano, S., Goodman, W., Tamura, R. and Gonzales, J. (2001). Long-term treatment of obsessive-compulsive disorder after an acute response: A comparison of fluoxetine versus placebo. *Journal of Clinical Psychopharmacology*, 21(1), 46–52.

Roose, S.P., Glassman, A.H., Attia, E., *et al.* (1998a). Cardiovascular effects of fluoxetine in depressed patients with heart disease. *American Journal of Psychiatry*, 155(5), 660–665.

Roose, S.P., Laghrissi-Thode, F., Kennedy, J.S., *et al.* (1998b). Comparison of paroxetine and nortriptyline in depressed patients with ischemic heart disease. *Journal of the American Medical Association*, 279(4), 287–291.

Roscoe, J.A., Morrow, G.R., Hickok, J.T., *et al.* (2005). Effect of paroxetine hydrochloride (Paxil) on fatigue and depression in breast cancer patients receiving chemotherapy. *Breast Cancer Research and Treatment*, 89(3), 243–249.

Rosenbaum, J.F., Fava, M., Hoog, S.L., *et al.* (1998). Selective serotonin reuptake inhibitor discontinuation syndrome: A randomized clinical trial. *Biological Psychiatry*, 44(2), 77–87.

Rosenbaum, J.F. and Zajecka, J. (1997). Clinical management of antidepressant discontinuation. *Journal of Clinical Psychiatry*, 58(Suppl 7), 37–40.

Rosenstein, D.L, Nelson, J.C. and Jacobs, S.C. (1993). Seizures associated with antidepressants: A review. *Journal of Clinical Psychiatry*, 54(8), 289–299.

Rothenhausler, H.B., Ehrentraut, S., von Degenfeld, G., *et al.* (2000). Treatment of depression with methylphenidate in patients difficult to wean from mechanical ventilation in the intensive care unit. *Journal of Clinical Psychiatry*, 61(10), 750–755.

Rothman, R.B. and Baumann, M.H. (2002). Serotonin releasing agents. Neurochemical, therapeutic and adverse effects. *Pharmacology, Biochemistry, and Behavior*, 71(4), 825–836.

Rothschild, A.J. (1995). Selective serotonin reuptake inhibitor-induced sexual dysfunction: Efficacy of a drug holiday. *American Journal of Psychiatry*, 152(10), 1514–1516.

Rothschild, A.J., Williamson, D.J., Tohen, M.F., *et al.* (2004). A double-blind, randomized study of olanzapine and olanzapine/fluoxetine combination for major depression with psychotic features. *Journal of Clinical Psychopharmacology*, 24(4), 365–373.

Roy, A. (1998). Placebo-controlled study of sertraline in depressed recently abstinent alcoholics. *Biological Psychiatry*, 44(7), 633–537.

Roy-Byrne, P.P., Pages, K.P., Russo, J.E., *et al.* (2000). Nefazodone treatment of major depression in alcohol-dependent patients: A double-blind, placebo-controlled trial. *Journal of Clinical Psychopharmacology*, 20(2), 129–136.

Rudberg, I., Hermann, M., Refsum, H. and Molden, E. (2008a). Serum concentrations of sertraline and N-desmethyl sertraline in relation to CYP2C19 genotype in psychiatric patients. *European Journal of Clinical Pharmacology*, 83(2), 322–327.

Rudberg, I., Hendset, M., Uthus, L.H., *et al.* (2008b). Heterozygous mutation in CYP2C19 significantly increases the concentration/dose ratio of racemic citalopram and escitalopram (S-citalopram). *Therapeutic Drug Monitoring*, 28(1), 102–105.

Rudberg, I., Mohebi, B., Hermann, M., *et al.* (2008c). Impact of the ultrarapid CYP2C19*17 allele on serum concentration of escitalopram in psychiatric patients. *Clinical Pharmacology and Therapeutics*, 83(2), 322–327.

Ruhé, H.G., Booij, J., Weert, H.C., *et al.* (2009a). Evidence why paroxetine dose escalation is not effective in major depressive disorder: A randomized controlled trial with assessment of serotonin transporter occupancy. *Neuropsychopharmacology*, 34(4), 999–1010.

Ruhé, H.G., Ooteman, W., Booij, J., *et al.* (2009b). Serotonin transporter gene promoter polymorphisms modify the association between paroxetine serotonin transporter occupancy and clinical response in major depressive disorder. *Pharmacogenetics and Genomics*, 19(1), 67–76.

Rush, A.J., Armitage, R., Gillin, J.C., *et al.* (1998). Comparative effects of nefazodone and fluoxetine on sleep in outpatients with major depressive disorder. *Biological Psychiatry*, 44(1), 3–14.

Sabelli, H.C., Fawcett, J., Gusovsky, F., *et al.* (1986). Clinical studies on the phenylethylamine hypothesis of affective disorder: Urine and blood phenylacetic acid and phenylalanine dietary supplements. *Journal of Clinical Psychiatry*, 47(2), 66–70.

Sachdev, M., Miller, W.C., Ryan, T. and Jollis, J.G. (2002). Effect of fenfluramine-derivative diet pills on cardiac valves: A meta-analysis of observational studies. *American Heart Journal*, 144(6), 1065–1073.

Sachs, G.S., Nierenberg, A.A., Calabrese, J.R., *et al.* (2007). Effectiveness of adjunctive antidepressant treatment for bipolar depression. *New England Journal of Medicine*, 356(17), 1711–1722.

Salva, M.A., Vanier, B., Laredo, J., *et al.* (2007). Major depressive disorder, sleep EEG and agomelatine: An open-label study. *International Journal of Neuropsychopharmacology*, 10(5), 691–696.

Saenz de Tejada, I., Ware, J.C., Blanco, R., *et al.* (1991). Pathophysiology of prolonged penile erection associated with trazodone use. *Journal of Urology*, 145(1), 60–64.

Sagud, M., Pivac, N., Muck-Seler, D., *et al.* (2002). Effects of sertraline treatment on plasma cortisol, prolactin and thyroid hormones in female depressed patients. *Neuropsychobiology*, 45(3), 139–143.

Salomon, R.M., Ripley, B., Kennedy, J.S., *et al.* (2003). Diurnal variation of cerebrospinal fluid hypocretin-1 (Orexin-A) levels in control and depressed subjects. *Biological Psychiatry*, 54(2), 96–104.

Salzman, C., Jimerson, D., Vasile, R., *et al.* (1993). Response to SSRI antidepressants correlates with reduction in plasma HVA: Pilot study. *Biological Psychiatry*, 34(8), 569–571.

Sanacora, G., Mason, G.F., Rothman, D.L. and Krystal, J.H. (2002). Increased occipital cortex GABA concentrations in depressed patients after therapy with selective serotonin reuptake inhibitors. *American Journal of Psychiatry*, 159(4), 663–665.

Sannicandro, T.J., Farrar, M.C. and Markowitz, J.S. (2002). Selective serotonin reuptake inhibitor-induced rash: Case report and review of the literature. *Pharmacotherapy*, 22(4), 516–518.

Sansone, R.A. and Sansone, L.A. (2003). Sertraline-induced hyperglycemia: Case report. *International Journal of Psychiatry in Medicine*, 33(1), 103–105.
Santos, R.P. and Pergolizzi, J.J. (2004). Transient neonatal jitteriness due to maternal use of sertraline (Zoloft). *Journal of Perinatology*, 24(6), 392–394.
Sanz, E.J., De-las-Cuevas, C., Kiuru, A., *et al.* (2005). Selective serotonin reuptake inhibitors in pregnant women and neonatal withdrawal syndrome: A database analysis. *The Lancet*, 365(9458), 482–487.
Saper, J.R., Lake, A.E. and Tepper, S.J. (2001). Nefazodone for chronic daily headache prophylaxis: An open-label study. *Headache*, 41(5), 465–474.
Saraf, M. and Schrader, G. (1999). Seizure associated with sertraline. *Australian and New Zealand Journal of Psychiatry*, 33(6), 944–945.
Sargent, P.A., Sharpley, A.L., Williams, C., *et al.* (1997). 5-HT2C receptor activation decreases appetite and body weight in obese subjects. *Psychopharmacology*, 133(3), 309–312.
Saunders, C., Ferrer, J.V., Shi, L., *et al.* (2000). Amphetamine-induced loss of human dopamine transporter activity: An internalization-dependent and cocaine-sensitive mechanism. *Proceedings of the National Academy of Sciences of the United States of America*, 97(12), 6850–6855.
Sayal, K.S., Duncan-McConnell, D.A., McConnell, H.W. and Taylor, D.M. (2000). Psychotropic interactions with warfarin. *Acta Psychiatrica Scandinavica*, 102(4), 250–255.
Scarzella, L., Scarzella, R., Mailland, F. and Bergamasco, B. (1985). Amineptine in the management of the depressive syndromes. *Progress in Neuropsychopharmacology and Biological Psychiatry*, 9(4), 429–439.
Schachter, M. and Parkes, J.D. (1980). Fluvoxamine and clomipramine in the treatment of cataplexy. *Journal of Neurology, Neurosurgery and Psychiatry*, 43(2), 171–174.
Schalekamp, T., Klungel, J.H., Souverein, P.C. and de Boer, A. (2008). Increased bleeding risk with concurrent use of selective serotonin reuptake inhibitors and coumarins. *Archives of Internal Medicine*, 168(2), 180–185.
Scharko, A.M. and Schumacher, J. (2008). Prolonged QTc interval in a 14-year-old girl with escitalopram overdose. *Journal of Child and Adolescent Psychopharmacology*, 18(3), 297–298.
Schattner, A. and Skurnik, Y. (1996). Fluoxetine-induced SIADH. *Journal of the American Geriatric Society*, 44(11), 1413.
Schechter, J.O. (1998). Treatment of disequilibrium and nausea in the SRI discontinuation syndrome. *Journal of Clinical Psychiatry*, 59(8), 431–432.
Schneeweiss, S. and Wang, P.S. (2004). Association between SSRI use and hip fractures and the effect of residual confounding bias in claims database studies. *Journal of Clinical Psychopharmacology*, 24(6), 632–638.

Schlosser, R., Wetzel, H., Dorr, H., *et al.* (2000). Effects of subchronic paroxetine administration on night-time endocrinological profiles in healthy male volunteers. *Psychoneuroendocrinology*, 25(4), 377–388.

Schmidt, M.E., Fava, M., Robinson, J.M. and Judge, R. (2000). The efficacy and safety of a new enteric-coated formulation of fluoxetine given once weekly during the continuation treatment of major depressive disorder. *Journal of Clinical Psychiatry*, 61(11), 851–857.

Schmitz, J.M., Averill, P., Stotts, A.L., *et al.* (2001). Fluoxetine treatment of cocaine-dependent patients with major depressive disorder. *Drug and Alcohol Dependence*, 63(3), 207–214.

Schneier, F.R., Garfinkel, R., Kennedy, B., *et al.* (1996). Ondansetron in the treatment of panic disorder. *Anxiety*, 2(4), 199–202.

Schneider, L.S., Nelson, J.C., Clary, C.M., *et al.* (2003). An 8-week multicenter, parallel-group, double-blind, placebo-controlled study of sertraline in elderly outpatients with major depression. *American Journal of Psychiatry*, 160(7), 1277–1285.

Schramm, T.M., Lawford, B.R., Macdonald, G.A. and Cooksley, W.G. (2000). Sertraline treatment of interferon-alfa-induced depressive disorder. *Medical Journal of Australia*, 173(7), 359–361.

Schreiber, S., Backer, M.M., Herman, I., *et al.* (2000). The antinociceptive effect of trazodone in mice is mediated through both mu-opioid and serotonergic mechanisms. *Behavior and Brain Research*, 114(1–2), 51–56.

Schwartz, G.E., Such, P. and Schatzberg, A. (2002). The reboxetine study group. Reboxetine vs. venlafaxine in the treatment of severe major depression. Presented at the 42nd Annual Meeting of the New Clinical Drug Evaluation Unit of the National Institute of Mental Health. Boca Raton, Florida.

Scordo, M.G., Spina, E., Dahl, M.L., *et al.* (2005). Influence of CYP2C9, 2C19 and 2D6 genetic polymorphisms on the steady-state plasma concentrations of the enantiomers of fluoxetine and norfluoxetine.*Basic and Clinical Pharmacology and Toxicology*, 97(5), 296–301.

Serebruany, V.L., Glassman, A.H., Malinin, A.I., *et al.* (2003). Platelet/endothelial biomarkers in depressed patients treated with the selective serotonin reuptake inhibitor sertraline after acute coronary events: The Sertraline AntiDepressant Heart Attack Randomized Trial (SADHART) Platelet Substudy. *Circulation*, 108(8), 939–944.

Service, J.A. and Waring, W.S. (2008). QT prolongation and delayed atrioventricular conduction caused by acute ingestion of trazodone. *Clinical Toxicology*, 46(1), 71–73.

Settle, E.C. Jr. (1993). Akathisia and sertraline. *Journal of Clinical Psychiatry*, 54(8), 321.

Shah, S.J., Gomberg-Maitland, M., Thenappan, T. and Rich, S. (2009). Selective serotonin reuptake inhibitors and the incidence and outcome of pulmonary hypertension. *Chest*, 136(3), 694–700.

Shapiro, P.A., Lesperance, F., Frasure-Smith, N., *et al.* (1999). An open-label preliminary trial of sertraline for treatment of major depression after acute myocardial infarction (the SADHAT Trial). Sertraline Anti-Depressant Heart Attack Trial. *American Heart Journal*, 137(6), 1100–1106.

Shaw, K., Turner, J. and Del Mar, C. (2002a). Are tryptophan and 5-hydroxytryptophan effective treatments for depression? A meta-analysis. *Australian and New Zealand Journal of Psychiatry*, 36(4), 488–491.

Shaw, K., Turner, J. and Del Mar, C. (2002b). Tryptophan and 5-hydroxytryptophan for depression. *Cochrane Database Syst Rev*, (1), CD003198.

Shelton, R.C., Winn, S., Ekhatore, N. and Loosen, P.T. (1993). The effects of antidepressants on the thyroid axis in depression. *Biological Psychiatry*, 33(2), 120–126.

Shihabuddin, L. and Rapport, D. (1994). Sertraline and extrapyramidal side effects. *American Journal of Psychiatry*, 151(2), 288.

Siah, S., Benziane, H., Dami, A., *et al.* (2007). Fluoxetine and inappropriate antidiuretic hormone secretion in elderly patients: A case report. *Annales de Biologie Clinique*, 65(4), 417–420.

Siddiqui, M.A. and Khan, I.A. (2004). Nefazodone-associated torsade de pointes. *International Journal of Cardiology*, 93(1), 85–86.

Simon, G.E., Heiligenstein, J.H., Grothaus, L., *et al.* (1998). Should anxiety and insomnia influence antidepressant selection: A randomized comparison of fluoxetine and imipramine. *Journal of Clinical Psychiatry*, 59(2), 49–55.

Sivojelezova, A., Shuhaiber, S., Sarkissian, L., *et al.* (2005). Citalopram use in pregnancy: Prospective comparative evaluation of pregnancy and fetal outcome. *American Journal of Obstetrics and Gynecology*, 193(6), 2004–2009.

Smeraldi, E. (1998). Amisulpride versus fluoxetine in patients with dysthymia or major depression in partial remission: A double-blind, comparative study. *Journal of Affective Disorders*, 48(1), 47–56.

Smith, D.L. and Wenegrat, B.G. (2000). A case report of serotonin syndrome associated with combined nefazodone and fluoxetine. *Journal of Clinical Psychiatry*, 61(2), 146.

Sonawalla, S., Chakraborty, N. and Parikh, R. (2003). Treatment of major depression and anxiety with the selective serotonin re-uptake enhancer tianeptine in the outpatient psychiatric care setting of India. *Journal of the Indian Medical Association*, 101(2), 116–117.

Sorkin, E.M. and Heel, R.C. (1986). Guanfacine. A review of its pharmacodynamic and pharmacokinetic properties, and therapeutic efficacy in the treatment of hypertension. *Drugs*, 31(4), 301–336.

Spigset, O. (1999). Adverse reactions of selective serotonin reuptake inhibitors: Reports from a spontaneous reporting system. *Drug Safety*, 20(3), 277–287.

Spigset, O., Hedenmalm, K., Dahl, M.L., *et al.* (1997). Seizures and myoclonus associated with antidepressant treatment: Assessment of potential risk factors, including CYP2D6 and CYP2C19 polymorphisms, and treatment with CYP2D6 inhibitors. *Acta Psychiatrica Scandinavica*, 96(5), 379–384.

Spigset, O. and Mjorndal, T. (1997). The effect of fluvoxamine on serum prolactin and serum sodium concentrations: Relation to platelet 5-HT2A receptor status. *Journal of Clinical Psychopharmacology*, 17(4), 292–297.

Spivey, K.M. and Wait, C.M. (1993). Perioperative seizures and fluvoxamine. *British Journal of Anaesthesia*, 71(2), 321.

Sporn, J., Ghaemi, S.N., Sambur, M.R., *et al.* (2000). Pramipexole augmentation in the treatment of unipolar and bipolar depression: A retrospective chart review. *Annals of Clinical Psychiatry*, 12(3), 137–140.

Sramek, J.J., Tansman, M., Suri, A., *et al.* (1996). Efficacy of buspirone in generalized anxiety disorder with coexisting mild depressive symptoms. *Journal of Clinical Psychiatry*, 57(7), 287–291.

Stahl, S.M., Kaiser, L., Roeschen, J., *et al.* (1998). Effectiveness of ipsapirone, a 5-HT-1A partial agonist, in major depressive disorder: Support for the role of 5-HT-1A receptors in the mechanism of action of serotonergic antidepressants. *International Journal of Neuropsychopharmcology*, 1(1), 11–18.

Stanislav, S.W. and Childs, N.L. (1999). Dystonia associated with sertraline. *Journal of Clinical Psychopharmacology*, 19(1), 98–100.

Staufenberg, E.F. and Tantam, D. (1989). Malignant hyperpyrexia syndrome in combined treatment. *British Journal of Psychiatry*, 154, 577–578.

Stein, D.J., Ahokas, A.A. and de Bodinat C. (2008). Efficacy of agomelatine in generalized anxiety disorder: A randomized, double-blind, placebo-controlled study. *Journal of Clinical Psychopharmacology*, 28(5), 561–566.

Stein, D.J., Seedat, S., van der Linden, G.J. and Zungu-Dirwayi, N. (2000). Selective serotonin reuptake inhibitors in the treatment of post-traumatic stress disorder: A meta-analysis of randomized controlled trials. *International Clinical Psychopharmacology*, 15(Suppl 2), S31–39.

Stein, D.J., Versiani, M., Hair, T. and Kumar, R. (2002). Efficacy of paroxetine for relapse prevention in social anxiety disorder: A 24-week study. *Archives of General Psychiatry*, 59(12), 1111–1118.

Stein, M.B., Chartier, M.J., Hazen, A.L., *et al.* (1996). Paroxetine in the treatment of generalized social phobia: Open-label treatment and double-blind placebo-controlled discontinuation. *Journal of Clinical Psychopharmacology*, 16(3), 218–222.

Steiner, W. and Fontaine, R. (1986). Toxic reaction following the combined administration of fluoxetine and L-tryptophan: Five case reports. *Biological Psychiatry*, 21(11), 1067–1071.

Steingart, A., Cotterchio, M., Kreiger, N. and Sloan, M. (2003). Antidepressant medication use and breast cancer risk: A case-control study.*International Journal of Epidemiology*, 32(6), 961–966.

Steur, E.N. (1993). Increase of Parkinson disability after fluoxetine medication. *Neurology*, 43(1), 211–213.

Stewart, D.E. (2002). Hepatic adverse reactions associated with nefazodone. *Canadian Journal of Psychiatry*, 47(4), 375–377.

Stinson, J.C., Murphy, C.M., Andrews, J.F. and Tomkin, G.H. (1992). An assessment of the thermogenic effects of fluoxetine in obese subjects. *International Journal of Obesity*, 16, 391–395.

Stoll, A.L., Pillay, S.S., Diamond, L., *et al.* (1996). Methylphenidate augmentation of serotonin selective reuptake inhibitors: A case series. *Journal of Clinical Psychiatry*, 57(2), 72–76.

Stone, M., Laughren, T., Jones, M.L., *et al.* (in press). Risk of suicidality in clinical trials of antidepressants in adults: Analysis of proprietary data submitted to US Food and Drug Administration. *British Medical Journal*.

Stormer, E., von Moltke, L.L., Perloff, M.D. and Greenblatt, D.J. (2001). P-glycoprotein interactions of nefazodone and trazodone in cell culture. *Journal of Clinical Pharmacology*, 41(7), 708–714.

Strauss, W.L. and Dager, S.R. (2001). Magnetization transfer of fluoxetine in the human brain using fluorine magnetic resonance spectroscopy. *Biological Psychiatry*, 49(9), 798–802.

Strauss, W.L., Layton, M.E. and Dager, S.R. (1998). Brain elimination half-life of fluvoxamine measured by 19F magnetic resonance spectroscopy. *American Journal of Psychiatry*, 155(3), 380–384.

Strauss, W.L:, Layton, M.E., Hayes, C.E. and Dager, S.R. (1997). 19F magnetic resonance spectroscopy investigation *in vivo* of acute and steady-state brain fluvoxamine levels in obsessive-compulsive disorder. *American Journal of Psychiatry*, 154(4), 516–522.

Strik, J.J., Honig, A., Lousberg, R., *et al.* (1998). Cardiac side-effects of two selective serotonin reuptake inhibitors in middle-aged and elderly depressed patients. *International Clinical Psychopharmacology*, 13(6), 263–267.

Strik, J.J., Honig, A., Lousberg, R., *et al.* (2000). Efficacy and safety of fluoxetine in the treatment of patients with major depression after first myocardial infarction: Findings from a double-blind, placebo-controlled trial. *Psychosomatic Medicine*, 62(6), 783–789.

Strouse, T.B., Fairbanks, L.A., Skotzko, C.E. and Fawzy, F.I. (1996). Fluoxetine and cyclosporine in organ transplantation. Failure to detect significant drug interactions or adverse clinical events in depressed organ recipients. *Psychosomatics*, 37(1), 23–30.

Suhara, T., Takano, A., Sudo, Y., *et al.* (2003). High levels of serotonin transporter occupancy with low-dose clomipramine in comparative occupancy study with fluvoxamine using positron emission tomography. *Archives of General Psychiatry*, 60(4), 386–391.

Sussman, N., Ginsberg, D.L. and Bikoff, J. (2001). Effects of nefazodone on body weight: A pooled analysis of selective serotonin reuptake inhibitor- and imipramine-controlled trials. *Journal of Clinical Psychiatry*, 62(4), 256–260.

Suzuki, E., Yoshida, Y., Shibuya, A. and Miyaoka, H. (2003). Nitric oxide involvement in depression during interferon-alpha therapy. *International Journal of Neuropsychopharmacology*, 6(4), 415–419.

Swenson, J.R., O'Connor, C.M., Barton, D., *et al.* (2003). Influence of depression and effect of treatment with sertraline on quality of life after hospitalization for acute coronary syndrome. *American Journal of Cardiology*, 92(11), 1271–1276.

Taddio, A., Ito, S. and Koren, G. (1996). Excretion of fluoxetine and its metabolite, norfluoxetine, in human breast milk. *Journal of Clinical Pharmacology*, 36(1), 42–47.

Takahashi, H., Yoshida, K., Higuchi, H., *et al.* (2003). Addition of a dopamine agonist, cabergoline, to a serotonin-noradrenalin reuptake inhibitor, milnacipran as a therapeutic option in the treatment of refractory depression: Two case reports. *Clinical Neuropharmacology*, 26(5), 230–232.

Takahashi, M., Sawayama, E., Sawayama, T. and Miyaoka, H. (2007). Reversible paroxetine-induced symptomatic hypothyroidism. *Pharmacopsychiatry*, 40(5), 201–202.

Takano, A., Suhara, T., Ichimiya, T., *et al.* (2006). Time course of *in vivo* 5-HTT transporter occupancy by fluvoxamine. *Journal of Clinical Psychopharmacology*, 26(2), 188–191.

Tamim, H.M., Mahmud, S., Hanley, J.A., *et al.* (2008). Antidepressants and risk of prostate cancer: A nested case-control study. *Prostate Cancer and Prostatic Diseases*, 11(1), 53–60.

Tarabar, A.F., Hoffman, R.S. and Nelson, L. (2008). Citalopram overdose: Late presentation of torsades de pointes (TdP) with cardiac arrest. *Journal of Medical Toxicology*, 4(2), 101–105.

Taylor, D.P., Carter, R.B., Eison, A.S., *et al.* (1995). Pharmacology and neurochemistry of nefazodone, a novel antidepressant drug. *Journal of Clinical Psychiatry*, 56 (Suppl 6), 3–11.

Taylor, F.B. and Russo, J. (2001). Comparing guanfacine and dextroamphetamine for the treatment of adult attention-deficit/hyperactivity disorder. *Journal of Clinical Psychopharmacology*, 21(2), 223–228.

Teicher, M.H., Glod, C. and Cole, J.O. (1990). Emergence of intense suicidal preoccupation during fluoxetine treatment. *American Journal of Psychiatry*, 147(2), 207–210.

Terra, J.L. and Montgomery, S.A. (1998). Fluvoxamine prevents recurrence of depression: Results of a long-term, double-blind, placebo-controlled study. *International Clinical Psychopharmacology*, 13(2), 55–62.

Terstappen, G.C., Pellacani, A., Aldegheri, L., *et al.* (2003). The antidepressant fluoxetine blocks the human small conductance calcium-activated potassium channels SK1, SK2 and SK3. *Neuroscience Letters*, 346(1–2), 85–88.

Tesei, S., Antonini, A., Canesi, M., *et al.* (2000). Tolerability of paroxetine in Parkinson's disease: A prospective study. *Movement Disorders*, 15(5), 986–989.

Thase, M.E. and Bartlett, C. (2001). Reboxetine does not cause weight gain during long-term therapy. *European Neuropsychopharmacology*, 11(3), S215.

Thase, M.E., Carpenter, D.J., Fong, R., *et al.* (2006). Suicidality in adult paroxetine depression studies. *Neuropsychopharmacology*, 31(s1), s224.

Thase, M.E., Fava, M., Halbreich, U., *et al.* (1996). A placebo-controlled, randomized clinical trial comparing sertraline and imipramine for the treatment of dysthymia. *Archives of General Psychiatry*, 53(9), 777–784.

Thedenat, B., Loche, F., Albes, B., *et al.* (2001). Acute generalized exanthematous pustulosis with photodistribution pattern induced by sertraline. *Dermatology*, 203(1), 87–88.

Theohar, C., Fischer-Cornelssen, K., Brosch, H., *et al.* (1982). A comparative, multicenter trial between bromocriptine and amitriptyline in the treatment of endogenous depression. *Arzneimittelforschung*, 32, 783–787.

Thirumalai, S.S. and Shubin, R.A. (2000). The use of citalopram in resistant cataplexy. *Sleep Medicine*, 1(4), 313–316.

Thomas, D., Gut, B., Wendt-Nordah, G. and Kiehn, J. (2002). The antidepressant drug fluoxetine is an inhibitor of human ether-a-go-go-related gene (HERG) potassium channels. *Journal of Pharmacology and Experimental Therapeutics*, 300(2), 543–548.

Thompson, J.W. Jr., Ware, M.R. and Blashfield, R.K. (1990). Psychotropic medication and priapism: A comprehensive review. *Journal of Clinical Psychiatry*, 51(10), 430–433.

Toh, S., García Rodríguez, L.A. and Hernández-Díaz, S. (2007). Use of antidepressants and risk of lung cancer. *Cancer Causes and Control*, 18(10), 1055–1064.

Toh, S., Mitchell, A.A., Louik, C., *et al.* (2009). Selective serotonin reuptake inhibitor use and risk of gestational hypertension. *American Journal of Psychiatry*, 166(3), 320–328.

Tohen, M., Vieta, E., Calabrese, J., *et al.* (2003). Efficacy of olanzapine and olanzapine-fluoxetine combination in the treatment of bipolar I depression. *Archives of General Psychiatry*, 60(11), 1079–1088.

Tollefson, G.D., Bosomworth, J.C., Heiligenstein, J.H., *et al.* (1995). A double-blind, placebo-controlled clinical trial of fluoxetine in geriatric patients with major depression. The fluoxetine collaborative study group. *International Psychogeriatrics*, 7(1), 89–104.

Tollefson, G.D., Greist, J.H., Jefferson, J.W., *et al.* (1994b). Is baseline agitation a relative contraindication for a selective serotonin reuptake inhibitor: A comparative trial of fluoxetine versus imipramine. *Journal of Clinical Psychopharmacology*, 14(6), 385–391.

Tollefson, G.D., Holman, S.L., Sayler, M.E. and Potvin, J.H. (1994a). Fluoxetine, placebo, and tricyclic antidepressants in major depression with and without anxious features. *Journal of Clinical Psychiatry*, 55(2), 50–59.

Toofanny, N. and Maddens, M.E. (2002). Reversible penile priapism associated with nefazodone. *Journal of the American Geriatric Society*, 50(9), 1610–1611.

Torta, R., Siri, I., Caldera, P. (2008). Sertraline effectiveness and safety in depressed oncological patients.*Supportive Care in Cancer*, 16(1), 83–91.

Tousoulis, D., Antoniades, C., Drolias, A., *et al.* (2008). Selective serotonin reuptake inhibitors modify the effect of beta-blockers on long-term survival of patients with end-stage heart failure and major depression. *Journal of Cardiac Failure*, 14(6), 456–464.

Trabert, W., Hohagen, F., Winkelmann, G. and Berger, M. (1995). A seizure, and electroencephalographic signs of a lowered seizure threshold, associated with fluvoxamine treatment of obsessive-compulsive disorder. *Pharmacopsychiatry*, 28(3), 95–97.

Trescoli-Serrano, C. and Smith, N.K. (1996). Sertraline-induced agranulocytosis. *Postgraduate Medical Journal*, 72(849), 446.

Uhr, M. and Grauer, M.T. (2003b). abcb1ab P-glycoprotein is involved in the uptake of citalopram and trimipramine into the brain of mice. *Journal of Psychiatric Research*, 37(3), 179–185.

Uhr, M., Grauer, M.T. and Holsboer, F. (2003a). Differential enhancement of antidepressant penetration into the brain in mice with abcb1ab (mdr1ab) P-glycoprotein gene disruption. *Biological Psychiatry*, 54(8), 840–846.

Uhr, M., Steckler, T., Yassouridis, A. and Holsboer, F. (2000). Penetration of amitriptyline, but not of fluoxetine, into brain is enhanced in mice with blood-brain barrier deficiency due to mdr1a P-glycoprotein gene disruption. *Neuropsychopharmacology*, 22(4), 380–397.

Urban, R.J. and Veldhuis, J.D. (1991). A selective serotonin reuptake inhibitor, fluoxetine hydrochloride, modulates the pulsatile release of prolactin in postmenopausal women. *American Journal of Obstetrics and Gynecology*, 164(1 Pt 1), 147–152.

van Amerongen, P. (1979). Double-blind clinical trial of the antidepressant action of amineptine. *Current Medical Research and Opinion*, 6(2), 93–100.

van de Merwe, T.J., Silverstone, T., Ankier, S.I., *et al.* (1984). A double-blind non-crossover placebo-controlled study between group comparison of trazodone and amitriptyline on cardiovascular function in major depressive disorder. *Psychopathology*, 17(Suppl 2), 64–76.

van de Vijver, D.A., Roos, R.A., Jansen, P.A., *et al.* (2002). Start of a selective serotonin reuptake inhibitor (SSRI) and increase of antiparkinsonian drug treatment in patients on levodopa. *British Journal of Clinical Pharmacology*, 54(2), 168–170.

Vanelle, J.M., Attar-Levy, D., Poirier, M.F., *et al.* (1997). Controlled efficacy study of fluoxetine in dysthymia. *British Journal of Psychiatry*, 170, 345–350.

van Praag, H.M. (1981). Management of depression with serotonin precursors. *Biological Psychiatry*, 16(3), 291–310.

van Praag, H.M., Lemus, C. and Kahn, R. (1986). The pitfalls of serotonin precursors as challengers in hormonal probes of central serotonin activity. *Psychopharmacology Bulletin*, 22(3), 565–570.

van Walraven, C., Mamdani, M.M., Wells, P.S. and Williams, J.I. (2001). Inhibition of serotonin reuptake by antidepressants and upper gastrointestinal bleeding in elderly patients: Retrospective cohort study. *British Medical Journal*, 323(7314), 655–658.

Vanpee, D., Laloyaux, P. and Gillet, J.B. (1999). Seizure and hyponatraemia after overdose of trazadone. *American Journal of Emergency Medicine*, 17(4), 430–431.

Vauterin, C. and Bazot, M. (1979). A double-blind controlled trial of amineptine versus trimipramine in depression. *Current Medical Research and Opinion*, 6(2), 101–106.

Versiani, M., Amin, M. and Chouinard, G. (2000). Double-blind, placebo-controlled study with reboxetine in inpatients with severe major depressive disorder. *Journal of Clinical Psychopharmacology*, 20(1), 28–34.

Versiani, M., Cassano, G., Perugi, G., *et al.* (2002). Reboxetine, a selective norepinephrine reuptake inhibitor, is an effective and well-tolerated treatment for panic disorder. *Journal of Clinical Psychiatry*, 63(1), 31–37.

Versiani, M., Ontiveros, A., Mazzotti, G., *et al.* (1999). Fluoxetine versus amitriptyline in the treatment of major depression with associated anxiety (anxious depression): A double-blind comparison. *International Clinical Psychopharmacology*, 14(6), 321–327.

Vestergaard, P., Rejnmark, L. and Mosekilde, L. (2008). Selective serotonin reuptake inhibitors and other antidepressants and risk of fracture. *Calcified Tissue International*, 82(2), 92–101.

Vidal, X., Ibáñez, L., Vendrell, L., *et al.* (2008). Risk of upper gastrointestinal bleeding and the degree of serotonin reuptake inhibition by antidepressants: A case-control study. *Drug Safety*, 31(2), 159–168.

Vieta, E., Martinez-Aran, A., Goikolea, J.M., *et al.* (2002). A randomized trial comparing paroxetine and venlafaxine in the treatment of bipolar depressed patients taking mood stabilizers. *Journal of Clinical Psychiatry*, 63(6), 508–512.

Vilinsky, F.D. and Lubin, A. (1997). Severe neutropenia associated with fluoxetine hydrochloride. *Annals of Internal Medicine*, 127(7), 573–574.

Visser, M., Seidell, J.C., Koppeschaar, H.P.F. and Smits, P. (1993). The effect of fluoxetine on body weight, body composition and visceral fat accumulation. *International Journal of Obesity*, 17, 247–253.

Vitullo, R.N., Wharton, J.M., Allen, N.B. and Pritchett, E.L. (1990). Trazodone-related exercise-induced nonsustained ventricular tachycardia. *Chest*, 98(1), 247–248.

Vlay, S.C. and Friedling, S. (1983). Trazodone exacerbation of VT.*American Heart Journal*, 106(3), 604.

Voineskos, A.N., Wilson, A.A., Boovariwala, A., *et al.* (2007). Serotonin transporter occupancy of high-dose selective serotonin reuptake inhibitors during major depressive disorder measured with [(11)C]DASB positron emission tomography. *Psychopharmacology*, 193(4), 539–545.

Volkow, N.D., Fowler, J.S., Wang, G., *et al.* (2002). Mechanism of action of methylphenidate: Insights from PET imaging studies. *Journal of Attention Disorders*, 6(Suppl 1), S31–43.

Wadsworth, E.J., Moss, S.C., Simpson, S.A. and Smith, A.P. (2005). SSRIs and cognitive performance in a working sample. *Human Psychopharmacology*, 20(8), 561–572.

Waehrens, J. and Gerlach, J. (1981). Bromocriptine and imipramine in endogenous depression. A double-blind controlled trial in out-patients. *Journal of Affective Disorders*, 3(2), 193–202.

Wagner, G.J. and Rabkin, R. (2000). Effects of dextroamphetamine on depression and fatigue in men with HIV: A double-blind, placebo-controlled trial. *Journal of Clinical Psychiatry*, 61(6), 436–440.

Wagner, K.D., Ambrosini, P., Rynn, M., *et al.* (2003). Efficacy of sertraline in the treatment of children and adolescents with major depressive disorder: Two randomized controlled trials. *Journal of the American Medical Association*, 290(8), 1033–1041.

Wagner, K.D., Robb, A.S., Findling, R.L., *et al.* (2004). A randomized, placebo-controlled trial of citalopram for the treatment of major depression in children and adolescents. *American Journal of Psychiatry*, 161(6), 1079–1083.

Wagstaff, A.J., Frampton, J.E. and Croom, K.F. (2003). Tegaserod: A review of its use in the management of irritable bowel syndrome with constipation in women. *Drugs*, 63(11), 1101–1020.

Waintraub, L., Septien, L. and Azoulay, P. (2002). Efficacy and safety of tianeptine in major depression: Evidence from a 3-month controlled clinical trial versus paroxetine. *CNS Drugs*, 16(1), 65–75.

Walker, J.R., Van Ameringen, M.A., Swinson, R., *et al.* (2000). Prevention of relapse in generalized social phobia: Results of a 24 week study in responders to 20 weeks of sertraline treatment. *Journal of Clinical Psychopharmacology*, 20(6), 636–644.

Walker, L. (2002). Sertraline-induced akathisia and dystonia misinterpreted as a panic attack. *Psychiatric Services*, 53(11), 1477–1478.

Wang, J.S., Zhu, H.J., Gibson, B.B., *et al.* (2008). Sertraline and its metabolite desmethylsertraline, but not bupropion or its three major metabolites, have high affinity for P-glycoprotein. *Biological & Pharmaceutical Bulletin*, 31(2), 231–234.

Wang, P.S., Walker, A.M., Tsuang, M.T., *et al.* (2001). Antidepressant use and the risk of breast cancer: A non-association. *Journal of Clinical Epidemiology*, 54(7), 728–734.

Wang, S.J., Su, C.F. and Kuo, Y.H. (2003). Fluoxetine depresses glutamate exocytosis in the rat cerebrocortical nerve terminals (synaptosomes) via inhibition of P/Q-type Ca^{2+} channels. *Synapse*, 48(4), 170–177.

Ware, M.R. and Stewart, R.B. (1989). Seizures associated with fluoxetine therapy. *DICP: The Annals of Pharmacotherapy*, 23(5), 428.

Warnock, C.A. and Azadian, A.G. (2002). Cross-sensitivity between paroxetine and sertraline. *Annals of Pharmacotherapy*, 36(4), 631–633.

Warnock, J.K. and Biggs, F. (1997). Nefazodone-induced hypoglycemia in a diabetic patient with major depression. *American Journal of Psychiatry*, 154(2), 288–299.

Warnock, J.K., Bundren, J.C. and Morris, D.W. (1988). Sertraline in the treatment of depression associated with gonadotropin-releasing hormone agonist therapy. *Biological Psychiatry*, 43(6), 464–465.

Warnock, J.K., Clayton, A.H., Shaw, H.A. and O'Donnell, T. (1995). Onset of menses in two adult patients with Prader-Willi syndrome treated with fluoxetine. *Psychopharmacology Bulletin*, 31(2), 239–242.

Watanabe, J., Suzuki, Y., Fukui, N., *et al.* (2008). Dose-dependent effect of the CYP2D6 genotype on the steady-state fluvoxamine concentration. *Therapeutic Drug Monitoring*, 30(6), 705–708.

Weber, C.C., Kressmann, S., Ott, M., *et al.* (2005). Inhibition of P-glycoprotein function by several antidepressants may not contribute to clinical efficacy. *Pharmacopsychiatry*, 38(6), 293–300.

Weinrieb, R.M., Auriacombe, M., Lynch, K.G., *et al.* (2003). A critical review of selective serotonin reuptake inhibitor–associated bleeding: Balancing the risk of treating hepatitis C-infected patients. *Journal of Clinical Psychiatry*, 64(12), 1502–1510.

Weiss, J., Dormann, S.M., Martin-Facklam, M., *et al.* (2003). Inhibition of P-glycoprotein by newer antidepressants. *Journal of Pharmacology and Experimental Therapeutics*, 305(1), 197–204.

Weissman, A.M., Levy, B.T., Hartz, A.J., *et al.* (2004). Pooled analysis of antidepressant levels in lactating mothers, breast milk, and nursing infants. *American Journal of Psychiatry*, 161(6), 1066–1078.

Weitzner, M.A., Moncello, J., Jacobsen, P.B. and Minton, S. (2002). A pilot trial of paroxetine for the treatment of hot flashes and associated symptoms in women with breast cancer. *Journal of Pain and Symptom Management*, 23(4), 337–345.

Wermuth, L., Sorensen, P.S., Timm, B., *et al.* (1998). Depression in idiopathic Parkinson's disease treated with citalopram — A placebo-controlled trial. *Nordic Journal of Psychiatry*, 52(2), 163–169.

Werneck, A.L., Rosso, A.L. and Vincent, M.B. (2009). The use of an antagonist 5-HT2a / c for depression and motor function in Parkinson's disease. *Arquivos de neuro-psiquiatria*, 67(2B), 407–412.

White, N., Litovitz, T. and Clancy, C. (2008). Suicidal antidepressant overdoses: A comparative analysis by antidepressant type. *Journal of Medical Toxicology*, 4(4), 238–250.

White, W.B. and Wong, S.H. (1985). Rapid atrial fibrillation associated with trazodone hydrochloride. *Archives of General Psychiatry*, 42(4), 424.

Whittington, C.J., Kendall, T., Fonagy, P., *et al.* (2004). Selective serotonin reuptake inhibitors in childhood depression: Systematic review of published versus unpublished data. *The Lancet*, 363(9418), 1341–1345.

Wiart, L., Petit, H., Joseph, P.A., *et al.* (2000). Fluoxetine in early post*Stroke* depression: A double-blind placebo-controlled study. *Stroke*, 31(8), 1829–1832.

Wichman, C.L., Moore, K.M., Lang, T.R., *et al.* (2009). Congenital heart disease associated with selective serotonin reuptake inhibitor use during pregnancy. *Mayo Clinic Proceedings*, 84(1), 23–27.

Wilcox, C.S., Ferguson, J.M., Dale, J.L. and Heiser, J.F. (1996). A double-blind trial of low- and high-dose ranges of gepirone-ER compared with placebo in the treatment of depressed outpatients. *Psychopharmacology Bulletin*, 32(3), 335–342.

Wilde, M.I. and Benfield, P. (1995). Tianeptine. A review of its pharmacodynamic and pharmacokinetic properties, and therapeutic efficacy in depression and coexisting anxiety and depression. *Drugs*, 49(3), 411–439.

Wilens, T.E., Biederman, J., March, J.S., *et al.* (1999). Absence of cardiovascular adverse effects of sertraline in children and adolescents. *Journal of the American Academy of Child and Adolescent Psychiatry*, 38(5), 573–577.

Williamson, B.L., Benson, L.M., Tomlinson, A.J., *et al.* (1997). On-line HPLC-tandem mass spectrometry analysis of contaminants of L-tryptophan associated with the onset of the eosinophilia-myalgia syndrome. *Toxicology Letters*, 92(2), 139–148.

Williamson, B.L., Tomlinson, A.J., Mishra, P.K., *et al.* (1998a). Structural characterization of contaminants found in commercial preparations of melatonin: Similarities to case-related compounds from L-tryptophan associated with eosinophilia-myalgia syndrome. *Chemical Research in Toxicology*, 11(3), 234–240.

Williamson, B.L., Klarskov, K., Tomlinson, A.J., *et al.* (1998b). Problems with over-the-counter 5-hydroxy-L-tryptophan. *Nature Medicine*, 4(9), 983.

Williamson, B.L., Tomlinson, A.J., Hurth, K.M., *et al.* (1998c). Rapid HPLC screening method for contaminants found in implicated L-tryptophan associated with eosinophilia myalgia syndrome and adulterated rapeseed oil associated with toxic oil syndrome. *Biomedical Chromatography*, 12(5), 255–261.

Williamson, B.L., Johnson, K.L., Tomlinson, A.J., *et al.* (1998d). On-line HPLC-tandem mass spectrometry structural characterization of case-associated contaminants of L-tryptophan implicated with the onset of eosinophilia myalgia syndrome. *Toxicology Letters*, 99(2), 139–150.

Winokur, A., Baker R.A., Simmons, J., *et al.* (2005). Comparative sleep improving effects of mirtazapine vs SSRIs in depressed patients: A meta-analysis of individual patient data. *World Journal of Biological Psychiatry*, 6(s1), s366.

Wise, M. (2001). Citalopram-induced bruxism. *British Journal of Psychiatry*, 178, 182.

Wise, S.D. (1992). Clinical studies with fluoxetine in obesity.*American Journal of Clinical Nutrition*, 55, 181s-184s.

Wisner, K.L., Perel, J.M. and Blumer, J. (1998). Serum sertraline and N-desmethylsertraline levels in breast-feeding mother-infant pairs. *American Journal of Psychiatry*, 155(5), 690–692.

Wisner, K.L., Perel, J.M. and Findling, R.L. (1996). Antidepressant treatment during breast-feeding. *American Journal of Psychiatry*, 153(9), 1132–1137.

Wisner, K.L., Perel, J.M., Peindl, K.S., *et al.* (2004). Prevention of postpartum depression: A pilot randomized clinical trial. *American Journal of Psychiatry*, 161(7), 1290–1292.

Wong, E.H., Sonders, M.S., Amara, S.G., *et al.* (2000). Reboxetine: A pharmacologically potent, selective, and specific norepinephrine reuptake inhibitor. *Biological Psychiatry*, 47(9), 818–829.

Woods, S.W., Tesar, G.E., Murray, G.B. and Cassem, N.H. (1986). Psychostimulant treatment of depressive disorders secondary to medical illness. *Journal of Clinical Psychiatry*, 47(1), 12–15.

Woolfrey, S., Gammack, N.S., Dewar, M.S. and Brown, P.J. (1993). Fluoxetine-warfarin interaction. *British Medical Journal*, 307(6898), 241.

Wysowski, D.K., Corken, A., Gallo-Torres, H., *et al.* (2001). Postmarketing reports of QT prolongation and ventricular arrhythmia in association with cisapride and Food and Drug Administration regulatory actions. *American Journal of Gastroenterology*, 96(6), 1698–1703.

Xu, W., Tamim, H., Shapiro, S., *et al.* (2006). Use of antidepressants and risk of colorectal cancer: A nested case-control study. *Lancet Oncology*, 7(4), 301–308.

Yamada, K., Yagi, G. and Kanba, S. (2003). Clinical efficacy of tandospirone augmentation in patients with major depressive disorder: A randomized controlled trial. *Psychiatry and Clinical Neurosciences*, 57(2), 183–187.

Yap, K.B. and Low, S.T. (1999). Interaction of fluvoxamine with warfarin in an elderly woman. *Singapore Medical Journal*, 40(7), 480–482.

Yeung, S.Y., Millar, J.A. and Mathie, A. (1999). Inhibition of neuronal KV potassium currents by the antidepressant drug, fluoxetine. *British Journal of Pharmacology*, 128(7), 1609–1615.

Yin, O.Q., Wing, Y.K., Cheung, Y., *et al.* (2006). Phenotype-genotype relationship and clinical effects of citalopram in Chinese patients. *Journal of Clinical Psychopharmacology*, 26(4), 367–372.

Yonkers, K.A., Lin, H., Howell, H.B., *et al.* (2008). Pharmacologic treatment of postpartum women with new-onset major depressive disorder: A randomized controlled trial with paroxetine. *Journal of Clinical Psychiatry*, 69(4), 659–665.

Yoon, Y.R., Cha, I.J., Shon, J.H., *et al.* (2000). Relationship of paroxetine disposition to metoprolol metabolic ratio and CYP2D6*10 genotype of Korean subjects. *Clinical Pharmacology and Therapeutics*, 67(5), 567–576.

Yu, A., Kneller, B.M., Rettie, A.E. and Haining, R.L. (2002). Expression, purification, biochemical characterization, and comparative function of human cytochrome P450 2D6.1, 2D6.2, 2D6.10, and 2D6.17 allelic isoforms. *Journal of Pharmacology and Experimental Therapeutics*, 303(3), 1291–1300.

Yu, B.N., Chen, G.L., He, N., *et al.* (2003). Pharmacokinetics of citalopram in relation to genetic polymorphism of CYP2C19. *Drug Metabolism and Disposition*, 31(10), 1255–1259.

Zajecka, J., Fawcett, J., Amsterdam, J., *et al.* (1998). Safety of abrupt discontinuation of fluoxetine: A randomized, placebo-controlled study. *Journal of Clinical Psychopharmacology*, 18(3), 193–197.

Ziegler, M., Castro-Caldas, A., Del Signore, S. and Rascol, O. (2003). Efficacy of piribedil as early combination to levodopa in patients with stable Parkinson's disease: A 6-month, randomized, placebo-controlled study. *Movement Disorders*, 18(4), 418–425.

Ziere, G., Dieleman, J.P., van der Cammen, T.J., *et al.* (2008). Selective serotonin reuptake inhibiting antidepressants are associated with an increased risk of nonvertebral fractures. *Journal of Clinical Psychopharmacology*, 28(4), 411–417.

Zisook, S., Peterkin, J., Goggin, K.J., *et al.* (1998). Treatment of major depression in HIV-seropositive men. HIV Neurobehavioral Research Center Group. *Journal of Clinical Psychiatry*, 59(5), 217–224.

Zisook, S., Trivedi, M.H., Warden, D., *et al.* (2009). Clinical correlates of the worsening or emergence of suicidal ideation during SSRI treatment of depression: An examination of citalopram in the STARD study. *Journal of Affective Disorders*, 117(1–2), 63–73.

Chapter 3

Abrahamian, H., Hofmann, P., Prager, R. and Toplak, H. (2009). Diabetes mellitus and co morbid depression: Treatment with milnacipran results in significant improvement of both diseases (results from the Austrian MDDM study group). *Neuropsychiatric Disease and Treatment*, 5, 261–266.

Acharya, N., Rosen, A.S., Polzer, J.P., *et al.* (2006). Duloxetine: Meta-analyses of suicidal behaviors and ideation in clinical trials for major depressive disorder. *Journal of Clinical Psychopharmacology*, 26(6), 587–594.

Achong, M.R. and Keane, P.M. (1981). Pheochromocytoma unmasked by desipramine therapy. *Annals of Internal Medicine*, 94(3), 358–359.

Adlakha, A., Manocha, A.P. and Bechard, D.L. (1991). Imipramine-induced syndrome of inappropriate antidiuretic hormone secretion. *Southern Medical Journal*, 84(12), 1507–1509.

Agundez, J.A., Ledesma, M.C., Ladero, J.M. and Benitez, J. (1995). Prevalence of CYP2D6 gene duplication and its repercussion on the oxidative phenotype in a white population. *Clinical Pharmacology and Therapeutics*, 57(3), 265–269.

Ahlfors, U.G., Elovaara, S., Harma, P., *et al.* (1988). Clinical multicentre study of citalopram compared double-blindly with mianserin in depressed patients in Finland. *Nordisk Psykiatrisk Tidsskrift*, 42(3), 201–210.

Ahmed, A. (2002). Neutropenia associated with mirtazapine use: Is a drop in the neutrophil count in a symptomatic older adults a cause for concern? *Journal of the American Geriatric Society*, 50(8), 1461–1463.

Aklillu, E., Persson, I., Bertilsson, L., *et al.* (1996). Frequent distribution of ultrarapid metabolizers of debrisoquine in an ethiopian population carrying duplicated and multiduplicated functional CYP2D6 alleles. *Journal of Pharmacology and Experimental Therapeutics*, 278(1), 441–446.

Allgulander, C., Nutt, D., Detke, M., *et al.* (2008). A non-inferiority comparison of duloxetine and venlafaxine in the treatment of adult patients with generalized anxiety disorder. *Journal of Psychopharmacology*, 22(4), 417–425.

Allgulander, C., Hartford, J., Russell, J., *et al.* (2007). Pharmacotherapy of generalized anxiety disorder: Results of duloxetine treatment from a pooled analysis of three clinical trials. *Current Medical and Research Opinion*, 23(6), 1245–1252.

Alonso-Navarro, H., Martín-Prieto, M., Ruiz-Ezquerro, J.J. and Jiménez-Jiménez, F.J. (2009). Bruxism possibly induced by venlafaxine. *Clinical Neuropharmacology*, 32(2), 111–112.

Amsterdam, J.D., Garcia-Espana, F., Goodman, D., *et al.* (1997). Breast enlargement during chronic antidepressant therapy. *Journal of Affective Disorders*, 46(2), 151–156.

Anand, V.S. (1995). Clomipramine–induced galactorrhoea and amenorrhoea. *British Journal of Psychiatry*, 147, 87–88.

Anderson, I.M. (2000). Selective serotonin reuptake inhibitors versus tricyclic antidepressants: A meta-analysis of efficacy and tolerability. *Journal of Affective Disorders*, 58(1), 19–36.

Anderson, I.M. and Tomenson, B.M. (1995). Treatment discontinuation with selective serotonin reuptake inhibitors compared with tricyclic antidepressants: A meta-analysis. *British Medical Journal*, 310(6992), 1433–1438.

Anderson, J.W., Greenway, F.L., Fujioka, K., *et al.* (2002). Bupropion SR enhances weight loss: A 48-week double-blind, placebo- controlled trial. *Obesity Research*, 10(7), 633–641.

Anghelescu, I., Klawe, C. and Dahmen, N. (2002). Venlafaxine in a patient with idiopathic leukopenia and mirtazapine-induced severe neutropenia. *Journal of Clinical Psychiatry*, 63(9), 838.

Ansseau, M., von Frenckell, R., Mertens, C., *et al.* (1989). Controlled comparison of two doses of milnacipran (F 2207) and amitriptyline in major depressive inpatients. *Psychopharmacology*, 98(2), 163–168.

Anttila, S.A. and Leinonen, E.V. (2001). A review of the pharmacological and clinical profile of mirtazapine. *CNS Drug Reviews*, 7(3), 249–264.

Archer, D.F., Dupont, C.M., Constantine, G.D., *et al.* (2009a). Desvenlafaxine for the treatment of vasomotor symptoms associated with menopause: A double-blind, randomized, placebo-controlled trial of efficacy and safety. *American Journal of Obstetrics and Gynecology*, 200(3), 238.

Archer, D.F., Seidman, L., Constantine, G.D., *et al.* (2009b). A double-blind, randomly assigned, placebo-controlled study of desvenlafaxine efficacy and safety for the treatment of vasomotor symptoms associated with menopause. *American Journal of Obstetrics and Gynecology*, 200(2), 172.

Arnold, L.M., Lu, Y., Crofford, L.J., *et al.* (2004). A double-blind, multicenter trial comparing duloxetine with placebo in the treatment of fibromyalgia patients with or without major depressive disorder. *Arthritis and Rheumatism*, 50(9), 2974–2984.

Arnold, L.M., Pritchett, Y.L., D'Souza, D.N., *et al.* (2007). Duloxetine for the treatment of fibromyalgia in women: Pooled results from two randomized, placebo-controlled clinical trials. *Journal of Womens Health (Larchmt)*, 16(8), 1145–1156.

Arnold, L.M., Rosen, A., Pritchett, Y.L., *et al.* (2005). A randomized, double-blind, placebo-controlled trial of duloxetine in the treatment of women with fibromyalgia with or without major depressive disorder. *Pain*, 119(1–3), 5–15.

Ascher, J.A., Cole, J.O., Colin, J.N., *et al.* (1995). Bupropion: A review of its mechanism of antidepressant activity. *Journal of Clinical Psychiatry*, 56(9), 395–401.

Atkin, D.H. and Fitzpatrick, R.E. (2000). Laser treatment of imipramine-induced hyperpigmentation. *Journal of the American Academy of Dermatology*, 43(1 Pt 1), 77–80.

Bagley, S.C. and Yaeger, D. (2005). Hyponatremia associated with bupropion, a case verified by rechallenge. *Journal of Clinical Psychopharmacology*, 25(1), 98–99.

Bagshaw, S.M., Cload, B., Gilmour, J., *et al.* (2003). Drug-induced rash with eosinophilia and systemic symptoms syndrome with bupropion administration. *Annals of Allergy, Asthma, and Immunology*, 90(5), 572–575.

Baker, G.B. and Prior, T.I. (2002). Stereochemistry and drug efficacy and development: Relevance of chirality to antidepressant and antipsychotic drugs. *Annals of Medicine*, 34(7–8), 537–543.

Balhara, Y., Sagar, R. and Varghese, S.T. (2007). Bleeding gums: Duloxetine may be the cause. *Journal of Postgraduate Medicine*, 53(1), 44–45.

Bavbek, N., Kargili, A., Akcay, A. and Kaya, A. (2006). Recurrent hyponatremia associated with citalopram and mirtazapine. *American Journal of Kidney Diseases*, 48(4), e61–62.

Beasley, C.M. Jr., Koke, S.C., Nilsson, M.E. and Gonzales, J.S. (2000). Adverse events and treatment discontinuations in clinical trials of fluoxetine in major depressive disorder: An updated meta-analysis. *Clinical Therapeutics*, 22(11), 1319–1330.

Becker, R.E. and Dufresne, R.L. (1982). Perceptual changes with bupropion, a novel antidepressant. *American Journal of Psychiatry*, 139(9), 1200–1201.

Behnke, K., Sogaard, J., Martin, S., *et al.* (2003). Mirtazapine orally disintegrating tablet versus sertraline: A prospective onset of action study. *Journal of Clinical Psychopharmacology*, 23(4), 358–364.

Bell, S. and Shipman, M. (2000). Reduced testosterone level in a venlafaxine treated patient. *Annals of Clinical Psychiatry*, 12(3), 171–173.

Benazzi, F. (1998b). Mirtazapine withdrawal symptoms. *Canadian Journal of Psychiatry*, 43(5), 525.

Benazzi, F. (1998a). Serotonin syndrome with mirtazapine-fluoxetine combination. *International Journal of Geriatric Psychiatry*, 13(7), 495–496.

Benkert, O., Grunder, G., Wetzel, H. and Hackett, D. (1996). A randomized, double-blind comparison of a rapidly escalating dose of venlafaxine and imipramine in inpatients with major depression and melancholia. *Journal of Psychiatric Research*, 30(6), 441–451.

Benkert, O., Szegedi, A. and Kohnen, R. (2000). Mirtazapine compared with paroxetine in major depression. *Journal of Clinical Psychiatry*, 61(9), 656–663.

Benkert, O., Szegedi, A., Philipp, M., *et al.* (2006). Mirtazapine orally disintegrating tablets versus venlafaxine extended release: A double-blind, randomized multicenter trial comparing the onset of antidepressant response in patients with major depressive disorder. *Journal of Clinical Psychopharmacology*, 26(1), 75–78.

Benson, E. (2001). Bupropion-induced hypersensitivity reactions. *Medical Journal of Australia*, 174(12), 650–651.

Bergman, B.R., Reynolds, H.R., Skolnick, A.H. and Castillo, D. (2008). A case of apical ballooning cardiomyopathy associated with duloxetine. *Annals of Internal Medicine*, 149(3), 218–219.

Bergmann, T.K., Bathum, L. and Brosen, K. (2001). Duplication of CYP2D6 predicts high clearance of desipramine but high clearance does not predict duplication of CYP2D6. *European Journal of Clinical Pharmacology*, 57(2), 123–127.

Berigan, T.R. (2002). Bupropion-associated withdrawal symptoms revisited: A case report. *Primary Care Companion of the Journal of Clinical Psychiatry*, 4(2), 78.

Berigan, T.R. (2001). Mirtazapine-associated withdrawal symptoms: A case report. *Primary Care Companion of the Journal of Clinical Psychiatry*, 3(3), 143.

Berigan, T.R. and Harazin, J.S. (1999). Bupropion-associated withdrawal symptoms: A case report. *Primary Care Companion of the Journal of Clinical Psychiatry*, 1(2), 50–51.

Berle, J.O., Steen, V.M., Aamo, T.O., *et al.* (2004). Breastfeeding during maternal antidepressant treatment with serotonin reuptake inhibitors: Infant exposure, Clinical symptoms, and cytochrome p450 genotypes. *Journal of Clinical Psychiatry*, 65(9), 1228–1234.

Bertilsson, L., Aberg-Wistedt, A., Gustafsson, L.L. and Nordin, C. (1985). Extremely rapid hydroxylation of debrisoquine: A case report with implication for treatment with nortriptyline and other tricyclic antidepressants. *Therapeutic Drug Monitoring*, 7(4), 478–480.

Bhatara, V.S., Magnus, R.D., Paul, K.L. and Preskorn, S.H. (1998). Serotonin syndrome induced by venlafaxine and fluoxetine: A case study in polypharmacy and potential pharmacodynamic and pharmacokinetic mechanisms. *Annals of Pharmacotherapy*, 32(4), 432–436.

Birkebaek, N.H. and Perrild, B.D. (1996). Pheochromocytoma diagnosed in an enuretic boy after imipramine-induced hypertension. *Pediatric Hematology and Oncology*, 3(3), 283–285.

Biswas, P.N., Wilton, L.V. and Shakir, S.A. (2003). The pharmacovigilance of mirtazapine: Results of a prescription event monitoring study on 13554 patients in England. *Journal of Psychopharmacology*, 17(1), 121–126.

Blanch, J., De Pablo, J., Rousaud, A., *et al.* (2001). Open trial of the efficacy and tolerability of mirtazapine in the treatment of major depression in HIV-1 infected outpatients. *European Neuropsychopharmacology*, 11(3), S228.

Bondarev, M.L., Bondareva, T.S., Young, R. and Glennon, R.A. (2003). Behavioral and biochemical investigations of bupropion metabolites. *European Journal of Pharmacology*, 474(1), 85–93.

Bonin, B., Vandel, P. and Kantelip, J.P. (2000). Mirtazapine and restless leg syndrome: A case report. *Therapie*, 55(5), 655–656.

Borderías Clau, L., Marigil Gómez, M.A., Val Adán, P., *et al.* (2008). Hypersensitivity pneumonitis due to venlafaxine. *Archivos de Bronconeumología*, 44(10), 571–573.

Borson, S., McDonald, G.J., Gayle, T., *et al.* (1992). Improvement in mood, physical symptoms, and function with nortriptyline for depression in patients with chronic obstructive pulmonary disease. *Psychosomatics*, 33(2), 190–201.

Boucher, N., Koren, G. and Beaulac-Baillargeon, L. (2009). Maternal use of venlafaxine near term: Correlation between neonatal effects and plasma concentrations. *Therapeutic Drug Monitoring*, 31(3), 404–409.

Bourgeois, J.A. (2005). Reversible hyponatremia and venlafaxine. *Psychosomatics*, 46(5), 495–496.

Boyer, P., Montgomery, S., Lepola, U., *et al.* (2008). Efficacy, safety, and tolerability of fixed-dose desvenlafaxine 50 and 100 mg/day for major depressive disorder in a placebo-controlled trial. *International Clinical Psychopharmacology*, 23(5), 243–253.

Bradley, R.H., Barkin, R.L., Jerome, J., *et al.* (2003). Efficacy of venlafaxine for the long term treatment of chronic pain with associated major depressive disorder. *American Journal of Therapeutics*, 10(5), 318–323.

Briggs, G.G., Samson, J.H., Ambrose, P.J. and Schroeder, D.H. (1993). Excretion of bupropion in breast milk. *Annals of Pharmacotherapy*, 27(4), 431–433.

Brisard, C., Zitek, B.E., Ninan, P.T., *et al.* (2007). Treating the painful physical symptoms of depression with desvenlafaxine succinate versus placebo in depressed outpatients. Presented at the 160th Annual Meeting of the American Psychiatric Association, San Diego, California.

Brosen, K., Klysner, R., Gram, L.F., *et al.* (1986a). Steady-state concentrations of imipramine and its metabolites in relation to the sparteine/debrisoquine polymorphism. *European Journal of Clinical Pharmacology*, 30(6), 679–684.

Brosen, K., Otton, S.V. and Gram, L.F. (1986b). Imipramine demethylation and hydroxylation: Impact of the sparteine oxidation phenotype. *Clinical Pharmacology and Therapeutics*, 40(5), 543–549.

Brown, E.S. and Hong, S.C. (1999). Antidepressant-induced bruxism successfully treated with gabapentin. *Journal of the American Dental Association*, 130(10), 1467–1469.

Brown, E.S., Vornik, L.A., Khan, D.A. and Rush, A.J. (2007). Bupropion in the treatment of outpatients with asthma and major depressive disorder. *International Journal of Psychiatry in Medicine*, 37(1), 23–28.

Brown, K., Ratner, M. and Stoll, M. (2003). Pheochromocytoma unmasked by imipramine in an 8-year-old girl. *Pediatric Emergency Care*, 19(3), 174–177.

Brubacher, J.R., Hoffman, R.S. and Lurin, M.J. (1996). Serotonin syndrome from venlafaxine-tranylcypromine interaction. *Veterinary and Human Toxicology*, 38(5), 358–361.

Brunnauer, A., Laux, G., Geiger, E., *et al.* (2006). Antidepressants and driving ability: Results from a clinical study. *Journal of Clinical Psychiatry*, 67(11), 1776–1781.

Brunnauer, A., Laux, G., David, I., *et al.* (2008). The impact of reboxetine and mirtazapine on driving simulator performance and psychomotor function in depressed patients. *Journal of Clinical Psychiatry*, 69(12), 1880–1886.

Bymaster, F.P., Dreshfield-Ahmad, L.J., Threlkeld, P.G., *et al.* (2001). Comparative affinity of duloxetine and venlafaxine for serotonin and norepinephrine transporters *in vitro* and *in vivo*, human serotonin receptor subtypes, and other neuronal receptors. *Neuropsychopharmacology*, 25(6), 871–880.

Casis, O. and Sanchez-Chapula, J.A. (1998). Mechanism of block of cardiac transient outward K+ current (I(to)) by antidepressant drugs. *Journal of Cardiovascular Pharmacology*, 32(4), 527–534.

Chang, T.T., Lêng, C.H., Wu, J.Y., *et al.* (2008). Lower side effects of milnacipran than paroxetine in the treatment of major depression disorder among Han Chinese in Taiwan. *Chinese Journal of Physiology*, 51(6), 387–393.

Chaudron, L.H. and Schoenecker, C.J. (2004). Bupropion and breastfeeding: A case of a possible infant seizure. *Journal of Clinical Psychiatry*, 65(6), 881–882.

Cheah, C.Y., Ladhams, B. and Fegan, P.G. (2008). Mirtazapine associated with profound hyponatremia: Two case reports. *American Journal of Geriatric Pharmacotherapy*, 6(2), 91–95.

Chiaverini, C., Baldin, B., Chichmanian, R.M., *et al.* (2003). Bupropion (Zyban) induced urticaria: 2 cases. *Annales de Dermatologie et de Vénéréologie*, 130(2 Pt 1), 208–209.

Choy, E.H., Mease, P.J., Kajdasz, D.K., *et al.* (2009). Safety and tolerability of duloxetine in the treatment of patients with fibromyalgia: Pooled analysis of data from five clinical trials. *Clinical Rheumatology*, 28(9), 1035–1044.

Chun-Fai-Chan, B., Koren, G., Fayez, I., *et al.* (2005). Pregnancy outcome of women exposed to bupropion during pregnancy: A prospective comparative study. *American Journal of Obstetrics and Gynecology*, 192(3), 932–936.

Clauw, D.J., Mease, P., Palmer, R.H., *et al.* (2008). Milnacipran for the treatment of fibromyalgia in adults: A 15-week, multicenter, randomized, double-blind, placebo-controlled, multiple-dose clinical trial. *Clinical Therapeutics*, 30(11), 1988–2004.

Clayton, A.H., Croft, H.A., Horrigan, J.P., *et al.* (2006). Bupropion extended release compared with escitalopram: Effects on sexual functioning and antidepressant efficacy in 2 randomized, double-blind, placebo-controlled studies. *Journal of Clinical Psychiatry*, 67(5), 736–746.

Clayton, A., Kornstein, S., Prakash, A., *et al.* (2007). Changes in sexual functioning associated with duloxetine, escitalopram, and placebo in the treatment of patients with major depressive disorder. *Journal of Sex Medicine*, 4(4i), 917–929.

Clayton, A.H., Kornstein, S.G., Rosas, G., *et al.* (2009). An integrated analysis of the safety and tolerability of desvenlafaxine compared with placebo in the treatment of major depressive disorder. *CNS Spectrums*, 14(4), 183–195.

Clayton, A.H., Pradko, J.F., Croft, H.A., *et al.* (2002). Prevalence of sexual dysfunction among newer antidepressants. *Journal of Clinical Psychiatry*, 63(4), 357–366.

Clerc, G. and Milnacipran/Fluvoxamine Study Group. (2001). Antidepressant efficacy and tolerability of milnacipran, a dual serotonin and noradrenaline reuptake inhibitor: A comparison with fluvoxamine. *International Clinical Psychopharmacology*, 16(3), 145–151.

Cohn, J.B., Collins, G., Ashbrook, E. and Wernicke, J.F. (1989). A comparison of fluoxetine imipramine and placebo in patients with bipolar depressive disorder. *International Clinical Psychopharmacology*, 4(4), 313–322.

Cole, J.A., Modell, J.G., Haight, B.R., *et al.* (2007). Bupropion in pregnancy and the prevalence of congenital malformations. *Pharmacoepidemiology and Drug Safety*, 16(5), 474–484.

Coleman, C.C., Cunningham, L.A., Foster, V.J., *et al.* (1999). Sexual dysfunction associated with the treatment of depression: A placebo-controlled comparison of bupropion sustained release and sertraline treatment. *Annals of Clinical Psychiatry*, 11(4), 205–215.

Colucci, V.J. and Berry, B.D. (2008). Heart failure worsening and exacerbation after venlafaxine and duloxetine therapy. *Annals of Pharmacotherapy*,42(6), 882–887.

Combes, A., Peytavin, G. and Theron, D. (2001). Conduction disturbances associated with venlafaxine. *Annals of Internal Medicine*, 134(2), 166–167.

Conners, C.K., Casat, C.D., Gualtieri, C.T., *et al.* (1996). Bupropion hydrochloride in attention deficit disorder with hyperactivity. *Journal of the American Academy of Child and Adolescent Psychiatry*, 35(10), 1314–1321.

Cooper, T.B., Suckow, R.F. and Glassman, A. (1984). Determination of bupropion and its major basic metabolites in plasma by liquid chromatography with dual-wavelength ultraviolet detection. *Journal of Pharmaceutical Sciences*, 73(8), 1104–1107.

Courtney, D.B. (2004). Selective serotonin reuptake inhibitor and venlafaxine use in children and adolescents with major depressive disorder: A systematic review of published randomized controlled trials. *Canadian Journal of Psychiatry*, 49(8), 557–563.

Cravello, L., Caltagirone, C. and Spalletta, G. (2009). The SNRI venlafaxine improves emotional unawareness in patients with post-stroke depression. *Human Psychopharmacology*, 24(4), 331–336.

Croft, H., Houser, T.L., Jamerson, B.D., *et al.* (2002). Effect on body weight of bupropion sustained-release in patients with major depression treated for 52 weeks. *Clinical Therapeutics*, 24(4), 662–672.

Croft, H., Settle, E. Jr., Houser, T., *et al.* (1999). A placebo-controlled comparison of the antidepressant efficacy and effects on sexual functioning of sustained-release bupropion and sertraline. *Clinical Therapeutics*, 21(4), 643–658.

Cunningham, L.A., Borison, R.L., Carman, J.S., *et al.* (1994). A comparison of venlafaxine, trazodone, and placebo in major depression. *Journal of Clinical Psychopharmacology*, 14(2), 99–106.

Currier, M.B., Molina, G. and Kato, M. (2003). A prospective trial of sustained-release bupropion for depression in HIV-seropositive and AIDS patients. *Psychosomatics*, 44(2), 120–125.

Dalery, J. and Aubin, V. (2001). Comparative study of paroxetine and mianserin in depression in elderly patients: Efficacy, tolerance, serotonin dependence. *Encephale*, 27(1), 71–81.

Danish University Antidepressant Group. (1986). Citalopram: Clinical effect profile in comparison with clomipramine. A controlled multicenter study. *Psychopharmacology*, 90(1), 131–138.

Danish University Antidepressant Group. (1990). Paroxetine: A selective serotonin reuptake inhibitor showing better tolerance, but weaker antidepressant effect than clomipramine in a controlled multicenter study. *Journal of Affective Disorders*, 18(4), 289–299.

Davidson, J., Baldwin, D., Stein, D.J., *et al.* (2006). Treatment of posttraumatic stress disorder with venlafaxine extended release: A 6-month randomized controlled trial. *Archives of General Psychiatry*, 63(10), 1158–1165.

Davidson, J., Watkins, L., Owens, M., *et al.* (2005). Effects of paroxetine and venlafaxine XR on heart rate variability in depression. *Journal of Clinical Psychopharmacology*, 25(5), 480–484.

Davidson, J.R., Meoni, P., Haudiquet, V., *et al.* (2002). Achieving remission with venlafaxine and fluoxetine in major depression: Its relationship to anxiety symptoms. *Depression and Anxiety*, 16(1), 4–13.

Davidson, J.R., Weisler, R.H., Butterfield, M.I., *et al.* (2003). Mirtazapine vs. placebo in posttraumatic stress disorder: A pilot trial. *Biological Psychiatry*, 53(2), 188–191.

Davis, J.S., Boyle, M.J., Hannaford, R. and Watson, A. (2001). Bupropion and serum sickness-like reaction. *Medical Journal of Australia*, 174(9), 479–480.

de Boer, T. (1996). The pharmacologic profile of mirtazapine. *Journal of Clinical Psychiatry*, 57(Suppl 4), 19–25.

de Boer, T.H., Maura, G., Raiteri, M., *et al.* (1988). Neurochemical and autonomic pharmacological profiles of the 6-aza-analogue of mianserin, Org 3770 and its enantiomers. *Neuropharmacology*, 27(4), 399–408.

De Santiago Hernando, M.L., Roldan San Juan, J., Gutierrez Agramunt, A. and Munoz Gomez, B. (2002). Serum sickness-like reaction induced by bupropion. *Medicina Clinica*, 119(2), 76.

de Vasconcelos Cunha, U.G., Lopes Rocha, F., Avila de Melo, R., *et al.* (2007). A placebo-controlled double-blind randomized study of venlafaxine in the treatment of depression in dementia. *Dementia and Geriatric Cognitive Disorders*, 24(1), 36–41.

Degner, D., Grohmann, R., Kropp, S., *et al.* (2004). Severe adverse drug reactions of antidepressants: Results of the German multicenter drug surveillance program AMSP. *Pharmacopsychiatry*, 37(Suppl 1), S39–45.

Deecher, D.C., Beyer, C.E., Johnston, G., *et al.* (2006). Desvenlafaxine succinate: A new serotonin and norepinephrine reuptake inhibitor. *Journal of Pharmacology and Experimental Therapeutics*, 318(2), 657–665.

Delgado, P.L., Brannan, S.K., Mallinckrodt, C.H., *et al.* (2005). Sexual functioning assessed in 4 double-blind placebo- and paroxetine-controlled trials of duloxetine for major depressive disorder. *Journal of Clinical Psychiatry*, 66(6), 686–692.

Delini-Stula, A. (2000). Milnacipran: An antidepressant with dual selectivity of action on noradrenaline and serotonin uptake. *Human Psychopharmacology*, 15(4), 255–260.

DeMartinis, N.A., Yeung, P.P., Entsuah, R. and Manley, A.L. (2007). A double-blind, placebo-controlled study of the efficacy and safety of desvenlafaxine succinate in the treatment of major depressive disorder. *Journal of Clinical Psychiatry*, 68(5), 677–688.

Demers, J.C. and Malone, M. (2001). Serotonin syndrome induced by fluvoxamine and mirtazapine. *Annals of Pharmacotherapy*, 35(10), 1217–1220.

Den Braber, E., Schutte, A.J. and Van der Flier, S. (2003). Tolerability of mirtazapine versus SSRIs in patients with major depression. *European Neuropsychopharmacology*, 13(4), S252.

Detke, M.J., Wiltse, C.G., Mallinckrodt, C.H., *et al.* (2004). Duloxetine in the acute and long-term treatment of major depressive disorder: A placebo- and paroxetine-controlled trial. *European Neuropsychopharmacology*, 14(6), 457–470.

Detweiler, M.B. and Harpold, G.J. (2002). Bupropion-induced acute dystonia. *Annals of Pharmacotherapy*, 36(2), 251–254.

Devanand, D.P., Juszczak, N., Nobler, M.S., *et al.* (2004). An open treatment trial of venlafaxine for elderly patients with dysthymic disorder. *Journal of Geriatric Psychiatry and Neurology*, 17(4), 219–224.

Diamond, S., Pepper, B.J., Diamond, M.L., *et al.* (1998). Serotonin syndrome induced by transitioning from phenelzine to venlafaxine: Four patient reports. *Neurology*, 51(1), 274–276.

Dimellis, D. (2002). Serotonin syndrome produced by a combination of venlafaxine and mirtazapine. *World J Biological Psychiatry*, 3(3), 167.

Dirks, A.C. and van Hyfte, D.M. (2007). Recurrent hyponatremia after substitution of citalopram with duloxetine. *Journal of Clinical Psychopharmacology*, 27(3), 313.

Djulus, J., Koren, G., Einarson, T.R., *et al.* (2006). Exposure to mirtazapine during pregnancy: A prospective, comparative study of birth outcomes. *Journal of Clinical Psychiatry*, 67(8), 1280–1284.

Dong, J. and Blier, P. (2001). Modification of norepinephrine and serotonin, but not dopamine, neuron firing by sustained bupropion treatment. *Psychopharmacology*, 155(1), 52–57.

Dorman, T. (1992). Sleep and paroxetine: A comparison with mianserin in elderly depressed patients. *International Clinical Psychopharmacology*, 6(s4), 53–58.

Dougherty, J.A., Young, H. and Shafi, T. (2002). Serotonin syndrome induced by amitriptyline, meperidine, and venlafaxine. *Annals of Pharmacotherapy*, 36(10), 1647–1648.

Dreixler, J.C., Bian, J., Cao, Y., *et al.* (2000). Block of rat brain recombinant SK channels by tricyclic antidepressants and related compounds. *European Journal of Pharmacology*, 401(1), 1–7.

Dunner, D.L., Zisook, S., Billow, A.A., *et al.* (1998). A prospective safety surveillance study for bupropion sustained-release in the treatment of depression. *Journal of Clinical Psychiatry*, 59(7), 366–373.

Egger, C., Muehlbacher, M., Nickel, M., *et al.* (2006). A case of recurrent hyponatremia induced by venlafaxine. *Journal of Clinical Psychopharmacology*. 2006, 26(4), 439.

Ehret, M.J., Levin, G.M., Narasimhan, M. and Rathinavelu, A. (2007). Venlafaxine induces P-glycoprotein in human Caco-2 cells. *Human Psychopharmacology*, 22(1), 49–53.

Einarson, A., Choi, J., Einarson, T.R. and Koren, G. (2009). Incidence of major malformations in infants following antidepressant exposure in pregnancy: Results of a large prospective cohort study. *Canadian Journal of Psychiatry*, 54(4), 242–246.

Einarson, A., Fatoye, B., Sarkar, M., *et al.* (2001). Pregnancy outcome following gestational exposure to venlafaxine: A Multicenter prospective controlled study. *American Journal of Psychiatry*, 158(10), 1728–1730.

Einarson, T.R. and Einarson, A. (2005). Newer antidepressants in pregnancy and rates of major malformations: A meta-analysis of prospective comparative studies. *Pharmacoepidemiology and Drug Safety*, 14(12), 823–827.

Emslie, G.J., Findling, R.L., Yeung, P.P., *et al.* (2007). Venlafaxine ER for the treatment of pediatric subjects with depression: Results of two placebo-controlled trials. *Journal of the American Academy of Child and Adolescent Psychiatry*, 46(4), 479–488.

Entsuah, A.R., Huang, H. and Thase, M.E. (2001). Response and remission rates in different subpopulations with major depressive disorder administered venlafaxine, selective serotonin reuptake inhibitors, or placebo. *Journal of Clinical Psychiatry*, 62(11), 869–877.

Entsuah, R., Rudolph, R.L., Hackett, D. and Miska, S. (1996). Efficacy of venlafaxine and placebo during long-term treatment of depression: A pooled analysis of relapse rates. *International Clinical Psychopharmacology*, 11(2), 137–145.

Ersoy, M.A., Noyan, A.M. and Elbi, H. (2008) An open-label long-term naturalistic study of mirtazapine treatment for depression in cancer patients. *Clinical Drug Investigation*, 28(2), 113–120.

Espeleta, V.J., Moore, W.H., Kane, P.B. and Baram, D. (2007). Eosinophilic pneumonia due to duloxetine. *Chest*, 131(3), 901–903.

Fabre, L.F., Brodie, H.K., Garver, D. and Zung, W.W. (1983). A multicenter evaluation of bupropion versus placebo in hospitalized depressed patients. *Journal of Clinical Psychiatry*, 44(5 Pt 2), 88–94.

Fava, M., Judge, R., Hoog, S.L., *et al.* (2000). Fluoxetine versus sertraline and paroxetine in major depressive disorder: Changes in weight with long-term treatment. *Journal of Clinical Psychiatry*, 61(11), 863–867.

Fava, M., Martinez, J.M., Greist, J., *et al.* (2007). The efficacy and tolerability of duloxetine in the treatment of anxious versus non-anxious depression: A post-hoc analysis of an open-label outpatient study. *Annals of Clinical Psychiatry*, 19(3), 187–195.

Fava, M., Mulroy, R., Alpert, J., *et al.* (1997). Emergence of adverse events following discontinuation of treatment with extended-release venlafaxine. *American Journal of Psychiatry*, 154(12), 1760–1762.

Fays, S., Trechot, P., Schmutz, J.L., *et al.* (2003). Bupropion and generalized acute urticaria: Eight cases. *British Journal of Dermatology*, 148(1), 177–178.

Feiger, A.D., Tourian, K.A., Rosas, G.R. and Padmanabhan, S.K. (2009). A placebo-controlled study evaluating the efficacy and safety of flexible-dose desvenlafaxine treatment in outpatients with major depressive disorder. *CNS Spectrums*, 14(1), 41–50.

Feighner, J.P. (1995). Cardiovascular safety in depressed patients: Focus on venlafaxine. *Journal of Clinical Psychiatry*, 56(12), 574–579.

Feighner, J.P., Gardner, E.A., Johnston, J.A., *et al.* (1991). Double-blind comparison of bupropion and fluoxetine in depressed outpatients. *Journal of Clinical Psychiatry*, 52(8), 329–335.

Ferguson, K.L. (1994). Imipramine-provoked paradoxical pheochromocytoma crisis: A case of cardiogenic shock. *American Journal of Emergency Medicine*, 12(2), 190–192.

Ferreira, E., Carceller, A.M., Agogue, C., *et al.* (2007). Effects of selective serotonin reuptake inhibitors and venlafaxine during pregnancy in term and preterm neonates. *Pediatrics*, 119(1), 52–59.

Flanagan, R.J. (2008). Fatal toxicity of drugs used in psychiatry. *Human Psychopharmacology*, 23(Suppl 1), 43–51.

Flemenbaum, A. (1976). Pavor nocturnus: A complication of single daily tricyclic or neuroleptic dosage. *American Journal of Psychiatry*, 133(5), 570–572.

Foley, K.F. and Cozzi, N.V. (2002). Inhibition of transport function and desipramine binding at the human noradrenaline transporter by N-ethylmaleimide and protection by substrate analogs. *Naunyn-Schmiedeberg's Archives of Pharmacology*, 365(6), 457–461.

Fowlie, S. and Burton, J. (1987). Hyperprolactinaemia and nonpuerperal lactation associated with clomipramine. *Scottish Medical Journal*, 32(2), 52.

Fric, M., Pfuhlmann, B., Laux, G., *et al.* (2008). The influence of smoking on the serum level of duloxetine. *Pharmacopsychiatry*, 41(4), 151–155.

Fryer, J.D. and Lukas, R.J. (1999). Noncompetitive functional inhibition at diverse, human nicotinic acetylcholine receptor subtypes by bupropion, phencyclidine, and ibogaine. *Journal of Pharmacology and Experimental Therapeutics*, 288(1), 88–92.

Fukuda, T., Nishida, Y., Imaoka, S., *et al.* (2000a). The decreased *in vivo* clearance of CYP2D6 substrates by CYP2D6*10 might be caused not only by the low-expression but also by low affinity of CYP2D6. *Archives of Biochemistry and Biophysics*, 380(2), 303–308.

Fukuda, T., Nishida, Y., Zhou, Q., *et al.* (2000b). The impact of the CYP2D6 and CYP2C19 genotypes on venlafaxine pharmacokinetics in a Japanese population. *European Journal of Clinical Pharmacology*, 56(2), 175–180.

Gadde, K.M., Parker, C.B., Maner, L.G., *et al.* (2001). Bupropion for weight loss: An investigation of efficacy and tolerability in overweight and obese women. *Obesity Research*, 2001, 9(9), 544–551.

Galeotti, N., Ghelardini, C. and Bartolini, A. (2001). Involvement of potassium channels in amitriptyline and clomipramine analgesia. *Neuropharmacology*, 40(1), 75–84.

Galeotti, N., Ghelardini, C., Capaccioli, S., *et al.* (1997). Blockade of clomipramine and amitriptyline analgesia by an antisense oligonucleotide to mKv1.1, a mouse Shaker-like K+ channel. *European Journal of Pharmacology*, 330(1), 15–25.

Garner, E.M., Kelly, M.W. and Thompson, D.F. (1993). Tricyclic antidepressant withdrawal syndrome. *Annals of Pharmacotherapy*, 27(9), 1068–1072.

Gendreau, R.M., Thorn, M.D., Gendreau, J.F., *et al.* (2005). Efficacy of milnacipran in patients with fibromyalgia. *Journal of Rheumatology*, 32(10), 1975–1985.

Gex-Fabry, M., Balant-Gorgia, A.E., Balant, L.P., *et al.* (2004). Time course of clinical response to venlafaxine: Relevance of plasma level and chirality. *European Journal of Clinical Pharmacology*, 59(12), 883–891.

Giers, G., Salama, A. and Mueller-Eckhardt, C. (1991). Follow-up study on 24 patients with nomifensine-induced immune haemolytic anaemia. *Transfusion Medicine*, 1(2), 115–119.

Girishchandra, B.G., Johnson, L., Cresp, R.M. and Orr, K.G. (2002). Mirtazapine-induced akathisia. *Medical Journal of Australia*, 176(5), 242.

Gitlin, M.J. (1997). Venlafaxine, monoamine oxidase inhibitors, and the serotonin syndrome. *Journal of Clinical Psychopharmacology*, 17(1), 66–67.

Glod, C.A., Lynch, A., Flynn, E., *et al.* (2003). Open trial of bupropion SR in adolescent major depression. *Journal of Child and Adolescent Psychiatric Nursing*, 16(3), 123–130.

Goetz, C.G., Tanner, C.M. and Klawans, H.L. (1984). Bupropion in Parkinson's disease. *Neurology*, 34(8), 1092–1094.

Golden, R.N., De Vane, C.L., Laizure, S.C., *et al.* (1988). Bupropion in depression. II. The role of metabolites in clinical outcome. *Archives of General Psychiatry*, 45(2), 145–149.

Goldstein, D.J., Lu, Y., Detke, M.J., *et al.* (2004). Duloxetine in the treatment of depression: A double-blind placebo-controlled comparison with paroxetine. *Journal of Clinical Psychopharmacology*, 24(4), 389–399.

Goldstein, D.J., Mallinckrodt, C., Lu, Y. and Demitrack, M.A. (2002). Duloxetine in the treatment of major depressive disorder: A double-blind clinical trial. *Journal of Clinical Psychiatry*, 63(3), 225–231.

Gonzalez, E., Sanguino, R.M. and Franco, M.A. (2006). Bupropion in atopic dermatitis. *Pharmacopsychiatry*, 39(6), 229.

Gonzalez-Pinto, A., Gutierrez, M., Gonzalez, N., *et al.* (2002). Efficacy and safety of venlafaxine-ECT combination in treatment-resistant depression. *Journal of Neuropsychiatry and Clinical Neurosciences*, 14(2), 206–209.

Goodnick, P.J. (2001). Use of antidepressants in treatment of comorbid diabetes mellitus and depression as well as in diabetic neuropathy. *Annals of Clinical Psychiatry*, 13(1), 31–41.

Gordon, G.H., Michiels, T.M., Mahutte, C.K. and Light, R.W. (1985). Effect of desipramine on control of ventilation and depression scores in patients with severe chronic obstructive pulmonary disease. *Psychiatry Research*, 15(1), 25–32.

Grasmader, K., Verwohlt, P.L., Rietschel, M., *et al.* (2004). Impact of polymorphisms of cytochrome-P450 isoenzymes 2C9, 2C19 and 2D6 on plasma concentrations and clinical effects of antidepressants in a naturalistic clinical setting. *European Journal of Clinical Pharmacology*, 60(5), 329–336.

Greenberg, H.E., Scharf, S.M. and Green, H. (1993). Nortriptyline-induced depression of ventilatory control in a patient with chronic obstructive pulmonary disease. *American Review of Respiratory Disease*, 147(5), 1303–1305.

Griffith, J.D., Carranza, J., Griffith, C. and Miller, L.L. (1983). Bupropion: Clinical assay for amphetamine-like abuse potential. *Journal of Clinical Psychiatry*, 44(5 Pt 2), 206–208.

Grunnet, M., Jespersen, T., Angelo, K., *et al.* (2001). Pharmacological modulation of SK3 channels. *Neuropharmacology*, 40(7), 879–887.

Guelfi, J.D., Ansseau, M., Timmerman, L., *et al.* (2001). Mirtazapine versus venlafaxine in hospitalized severely depressed patients with melancholic features. *Journal of Clinical Psychopharmacology*, 21(4), 425–431.

Gupta, A.K. and Saravay, S.M. (1997). Venlafaxine-induced hyponatremia. *Journal of Clinical Psychopharmacology*, 17(3), 223–225.

Haddjeri, N., Blier, P. and de Montigny, C. (1995). Noradrenergic modulation of central serotonergic neurotransmission: Acute and long-term actions of mirtazapine. *International Clinical Psychopharmacology*, 10(Suppl 4), 11–17.

Halikas, J.A. (1995). Org 3770 (Mirtazapine) versus trazodone: A placebo-controlled trial in depressed elderly patients. *Human Psychopharmacology*, 10, S125–133.

Hanje, A.J., Pell, L.J., Votolato, N.A., *et al.* (2006). Case report: Fulminant hepatic failure involving duloxetine hydrochloride. *Clinical Gastroenterology and Hepatology*, 4(7), 912–917.

Hanna, G.L., McCracken, J.T. and Cantwell, D.P. (1991). Prolactin in childhood obsessive-compulsive disorder: Clinical correlates and response to clomipramine. *Journal of the American Academy of Child and Adolescent Psychiatry*, 30(2), 173–178.

Harrigan, R.A and Brady, W.J. (1999). ECG abnormalities in tricyclic antidepressant ingestion. *American Journal of Emergency Medicine*, 17(4), 387–393.

Harvey, A.T., Rudolph, RL. and Preskorn, S.H. (2000). Evidence of the dual mechanisms of action of venlafaxine. *Archives of General Psychiatry*, 57(5), 503–509.

Hayashi, Y., Ohyagi, Y., Inoue, I., *et al.* (2000). A case of amoxapine-induced tardive dystonia successfully treated with a low dose anti-cholinergic agent. *Rinsho Shinkeigaku*, 40(4), 367–371.

Heisler, M.A., Guidry, J.R. and Arnecke, B. (1996). Serotonin syndrome induced by administration of venlafaxine and phenelzine. *Annals of Pharmacotherapy*, 30(1), 84.

Henry, J.A., Alexander, C.A. and Sener, E.K. (1995). Relative mortality from overdose of antidepressants. *British Medical Journal*, 310(6974), 221–224.

Hermann, M., Hendset, M., Fosaas, K., *et al.* (2008). Serum concentrations of venlafaxine and its metabolites *O*-desmethylvenlafaxine and N-desmethylvenlafaxine in heterozygous carriers of the CYP2D6*3, *4 or *5 allele. *European Journal of Clinical Pharmacology*, 64(5), 483–487.

Hernandez, J.L., Ramos, F.J., Infante, J., *et al.* (2002). Severe serotonin syndrome induced by mirtazapine monotherapy. *Annals of Pharmacotherapy*, 36(4), 641–643.

Hesse, L.M., Venkatakrishnan, K., Court, M.H., *et al.* (2000). CYP2B6 mediates the *in vitro* hydroxylation of bupropion: Potential drug interactions with other antidepressants. *Drug Metabolism and Disposition*, 28(10), 1176–1183.

Hewett, K., Chrzanowski, W., Jokinen, R., *et al.* (in press). Double-blind, placebo-controlled evaluation of extended-release bupropion in elderly patients with major depressive disorder. *Journal of Psychopharmacology*.

Hewett, K., Chrzanowski, W., Schmitz, M., *et al.* (2009). Eight-week, placebo-controlled, double-blind comparison of the antidepressant efficacy and tolerability of bupropion XR and venlafaxine XR. (in press). *Journal of Psychopharmacology*, 23(5), 531–538.

Hildebrandt, M.G., Steyerberg, E.W., Stage, K.B., *et al.* (2003). Danish University Antidepressant Group. Are gender differences important for the clinical effects of antidepressants? *American Journal of Psychiatry*, 160(9), 1643–1650.

Hinze-Selch, D., Schuld, A., Kraus, T., *et al.* (2000). Effects of antidepressants on weight and on the plasma levels of leptin, TNF-alpha and soluble TNF receptors: A longitudinal study in patients treated with amitriptyline or paroxetine. *Neuropsychopharmacology*, 23(1), 13–19.

Hodgman, M.J., Martin, T.G. and Krenzelok, E.P. (1997). Serotonin syndrome due to venlafaxine and maintenance tranylcypromine therapy. *Human and Experimental Toxicology*, 16(1), 14–17.

Höjer, J., Hulting, J. and Salmonson, H. (2008). Fatal cardiotoxicity induced by venlafaxine overdosage. *Clinical Toxicology*, 46(4), 336–337.

Hong, C.J., Hu, W.H., Chen, C.C., *et al.* (2003). A double-blind, randomized, group-comparative study of the tolerability and efficacy of 6 weeks' treatment with mirtazapine or fluoxetine in depressed chinese patients. *Journal of Clinical Psychiatry*, 64(8), 921–926.

Honig, A., Kuyper, A.M., Schene, A.H., *et al.* (2007). Treatment of post-myocardial infarction depressive disorder: A randomized, placebo-controlled trial with mirtazapine.*Psychosomatic Medicine*, 69(7), 606–613.

Horne, R.L., Ferguson, J.M., Pope, H.G. Jr., *et al.* (1988). Treatment of bulimia with bupropion: A multicenter controlled trial. *Journal of Clinical Psychiatry*, 49(7), 262–266.

Hornig-Rohan, M. and Amsterdam, J.D. (2002). Venlafaxine versus stimulant therapy in patients with dual diagnosis ADD and depression. *Progress in Neuropsychopharmacology and Biological Psychiatry*, 26(3), 585–589.

Howell, C., Wilson, A.D. and Waring, W.S. (2007). Cardiovascular toxicity due to venlafaxine poisoning in adults: A review of 235 consecutive cases. *British Journal of Clinical Pharmacology*, 64(2), 192–197.

Huang, C.C. (1986). Persistent tardive dyskinesia associated with amoxapine therapy. *American Journal of Psychiatry*, 143(8), 1069–1070.

Humayun, F., Shehab, T.M., Tworek, J.A. and Fontana, R.J. (2007). A fatal case of bupropion (Zyban) hepatotoxicity with autoimmune features: A case report. *Journal of Medical Case Reports*, 1(1), 88.

Hussain, A. and Burke, J. (2008) Mirtazapine associated with recurrent pancreatitis — a case report. *Journal of Psychopharmacology*, 22(3), 336–337.

Hutchison, L.C. (2001). Mirtazapine and bone marrow suppression: A case report. *Journal of the American Geriatric Society*, 49(8), 1129–1130.

Ilett, K.F., Hackett, L.P., Dusci, L.J., *et al.* (1998). Distribution and excretion of venlafaxine and O-desmethylvenlafaxine in human milk. *British Journal of Clinical Pharmacology*, 45(5), 459–462.

Ilett, K.F., Kristensen, J.H., Hackett, L.P., *et al.* (2002). Distribution of venlafaxine and its O-desmethyl metabolite in human milk and their effects in breastfed infants. *British Journal of Clinical Pharmacology*, 53(1), 17–22.

Isbister, G.K. and Balit, C.R. (2003). Bupropion overdose: QTc prolongation and its clinical significance. *Annals of Pharmacotherapy*, 37(7–8), 999–1002.

Iwamoto, K., Takahashi, M., Nakamura, Y., *et al.* (2008). The effects of acute treatment with paroxetine, amitriptyline, and placebo on driving performance and cognitive function in healthy Japanese subjects: A double-blind crossover trial. *Human Psychopharmacology*, 23(5), 399–407.

Iwashita, T. and Shimizu, T. (1992). Imipramine inhibits intrathecal substance P-induced behavior and blocks spinal cord substance P receptors in mice. *Brain Research*, 581(1), 59–66.

Jaffee, M.S. and Bostwick, J.M. (2000). Buspirone as an antidote to venlafaxine-induced bruxism. *Psychosomatics*, 41(6), 535–536.

Jain, A.K., Kaplan, R.A., Gadde, K.M., *et al.* (2002). Bupropion SR vs. placebo for weight loss in obese patients with depressive symptoms. *Obesity Research*, 10(10), 1049–1056.

Jo, S.H., Youm, J.B., Lee, C.O., *et al.* (2000). Blockade of the HERG human cardiac K(+) channel by the antidepressant drug amitriptyline. *British Journal of Pharmacology*, 129(7), 1474–1480.

Joffe, H., Groninger, H., Soares, C.N., *et al.* (2001). An open trial of mirtazapine in menopausal women with depression unresponsive to estrogen replacement therapy. *Journal of Women's Health and Gender-Based Medicine*, 10(10), 999–1004.

Johnson, E.M., Whyte, E., Mulsant, B.H., *et al.* (2006). Cardiovascular changes associated with venlafaxine in the treatment of late-life depression. *American Journal of Geriatric Psychiatry*, 14(9), 796–802.

Johnson, E.R., Jones, M.D. and Stewart, J.N. (1979). Occurrence of a pheochromocytoma after ingestion of imipramine. *Journal of the American Osteopathathic Association*, 78(5), 332–335.

Johnston, J.A., Lineberry, C.G., Ascher, J.A., *et al.* (1991). A 102-center prospective study of seizure in association with bupropion. *Journal of Clinical Psychiatry*, 52(11), 450–456.

Joo, J.H., Lenze, E.J., Mulsant, B.H., *et al.* (2002). Risk factors for falls during treatment of late-life depression. *Journal of Clinical Psychiatry*, 63(10), 936–941.

Joyce, P.R., Mulder, R.T., Luty, S.E., *et al.* (2003). Age-dependent antidepressant pharmacogenomics: Polymorphisms of the serotonin transporter and G protein beta3 subunit as predictors of response to fluoxetine and nortriptyline. *International Journal of Neuropsychopharmacology*, 6(4), 339–346.

Kapur, S., Cho, R., Jones, C., *et al.* (1999). Is amoxapine an atypical antipsychotic? Positron-emission tomography investigation of its dopamine2 and serotonin2 occupancy. *Biological Psychiatry*, 45(9), 1217– 1220.

Karlsson, I., Godderis, J., Augusto De Mendonca Lima, C., *et al.* (2000). A randomised, double-blind comparison of the efficacy and safety of citalopram compared to mianserin in elderly, depressed patients with or without mild to moderate dementia. *International Journal of Geriatric Psychiatry*, 15(4), 295–305.

Kasper, S., Pletan, Y., Solles, A. and Tournoux, A. (1996). Comparative studies with milnacipran and tricyclic antidepressants in the treatment of patients with major depression: A summary of clinical trial results. *International Clinical Psychopharmacology*, 11(Suppl 4), 35–39.

Kasper, S., Praschak-Rieder, N., Tauscher, J. and Wolf, R. (1997). A risk-benefit assessment of mirtazapine in the treatment of depression. *Drug Safety*, 17(4), 251–264.

Kasper, S., Zivkov, M., Roes, K.C. and Pols, A.G. (1997). Pharmacological treatment of severely depressed patients: A meta-analysis comparing efficacy of mirtazapine and amitriptyline. *European Neuropsychopharmacology*, 7(2), 115–124.

Katz, I.R., Reynolds, C.F. 3rd, Alexopoulos, G.S. and Hackett, D. (2002). Venlafaxine ER as a treatment for generalized anxiety disorder in older adults: Pooled analysis of five randomized placebo-controlled clinical trials. *Journal of the American Geriatric Society*, 50(1), 18–25.

Kavoussi, R.J., Segraves, R.T., Hughes, A.R., *et al.* (1997). Double-blind comparison of bupropion sustained release and sertraline in depressed outpatients. *Journal of Clinical Psychiatry*, 58(12), 532–537.

Keller, M.B., Trivedi, M.H., Thase, M.E., *et al.* (2007). The prevention of recurrent episodes of depression with venlafaxine for two years (PREVENT) study: Outcomes from the 2-year and combined maintenance phases. *Journal of Clinical Psychiatry*, 68(8), 1246–1256.

Khalifa, M., Daleau, P. and Turgeon, J. (1999). Mechanism of sodium channel block by venlafaxine in guinea pig ventricular myocytes. *Journal of Pharmacology and Experimental Therapeutics*, 291(1), 280–284.

Khan, A., Bose, A., Alexopoulos, G.S., *et al.* (2007). Double-blind comparison of escitalopram and duloxetine in the acute treatment of major depressive disorder. *Clinical Drug Investigation*, 27(7), 481–492.

Khazaal, Y., Krenz, S. and Zullino, D.F. (2003). Bupropion-induced somnambulism. *Addiction Biology*, 8(3), 359–362.

Kiev, A., Masco, H.L., Wenger, T.L., *et al.* (1994). The cardiovascular effects of bupropion and nortriptyline in depressed outpatients. *Annals of Clinical Psychiatry*, 6(2), 107–115.

Kinney, J.L. (1985). Nomifensine maleate: A new second-generation antidepressant. *Clinical Pharmacy*, 4(6), 625–636.

Kirby, D., Harrigan, S. and Ames, D. (2002). Hyponatraemia in elderly psychiatric patients treated with Selective Serotonin Reuptake Inhibitors and venlafaxine: A retrospective controlled study in an inpatient unit. *International Journal of Geriatric Psychiatry*, 17(3), 231–237.

Kirchheiner, J., Klein, C., Meineke, I., *et al.* (2003). Bupropion and 4-OH-bupropion pharmacokinetics in relation to genetic polymorphisms in CYP2B6. *Pharmacogenetics*, 13(10), 619–626.

Klein, J.J., Segal, R.L. and Warner, R.R. (1964). Galactorrhea due to Imipramine. Report of a case. *New England Journal of Medicine*, 271, 510–512.

Kluge, M., Schussler, P. and Steiger, A. (2007). Duloxetine increases stage 3 sleep and suppresses rapid eye movement (REM) sleep in patients with major depression. *European Neuropsychopharmacology*, 17(8), 527–531.

Knowles, S.R., Shapiro, L.E. and Shear, N.H. (2003). Reactive metabolites and adverse drug reactions: Clinical considerations. *Clinical Review of Allergy and Immunology*, 24(3), 229–238.

Kohn, S. and Labbate, L.A. (1997). Venlafaxine and ecchymosis. *Canadian Journal of Psychiatry*, 42(1), 91.

Kolecki, P. (1997a). Isolated venlafaxine-induced serotonin syndrome. *Journal of Emergency Medicine*, 15(4), 491–493.

Kolecki, P. (1997b). Venlafaxine induced serotonin syndrome occurring after abstinence from phenelzine for more than two weeks. *Journal of Toxicology. Clinical Toxicology*, 35(2), 211–212.

Koran, L.M., Aboujaoude, E.N. and Gamel, N.N. (2007). Duloxetine treatment of dysthymia and double depression: An open-label trial. *Journal of Clinical Psychiatry*, 68(5), 761–765.

Kornstein, S.G., Li, D., Mao, Y., *et al.* (2009). Escitalopram versus SNRI antidepressants in the acute treatment of major depressive disorder. *CNS Spectrums*, 14(6), 326–333.

Kornstein, S.G., Schatzberg, A.F., Thase, M.E., *et al.* (2000). Gender differences in treatment response to sertraline versus imipramine in chronic depression. *American Journal of Psychiatry*, 157(9), 1445–1452.

Korzets, A., Floro, S., Ori, Y., *et al.* (1997). Clomipramine-induced pheochromocytoma crisis: A near fatal complication of a tricyclic antidepressant. *Journal of Clinical Psychopharmacology*, 17(5), 428–430.

Kraus, T., Haack, M., Schuld, A., *et al.* (2002). Body weight, the tumor necrosis factor system, and leptin production during treatment with mirtazapine or venlafaxine. *Pharmacopsychiatry*, 35(6), 220–225.

Krebs, E.E., Gaynes, B.N., Gartlehner, G., *et al.* (2008). Treating the physical symptoms of depression with second-generation antidepressants: A systematic review and metaanalysis. *Psychosomatics*, 49(3), 191–198.

Kristensen, J.H., Ilett, K.F., Rampono, J., *et al.* (2007). Transfer of the antidepressant mirtazapine into breast milk. *British Journal of Clinical Pharmacology*, 63(3), 322–327.

Kruger, S. and Lindstaedt, M. (2007). Duloxetine and hyponatremia: A report of 5 cases. *Journal of Clinical Psychopharmacology*, 27(1), 101–104.

Kuhs, H. (1998). Unmasking pheochromocytoma by amitriptyline. *Nervenarzt*, 69(1), 76–77.

Kuhn, K.U., Quednow, B.B., Thiel, M., *et al.* (2003). Antidepressive treatment in patients with temporal lobe epilepsy and major depression: A prospective study with three different antidepressants. *Epilepsy and Behavior*, 4(6), 674–679.

Kucukalic, A., Bravo-Mehmedbasic, A., Kulenovic, A.D. and Suljic-Mehmedika, E. (2007). Venlafaxine eficacy and tolerability in the treatment of post-stroke depression. *Psychiatria Danubina*, 19(1–2), 56–60.

Kusalic, M., Engelsmann, F. and Bradwejn, J. (1993). Thyroid functioning during treatment for depression. *Journal of Psychiatry and Neuroscience*, 18(5), 260–263.

Ladino, M., Guardiola, V.D. and Paniagua, M. (2006). Mirtazapine-induced hyponatremia in an elderly hospice patient. *Journal of Palliative Medicine*, 9(2), 258–260.

La Pia, S., Giorgio, D., Ciriello, R., *et al.* (1992). Evaluation of the efficacy, tolerability and therapeutic profile of fluoxetine versus mianserin in the treatment of depressive disorders in the elderly. *Current Therapeutic Research*, 52(6), 847–858.

Lam, R.W., Andersen, H.F. and Wade, A.G. (2008). Escitalopram and duloxetine in the treatment of major depressive disorder: A pooled analysis of two trials. *International Clinical Psychopharmacology*, 23(4), 181–187.

Learned-Coughlin, S.M., Bergstrom, M., Savitcheva, I., *et al.* (2003). *In vivo* activity of bupropion at the human dopamine transporter as measured by positron emission tomography. *Biological Psychiatry*, 54(8), 800–805.

Lecrubier, Y., Pletan, Y., Solles, A., *et al.* (1996). Clinical efficacy of milnacipran: Placebo-controlled trials. *International Clinical Psychopharmacology*. 1996, 11(Suppl 4), 29–33.

Lee, I., Chung, S., Lee, S., *et al.* (2007). Mirtazapine versus venlafaxine for the treatment of depressive and physical symptoms in major depressive disorder. Presented at the 160th Annual Meeting of the American Psychiatric Association. San Diego, California.

Lee, P., Shu, L., Xu, X., *et al.* (2007). Once-daily duloxetine 60 mg in the treatment of major depressive disorder: Multicenter, double-blind, randomized, paroxetine-controlled, non-inferiority trial in China, Korea, Taiwan and Brazil. *Psychiatry and Clinical Neuroscience*, 61(3), 295–307.

Leinonen, E., Skarstein, J., Behnke, K., *et al.* (1999). Efficacy and tolerability of mirtazapine versus citalopram: A double-blind, randomized study in patients with major depressive disorder. Nordic Antidepressant Study Group. *International Clinical Psychopharmacology*, 14(6), 329–337.

Leipzig, R.M., Cumming, R.G. and Tinetti, M.E. (1999). Drugs and falls in older people: A systematic review and meta-analysis: I. Psychotropic drugs. *Journal of the American Geriatric Society*, 47(1), 30–39.

Lessard, E., Yessine, M.A., Hamelin, B.A., *et al.* (1999). Influence of CYP2D6 activity on the disposition and cardiovascular toxicity of the antidepressant agent venlafaxine in humans. *Pharmacogenetics*, 9(4), 435–443.

Letsas, K., Korantzopoulos, P., Pappas, L., *et al.* (2006). QT interval prolongation associated with venlafaxine administration. *International Journal of Cardiology*, 109(1), 116–117.

Levin, A. (1982). Nomifensine and maprotiline in endogenous depression: Comparative efficacy and side effects. *International Pharmacopsychiatry*, 17(Suppl 1), 89–96.

Levinson-Castiel, R., Merlob, P., Linder, N., *et al.* (2006). Neonatal abstinence syndrome after in utero exposure to selective serotonin reuptake inhibitors in term infants. *Archives of Pediatric and Adolescent Medicine*, 160(2), 173–176.

Lewis-Hall, F.C., Wilson, M.G., Tepner, R.G. and Koke, S.C. (1997). Fluoxetine vs. tricyclic antidepressants in women with major depressive disorder. *Journal of Women's Health*, 6(3), 337–343.

Li, S.X., Perry, K.W. and Wong, D.T. (2002). Influence of fluoxetine on the ability of bupropion to modulate extracellular dopamine and norepinephrine concentrations in three mesocorticolimbic areas of rats. *Neuropharmacology*, 42(2), 181–190.

Lieberman, D.Z., Montgomery, S.A., Tourian, K.A., *et al.* (2008). A pooled analysis of two placebo-controlled trials of desvenlafaxine in major depressive disorder. *International Clinical Psychopharmacology*, 23(4), 188–197.

Liebowitz, M.R., Gelenberg, A.J. and Munjack, D. (2005). Venlafaxine extended release vs placebo and paroxetine in social anxiety disorder. *Archives of General Psychiatry*, 62(2), 190–198.

Liebowitz, M.R., Manley, A.L., Padmanabhan, S.K., *et al.* (2008). Efficacy, safety, and tolerability of desvenlafaxine 50 mg/day and 100 mg/day in outpatients with major depressive disorder. *Current Medical and Research Opinion*, 24(7), 1877–1890.

Liebowitz, M.R., Yeung P.P. and Entsuah, R. (2007). A randomized, double-blind, placebo-controlled trial of desvenlafaxine succinate in adult outpatients with major depressive disorder. *Journal of Clinical Psychiatry*, 68(11), 1663–1672.

Lineberry, T.W., Peters, G.E. Jr. and Bostwick, J.M. (2001). Bupropion-induced erythema multiforme. *Mayo Clinic Proceedings*, 76(6), 664–666.

Linnebur, S.A., Saseen, J.J. and Pace, W.D. (2002). Venlafaxine-associated vaginal bleeding. *Pharmacotherapy*, 22(5), 652–655.

Linnoila, M., Gold, P., Potter, W.Z. and Wehr, T.A. (1981). Tricyclic antidepressants do not alter thyroid hormone levels in patients suffering from a major affective disorder. *Psychiatry Research*, 4(3), 357–360.

Liskin, B., Walsh, B.T., Roose, S.P. and Jackson, W. (1984). Imipramine-induced inappropriate ADH secretion. *Journal of Clinical Psychopharmacology*, 4(3), 146–147.

Liu, X. and Sahud, M.A. (2003). Glycoprotein IIb/IIIa complex is the target in mirtazapine-induced immune thrombocytopenia. *Blood Cells, Molecules and Diseases*, 30(3), 241–245.

Loo, W.J., Alexandroff, A. and Flanagan, N. (2003). Bupropion and generalized acute urticaria: A further case. *British Journal of Dermatology*, 149(3), 660.

Lu, R., Hurley, A.D. and Gourley, M. (2002). Dystonia induced by mirtazapine. *Journal of Clinical Psychiatry*, 63(5), 452–453.

Lustman, P.J., Griffith, L.S., Clouse, R.E., *et al.* (1997). Effects of nortriptyline on depression and glycemic control in diabetes: Results of a double-blind, placebo-controlled trial. *Psychosomatic Medicine*, 59(3), 241–250.

Lyons, J.E. and Symon, J. (2008). Asystole during electroconvulsive therapy in an elderly woman treated concomitantly with venlafaxine. *Australian and New Zealand Journal of Psychiatry*, 42(3), 255.

MacCall, C. and Callender, J. (1999). Mirtazapine withdrawal causing hypomania. *British Journal of Psychiatry*, 175, 390.

Macher, J.P., Sichel, J.P., Serre, C., *et al.* (1989). Double-blind placebo-controlled study of milnacipran in hospitalized patients with major depressive disorders. *Neuropsychobiology*, 22(2), 77–82.

Madhusoodanan, S. and Osnos, R. (1981). Amitriptyline induced hyponatremia: A case report. *Mount Sinai Journal of Medicine*, 48(5), 431–433.

Mago, R., Sadowski, S.D., Daskalakis, C., *et al.* (2008). Bupropion extended release for major depressive disorder in women with breast cancer: A pilot study. American Psychiatric Association Annual Meeting.

Maier, U. and Koinig, G. (1994). Andrological findings in young patients under long-term antidepressive therapy with clomipramine. *Psychopharmacology*, 116(3), 357–359.

Malesker, M.A., Soori, G.S., Malone, P.M., *et al.* (1995). Eosinophilia associated with bupropion. *Annals of Pharmacotherapy*, 29(9), 867–869.

Malt, U.F., Robak, O.H., Madsbu, H.P., *et al.* (1999). The Norwegian naturalistic treatment study of depression in general practice (NORDEP)-I: Randomised double blind study. *BMJ*, 318(7192), 1180–1184.

Mandoki, M.W., Tapia, M.R., Tapia, M.A., *et al.* (1997). Venlafaxine in the treatment of children and adolescents with major depression. *Psychopharmacology Bulletin*, 33(1), 149–154.

Maramattom, B.V. (2006). Duloxetine-induced syndrome of inappropriate antidiuretic hormone secretion and seizures. *Neurology*, 66(5), 773–774.

Martenyi, F., Dossenbach, M., Mraz, K. and Metcalfe, S. (2001). Gender differences in the efficacy of fluoxetine and maprotiline in depressed patients: A double-blind trial of antidepressants with serotonergic or norepinephrinergic reuptake inhibition profile. *European Neuropsychopharmacology*, 11(3), 227–232.

Marttila, M., Jääskeläinen, J., Järvi, R., *et al.* (1995). A double-blind study comparing the efficacy and tolerability of mirtazapine and doxepin in patients with major depression. *European Neuropsychopharmacology*, 5(4), 441–446.

Mbaya, P., Alam, F., Ashim, S. and Bennett, D. (2007). Cardiovascular effects of high dose venlafaxine XL in patients with major depressive disorder. *Human Psychopharmacology*, 22(3), 129–133.

McCollom, R.A., Elbe, D.H. and Ritchie, A.H. (2000). Bupropion-induced serum sickness-like reaction. *Annals of Pharmacotherapy*, 34(4), 471–473.

McCue, R.E. and Joseph, M. (2001). Venlafaxine- and trazodone-induced serotonin syndrome. *American Journal of Psychiatry*, 158(12), 2088–2089.

McLaughlin, T., Hogue, S.L. and Stang, P.E. (2007). Once-daily bupropion associated with improved patient adherence compared with twice-daily bupropion in treatment of depression, *American Journal of therapeutics*, 14(2), 221–225.

Mekler, G. and Woggon, B. (1997). A case of serotonin syndrome caused by venlafaxine and lithium. *Pharmacopsychiatry*, 30(6), 272–273.

Meltzer, H.Y., Piyakalmala, S., Schyve, P. and Fang, V.S. (1977). Lack of effect of tricyclic antidepressants on serum prolactin levels. *Psychopharmacology*, 51(2), 185–187.

Menza, M., Defronzo Dobkin, R., Marin, H., *et al.* (2009). A controlled trial of antidepressants in patients with Parkinson disease and depression. *Neurology*, 72(10), 886–892.

Mercuri, N.B., Calabresi, P. and Bernardi, G. (1992). The electrophysiological actions of dopamine and dopaminergic drugs on neurons of the substantia nigra pars compacta and ventral tegmental area. *Life Sciences*, 51(10), 711–718.

Mertens, C. and Pintens, H. (1988). Paroxetine in the treatment of depression. A double-blind multicenter study versus mianserin. *Acta Psychiatrica Scandinavica*, 77(6), 683–688.

Meyer, J.H., Goulding, V.S., Wilson, A.A., *et al.* (2002). Bupropion occupancy of the dopamine transporter is low during clinical treatment. *Psychopharmacology*, 163(1), 102–105.

Meyer, J.H., Wilson, A.A., Sagrati, S., *et al.* (2004). Serotonin transporter occupancy of five selective serotonin reuptake inhibitors at different doses: An [11C]DASB positron emission tomography study. *American Journal of Psychiatry*, 161(5), 826–835.

Meyers, B.S., Mattis, S., Gabriele, M. and Kakuma, T. (1991). Effects of nortriptyline on memory self-assessment and performance in recovered elderly depressives. *Psychopharmacology Bulletin*, 27(3), 295–299.

Meynaar, I.A., Peeters, A.J., Mulder, A.H. and Ottervanger, J.P. (1997). Syndrome of inappropriate ADH secretion attributed to the serotonin re-uptake inhibitors, venlafaxine and paroxetine. *Netherlands Journal of Medicine*, 50(6), 243–245.

Michelson, D., Amsterdam, J.D., Quitkin, F.M., *et al.* (1999). Changes in weight during a 1-year trial of fluoxetine. *American Journal of Psychiatry*, 156(8), 1170–1176.

Miller, D.K., Sumithran, S.P. and Dwoskin, L.P. (2002). Bupropion inhibits nicotine-evoked [(3)H]overflow from rat striatal slices preloaded with [(3)H]dopamine and from rat hippocampal slices preloaded with [(3)H]norepinephrine. *Journal of Pharmacology and Experimental Therapeutics*, 302(3), 1113–1122.

Miller, L. and Griffith, J. (1983). A comparison of bupropion, dextroamphetamine, and placebo in mixed-substance abusers. *Psychopharmacology*, 80(3), 199–205.

Ming, M.E., Bhawan, J., Stefanato, C.M., *et al.* (1999). Imipramine-induced hyperpigmentation: Four cases and a review of the literature. *Journal of the American Academy of Dermatology*, 40(2 Pt 1), 159–166.

Mizukami, K., Hatanaka, K., Tanaka, Y., *et al.* (2009). Therapeutic effects of the selective serotonin noradrenaline reuptake inhibitor milnacipran on depressive symptoms in patients with Alzheimer's disease. *Progress in Neuropsychopharmacology and Biological Psychiatry*, 33(2), 349–352.

Mochizuki, D., Tsujita, R., Yamada, S., *et al.* (2002). Neurochemical and behavioural characterization of milnacipran, a serotonin and noradrenaline reuptake inhibitor in rats. *Psychopharmacology*, 162(3), 323–332.

Modell, J.G., Rosenthal, N.E., Harriett, A.E., *et al.* (2005). Seasonal affective disorder and its prevention by anticipatory treatment with bupropion XL. *Biological Psychiatry*, 58(8), 658–667.

Mok, J. and Swann, I. (1978). Diagnosis of phaeochromocytoma after ingestion of imipramine. *Archives of Disease in Childhood*, 53(8), 676–677.

Moller, H.J., Kasper, S., Muller, H., *et al.* (1995). A controlled study of the efficacy and safety of mianserin and amitriptyline in depressive inpatients. *Pharmacopsychiatry*, 28(6), 249–252.

Moller, H.J., Riehl, T., Dietzfelbinger, T. and Wernicke, T. (1991). A controlled study of the efficacy and safety of mianserin and maprotiline in outpatients with major depression. *International Clinical Psychopharmacology*, 6(3), 179–192.

Montejo, A.L., Llorca, G., Izquierdo, J.A. and Rico-Villademoros, F. (2001). Incidence of sexual dysfunction associated with antidepressant agents: A prospective multicenter study of 1022 outpatients. Spanish Working Group for the Study of Psychotropic-Related Sexual Dysfunction. *Journal of Clinical Psychiatry*, 62(Suppl 3), 10–21.

Montgomery, S.A. and Andersen, H.F. (2006). Escitalopram versus venlafaxine XR in the treatment of depression. *International Clinical Psychopharmacology*, 21(5), 297–309.

Montgomery, S.A., Entsuah, R., Hackett, D., *et al.* (2004a). Venlafaxine 335 Study Group. Venlafaxine versus placebo in the preventive treatment of recurrent major depression. *Journal of Clinical Psychiatry*, 65(3), 328–336.

Montgomery, S.A., Fava, M., Padmanabhan, S.K., *et al.* (2009). Discontinuation symptoms and taper/poststudy-emergent adverse events with desvenlafaxine treatment for major depressive disorder. *International Clinical Psychopharmacology*, 24(6), 296–305.

Montgomery, S.A., Huusom, A.K. and Bothmer, J. (2004b). A randomised study comparing escitalopram with venlafaxine XR in primary care patients with major depressive disorder. *Neuropsychobiology*, 50(1), 57–64.

Montgomery, S.A., Mahé, V., Haudiquet, V. and Hackett, D. (2002a). Effectiveness of venlafaxine, extended release formulation, in the short-term and long-term treatment of generalized anxiety disorder: Results of a survival analysis. *Journal of Clinical Psychopharmacology*, 22(6), 561–567.

Montgomery, S.A., Reimitz, P.E. and Zivkov, M. (1998). Mirtazapine versus amitriptyline in the long-term treatment of depression: A double-blind placebo-controlled study. *International Clinical Psychopharmacology*, 13(2), 63–73.

Montgomery, S.A., Sheehan, D.V., Meoni, P., *et al.* (2002b). Characterization of the longitudinal course of improvement in generalized anxiety disorder during long-term treatment with venlafaxine XR. *Journal of Psychiatric Research*, 36(4), 209–217.

Moon, C.A. and Jesinger, D.K. (1991). The effects of psychomotor performance of fluvoxamine versus mianserin in depressed patients in general practice. *British Journal of Clinical Practice*, 45(4), 259–262.

Moosa, M.Y., Panz, V.R., Jeenah, F.Y. and Joffe, B.I. (2003). African women with depression: The effect of imipramine and fluoxetine on body mass index and leptin secretion. *Journal of Clinical Psychopharmacology*, 23(6), 549–552.

Morazin, F., Lumbroso, A., Harry, P., *et al.* (2007) Cardiogenic shock and status epilepticus after massive bupropion overdose. *Clinical Toxicology*, 45(7), 794–797.

Muehlbacher, M., Nickel, M.K., Nickel, C., *et al.* (2005). Mirtazapine treatment of social phobia in women: A randomized, double-blind, placebo-controlled study. *Journal of Clinical Psychopharmacol*, 25(6), 580–583.

Muijen, M., Roy, D., Silverstone, T., *et al.* (1988). A comparative clinical trial of fluoxetine, mianserin and placebo in depressed outpatients. *Acta Psychiatrica Scandinavica*, 78(3), 384–390.

Mulsant, B.H., Pollock, B.G., Nebes, R.D., *et al.* (1999). A double-blind randomized comparison of nortriptyline and paroxetine in the treatment of late-life depression: 6-week outcome. *Journal of Clinical Psychiatry*, 60(Suppl 20), 16–20.

Müssig, K., Mörike, K. and Häring, H.U. (2009). Severe and symptomatic hyponatremia following duloxetine treatment. *Journal of Psychopharmacology*, 23(3), 338–339.

Navarro, V., Gasto, C., Torres, X., Marcos, T. and Pintor, L. (2001). Citalopram versus nortriptyline in late-life depression: A 12-week randomized single-blind study. *Acta Psychiatrica Scandinavica*, 103(6), 435–440.

Nelson, J.C., Kennedy, J.S., Pollock, B.G., *et al.* (1999). Treatment of major depression with nortriptyline and paroxetine in patients with ischemic heart disease. *American Journal of Psychiatry*, 156(7), 1024–1028.

Nelson, J.C., Lu Pritchett, Y., Martynov, O., *et al.* (2006). The safety and tolerability of duloxetine compared with paroxetine and placebo: A pooled analysis of 4 clinical trials. *Primary Care Companion of the Journal of Clinical Psychiatry*, 8(4), 212–219.

Nemeroff, C.B., Entsuah, R., Benattia, I., *et al.* (2008). Comprehensive analysis of remission (COMPARE) with venlafaxine versus SSRIs. *Biological Psychiatry*, 63(4), 424–434.

Nemeroff, C.B., Evans, D.L., Gyulai, L., *et al.* (2001). Double-blind, placebo-controlled comparison of imipramine and paroxetine in the treatment of bipolar depression. *American Journal of Psychiatry*, 158(6), 906–912.

Newport, D.J., Ritchie, J.C., Knight, B.T., *et al.* (2009). Venlafaxine in human breast milk and nursing infant plasma: Determination of exposure. *Journal of Clinical Psychiatry*, 70(9), 1304–1310.

Nicholas, L.M., Ford, A.L., Esposito, S.M., *et al.* (2003). The effects of mirtazapine on plasma lipid profiles in healthy subjects. *Journal of Clinical Psychiatry*, 64(8), 883–889.

Niedermaier, N., Bohrer, E., Schulte, K., *et al.* (2004). Prevention and treatment of poststroke depression with mirtazapine in patients with acute stroke. *Journal of Clinical Psychiatry*, 65(12), 1619–1623.

Nielsen, J.L. (1980). Plasma prolactin during treatment with nortriptyline. *Neuropsychobiology*, 6(1), 52–55.

Nierenberg, A.A., Greist, J.H., Mallinckrodt, C.H., *et al.* (2007). Duloxetine versus escitalopram and placebo in the treatment of patients with major depressive disorder: Onset of antidepressant action, a non-inferiority study. *Current Medical and Research Opinion*, 23(2), 401–416.

Nofzinger, E.A., Reynolds, C.F. 3rd, Thase, M.E., *et al.* (1995). REM sleep enhancement by bupropion in depressed men. *American Journal of Psychiatry*, 152(2), 274–276.

Nomikos, G.G., Damsma, G., Wenkstern, D. and Fibiger, H.C. (1989). Acute effects of bupropion on extracellular dopamine concentrations in rat striatum and nucleus accumbens studied by *in vivo* microdialysis. *Neuropsychopharmacology*, 2(4), 273–279.

Nonacs, R.M., Soares, C.N., Viguera, A.C., *et al.* (2005). Bupropion SR for the treatment of postpartum depression: A pilot study. *International Journal of Neuropsychopharmacology*, 8(3), 445–449.

Nordgren, L. and von Scheele, C. (1981). Nortriptyline and pituitary-thyroid function in affective disorder. *Pharmacopsychiatria*, 14(2), 61–65.

Nunez, E., Lopez-Corcuera, B., Vazquez, J., *et al.* (2000). Differential effects of the tricyclic antidepressant amoxapine on glycine uptake mediated by the recombinant GLYT1 and GLYT2 glycine transporters. *British Journal of Pharmacology*, 129(1), 200–206.

O'Malley, P.G., Jackson, J.L., Santoro, J., *et al.* (1999). Antidepressant therapy for unexplained symptoms and symptom syndromes. *Journal of Family Practice*, 48(12), 980–990.

Olusi, S.O. and Fido, A.A. (1996). Serum lipid concentrations in patients with major depressive disorder. *Biological Psychiatry*, 40(11), 1128–1131.

Oshika, T. (1995). Ocular adverse effects of neuropsychiatric agents. Incidence and management. *Drug Safety*, 12(4), 256–263.

Otton, S.V., Ball, S.E., Cheung, S.W., *et al.* (1996). Venlafaxine oxidation *in vitro* is catalysed by CYP2D6. *British Journal of Clinical Pharmacology*, 41(2), 149–156.

Pan, J.J. and Shen, W.W. (2003). Serotonin syndrome induced by low-dose venlafaxine. *Annals of Pharmacotherapy*, 37(2), 209–211.

Pancrazio, J.J., Kamatchi, G.L., Roscoe, A.K. and Lynch, C. 3rd. (1998). Inhibition of neuronal Na^+ channels by antidepressant drugs. *Journal of Pharmacology and Experimental Therapeutics*, 284(1), 208–214.

Papakostas, G.I. (2007). Current limitations of antidepressant monotherapy: Tolerability. *Journal of Clinical Psychiatry*, 68(Suppl 10), 11–17.

Papakostas, G.I. (2006). Dopaminergic-based pharmacotherapies for depression. *European Neuropsychopharmacology*, 16(6), 391–402.

Papakostas, G.I. and Fava, M. (2007). A meta-analysis of clinical trials comparing milnacipran, a serotonin–norepinephrine reuptake inhibitor, with a selective serotonin reuptake inhibitor for the treatment of major depressive disorder. *European Neuropsychopharmacology*, 17(1), 32–36.

Papakostas, G.I., Homberger, C.H. and Fava, M. (2008a). A meta-analysis of clinical trials comparing mirtazapine with a selective serotonin reuptake inhibitor for the treatment of major depressive disorder. *Journal of Psychopharmacology*, 22(8), 843–848.

Papakostas, G.I., Kornstein, S.G., Clayton, A.H., *et al.* (2007b). Relative antidepressant efficacy of bupropion and the selective serotonin reuptake inhibitors in major depressive disorder: Gender-age interactions. *International Clinical Psychopharmacology*, 22(4), 226–229.

Papakostas, G.I., Montgomery, S.A., Thase, M.E., *et al.* (2007c) Comparing the rapidity of response during treatment of major depressive disorder with bupropion and the SSRIs: A survival analysis-based meta-analysis of individual patient data from 7 double-blind, randomized clinical trials. *Journal of Clinical Psychiatry*, 68(12), 1907–1912.

Papakostas, G.I., Nutt, D.J., Hallett, L.A., *et al.* (2006). Resolution of sleepiness and fatigue in major depressive disorder: A comparison of bupropion and the selective serotonin reuptake inhibitors. *Biological Psychiatry*, 60(12), 1350–1355.

Papakostas, G.I., Stahl, S.M., Krishen, A., *et al.* (2008c). Efficacy of bupropion and the selective serotonin reuptake inhibitors in the treatment of major depressive disorder with high levels of anxiety (anxious depression). *Journal of Clinical Psychiatry*, 69(8), 1287–1292.

Papakostas, G.I., Thase, M.E., Fava, M., *et al.* (2007a). Are antidepressants that combine serotonergic and noradrenergic mechanisms of action more effective than the selective serotonin reuptake inhibitors in treating major depressive disorder? A meta-analysis of studies of newer agents. *Biological Psychiatry*, 62(11), 1217–1227.

Papakostas, G.I., Trivedi, M.H., Alpert, J.E., *et al.* (2008b). Efficacy of bupropion and the selective serotonin reuptake inhibitors in the treatment of anxiety symptoms in major depressive disorder. A meta-analysis of individual patient data from 10 double-blind, randomized clinical trials. *Journal of Psychiatric Research*, 42(2), 134–140.

Paris, P.A. and Saucier, J.R. (1998). ECG conduction delays associated with massive bupropion overdose. *Journal of Toxicology. Clinical Toxicology*, 36(6), 595–598.

Parker, W.A. (1984). Imipramine-induced syndrome of inappropriate antidiuretic hormone secretion. *Drug Intelligence and Clinical Pharmacy*, 18(11), 890–894.

Patroneva, A., Zitek, B, Ninan, P.T., *et al.* (2007). Analysis of weight change with short- and longer-term treatment with desvenlafaxine succinate for major depressive disorder. Presented at the 160th Annual Meeting of the American Psychiatric Association. Diego, California.

Peeters, F.P., deVries, M.W. and Vissink, A. (1998). Risks for oral health with the use of antidepressants. *General Hospital Psychiatry*, 20(3), 150–154.

Peloso, P.M., Baillie and C. (1999). Serum sickness-like reaction with bupropion. *Journal of the American Medical Association*, 282(19), 1817.

Perahia, D., Acharya, N., Wang, F., *et al.* (2007). Duloxetine hepatic effects: 2006 review. *European Neuropsychopharmacology*, 17(s4), s356.

Perahia, D.G., Gilaberte, I., Wang, F., *et al.* (2006b). Duloxetine in the prevention of relapse of major depressive disorder: Double-blind placebo-controlled study. *British Journal of Psychiatry*, 188, 346–353.

Perahia, D.G., Kajdasz, D.K., Desaiah, D. and Haddad, P.M. (2005). Symptoms following abrupt discontinuation of duloxetine treatment in patients with major Depressive disorder. *Journal of Affective Disorders*, 89(1–3), 207–212.

Perahia, D.G., Pritchett, Y.L., Kajdasz, D.K., *et al.* (2008). A randomized, double-blind comparison of duloxetine and venlafaxine in the treatment of patients with major depressive disorder. *Journal of Psychiatric Research*, 42(1), 22–34.

Perahia, D.G., Wang, F., Mallinckrodt, C.H., *et al.* (2006a). Duloxetine in the treatment of major depressive disorder: A placebo- and paroxetine-controlled trial. *European Psychiatry*, 21(6), 367–378.

Pereira, C.E. and Goldman-Levine, J.D. (2007). Extended-release Venlafaxine-Induced Alopecia. *Annals of Pharmacotherapy*, 41(6), 1084.

Perez, A. and Ashford, J.J. (1990). A double-blind, randomized comparison of fluvoxamine with mianserin in depressive illness. *Current Medical and Research Opinion*, 12(4), 234–241.

Perry, N.K. (2000). Venlafaxine-induced serotonin syndrome with relapse following amitriptyline. *Postgraduate Medical Journal*, 76(894), 254–256.

Perry, P.J., Zeilmann, C. and Arndt, S. (1994). Tricyclic antidepressant concentrations in plasma: An estimate of their sensitivity and specificity as a predictor of response. *Journal of Clinical Psychopharmacology*, 14(4), 230–240.

Petersen, T., Dording, C., Neault, N.B., *et al.* (2002). A survey of prescribing practices in the treatment of depression. *Progress in Neuropsychopharmacology and Biological Psychiatry*, 26(1), 177–187.

Phanjoo, A.L., Wonnacott, S. and Hodgson, A. (1991). Double-blind comparative multicentre study of fluvoxamine and mianserin in the treatment of major depressive episode in elderly people. *Acta Psychiatrica Scandinavica*, 83(6), 476–479.

Philipp, M., Tiller, J.W., Baier, D. and Kohnen, R. (2000). Comparison of moclobemide with selective serotonin reuptake inhibitors (SSRIs) on sexual function in depressed adults. The Australian and German Study Groups. *European Neuropsychopharmacology*, 10(5), 305–314.

Phillips, B.B., Digmann, R.R. and Beck, M.G. (2006). Hepatitis associated with low-dose venlafaxine for postmenopausal vasomotor symptoms. *Annals of Pharmacotherapy*, 40(2), 323–327.

Pigott, T.A., Prakash, A., Arnold, L.M., *et al.* (2007). Duloxetine versus escitalopram and placebo: An 8-month, double-blind trial in patients with major depressive disorder. *Current Medical and Research Opinion*, 23(6), 1303–1318.

Pisani, F., Oteri, G., Costa, C., *et al.* (2002). Effects of psychotropic drugs on seizure threshold. *Drug Safety*, 25(2), 91–110.

Pitchot, W. and Ansseau, M. (2001). Venlafaxine-induced hair loss. *American Journal of Psychiatry*, 158(7), 1159–1160.

Pjrek, E., Willeit, M., Praschak-Rieder, N., *et al.* (2008). Treatment of seasonal affective disorder with duloxetine: An open-label study. *Pharmacopsychiatry*, 41(3), 100–105.

Pollack, M., Mangano, R., Entsuah, R., *et al.* (2007). A randomized controlled trial of venlafaxine ER and paroxetine in the treatment of outpatients with panic disorder. *Psychopharmacology*, 194(2), 233–242.

Pollock, B.G., Perel, J.M., Paradis, C.F., *et al.* (1994). Metabolic and physiologic consequences of nortriptyline treatment in the elderly. *Psychopharmacology Bulletin*, 30(2), 145–150.

Pollock, B.G., Sweet, R.A., Kirshner, M. and Reynolds, C.F. 3rd. (1996). Bupropion plasma levels and CYP2D6 phenotype. *Therapeutic Drug Monitoring*, 18(5), 581–585.

Pomara, N., Willoughby, L.M., Wesnes, K. and Sidtis, J.J. (2004). Increased anticholinergic challenge-induced memory impairment associated with the APOE-epsilon4 allele in the elderly: A controlled pilot study. *Neuropsychopharmacology*, 29(2), 403–409.

Post, R.M., Altshuler, L.L., Leverich, G.S., *et al.* (2006). Mood switch in bipolar depression: Comparison of adjunctive venlafaxine, bupropion and sertraline. *British Journal of Psychiatry*, 189, 124–131.

Preskorn, S.H. (1983). Antidepressant response and plasma concentrations of bupropion. *Journal of Clinical Psychiatry*, 44(5 Pt 2), 137–139.

Preskorn, S., Patroneva, A., Silman, H., *et al.* (2009). Comparison of the pharmacokinetics of venlafaxine extended release and desvenlafaxine in extensive and poor cytochrome P450 2D6 metabolizers. *Journal of Clinical Psychopharmacology*, 29(1), 39–43.

Prior, F.H., Isbister, G.K., Dawson, A.H. and Whyte, I.M. (2002). Serotonin toxicity with therapeutic doses of dexamphetamine and venlafaxine. *Medical Journal of Australia*, 176(5), 240–241.

Pritchett, Y.L., Marciniak, M.D., Corey-Lisle, P.K., *et al.* (2007). Use of effect size to determine optimal dose of duloxetine in major depressive disorder. *Journal of Psychiatric Research*, 41(3–4), 311–318.

Raji, M.A., Barnum, P.D., Freeman, J. and Markowitz, A.B. (2007). Mirtazapine for depression and comorbidities in older patients with cancer. *Annals of Pharmacotherapy*, 41(9), 1548–1549.

Ramaekers, J.G. (2003). Antidepressants and driver impairment: Empirical evidence from a standard on-the-road test. *Journal of Clinical Psychiatry*, 64(1), 20–29.

Ranieri, P., Franzoni, S., Rozzini, R. and Trabucchi, M. (1997). Venlafaxine-induced reset osmostat syndrome: Case of a 79-year-old depressed woman. *Journal of Geriatric Psychiatry and Neurology*, 10(2), 75–78.

Raskin, J., Wiltse, C.G., Siegal, A., *et al.* (2007). Efficacy of duloxetine on cognition, depression, and pain in elderly patients with major depressive disorder: An 8-week, double-blind, placebo-controlled trial. *American Journal of Psychiatry*, 164(6), 900–909.

Ravindran, A.V., Charbonneau, Y., Zaharia, M.D., *et al.* (1998). Efficacy and tolerability of venlafaxine in the treatment of primary dysthymia. *Journal of Psychiatry and Neuroscience*, 23(5), 288–292.

Ray, W.A., Fought, R.L. and Decker, M.D. (1992). Psychoactive drugs and the risk of injurious motor vehicle crashes in elderly drivers. *American Journal of Epidemiology*, 136(7), 873–883.

Ray, W.A., Griffin, M.R. and Malcolm, E. (1991). Cyclic antidepressants and the risk of hip fracture. *Archives of Internal Medicine*, 151(4), 754–756.

Richelson, E. and Nelson, A. (1984). Antagonism by antidepressants of neurotransmitter receptors of normal human brain *in vitro*. *Journal of Pharmacology and Experimental Therapeutics*, 230, 94–102.

Richou, H. (1995). A multicentre, double-blind, clomiprapharmacolmine-controlled efficacy and safety study of Org 3770. *Human Psychopharmacology*. 10, 263–271.

Roberts, R.L., Joyce, P.R., Mulder, R.T., *et al.* (2002). A common P-glycoprotein polymorphism is associated with nortriptyline-induced postural hypotension in patients treated for major depression. *Pharmacogenomics Journal*, 2(3), 191–196.

Robinson, R.G., Schultz, S.K., Castillo, C., *et al.* (2000). Nortriptyline versus fluoxetine in the treatment of depression and in short-term recovery after stroke: A placebo-controlled, double-blind study. *American Journal of Psychiatry*, 157(3), 351–359.

Romero, S., Pintor, L., Serra, M., *et al.* (2007). Syndrome of inappropriate secretion of antidiuretic hormone due to citalopram and venlafaxine. *General Hospital Psychiatry*, 29(1), 81–84.

Roose, S.P., Dalack, G.W., Glassman, A.H., *et al.* (1991). Cardiovascular effects of bupropion in depressed patients with heart disease. *American Journal of Psychiatry*, 148(4), 512–516.

Roose, S.P., Glassman, A.H., Attia, E. and Woodring, S. (1994). Comparative efficacy of selective serotonin reuptake inhibitors and tricyclics in the treatment of melancholia. *American Journal of Psychiatry*, 151(12), 1735–1739.

Roose, S.P., Glassman, A.H., Giardina, E.G., *et al.* (1987b). Cardiovascular effects of imipramine and bupropion in depressed patients with congestive heart failure. *Journal of Clinical Psychopharmacology*, 7(4), 247–251.

Roose, S.P., Glassman, A.H., Giardina, E.G., *et al.* (1987a). Tricyclic antidepressants in depressed patients with cardiac conduction disease. *Archives of General Psychiatry*, 44(3), 273–275.

Roseboom, P.H. and Kalin, N.H. (2000). Neuropharmacology of venlafaxine. *Depression and Anxiety*, 12(Suppl 1), 20–29.

Rowland, D.L., Myers, L., Culver, A. and Davidson, J.M. (1997). Bupropion and sexual function: A placebo-controlled prospective study on diabetic men with erectile dysfunction. *Journal of Clinical Psychopharmacology*, 17(5), 350–357.

Roxanas, M.G. (2003). Mirtazapine-induced hyponatraemia. *Medical Journal of Australia*, 179(8), 453–454.

Roxanas, M., Hibbert, E. and Field, M. (2007). Venlafaxine hyponatraemia: Incidence, mechanism and management. *Australian and New Zealand Journal of Psychiatry*, 41(5), 411–418.

Roxanas, M.G. and Machado, J.F. (1998). Serotonin syndrome in combined moclobemide and venlafaxine ingestion. *Medical Journal of Australia*, 168(10), 523–524.

Rudolph, R.L. (2002). Achieving remission from depression with venlafaxine and venlafaxine extended release: A literature review of comparative studies with selective serotonin reuptake inhibitors. *Acta Psychiatrica Scandinavica, Supplementum*, (415), 24–30.

Rudolph, R.L. and Derivan, A.T. (1996). The safety and tolerability of venlafaxine hydrochloride: Analysis of the clinical trials database. The safety and tolerability of venlafaxine hydrochloride: Analysis of the clinical trials database. *Journal of Clinical Psychopharmacology*, 163(Suppl 2), 54S–59S.

Russell, I.J., Mease, P.J., Smith, T.R., *et al.* (2008). Efficacy and safety of duloxetine for treatment of fibromyalgia in patients with or without major depressive disorder: Results from a 6-month, randomized, double-blind, placebo-controlled, fixed-dose trial. *Pain*, 136(3), 432–444.

Russo, S., Boon, J.C., Korf, J. and Haagsm, E.B. (2003). Mirtazapine for the treatment of interferon-induced psychopathology. *General Hospital Psychiatry*, 25, 497.

Rye, D.B., Dihenia, B. and Bliwise, D.L. (1998). Reversal of atypical depression, sleepiness, and REM-sleep propensity in narcolepsy with bupropion. *Depression and Anxiety*, 7(2), 92–95.

Sa, D.S., Kapur, S. and Lang, A.E. (2001). Amoxapine shows an antipsychotic effect but worsens motor function in patients with Parkinson's disease and psychosis. *Clinical Neuropharmacology*, 24(4), 242–244.

Sachs, G.S., Lafer, B., Stoll, A.L., *et al.* (1994). A double-blind trial of bupropion versus desipramine for bipolar depression. *Journal of Clinical Psychiatry*, 55(9), 391–393.

Sachs, G.S., Nierenberg, A.A., Calabrese, J.R., *et al.* (2007). Effectiveness of adjunctive antidepressant treatment for bipolar depression. *New England Journal of Medicine*, 356(17), 1711–1722.

Safdieh, J.E. and Rudominer, R. (2006). A case of hyponatremia induced by duloxetine. *Journal of Clinical Psychopharmacology*, 26(6), 675–676

Salin-Pascual, R.J., Galicia-Polo, L. and Drucker-Colin, R. (1997). Sleep changes after 4 consecutive days of venlafaxine administration in normal volunteers. *Journal of Clinical Psychiatry*, 58(8), 348–350.

Salomon, R.M., Ripley, B., Kennedy, J.S., *et al.* (2003). Diurnal variation of cerebrospinal fluid hypocretin-1 (Orexin-A) levels in control and depressed subjects. *Biological Psychiatry*, 54(2), 96–104.

Sanchez, C. and Hyttel, J. (1999). Comparison of the effects of antidepressants and their metabolites on reuptake of biogenic amines and on receptor binding. *Cellular and Molecular Neurobiology*, 19(4), 467–489.

Sandor, P., Baker, B., Irvine, J., *et al.* (1998). Effectiveness of fluoxetine and doxepin in treatment of melancholia in depressed patients. *Depression and Anxiety*, 7(2), 69–72.

Sarma, A. and Horne, M.K. 3rd. (2006). Venlafaxine-induced ecchymoses and impaired platelet aggregation. *European Journal of Haematology*, 77(6), 533–537.

Schatzberg, A. and Roose, S. (2006). A double-blind, placebo-controlled study of venlafaxine and fluoxetine in geriatric outpatients with major depression. *American Journal of Geriatric Psychiatry*, 14(4), 361–370.

Schatzberg, A.F., Kremer, C., Rodrigues, H.E. and Murphy, G.M. Jr. (2002). Mirtazapine vs. Paroxetine Study Group. Double-blind, randomized comparison of mirtazapine and paroxetine in elderly depressed patients. *American Journal of Geriatric Psychiatry*, 10(5), 541–550.

Schilling, A.D., Yung-Sciame, R. and Leung, L. (2005). Comparison of inhibitory effects of desvenlafaxine succinate, venlafaxine, duloxetine, paroxetine, sertraline, and bupropion in human cytochrome P450 activities. Presented at the 6th Annual Meeting of the International Society for the Study of Xenobiotics. Munich, Germany.

Schinkel, A.H., Mol, C.A., Wagenaar, E., *et al.* (1995). Multidrug resistance and the role of P-glycoprotein knockout mice. *European Journal of Cancer*, 31A(7–8), 1295–1298.

Schinkel, A.H., Wagenaar, E., Mol, C.A. and van Deemter, L. (1996). P-glycoprotein in the blood-brain barrier of mice influences the brain penetration and pharmacological activity of many drugs. *Journal of Clinical Investigation*, 97(11), 2517–2524.

Schlienger, J.L., Kapfer, M.T., Singer, L. and Stephan, F. (1980). The action of clomipramine on thyroid function. *Horm Metab Res*, 12(9), 481–482.

Schmitt, A.B., Bauer, M., Volz, H.P., *et al.* (2009). Differential effects of venlafaxine in the treatment of major depressive disorder according to baseline severity. *European Archives of Psychiatry and Clinical Neurosciences*, 259(6), 329–339.

Septien-Velez, L., Pitrosky, B., Padmanabhan, S.K., *et al.* (2007). A randomized, double-blind, placebo-controlled trial of desvenlafaxine succinate in the treatment of major depressive disorder. *International Clinical Psychopharmacology*, 22(6), 338–347.

Settle, E.C., Stahl, S.M., Batey, S.R., *et al.* (1999). Safety profile of sustained-release bupropion in depression: Results of three clinical trials. *Clinical Therapeutics*, 21(3), 454–463.

Shams, M.E., Arneth, B., Hiemke, C., *et al.* (2006). CYP2D6 polymorphism and clinical effect of the antidepressant venlafaxine. *J Clinical Pharmacy Ther*, 31(5), 493–502.

Shang, C.Y., Soong, W.T. and Lin, H.N. (2002). Hypokalemia with venlafaxine. *Journal of Clinical Psychiatry*, 63(11), 1049–1050.

Shelton, R.C., Winn, S., Ekhatore, N. and Loosen, P.T. (1993). The effects of antidepressants on the thyroid axis in depression. *Biological Psychiatry*, 33(2), 120–126.

Shrivastava, R.K., Cohn, C., Crowder, J., *et al.* (1994). Long-term safety and clinical acceptability of venlafaxine and imipramine in outpatients with major depression. *Journal of Clinical Psychopharmacology*, 14(5), 322–329.

Simon, J.S., Aguiar, L.M., Kunz, N.R. and Lei, D. (2004). Extended-release venlafaxine in relapse prevention for patients with major depressive disorder. *Journal of Psychiatric Research*, 38(3), 249–257.

Sindrup, S.H. and Jensen, T.S. (1999). Efficacy of pharmacological treatments of neuropathic pain: An update and effect related to mechanism of drug action. *Pain*, 83(3), 389–400.

Sir, A., D'Souza, R.F., Uguz, S., *et al.* (2005). Randomized trial of sertraline versus venlafaxine XR in major depression: Efficacy and discontinuation symptoms. *Journal of Clinical Psychiatry*, 66(10), 1312–1320.

Slemmer, J.E., Martin, B.R. and Damaj, M.I. (2000). Bupropion is a nicotinic antagonist. *Journal of Pharmacology and Experimental Therapeutics*, 295(1), 321–327.

Smith, D., Dempster, C., Glanville, J., *et al.* (2002). Efficacy and tolerability of venlafaxine compared with selective serotonin reuptake inhibitors and other antidepressants: A meta-analysis. *British Journal of Psychiatry*, 180, 396–404.

Sommer, M., Dieterich, A., Krause, C., *et al.* (2001). Subclinical pancreatitis related to mirtazapine — a case report. *Pharmacopsychiatry*, 34(4), 158–159.

Sonntag, A., Rothe, B., Guldner, J., *et al.* (1996). Trimipramine and imipramine exert different effects on the sleep EEG and on nocturnal hormone secretion during treatment of major depression. *Depression*, 4(1), 1–13.

Spina, E., Birgersson, C., von Bahr, C., *et al.* (1984). Phenotypic consistency in hydroxylation of desmethylimipramine and debrisoquine in healthy subjects and in human liver microsomes. *Clinical Pharmacology and Therapeutics*, 36(5), 677–682.

Stahl, S.M., Entsuah, R. and Rudolph, R.L. (2002). Comparative efficacy between venlafaxine and SSRIs: A pooled analysis of patients with depression. *Biological Psychiatry*, 52(12), 1166–1174.

Stang, P., Suppapanaya, N., Hogue, S.L., *et al.* (2007a). Persistence with once-daily versus twice-daily bupropion for the treatment of depression in a large managed-care population. *American Journal of Therapeutics*, 14(3), 241–246.

Stang, P., Young, S. and Hogue, S. (2007b). Better patient persistence with once-daily bupropion compared with twice-daily bupropion. *American Journal of Therapeutics*, 14(1), 20–24.

Sternbach, H. (2003). Venlafaxine-induced galactorrhea. *Journal of Clinical Psychopharmacology*, 23(1), 109–110.

Stone, T.E., Swanson, C. and Feldman, M.D. (2007). Venlafaxine discontinuation syndrome and suicidal ideation: A case series. *Journal of Clinical Psychopharmacology*, 27(1), 94–95.

Strayhorn, J.M. and Nash, J.L. (1978). Frightening dreams and dosage schedule of tricyclic and neuroleptic drugs. *Journal of Nervous and Mental Disease*, 166(12), 878–880.

Suckow, R.F., Zhang, M.F. and Cooper, T.B. (1997). Enantiomeric determination of the phenylmorpholinol metabolite of bupropion in human plasma using coupled achiral-chiral liquid chromatography. *Biomedical Chromatography*, 11(3), 174–179.

Suhara, T., Takano, A., Sudo, Y., *et al.* (2003). High levels of serotonin transporter occupancy with low-dose clomipramine in comparative occupancy study with fluvoxamine using positron emission tomography. *Archives of General Psychiatry*, 60(4), 386–391.

Sussman, N., Ginsberg, D.L. and Bikoff, J. (2001). Effects of nefazodone on body weight: A pooled analysis of selective serotonin reuptake inhibitor- and imipramine-controlled trials. *Journal of Clinical Psychiatry*, 62(4), 256–260.

Szabo, Z., Argyelan, M., Kanyo, B., *et al.* (2004). Change of dopamine transporter activity (DAT) during the action of bupropion (in depression). *Neuropsychopharmacologica Hungarica*, 6(2), 79–81.

Tackett, A.E. and Smith, K.M. (2008). Bupropion-induced angioedema. *American Journal of Health Systems Pharmacy*, 65(17), 1627–1630.

Takano, A., Suzuki, K., Kosaka, J., *et al.* (2006). A dose-finding study of duloxetine based on serotonin transporter occupancy. *Psychopharmacology*, 185(3), 395–399.

Taylor, D., Stewart, S. and Connolly, A. (2006). Antidepressant withdrawal symptoms-telephone calls to a national medication helpline. *Journal of Affective Disorders*, 95(1–3), 129–133.

Teschemacher, A.G., Seward, E.P., Hancox, J.C. and Witchel, H.J. (1999). Inhibition of the current of heterologously expressed HERG potassium channels by imipramine and amitriptyline. *British Journal of Pharmacology*, 128(2), 479–485.

Thase, M.E. (1998). Effects of venlafaxine on blood pressure: A meta-analysis of original data from 3744 depressed patients. *Journal of Clinical Psychiatry*, 59(10), 502–508.

Thase, M.E., Clayton, A.H., Haight, B.R., *et al.* (2006). A double-blind comparison between bupropion XL and venlafaxine XR: Sexual functioning, antidepressant efficacy, and tolerability. *Journal of Clinical Psychopharmacology*, 26(5), 482–488.

Thase, M.E., Entsuah, R., Cantillon, M. and Kornstein, S.G. (2005a). Relative antidepressant efficacy of venlafaxine and SSRIs: Sex-age interactions. *Journal of Women's Health*, 14(7), 609–616.

Thase, M.E., Entsuah, A.R. and Rudolph, R.L. (2001a). Remission rates during treatment with venlafaxine or selective serotonin reuptake inhibitors. *British Journal of Psychiatry*, 178, 234–441.

Thase, M.E., Entsuah, R., Sloan, D.M. and Nemeroff, C.B. (2005a). Meta-analysis of randomized controlled trials comparing venlafaxine and SSRIs: The evidence revisited. Presented at the 158th Annual Meeting of the American Psychiatric Association. Atlanta, Georgia.

Thase, M.E., Haight, B.R., Richard, N., *et al.* (2005d). Remission rates following antidepressant therapy with bupropion or selective serotonin reuptake inhibitors: A meta-analysis of original data from 7 randomized controlled trials. *Journal of Clinical Psychiatry*, 66(8), 974–81.

Thase, M.E., Kornstein, S.G., Germain, J.G., *et al.* (2009). An integrated analysis of the efficacy of desvenlafaxine compared with placebo in patients with major depressive disorder. *CNS Spectrums*, 14(3), 144–154.

Thase, M.E., Kremer, C. and Rodrigues, H (2001b). Mirtazapine versus sertraline after SSRI non-response. Presented at the 41st Annual Meeting of the New Clinical Drug Evaluation Unit of the National Institute of Mental Health. Boca Raton, Florida.

Thase, M.E., Nierenberg, A.A., Keller, M.B., *et al.* (2001c). Efficacy of mirtazapine for prevention of depressive relapse: A placebo-controlled double-blind trial of recently remitted high-risk patients. *Journal of Clinical Psychiatry*, 62(10), 782–788.

Thase, M.E., Pritchett, Y.L., Ossanna, M.J., *et al.* (2007b). Efficacy of duloxetine and selective serotonin reuptake inhibitors: Comparisons as assessed by remission rates in patients with major depressive disorder. *Journal of Clinical Psychopharmacology*, 27(6), 672–676.

Thase, M.E., Tran, P.V., Wiltse, C., *et al.* (2005c). Cardiovascular profile of duloxetine, a dual reuptake inhibitor of serotonin and norepinephrine. *Journal of Clinical Psychopharmacology*, 25(2), 132–140.

Thayssen, P., Bjerre, M., Kragh-Sorensen, P., *et al.* (1981). Cardiovascular effect of imipramine and nortriptyline in elderly patients. *Psychopharmacology*, 74(4), 360–364.

Tourian, K.A., Ahmed, S., Patroneva, A., *et al.* (2007). Improvement of anxiety symptoms in patients with major depressive disorder treated with desvenlafaxine succinate: A pooled analysis. Presented at the 160th Annual Meeting of the American Psychiatric Association, San Diego, California.

Tourian, K.A., Padmanabhan, S.K., Groark, J., *et al.* (2009). Desvenlafaxine 50 and 100 mg/d in the treatment of major depressive disorder: An 8-week, phase III, multicenter, randomized, double-blind, placebo-controlled, parallel-group trial and a post hoc pooled analysis of three studies. *Clinical Therapeutics*, 31(Pt 1), 1405–1423.

Tripathi, A. and Greenberger, P.A. (1999). Bupropion hydrochloride induced serum sickness-like reaction. *Annals of Allergy, Asthma, and Immunology*, 83(2), 165–166.

Trivedi, M.H., Rush, A.J., Carmody, T.J., *et al.* (2001). Do bupropion SR and sertraline differ in their effects on anxiety in depressed patients? *Journal of Clinical Psychiatry*, 62(10), 776–781.

True, B.L., Perry, P.J. and Burns, E.A. (1987). Profound hypoglycemia with the addition of a tricyclic antidepressant to maintenance sulfonylurea therapy. *American Journal of Psychiatry*, 144(9), 1220–1221.

Turkel, S.B., Nadala, J.G. and Wincor, M.Z. (2001). Possible serotonin syndrome in association with 5-HT(3) antagonist agents. Psychosomatics, 42(3), 258–260.

Ubogu, E.E., Katirji, B. (2003). Mirtazapine-induced serotonin syndrome. *Clinical Neuropharmacology*, 26(2), 54–57.

Uhr, M. and Grauer, M.T. (2003b). abcb1ab P-glycoprotein is involved in the uptake of citalopram and trimipramine into the brain of mice. *Journal of Psychiatric Research*, 37(3), 179–185.

Uhr, M., Grauer, M.T. and Holsboer, F. (2003a). Differential enhancement of antidepressant penetration into the brain in mice with abcb1ab (mdr1ab) P-glycoprotein gene disruption. *Biological Psychiatry*, 54(8), 840–846.

Uhr, M., Steckler, T., Yassouridis, A. and Holsboer, F. (2000). Penetration of amitriptyline, but not of fluoxetine, into brain is enhanced in mice with blood-brain barrier deficiency due to mdr1a P-glycoprotein gene disruption. *Neuropsychopharmacology*, 22(4), 380–387.

Veefkind, A.H., Haffmans, P.M. and Hoencamp, E. (2000). Venlafaxine serum levels and CYP2D6 genotype. *Therapeutic Drug Monitoring*, 22(2), 202–208.

Versiani, M., Moreno, R., Ramakers-van Moorsel, C.J. and Schutte, A.J. (2005). Comparative Efficacy Antidepressants Study Group. Comparison of the effects of mirtazapine and fluoxetine in severely depressed patients. *CNS Drugs*, 19(2), 137–146.

Vieta, E., Martinez-Aran, A., Goikolea, J.M., *et al.* (2002). A randomized trial comparing paroxetine and venlafaxine in the treatment of bipolar depressed patients taking mood stabilizers. *Journal of Clinical Psychiatry*, 63(6), 508–512.

Vitton, O., Gendreau, M., Gendreau, J., *et al.* (2004). A double-blind placebo-controlled trial of milnacipran in the treatment of fibromyalgia. *Human Psychopharmacology*, 19(Suppl 1), S27–35.

Voineskos, A.N., Wilson, A.A., Boovariwala, A., *et al.* (2007). Serotonin transporter occupancy of high-dose selective serotonin reuptake inhibitors during major depressive disorder measured with [(11)C]DASB positron emission tomography. *Psychopharmacology*, 193(4), 539–545.

Volkow, N.D., Wang, G.J., Fischman, M.W., *et al.* (1997). Relationship between subjective effects of cocaine and dopamine transporter occupancy. *Nature*, 386(6627), 827–830.

Volkow, N.D., Wang, G.J., Fowler, J.S., *et al.* (1998). Dopamine transporter occupancies in the human brain induced by therapeutic doses of oral methylphenidate. *American Journal of Psychiatry*, 155(10), 1325–1331.

Volkow, N.D., Wang, G.J., Fowler, J.S., *et al.* (1999). Reinforcing effects of psychostimulants in humans are associated with increases in brain dopamine and occupancy of D(2) receptors. *Journal of Pharmacology and Experimental Therapeutics*, 291(1), 409–415.

Volkow, N.D., Wang, G.J., Fowler, J.S., *et al.* (2003). Cardiovascular effects of methylphenidate in humans are associated with increases of dopamine in brain and of epinephrine in plasma. *Psychopharmacology*, 166(3), 264–270.

Vormfelde, S.V., Bitsch, A., Meineke, I., *et al.* (1997). Non-response to maprotiline caused by ultra-rapid metabolism that is different from CYP2D6? *European Journal of Clinical Pharmacology*, 52(5), 387–390.

Wade, A., Crawford, G.M., Angus, M., *et al.* (2003). A randomized, double-blind, 24-week study comparing the efficacy and tolerability of mirtazapine and paroxetine in depressed patients in primary care. *International Clinical Psychopharmacology*, 18(3), 133–141.

Wade, A., Gembert, K. and Florea, I. (2007). A comparative study of the efficacy of acute and continuation treatment with escitalopram versus duloxetine in patients with major depressive disorder. *Current Medical and Research Opinion*, 23(7), 1605–1614.

Wang, J.S., Zhu, H.J., Gibson, B.B., *et al.* (2008). Sertraline and its metabolite desmethylsertraline, but not bupropion or its three major metabolites, have high affinity for P-glycoprotein. *Biological & pharmaceutical bulletin*, 31(2), 231–234.

Wedin, G.P., Oderda, G.M., Klein-Schwartz, W. and Gorman, R.L. (1986). Relative toxicity of cyclic antidepressants. *Annals of Emergency Medicine*, 15(7), 797–804.

Weihs, K.L., Houser, T.L., Batey, S.R., *et al.* (2002). Continuation phase treatment with bupropion SR effectively decreases the risk for relapse of depression. *Biological Psychiatry*, 51(9), 753–761.

Weihs, K.L., Settle, E.C. Jr., Batey, S.R., *et al.* (2000). Bupropion sustained release versus paroxetine for the treatment of depression in the elderly. *Journal of Clinical Psychiatry*, 61(3), 196–202.

Weiner, L.A., Smythe, M. and Cisek, J. (1998). Serotonin syndrome secondary to phenelzine-venlafaxine interaction. *Pharmacotherapy*, 18(2), 399–403.

Weiss, J., Dormann, S.M., Martin-Facklam, M., *et al.* (2003). Inhibition of P-glycoprotein by newer antidepressants. *Journal of Pharmacology and Experimental Therapeutics*, 305(1), 197–204.

Wellington, K. and Perry, C.M. (2001). Venlafaxine extended-release: A review of its use in the management of major depression. *CNS Drugs*, 15(8), 643–669.

Wenger, T.L., Cohn, J.B. and Bustrack, J. (1983). Comparison of the effects of bupropion and amitriptyline on cardiac conduction in depressed patients. *Journal of Clinical Psychiatry*, 44(5 Pt 2), 174–175.

Wermuth, L., Sorensen, P.S., Timm, B., *et al.* (1998). Depression in idiopathic Parkinson's disease treated with citalopram — A placebo-controlled trial. *Nordic Journal of Psychiatry*, 52(2), 163–169.

Wernicke, J., Acharya, N., Strombom, I., *et al.* (2008). Hepatic effects of duloxetine-II: Spontaneous reports and epidemiology of hepatic events. *Current Drug Safety*, 3(2), 143–153.

Wernicke, J., Lledo, A., Raskin, J., *et al.* (2007). An evaluation of the cardiovascular safety profile of duloxetine: Findings from 42 placebo-controlled studies. *Drug Safety*, 30(5), 437–455.

Wernicke, J.F., Gahimer, J., Yalcin, I., *et al.* (2005). Safety and adverse event profile of duloxetine. *Expert Opinion on Drug Safety*, 4(6), 987–993.

Wernicke, J., Pangallo, B., Wang, F., *et al.* (2008). Hepatic effects of duloxetine-I: Non-clinical and clinical trial data. *Current Drug Safety*, 3(2), 132–142.

White, N., Litovitz, T. and Clancy, C. (2008). Suicidal antidepressant overdoses: A comparative analysis by antidepressant type. *Journal of Medical Toxicology*, 4(4), 238–250.

Whiteman, P.D., Peck, A.W., Fowle, A.S. and Smith, P. (1982). Bupropion fails to affect plasma prolactin and growth hormone in normal subjects. *British Journal of Clinical Pharmacology*, 13(5), 743–745.

Whiteman, P.D., Peck, A.W., Fowle, A.S. and Smith, P.R. (1983). Failure of bupropion to affect prolactin or growth hormone in man. *Journal of Clinical Psychiatry*, 44(5 Pt 2), 209–210.

Whitmyer, V.G., Dunner, D.L., Kornstein, S.G., *et al.* (2007). A comparison of initial duloxetine dosing strategies in patients with major depressive disorder. *Journal of Clinical Psychiatry*, 68(12), 1921–1930.

Whittington, C.J., Kendall, T., Fonagy, P., *et al.* (2004). Selective serotonin reuptake inhibitors in childhood depression: Systematic review of published versus unpublished data. *The Lancet*, 363(9418), 1341–1345.

Whyte, E.M., Romkes, M., Mulsant, B.H., *et al.* (2006). CYP2D6 genotype and venlafaxine-XR concentrations in depressed elderly. *International Journal of Geriatric Psychiatry*, 21(6), 542–549.

Wichman, C.L. and Cunningham, J.L. (2008). A case of venlafaxine-induced galactorrhea? *Journal of Clinical Psychopharmacology*, 28(5), 580–581.

Widerlov, E., Wide, L. and Sjostrom, R. (1978). Effects of tricyclic antidepressants on human plasma levels of TSH, GH and prolactin. *Acta Psychiatrica Scandinavica*, 58(5), 449–456.

Wijkstra, J., Burger, H., van den Broek, W.W., *et al.* (in press). Treatment of unipolar psychotic depression: A randomized, double-blind study comparing imipramine, venlafaxine, and venlafaxine plus quetiapine. *Acta Psychiatrica Scandinavica*.

Wilcox, C.S., Cohn, J.B., Katz, B.B., *et al.* (1994). A double-blind, placebo-controlled study comparing mianserin and amitriptyline in moderately depressed outpatients. *International Clinical Psychopharmacology*, 9(4), 271–279.

Wilens, T.E., Haight, B.R., Horrigan, J.P., *et al.* (2005). Bupropion XL in adults with attention-deficit/hyperactivity disorder: A randomized, placebo-controlled study. *Biological Psychiatry*, 57(7), 793–801.

Wills, B.K., Zell-Kanter, M. and Aks, S.E. (2009). Bupropion-associated QRS prolongation unresponsive to sodium bicarbonate therapy. *American Journal of Therapeutics*, 16(2), 193–196.

Wilson, A.D., Howell, C. and Waring, W.S. (2007). Venlafaxine ingestion is associated with rhabdomyolysis in adults: A case series. *Journal of Toxicological Sciences*, 32(1), 97–101.

Wingen, M., Bothmer, J., Langer, S. and Ramaekers, J.G. (2005). Actual driving performance and psychomotor function in healthy subjects after acute and subchronic treatment with escitalopram, mirtazapine, and placebo: A crossover trial. *Journal of Clinical Psychiatry*, 66(4), 436–443.

Winokur, A., Baker R.A., Simmons, J., *et al.* (2005). Comparative sleep improving effects of mirtazapine vs SSRIs in depressed patients: A meta-analysis of individual patient data. *World Journal of Biological Psychiatry*, 6(s1), s366.

Winokur, A., DeMartinis, N.A., McNally, D.P., *et al.* (2003). Comparative effects of mirtazapine and fluoxetine on sleep physiology measures in patients with major depression and insomnia. *Journal of Clinical Psychiatry*, 64(10), 1224–1229.

Winokur, A., Gary, K.A., Rodner, S., *et al.* (2001). Depression, sleep physiology, and antidepressant drugs. *Depression and Anxiety*, 14(1), 19–28.

Winokur, A., Sateia, M.J., Hayes, J.B., *et al.* (2000). Acute effects of mirtazapine on sleep continuity and sleep architecture in depressed patients: A pilot study. *Biological Psychiatry*, 48(1), 75–78.

Wise, T.N., Perahia, D.G., Pangallo, B.A., *et al.* (2006). Effects of the antidepressant duloxetine on body weight: Analyses of 10 clinical studies. *Primary Care Companion of the Journal of Clinical Psychiatry*, 8(5), 269–278.

Wong, D.T., Bymaster, F.P., Mayle, D.A., *et al.* (1993). LY248686, a new inhibitor of serotonin and norepinephrine uptake. *Neuropsychopharmacology*, 8(1), 23–33.

Wooltorton, E. (2002). Bupropion (Zyban, Wellbutrin SR): Reports of deaths, seizures, serum sickness. *Candian Medical Association Journal*, 166(1), 68.

Yang, M.S., Cheng, W.J. and Huang, M.C. (2009). Dose-related hyperprolactinemia induced by venlafaxine. *Progress in Neuropsychopharmacology and Biological Psychiatry*, 33(4), 733–734.

Yolles, J.C., Armenta, W.A. and Alao, A.O. (1999). Serum sickness induced by bupropion. *Annals of Pharmacotherapy*, 33(9), 931–933.
Zivkov, M., Roes, K.C.B. and Pols, A.G. (1995). Efficacy of Org 3770 and amitriptyline in patients with major depressive disorder: A meta analysis. *Human Psychopharmacology*, 10(Suppl 2), s135–s145.

Chapter 4

Absher, J.R. and Black, D.W. (1998). Tranylcypromine withdrawal delirium. *Journal of Clinical Psychopharmacology*, 8(5), 379–380.

Adnitt, P.I. (1968). Monoamineoxidase inhibition and insulin sensitivity. *Journal of Endocrinology*, 42(3), 417–423.

Adnitt, P.I., Oleesky, S. and Schneiden, H. (1966). Potentiation of insulin hypoglycemia. *The Lancet*, 1(7440), 770.

Amsterdam, J.D. (2003). A double-blind, placebo-controlled trial of the safety and efficacy of selegiline transdermal system without dietary restrictions in patients with major depressive disorder. *Journal of Clinical Psychiatry*, 64(2), 208–214.

Amsterdam, J.D., Campbell, B.J. and Moonsammy, G. (2006). Sexual dysfunction in patients with major depressive disorder: A comparison between Selegiline transdermal system 6 mg/24 hr and placebo using a patient-rated scale. Presented at the 160th Annual Meeting of the American Psychiatric Association. San Diego, California.

Appolinario, J.C., Godoy-Matos, A., Fontenelle, L.F., *et al.* (2002). An open-label trial of sibutramine in obese patients with binge-eating disorder. *Journal of Clinical Psychiatry*, 63(1), 28–30.

Baker, G.B. and Prior, T.I. (2002). Stereochemistry and drug efficacy and development: Relevance of chirality to antidepressant and antipsychotic drugs. *Annals of Medicine*, 34(7–8), 537–543.

Baker, G.B., Urichuk, L.J., McKenna, K.F. and Kennedy, S.H. (1999). Metabolism of monoamine oxidase inhibitors. *Cellular and Molecular Neurobiology*, 19(3), 411–426.

Beasley, C.M. Jr., Masica, D.N., Heiligenstein, J.H., *et al.* (1993). Possible monoamine oxidase inhibitor-serotonin uptake inhibitor interaction: Fluoxetine clinical data and preclinical findings. *Journal of Clinical Psychopharmacology*, 13(5), 312–320.

Ben-Arie, O. and George, G.C. (1979). A case of tranylcypromine ('Parnate') addiction. *British Journal of Psychiatry*, 135, 273–274.

Bodkin, J.A. and Amsterdam, J.D. (2002). Transdermal selegiline in major depression: A double-blind, placebo-controlled, parallel-group study in outpatients. *American Journal of Psychiatry*, 159(11),1869–1875.

Bonkovsky, H.L., Blanchette, P.L. and Schned, A.R. (1986). Severe liver injury due to phenelzine with unique hepatic deposition of extracellular material. *American Journal of Medicine*, 80(4), 689–692.

Bonnet, U. (2003). Moclobemide: Therapeutic use and clinical studies. *CNS Drug Review*, 9(1), 97–140.

Brady, K.T., Lydiard, R.B. and Kellner, C. (1991). Tranylcypromine abuse. *American Journal of Psychiatry*, 148(9), 1268–1269.

Bressler, R., Vargas-Cord, M. and Lebovitz, H.E. (1968). Tranylcypromine: A potent insulin secretagogue and hypoglycemic agent. *Diabetes*, 17(10), 617–624.

Cantini, F., Bellandi, F., Niccoli, L. and Di Munno, O. (1994). Fluoxetine associated with cyclobenzaprine in the treatment of primary fibromyalgia. *Minerva Medica*, 85, 97–100.

Ceravolo, R., Piccini, P., Bailey, D.L., *et al.* (2002). 18F-dopa PET evidence that tolcapone acts as a central COMT inhibitor in Parkinson's disease. *Synapse*, 43(3), 201–207.

Chatterjee, A. and Tosyali, M.C. (1995). Thrombocytopenia and delirium associated with tranylcypromine overdose. *Journal of Clinical Psychopharmacology*, 15(2), 143–144.

Clayton, A.H., Campbell, B.J., Favit, A., *et al.* (2007). Symptoms of sexual dysfunction in patients treated for major depressive disorder: A meta-analysis comparing selegiline transdermal system and placebo using a patient-rated scale. *Journal of Clinical Psychiatry*, 68(12), 1860–1866.

Cooper, A.J. and Ashcroft, G. (1966). Potentiation of insulin hypoglycaemia by M.A.O.I. antidepressant drugs. *The Lancet*, 1(7434), 407–409.

Coulter, D.M. and Pillans, P.I. (1995). Hypertension with moclobemide. *The Lancet*, 346(8981), 1032.

Curtin, F., Berney, P. and Kaufmann, C. (2002). Moclobemide discontinuation syndrome predominantly presenting with influenza-like symptoms. *Journal of Psychopharmacology*, 16(3), 271–272.

Dams, R., Benijts, T.H., Lambert, W.E., *et al.* (2001). A fatal case of serotonin syndrome after combined moclobemide-citalopram intoxication. *Journal of Analytical Toxicology*, 25(2), 147–151.

Dardennes, R.M., Even, C., Ballon, N. and Bange, F. (1998). Serotonin syndrome caused by a clomipramine-moclobemide interaction. *Journal of Clinical Psychiatry*, 59(7), 382–383.

Davids, E., Roschke, J., Klawe, C., *et al.* (2000). Tranylcypromine abuse associated with delirium and thrombocytopenia. *Journal of Clinical Psychopharmacology*, 20(2), 270–271.

Delini-Stula, A., Baier, D., Kohnen, R., *et al.* (1999). Undesirable blood pressure changes under naturalistic treatment with moclobemide, a reversible MAO-A inhibitor — results of the drug utilization observation studies. *Pharmacopsychiatry*, 32(2), 61–67.

Dingemanse, J., Wallnofer, A., Gieschke, R., *et al.* (1998). Pharmacokinetic and pharmacodynamic interactions between fluoxetine and moclobemide in the investigation of development of the "serotonin syndrome". *Clinical Pharmacology and Therapeutics*, 63(4), 403–413.

Ebert, D., Albert, R., May, A., *et al.* (1995). Combined SSRI-RIMA treatment in refractory depression. Safety data and efficacy. *Psychopharmacology*, 119(3), 342–344.

Fava, M. and Rosenbaum, J.F. (1995a). Pharmacotherapy and somatic therapies. In E.E. Beckham and W.R. Leber (Eds.), *Handbook of Depression*, 1st ed., pp.280–301. New York: Guilford Publications.

Fava, M., Rosenbaum, J.F., Kolsky, A.R., *et al.* (1999). Open study of the catechol-O-methyltransferase inhibitor tolcapone in major depressive disorder. *Journal of Clinical Psychopharmacology*, 19(4), 329–335.

Feighner, J.P., Boyer, W.F., Tyler, D.L. and Neborsky, R.J. (1990). Adverse consequences of fluoxetine-MAOI combination therapy. *Journal of Clinical Psychiatry*, 51(6), 222–225.

Feiger, A.D., Rickels, K., Rynn, M.A., *et al.* (2006). Selegiline transdermal system for the treatment of major depressive disorder: An 8-week, double-blind, placebo-controlled, flexible-dose titration trial. *Journal of Clinical Psychiatry*, 67(9), 1354–1361.

Finge, T., Malavialle, C. and Lambert, J. (1997). Fatal form of serotonin syndrome. *Annales Françaises d'anesthèsie et de Rèanimation*, 16(1), 80–81.

Fowler, J.S., Volkow, N.D., Logan, J., *et al.* (2001). Evidence that L-deprenyl treatment for one week does not inhibit MAO A or the dopamine transporter in the human brain. *Life Sciences*, 68(24), 2759–2768.

Fowler, J.S., Volkow, N.D., Logan, J., *et al.* (1994). Slow recovery of human brain MAO B after L-deprenyl (Selegeline) withdrawal. *Synapse*, 18(2), 86–93.

Georgotas, A., McCue, R.E., Friedman, E. and Cooper, T.B. (1987). Electrocardiographic effects of nortriptyline, phenelzine, and placebo under optimal treatment conditions. *American Journal of Psychiatry*, 144(6), 798–801.

Giménez-Roldán, S., Dobato, J.L. and Mateo, D. (1997). Treatment of depression in Parkinson's disease with moclobemide: A pilot open-label study. *Parkinsonism and Related Disorders*, 3(4), 219–225.

Glick, S.D., Haskew, R.E., Maisonneuve, I.M., *et al.* (2000). Enantioselective behavioral effects of sibutramine metabolites. *European Journal of Pharmacology*, 397(1), 93–102.

Goldenberg, D., Mayskiy, M., Mossey, C., *et al.* (1996). A randomized, double-blind, crossover trial of fluoxetine and amitriptyline in the treatment of fibromyalgia. *Arthritis and Rheumatism*, 39, 1852–1859.

Gomez-Gil, E., Salmeron, J.M. and Mas, A. (1996). Phenelzine-induced fulminant hepatic failure. *Annals of Internal Medicine*, 124(7), 692–693.

Griffin, N., Draper, R.J. and Webb, M.G. (1981). Addiction to tranylcypromine. *British Medical Journal (Clinical Research Edition)*, 283(6287), 346.

Halle, M.T. and Dilsaver, S.C. (1993). Tranylcypromine withdrawal phenomena. *Journal of Psychiatry and Neuroscience*, 1993, 18(1), 49–50.

Hannonen, P., Malminiemi, K., Yli-Kerttula, U., *et al.* (1998). A randomized, double-blind, placebo-controlled study of moclobemide and amitriptyline in the treatment of fibromyalgia in females without psychiatric disorder. *British Journal of Rheumatology*, 37, 1279–1286.

Harrison, W., Stewart, J., Lovelace, R. and Quitkin, F. (1983). Case report of carpal tunnel syndrome associated with tranylcypromine. *American Journal of Psychiatry*, 140(9), 1229–1230.

Hasan, F., McCrodden, J.M., Kennedy, N.P. and Tipton, K.F. (1988). The involvement of intestinal monoamine oxidase in the transport and metabolism of tyramine. *Journal of Neural Transmission. Supplementum*, 26, 1–9.

Heal, D.J., Aspley, S., Prow, M.R., *et al.* (1998). Sibutramine: A novel anti-obesity drug. A review of the pharmacological evidence to differentiate it from d-amphetamine and d-fenfluramine. *International Journal of Obesity and Related Metabolic Disorders*, 22(Suppl 1), S18–28.

Hickie, I.B., Wilson, A.J., Wright, J.M., *et al.* (2000). A randomized, double-blind placebo-controlled trial of moclobemide in patients with chronic fatigue syndrome. *Journal of Clinical Psychiatry*, 61(9), 643–648.

Hilton, S.E., Maradit, H. and Moller, H.J. (1997). Serotonin syndrome and drug combinations: Focus on MAOI and RIMA. *European Archives of Psychiatry and Clinical Neuroscience*, 247(3), 113–119.

Hirvonen, J., Kailajärvi, M., Haltia, T., *et al.* (2009). Assessment of MAO-B occupancy in the brain with PET and [(11)C]-L-deprenyl-D(2): A dose-finding study with a novel MAO-B inhibitor, EVT 301. *Clinical Pharmacology and Therapeutics*, 85(5), 506–512.

Hojer, J., Personne, M., Skagius, A.S. and Hansson, O. (2002). Serotonin syndrome–several cases of this often overlooked diagnosis. *Tidsskrift for den Norske Laegeforening*, 122(17), 1660–1663.

Isbister, G.K., McGettigan, P. and Dawson, A. (2001). A fatal case of moclobemide-citalopram intoxication. *Journal of Analytical Toxicology*, 25(8), 716–717.

Joffe, R.T. and Bakish, D. (1994). Combined SSRI-moclobemide treatment of psychiatric illness. *Journal of Clinical Psychiatry*, 55(1), 24–25.

Joffe, R.T. and Singer, W. (1987). Effect of phenelzine on thyroid function in depressed patients. *Biological Psychiatry*, 22(8), 1033–1035.

Joyce, P.R. and Walshe, J. (1983). Nightmares during phenelzine withdrawal. *Journal of Clinical Psychopharmacology*, 3(2), 121.

Kłys, M., Kowalski, P., Rojek, S. and Gross, A. (2009). Death of a female cocaine user due to the serotonin syndrome following moclobemide-venlafaxine overdose. *Forensic Science International*, 184(1–3), e16–e20.

Kusalic, M., Engelsmann, F. and Bradwejn, J. (1993). Thyroid functioning during treatment for depression. *Journal of Psychiatry and Neuroscience*, 18(5), 260–263.

Laine, K., Anttila, M., Nyman, L., *et al.* (2001). CYP2C19 polymorphism is not important for the *in vivo* metabolism of selegiline. *European Journal of Clinical Pharmacology*, 57(2), 137–142.

Landolt, H.P., Raimo, E.B., Schnierow, B.J., *et al.* (2001). Sleep and sleep electroencephalogram in depressed patients treated with phenelzine. *Archives of General Psychiatry*, 58(3), 268–276.

Lane, R. and Baldwin, D. (1997). Selective serotonin reuptake inhibitor-induced serotonin syndrome: Review. *Journal of Clinical Psychopharmacology*, 17(3), 208–221.

Larsen, J.K., Gjerris, A., Holm, P., *et al.* (1991). Moclobemide in depression: A randomized, multicentre trial against isocarboxazide and clomipramine emphasizing atypical depression. *Acta Psychiatrica Scandinavica*, 84(6), 564–570.

Lavin, M.R., Mendelowitz, A. and Kronig, M.H. (1993). Spontaneous hypertensive reactions with monoamine oxidase inhibitors. *Biological Psychiatry*, 34(3), 146–151.

Levant, B. and Bancroft, G.N. (1998). Inhibition of [3H]quinpirole binding by a monoamine oxidase inhibitor in subcellular fractions of rat striatum. *Life Sciences*, 63(18), 1643–1651.

Levant, B., Moehlenkamp, J.D., Morgan, K.A., *et al.* (1996). Modulation of [3H]quinpirole binding in brain by monoamine oxidase inhibitors: Evidence for a potential novel binding site. *Journal of Pharmacology and Experimental Therapeutics*, 278(1), 145–153.

Liebowitz, M.R., Quitkin, F.M., Stewart, J.W., *et al.* (1988). Antidepressant specificity in atypical depression. *Archives of General Psychiatry*, 45(2), 129–137.

Lingjaerde, O., Reichborn-Kjennerud, T., Haggag, A., *et al.* (1993). Treatment of winter depression in Norway. II. A comparison of the selective monoamine oxidase A inhibitor moclobemide and placebo. *Acta Psychiatrica Scandinavica*, 88(5), 372–380.

Lonnqvist, J., Sihvo, S., Syvalahti, E. and Kiviruusu, O. (1994). Moclobemide and fluoxetine in atypical depression: A double-blind trial. *Journal of Affective Disorders*, 32(3), 169–177.

Markianos, M., Alevizos, B. and Hatzimanolis, J. (1988). Effect of moclobemide on clinical and neurochemical variables in depressed patients (preliminary findings). *Journal of Neural Transmission. Supplementum*, 26, 87–95.

Markianos, M., Alevizos, V. and Hatzimanolis, J. (1991). Plasma sex hormones and urinary biogenic amine metabolites during treatment of male depressed patients with the monoamine oxidase inhibitor moclobemide. *Neuroendocrinology Letters*, 13, 49–55.

Mawhinney, M., Cole, D. and Azzaro, A.J. (2003). Daily transdermal administration of selegiline to guinea-pigs preferentially inhibits monoamine oxidase activity in brain when compared with intestinal and hepatic tissues. *Journal of Pharmacy and Pharmacology*, 55(1), 27–34.

McGrath, P.J., Blood, D.K., Stewart, J.W., *et al.* (1987). A comparative study of the electrocardiographic effects of phenelzine, tricyclic antidepressants, mianserin, and placebo. *Journal of Clinical Psychopharmacology*, 7(5), 335–339.

Moll, E., Neumann, N., Schmid-Burgk, W., *et al.* (1994). Safety and efficacy during long-term treatment with moclobemide. *Clinical Neuropharmacology*, 17(Suppl 1), S74–87.

Murphy, D.L., Tamarkin, L., Sunderland, T., *et al.* (1986). Human plasma melatonin is elevated during treatment with the monoamine oxidase inhibitors clorgyline and tranylcypromine but not deprenyl. *Psychiatry Research*, 17(2), 119–127.

Natelson, B.H., Cheu, J., Hill, N., *et al.* (1998). Single-blind, placebo phase-in trial of two escalating doses of selegiline in the chronic fatigue syndrome. *Neuropsychobiology*, 37(3), 150–154.

Natelson, B.H., Cheu, J., Pareja, J., *et al.* (1996). Randomized, double blind, controlled placebo-phase in trial of low dose phenelzine in the chronic fatigue syndrome. *Psychopharmacology*, 124(3), 226–230.

Neusch, C., Schnierle, S. and Moser, A. (1997). Selegiline induces dopamine release through ATP-sensitive potassium channels in the rat caudate-putamen *in vitro*. *Neurochemistry International*, 31(2), 307–311.

Nisoli, E. and Carruba, M.O. (2003). A benefit-risk assessment of sibutramine in the management of obesity. *Drug Safety*, 26(14), 1027–1048.

Norregaard, J., Volkmann, H. and Danneskiold-Samsoe, B. (1995). A randomized controlled trial of citalopram in the treatment of fibromyalgia. *Pain*, 61, 445–449.

Nutt, D., Montgomery, S.A. (1996). Moclobemide in the treatment of social phobia. *International Clinical Psychopharmacology*, 11(Suppl 3), 77–82.

O'Brien, S., McKeon, P. and O'Regan, M. (1991). A comparative study of the electrocardiographic effects of tranylcypromine and amitriptyline when prescribed singly and in combination. *International Clinical Psychopharmacology*, 6(1), 11–17.

O'Grady, P. and Carney, P.A. (1997). Recurrent life-threatening thrombocytopenia in a patient with chronic "Parstelin" dependence. *Irish Medical Journal*, 90(1), 25.

Palladino, A. Jr. (1983). Adverse reactions to abrupt discontinuation of phenelzine. *Journal of Clinical Psychopharmacology*, 3(3), 206–207.

Pande, A.C., Birkett, M., Fechner-Bates, S., *et al.* (1996). Fluoxetine versus phenelzine in atypical depression. *Biological Psychiatry*, 40(10), 1017–1020.

Papakostas, G.I. and Fava, M. (2006). A metaanalysis of clinical trials comparing moclobemide with selective serotonin reuptake inhibitors for the treatment of major depressive disorder. *Canadian Journal of Psychiatry*, 51(12), 783–790.

Paykel, E.S., Rowan, P.R., Parker, R.R. and Bhat, A.V. (1982). Response to phenelzine and amitriptyline in subtypes of outpatient depression. *Archives of General Psychiatry*, 39(9), 1041–1049.

Pennings, E.J., Verkes, R.J., de Koning, J., *et al.* (1997). Tranylcypromine intoxication with malignant hyperthermia, delirium, and thrombocytopenia. *Journal of Clinical Psychopharmacology*, 17(5), 430–432.

Petersen, T., Dording, C., Neault, N.B., *et al.* (2002a). A survey of prescribing practices in the treatment of depression. *Progress in Neuropsychopharmacology and Biological Psychiatry*, 26(1), 177–187.

Peterson, J.C., Pollack, R.W., Mahoney, J.J. and Fuller, T.J. (1978). Inappropriate antidiuretic hormone secondary to a monamine oxidase inhibitor. *Journal of the American Medical Association*, 239(14), 1422–1423.

Philipp, M., Tiller, J.W., Baier, D. and Kohnen, R. (2000). Comparison of moclobemide with selective serotonin reuptake inhibitors (SSRIs) on sexual function in depressed adults. The Australian and German Study Groups. *European Neuropsychopharmacology*, 10(5), 305–314.

Potter, W.Z., Zaharko, D.S. and Beck, L.V. (1969). Possible role of hydrazine group in hypoglycemia associated with the use of certain monoamine-oxidase inhibitors (MAOI's). *Diabetes*, 18(8), 538–541.

Quitkin, F.M., Harrison, W., Stewart, J.W., *et al.* (1991). Response to phenelzine and imipramine in placebo nonresponders with atypical depression. A new application of the crossover design. *Archives of General Psychiatry*, 48(4), 319–323.

Quitkin, F.M., McGrath, P.J., Stewart, J.W., *et al.* (1990). Atypical depression, panic attacks, and response to imipramine and phenelzine. A replication. *Archives of General Psychiatry*, 47(10), 935–941.

Richard, I.H., Kurlan, R., Tanner, C., *et al.* (1997). Serotonin syndrome and the combined use of deprenyl and an antidepressant in Parkinson's disease. Parkinson Study Group. *Neurology*, 48(4), 1070–1077.

Robinson, D.S. and Amsterdam, J.D. (2008). The selegiline transdermal system in major depressive disorder: A systematic review of safety and tolerability. *Journal of Affective Disorders*, 105(1–3), 15–23.

Robinson, D.S., Kayser, A., Corcella, J., *et al.* (1985). Panic attacks in outpatients with depression: Response to antidepressant treatment. *Psychopharmacology Bulletin*, 21(3), 562–567.

Rodrigues, A.M., Radominski, R.B., Suplicy Hde, L., *et al.* (2002). The cerebrospinal fluid/serum leptin ratio during pharmacological therapy for obesity. *Journal of Clinical Endocrinology and Metabolism*, 87(4), 1621–1626.

Rogde, S., Hilberg, T. and Teige, B. (1999). Fatal combined intoxication with new antidepressants. Human cases and an experimental study of postmortem moclobemide redistribution. *Forensic Science International*, 100(1–2), 109–116.

Rowland, M.J., Bransome, E.D. Jr. and Hendry, L.B. (1994). Hypoglycemia caused by selegiline, an antiparkinsonian drug: Can such side effects be predicted? *Journal of Clinical Pharmacology*, 34(1), 80–85.

Ruggieri, S., Denaro, A., Meco, G., *et al.* (1986). Multicenter trial of L-Deprenyl in Parkinson disease. *Italian Journal of Neurological Sciences*, 7(1), 133–137.

Scheinin, H., Anttila, M., Dahl, M.L., *et al.* (1998). CYP2D6 polymorphism is not crucial for the disposition of selegiline. *Clinical Pharmacology Therapeutics*, 64(4), 402–411.

Singer, P.P. and Jones, G.R. (1997). An uncommon fatality due to moclobemide and paroxetine. *Journal of Analytical Toxicology*, 21(6), 518–520.

Slawson, M.H., Taccogno, J.L., Foltz, R.L. and Moody, D.E. (2002). Quantitative analysis of selegiline and three metabolites (N-desmethylselegiline, methamphetamine, and amphetamine) in human plasma by high-performance liquid chromatography-atmospheric pressure chemical ionization-tandem mass spectrometry. *Journal of Analytical Toxicology*, 26(7), 430–437.

Sogaard, J., Lane, R., Latimer, P., *et al.* (1999). A 12-week study comparing moclobemide and sertraline in the treatment of outpatients with atypical depression. *Journal of Psychopharmacology*, 13(4), 406–414.

Steiger, A., Benkert, O. and Holsboer, F. (1994). Effects of long-term treatment with the MAO-A inhibitor moclobemide on sleep EEG and nocturnal hormonal secretion in normal men. *Neuropsychobiology*, 30(2–3), 101–105.

Steiger, A., Holsboer, F. and Benkert, O. (1987). Effects of brofaromine (CGP 11 305A), a short-acting, reversible, and selective inhibitor of MAO-A on sleep, nocturnal penile tumescence and nocturnal hormonal secretion in three healthy volunteers. *Psychopharmacology*, 92(1), 110–114.

Stewart, J.W. and Halbreich, U. (1989). Plasma melatonin levels in depressed patients before and after treatment with antidepressant medication. *Biological Psychiatry*, 25(1), 33–38.

Stewart, J.W., Harrison, W., Quitkin, F., Liebowitz, M.R. (1984). Phenelzine-induced pyridoxine deficiency. *Journal of Clinical Psychopharmacology*, 4(4), 225–226.

Stewart, J.W., McGrath, P.J. and Quitkin, F.M. (2002). Do age of onset and course of illness predict different treatment outcome among DSM IV depressive disorders with atypical features? *Neuropsychopharmacology*, 26(2), 237–245.

Szelenyi, A. and Albrecht, J. (1998). Tranylcypromine abuse associated with an isolated thrombocytopenia. Pharmacopsychiatry, 31(6), 238–240.

Thase, M.E., Trivedi, M.H. and Rush, A.J. (1995). MAOIs in the contemporary treatment of depression. *Neuropsychopharmacology*, 12(3), 185–219.

Timmings, P. and Lamont, D. (1996). Intrahepatic cholestasis associated with moclobemide leading to death. *The Lancet*, 347(9003), 762–763.

Tipermas, A., Gilman, H.E. and Russakoff, L.M. (1984). A case report of leukopenia associated with phenelzine. *American Journal of Psychiatry*, 141(6), 806–807.

Tyrer, P. (1984). Clinical effects of abrupt withdrawal from tri-cyclic antidepressants and monoamine oxidase inhibitors after long-term treatment. *Journal of Affective Disorders*, 6(1), 1–7.

Vercoulen, J.H., Swanink, C.M., Zitman, F.G., *et al.* (1996). Randomized double-blind placebo-controlled study of fluoxetine in chronic fatigue syndrome. *The Lancet*, 347(9005), 858–861.

Versiani, M., Amrein, R. and Stabl, M. (1997). Moclobemide and imipramine in chronic depression (dysthymia): An international double-blind, placebo-controlled trial. International Collaborative Study Group. *International Clinical Psychopharmacology*, 12(4), 183–193.

Waring, W.S. and Wallace, W.A. (2007). Acute myocarditis after massive phenelzine overdose. *European Journal of Clinical Pharmacology*, 63(11), 1007–1009.

Wecker, L., James, S., Copeland, N. and Pacheco, M.A. (2003). Transdermal selegiline: Targeted effects on monoamine oxidases in the brain. *Biological Psychiatry*, 54(10), 1099–1104.

White, P.D. and Cleary, K.J. (1997). An open study of the efficacy and adverse effects of moclobemide in patients with the chronic fatigue syndrome. *International Clinical Psychopharmacology*, 12(1), 47–52.

Winokur, A., Gary, K.A., Rodner, S., *et al.* (2001). Depression, sleep physiology, and antidepressant drugs. *Depression and Anxiety*, 14(1), 19–28.

Wolfe, F., Cathey, M.A. and Hawley, D.J. (1994). A double-blind placebo controlled trial of fluoxetine in fibromyalgia. *Scandinavian Journal of Rheumatology*, 23, 255–259.

Chapter 5

Altshuler, L.L., Bauer, M., Frye, M.A., *et al.* (2001). Does thyroid supplementation accelerate tricyclic antidepressant response? A review and meta-analysis of the literature. *American Journal of Psychiatry*, 158(10), 1617–1622.

Amsterdam, J., Garcia-Espana, F., Fawcett, J., *et al.* (1999). Fluoxetine efficacy in menopausal women with and without estrogen replacement. *Journal of Affective Disorders*, 55(1), 11–17.

Anderson, J., Lambert, N.G. and Pigott, P.V. (1972). An evaluation of fluphenazine with nortriptyline in anxiety and depression. *Practitioner*, 208(246), 511–517.

Appelhof, B.C., Brouwer, J.P., van Dyck, R., *et al.* (2004). Triiodothyronine addition to paroxetine in the treatment of major depressive disorder. *Journal of Clinical Endocrinology and Metabolism*, 89(12), 6271– 6276.

Artigas, F., Perez, V. and Alvarez, E. (1994). Pindolol induces a rapid improvement of depressed patients treated with serotonin reuptake inhibitors. *Archives of General Psychiatry*, 51(3), 248–251.

Ayuso Gutierrez, J.L. and Alino, J.J. (1971). Tryptophan and an MAOI (nialamide) in the treatment of depression. A double-blind study. *International Pharmacopsychiatry*, 6(2), 92–97.

Bailey, H.R., Davies, E. and Morrison, I.J. (1981). Oxazepam in the treatment of anxiety associated with depression: Results of treatment in 1600 cases (Studies in depression, VI). *Current Medical and Research Opinion*, 7(3), 156–163.

Bakish, D., Hooper, C.L., Thornton, M.D., *et al.* (1997). Fast onset: An open study of the treatment of major depressive disorder with nefazodone and pindolol combination therapy. *International Clinical Psychopharmacology*, 12(2), 91–97.

Ballestros, J. and Callado, L.F. (2004). Effectiveness of pindolol plus serotonin uptake inhibitors in depression: A meta analysis of early and late outcomes from randomized controlled trials. *Journal of Affective Disorders*, 79, 137–147.

Baune, B.T., Caliskan, S. and Todder, D. (2006). Effects of adjunctive antidepressant therapy with quetiapine on clinical outcome, quality of sleep and daytime motor activity in patients with treatment-resistant depression. *Human Psychopharmacology*, 22(1), 1–9.

Beber, C.R. (1971). Treating anxiety and depression in the elderly. A double blind crossover evaluation of two widely used tranquilizers. *Journal of the Florida Medical Association*, 58(3), 35–38.

Bennett, J.A., Hirschowitz, J., Zemlan, F., *et al.* (1984). Combined thioridazine and desipramine: Early antidepressant response. *Psychopharmacology*, 82(3), 263–265.

Bennie, E.H. and Schiff, A.A. (1976). A comparison of amitriptyline and a fluphenazine/nortriptyline preparation in anxiety-depressive states. *Scottish Medical Journal*, 21(4), 204–209.

Berlanga, C., Mendieta, D., Alva, G. and del Carmen Lara, M. (2003). Failure of tibolone to potentiate the pharmacological effect of fluoxetine in postmenopausal major depression. *Journal of Women's Health*, 12(1), 33–39.

Berlanga, C., Ortega-Soto, H.A., Ontiveros, M. and Senties, H. (2001). Efficacy of s-adenosyl-L-methionine in speeding the onset of action of imipramine. *Psychiatry Research*, 44, 257–262.

Berman, R.M., Anand, A., Cappiello, A., *et al.* (1999). The use of pindolol with fluoxetine in the treatment of major depression: Final results from a double-blind, placebo-controlled trial. *Biological Psychiatry*, 45(9), 1170–1177.

Berman, R.M., Darnell, A.M., Miller, H.L., *et al.* (1997). Effect of pindolol in hastening response to fluoxetine in the treatment of major depression: A double-blind, placebo-controlled trial. *American Journal of Psychiatry*, 154(1), 37–43.

Berney, A., Nishikawa, M., Benkelfat, C., *et al.* (2008). An index of 5-HT synthesis changes during early antidepressant treatment: Alpha-[(11)C]methyl-l-tryptophan PET study. *Neurochemistry International*, 52(4–5), 701–708.

Blier, P. and Bergeron, R. (1995). Effectiveness of pindolol with selected antidepressant drugs in the treatment of major depression. *Journal of Clinical Psychopharmacology*, 15(3), 217–222.

Blier, P., Gobbi, G., Turcotte, J.E., *et al.* (2009). Mirtazapine and paroxetine in major depression: A comparison of monotherapy versus their combination from treatment initiation. *European Neuropsychopharmacology*, 19(7), 457–465.

Bordet, R., Thomas, P. and Dupuis, B. (1998). Effect of pindolol on onset of action of paroxetine in the treatment of major depression: Intermediate analysis of a double-blind, placebo-controlled trial. Reseau de Recherche et d'Experimentation Psychopharmacologique. *American Journal of Psychiatry*, 155(10), 1346–1351.

Bowden, C.L., Brugger, A.M., Swann, A.C., *et al.* (1994). Efficacy of divalproex vs lithium and placebo in the treatment of mania. The Depakote Mania Study Group. *Journal of the American Medical Association*, 271(12), 918–924.

Bowden, C.L., Calabrese, J.R., McElroy, S.L., *et al.* (2000). A randomized, placebo-controlled 12-month trial of divalproex and lithium in treatment of outpatients with bipolar I disorder. Divalproex Maintenance Study Group. *Archives of General Psychiatry*, 57(5), 481–489.

Bowden, C.L., Grunze, H., Mullen, J., *et al.* (2005). A randomized, double-blind, placebo-controlled efficacy and safety study of quetiapine or lithium as monotherapy for mania in bipolar disorder. *Journal of Clinical Psychiatry*, 66(1), 111–121.

Bowden, C.L., Swann, A.C., Calabrese, J.R., *et al.* (2006). A randomized, placebo-controlled, multicenter study of divalproex sodium extended release in the treatment of acute mania. *Journal of Clinical Psychiatry*, 67(10), 1501–1510.

Browne, M.W. (1966). Amitriptyline + perphenazine in depressive illness — a preliminary report. *Journal of the Irish Medical Association*, 59(352), 129–130.

Calabrese, J.R., Bowden, C.L, Sachs, G.S., *et al.* (1999). A double-blind placebo-controlled study of lamotrigine monotherapy in outpatients with bipolar I depression. Lamictal 602 Study Group. *Journal of Clinical Psychiatry*, 60(2), 79–88.

Calabrese, J.R., Keck, P.E. Jr., Macfadden, W., *et al.* (2005). A randomized, double-blind, placebo-controlled trial of quetiapine in the treatment of bipolar I or II depression. *American Journal of Psychiatry*, 162(7), 1351–1360.

Calcedo Ordonez, A., Arosamene, X., Otero Perez, F.J., *et al.* (1992). Clomipramine/bentazepam combination in the treatment of major depressive disorders. *Human Psychopharmacology*, 7, 115–122.

Camarasa, X., Lopez-Martinez, E., Duboc, A., *et al.* (2005). Escitalopram/reboxetine combination in depressed patients with substance use disorder. *Progress in Neuropsychopharmacology and Biological Psychiatry*, 29(1), 165–168.

Cappiello, A., McDougle, C.J., Delgado, P.L., *et al.* (1998). Lithium and desipramine versus desipramine alone in the treatment of severe major depression: A preliminary study. *International Clinical Psychopharmacology*, 13(5), 191–198.

Chacon, C. and Downham, E.T. (1967). Amitriptyline and amitriptyline-with-perphenazine in depression — a retrospective study. *British Journal of Psychiatry*, 113(495), 201–207.

Chengappa, K.N., Levine, J., Gershon, S., *et al.* (2000). Inositol as an add-on treatment for bipolar depression. *Bipolar Disorder*, 2(1), 47–55.

Chouinard, G., Young, S.N., Annable, L. and Sourkes, T.L. (1979). Tryptophan-nicotinamide, imipramine and their combination in depression. A controlled study. *Acta Psychiatrica Scandinavica*, 59(4), 395–414.

Chung, S.K., Hwang, I.K. and Lim, E.S. (2007). Are mirtazapine and venlafaxine combination therapy effective and safe in major depressive disorder? *European Neuropsychopharmacology*, 17(s4), S361.

Coffee, H.L. (1964). Combined amitriptyline and perphenazine in combined depression and anxiety. *Journal of the Medical Association of Georgia*, 53, 107–109.

Cooper-Kazaz, R., Apter, J.T., Cohen, R., *et al.* (2007). Combined treatment with sertraline and liothyronine in major depression: A randomized, double-blind, placebo-controlled trial. *Archives of General Psychiatry*, 64(6), 679–688.

Coppen, A. and Bailey, J. (2000). Enhancement of the antidepressant action of fluoxetine by folic acid: A randomised, placebo controlled trial. *Journal of Affective Disorders*, 60(2), 121–130.

Coppen, A., Montgomery, S., Peet, M., *et al.* (1974). Thyrotrophin-releasing hormone in the treatment of depression. *The Lancet*, 2(7878), 433–434.

Coppen, A., Shaw, D.M. and Farrell, J.P. (1963). Potentiation of the antidepressive effect of a monoamine-oxidase inhibitor by tryptophan. *The Lancet*, 1, 79–81.

Corya, S.A., Andersen, S.W., Detke, H.C., *et al.* (2003). Long-term antidepressant efficacy and safety of olanzapine/fluoxetine combination: A 76-week open-label study. *Journal of Clinical Psychiatry*, 64(11), 1349–1356.

Dam, J., Ryde, L., Svejso, J., *et al.* (1998). Morning fluoxetine plus evening mianserin versus morning fluoxetine plus evening placebo in the acute treatment of major depression. *Pharmacopsychiatry*, 31(2), 48–54.

Davis, W.G. (1968). Treating psychical disturbances induced by physical disorders: A double-blind study of perphenazine-amitriptyline in anxiety and depression. *Psychosomatics*, 9(1), 44–46.

De Montigny, C., Grunberg, F., Mayer, A. and Descenes, J.P. (1981). Lithium induces rapid relief of depression in tricyclic antidepressant drug nonresponders. *British Journal of Psychiatry*, 138, 252–256.

Delbello, M.P., Schwiers, M.L., Rosenberg, H.L. and Strakowski, S.M. (2002). A double-blind, randomized, placebo-controlled study of quetiapine as adjunctive treatment for adolescent mania. *Journal of the American Academy of Child and Adolescent Psychiatry*, 41(10), 1216–1223.

Desilverio, R.V., Rickels, K., Weise, C.C., *et al.* (1970). Perphenazine-amitriptyline in neurotic depressed outpatients: A controlled collaborative study. *American Journal of Psychiatry*, 127(3), 322–329.

Diamond, S. (1966). Double-blind controlled study of amitriptyline-perphenazine combination in medical office patients with depression and anxiety. *Psychosomatics*, 7, 371–375.

Dias, R.S., Kerr-Correa, F., Moreno, R.A., *et al.* (2006). Efficacy of hormone therapy with and without methyltestosterone augmentation of venlafaxine in the treatment of postmenopausal depression: A double-blind controlled pilot study. *Menopause*, 13(2), 202–211.

Dolberg, O.T., Hirschmann, S. and Grunhaus, L. (1998). Melatonin for the treatment of sleep disturbances in major depressive disorder. *American Journal of Psychiatry*, 155(8), 1119–1121.

Dominguez, R.A., Jacobson, A.F., Goldstein, B.J. and Steinbrook, R.M. (1984). Comparison of triazolam and placebo in the treatment of insomnia in depressed patients. *Current Therapeutic Research*, 36(5), 856–865.

Dorfman, W. (1966). Combined use of an anti-depressant with tranquilizer in the management of depression. *Diseases of the Nervous System*, (Suppl 7), 71–73.

Dunlop, B.W., Crits-Christoph, P., Evans, D.L., *et al.* (2007). Coadministration of modafinil and a selective serotonin reuptake inhibitor from the initiation of treatment of major depressive disorder with fatigue and sleepiness: A double-blind, placebo controlled study. *Journal of Clinical Psychopharmacology*, 27(6), 614–619.

Eden Evins, A., Demopulos, C., Yovel, I., *et al.* (2006). Inositol augmentation of lithium or valproate for bipolar depression. *Bipolar Disorder*, 8(2), 168–174.

Faleni, R. and Cia, A. (1972). Motival in the treatment of anxious depression. *Current Therapeutic Research, Clinical and Experimental*, 14(8), 461–469.

Fava, M. (2007). The combination of buspirone and bupropion in the treatment of depression. *Psychotherapy and Psychosomatics*, 76(5), 311–312.

Fava, M., Asnis, G., Shrivastava, R., *et al.* (2008). Zolpidem extended-release, co-administered with escitalopram, improves insomnia in patients with comorbid insomnia and major depressive disorder. APA 2008.

Fava, M., McCall, W.V., Krystal, A., *et al.* (2006). Eszopiclone co-administered with fluoxetine in patients with insomnia coexisting with major depressive disorder. *Biological Psychiatry*, 59(11), 1052–1060.

Fawcett, J., Edwards, J.H., Kravitz, H.M. and Jeffriess, H. (1987). Alprazolam: An antidepressant? Alprazolam, desipramine, and an alprazolam-desipramine combination in the treatment of adult depressed outpatients. *Journal of Clinical Psychopharmacology*, 7(5), 295–310.

Feet, P.O., Larsen, S. and Robak, O.H. (1985). A double blind study in outpatients with primary non-agitated depression treated with imipramine in combination with placebo, diazepam or dixyrazine. *Acta Psychiatrica Scandinavica*, 72(4), 334–340.

Feighner, J.P., Brauzer, B., Gelenberg, A.J., *et al.* (1979). A placebo-controlled multicenter trial of Limbitrol versus its components (amitriptyline and chlordiazepoxide) in the symptomatic treatment of depressive illness. *Psychopharmacology*, 61(2), 217–225.

Feighner, J.P., King, L.J., Schuckit, M.A., *et al.* (1972). Hormonal potentiation of imipramine and ECT in primary depression. *American Journal of Psychiatry*, 128(10), 1230–1238.

Feldman, P.E. (1965). Combined antidepressant-tranquilizer therapy of mixed psychiatric syndromes. *Psychosomatics*, 6(5), 312.

Feldmesser-Reiss, E.E. (1958). The application of triiodothyronine in the treatment of mental disorders. *Journal of Nervous and Mental Disease*, 127(6), 540–545.

Flach, F.F., Celian, C.I. and Rawson, R.W. (1958). Treatment of psychiatric disorders with triiodothyronine. *American Journal of Psychiatry*, 114(9), 841–842.

Frangou, S., Lewis, M. and McCrone, P. (2006). Efficacy of ethyl-eicosapentaenoic acid in bipolar depression: Randomized double-blind placebo-controlled study. *British Journal of Psychiatry*, 188, 46–50.

Frye, M.A., Ketter, T.A., Kimbrell, T.A., *et al.* (2000). A placebo-controlled study of lamotrigine and gabapentin monotherapy in refractory mood disorders. *Journal of Clinical Psychopharmacology*, 20(6), 607–614.

Furukawa, T.A., Streiner, D.L. and Young, L.T. (2001). Is antidepressant-benzodiazepine combination therapy clinically more useful? A meta-analytic study. *Journal of Affective Disorders*, 65(2), 173–177.

Garakani, A., Martinez, J.M., Marcus, S., *et al.* (2008). A randomized, double-blind, and placebo-controlled trial of quetiapine augmentation of fluoxetine in major depressive disorder. *International Clinical Psychopharmacology*, 23(5), 269–275.

Garlow, S.J., Dunlop, B., Ninan, P.T. and Nemeroff, C.B. (2007). Addition of tri-iodothyronine (T3) to sertraline does not impact treatment response in patients with major depressive disorder. Annual Meeting of the American College of Neuropsychopharmacology (ACNP).

Geddes, J.R., Burgess, S., Hawton, K., *et al.* (2004). Long-term lithium therapy for bipolar disorder: Systematic review and meta-analysis of randomized controlled trials. *American Journal of Psychiatry*, 161(2), 217–222.

Geddes, J.R., Calabrese, J.R., Goodwin, G.M. (2009). Lamotrigine for treatment of bipolar depression: Independent meta-analysis and meta-regression of individual patient data from five randomised trials. *British Journal of Psychiatry*, 194, 4–199.

General Practitioner Research Group (1969). General practitioner clinical trials. Chlordiazepoxide with amitriptyline in neurotic depression. *Practitioner*, 202(209), 437–440.

Geretsegger, C., Bitterluch, W., Stelzig, R., *et al.* (2008). Paroxetine with pindolol augmentation: A double-blind, randomized, placebo-controlled study in depressed in-patients. *European Neuropsychopharmacology*, 18(2), 141–146.

Glassman, A.H. and Platman, S.R. (1969). Potentiation of a monoamine oxidase inhibitor by tryptophan. *Journal of Psychiatric Research*, 7(2), 83–88.

Godfrey, P.S., Toone, B.K., Carney, M.W., *et al.* (1990). Enhancement of recovery from psychiatric illness by methylfolate. *The Lancet*, 336(8712), 392–395.

Goodnick, P.J. (2007). Bipolar depression: A review of randomised clinical trials. *Expert Opinion in Pharmacotherapy*, 8(1), 13–21.

Grainger, G.J. (1972). A clinical study of 'limbitrol' in the treatment of anxiety-depression in general practice. *Practitioner*, 208(248), 807–809.

Gwirtsman, H.E., Szuba, M.P., Toren, L. and Feist, M. (1994). The antidepressant response to tricyclics in major depressives is accelerated with adjunctive use of methylphenidate. *Psychopharmacology Bulletin*, 30(2), 157–164.

Haider, I. (1967b). A comparative trial of Ro 4-6270 and amitriptyline in depressive illness. *British Journal of Psychiatry*, 113(502), 993–998.

Haider, I. (1967a). Combination of amitriptyline and chlordiazepoxide in depressive states. *British Journal of Clinical Practice*, 21(1), 39–40.

Hannan, N., Hamzah, Z., Omoniyi Akinpeloye, H. and Meagher, D. (2007). Venlafaxine-mirtazapine combination in the treatment of persistent depressive illness. *Journal of Psychopharmacology*, 21(2), 161–164.

Hare, H.P. Jr. (1971). Comparison of chlordiazepoxide-amitriptyline combination with amitriptyline alone in anxiety-depressive states. *Journal of Clinical Pharmacology and New Drugs*, 11(6), 456–460.

Hirose, S. and Ashby, C.R. Jr. (2002). An open pilot study combining risperidone and a selective serotonin reuptake inhibitor as initial antidepressant therapy. *Journal of Clinical Psychiatry*, 63(8), 733–736.

Hirschfeld, R.M., Baker, J.D., Wozniak, P., *et al.* (2003). The safety and early efficacy of oral-loaded divalproex versus standard-titration divalproex, lithium, olanzapine, and placebo in the treatment of acute mania associated with bipolar disorder. *Journal of Clinical Psychiatry*, 64(7), 841–846.

Hirschfeld, R.M., Keck, P.E., Jr., Kramer, M., *et al.* (2004). Rapid antimanic effect of risperidone monotherapy: A 3-week multicenter, double-blind, placebo-controlled trial. *American Journal of Psychiatry*, 161(6), 1057–1065.

Hollister, L.E., Overall, J.E., Johnson, M.H., *et al.* (1966). Amitryptiline alone and combined with perphenazine in newly admitted depressed patients. *Journal of Nervous and Mental Disease*, 142(5), 460–469.

Hollister, L.E., Overall, J.E., Shelton, J., *et al.* (1967). Drug therapy of depression. Amitriptyline, perphenazine, and their combination in different syndromes. *Archives of General Psychiatry*, 17(4), 486–493.

Holtzheimer, P.E. 3rd., Meeks, T.W., Kelley, M.E., *et al.* (2008). A double-blind, placebo-controlled pilot study of galantamine augmentation of antidepressant treatment in older adults with major depression. *International Journal of Geriatric Psychiatry*, 23(6), 625–631.

Houck, J. (1970). Combined therapy in anxiety-depressive syndromes. II. Comparative effects of amitriptyline and limbitrol (chlordiazepoxide-amitriptyline). *Diseases of the Nervous System*, 31(6), 421–426.

Hussain, M.Z., Waheed, W. and Hussain, S. (2006). A comparison of unipolar depression treatment using antidepressants alone versus using antidepressants in combination with quetiapine (4 year follow-up). *European Neuropsychopharmacology*, 16(s4), S325.

Isaac, M.T., Isaac, M.B., Gallo, F. and Tournoux, A. (2003). Milnacipran and pindolol: A randomized trial of reduction of antidepressant latency. *Human Psychopharmacology*, 18(8), 595–601.

Jacobson, A.F. (1978). Doctor-patient concordance in a placebo-controlled trial of limbitrol versus its components. *Psychopharmacology Bulletin*, 14(3), 61–63.

Jahn, H., Schick, M., Kiefer, F., *et al.* (2004). Metyrapone as additive treatment in major depression: A double-blind and placebo-controlled trial. *Archives of General Psychiatry*, 61(12), 1235–1244.

James, R.T. and Dean, B.C. (1985). Comparison of limbitrol (chlordiazepoxide/amitriptyline) and amitriptyline alone as a single night-time dose for the treatment of depression with anxiety. *Journal of International Medical Research*, 13(2), 84–87.

Januel, D., Poirier, M.F., D'alche-Biree, F., *et al.* (2003). Multicenter double-blind randomized parallel-group clinical trial of efficacy of the combination clomipramine (150 mg/day) plus lithium carbonate (750 mg/day) versus clomipramine (150 mg/day) plus placebo in the treatment of unipolar major depression. *Journal of Affective Disorders*, 76(1–3), 191–200.

Jazayeri, S., Tehrani-Doost, M., Keshavarz, S.A., *et al.* (2008). Comparison of therapeutic effects of omega-3 fatty acid eicosapentaenoic acid and fluoxetine, separately and in combination, in major depressive disorder. *Australian and New Zealand Journal of Psychiatry*, 42(3), 192–198.

Ji, J.L., Liu, W.J., Zhang, N., *et al.* (2007). Effects of paroxetine with or without zolpidem on depression with insomnia: A multi-center randomized comparative study. *Zhonghua Yi Xue Za Zhi*, 87(23), 1585–1589.

Keck, P.E. Jr., Calabrese, J.R., McIntyre, R.S., *et al.* (2007). Aripiprazole monotherapy for maintenance therapy in bipolar I disorder: A 100-week, double-blind study versus placebo. *Journal of Clinical Psychiatry*, 68(10), 1480–1491.

Keck, P.E. Jr., Marcus, R., Tourkodimitris, S., *et al.* (2003a). A placebo-controlled, double-blind study of the efficacy and safety of aripiprazole in patients with acute bipolar mania. *American Journal of Psychiatry*, 160(9), 1651–1658.

Keck, P.E. Jr., Mintz, J., McElroy, S.L., *et al.* (2006). Double-blind, randomized, placebo-controlled trials of ethyl-eicosapentanoate in the treatment of bipolar depression and rapid cycling bipolar disorder. *Biological Psychiatry*, 60(9), 1020–1022.

Keck, P.E. Jr., Versiani, M., Potkin, *et al.* (2003b). Ziprasidone in the treatment of acute bipolar mania: A three-week, placebo-controlled, double-blind, randomized trial. *American Journal of Psychiatry*, 160(4), 741–748.

Kinzie, J.D. and Leung, P. (1989). Clonidine in Cambodian patients with posttraumatic stress disorder. *Journal of Nervous and Mental Disease*, 177(9), 546–550.

Krakowski, A.J. (1962). Treatment of depression with imipramine (Tofranil) and imipramine combined with promazine. *Journal of New Drugs*, 2, 56–62.

Kris, E.B. and Gerst, D. (1964). Combined perphenazine-amitriptyline as adjuvant therapy in psychiatric aftercare. *American Journal of Psychiatry*, 121, 498–501.

Lauritzen, L., Clemmesen, L., Klysner, R., *et al.* (1992). Combined treatment with imipramine and mianserin. A controlled pilot study. *Pharmacopsychiatry*, 25(4), 182–186.

Lavretsky, H., Kim, M.D., Kumar, A. and Reynolds, C.F. 3rd. (2003). Combined treatment with methylphenidate and citalopram for accelerated response in the elderly: An open trial. *Journal of Clinical Psychiatry*, 64(12), 1410–1414.

Lavretsky, H. and Kumar, A. (2001). Methylphenidate augmentation of citalopram in elderly depressed patients. *American Journal of Geriatric Psychiatry*, 9(3), 298–303.

Lavretsky, H., Park, S., Siddarth, P., *et al.* (2006). Methylphenidate-enhanced antidepressant response to citalopram in the elderly: A double-blind, placebo-controlled pilot trial. *American Journal of Geriatric Psychiatry*, 14(2), 181–185.

Leuchter, A.F., Lesser, I.M., Trivedi, M.H., *et al.* (2008). An open pilot study of the combination of escitalopram and bupropion-SR for outpatients with major depressive disorder. *Journal of Psychiatric Practice*, 14(5), 271–280.

Levine, J., Mishori, A., Susnosky, M., *et al.* (1999). Combination of inositol and serotonin reuptake inhibitors in the treatment of depression. *Biological Psychiatry*, 45(3), 270–273.

Levitan, R.D., Shen, J.H., Jindal, R., *et al.* (2000). Preliminary randomized double-blind placebo-controlled trial of tryptophan combined with fluoxetine to treat major depressive disorder: Antidepressant and hypnotic effects. *Journal of Psychiatry and Neuroscience*, 25(4), 337–346.

Lopez-Ibor Alino, J.J., Auyso Gutierrez, J.L. and Montejo Iglesias, M.L. (1973). Tryptophan and amitriptyline in the treatment of depression: A double-blind study. *International Pharmacopsychiatry*, 8, 145–151.

Lowney, J.F. Jr. and Cedarleaf, C.B. (1969). Double-blind evaluation of an amitriptyline-fluphenazine combination. *Current Therapeutic Research Clinical and Experimental*, 11(5), 271–277.

Maes, M., Vandoolaeghe, E. and Desnyder, R. (1996). Efficacy of treatment with trazodone in combination with pindolol or fluoxetine in major depression. *Journal of Affective Disorders*, 41(3), 201–210.

Malhi, G.S., Ng, F. and Berk, M. (2008). Dual-dual action? Combining venlafaxine and mirtazapine in the treatment of depression. *Australian and New Zealand Journal of Psychiatry*, 42(4), 346–349.

Mattey, W.E. (1963). Combination therapy for relief of anxiety and depression. *Current Therapeutic Research, Clinical and Experimental*, 5, 310–318.

McElroy, S., Young, A.H., Carlsson, A., *et al.* (2008). A double-blind, placebo-controlled study with acute and continuation phase of quetiapine and paroxetine in adults with bipolar depression (Embolden II). Annual Meeting of the Association of European Psychiatrists (AEP).

McGrath, P.J., Stewart, J.W., Fava, M., *et al.* (2006). Tranylcypromine versus venlafaxine plus mirtazapine following three failed antidepressant medication trials for depression: A STAR*D report. *American Journal of Psychiatry*, 163(9), 1531–1541.

McIntyre, R.S., Brecher, M., Paulsson, B., (2005). Quetiapine or haloperidol as monotherapy for bipolar mania — a 12-week, double-blind, randomised, parallel-group, placebo-controlled trial. *European Neuropsychopharmacology*, 15(5), 573–585.

Moller, H.J., Kissling, W., Herberger, B., *et al.* (1986). Controlled trial on the possible advantages of a combined therapy with maprotiline and haloperidol in endogenous depression. *Pharmacopsychiatry*, 19(5), 362–364.

Morakinyo, V.O. (1970). Amytriptyline and chlordiazepoxide (Limbitrol) in depressive states in Nigerians — a double-blind study. *African Journal of Medical Sciences*, 1(4), 409–414.

Muller, N., Schwarz, M.J., Dehning, S., (2006). The cyclooxygenase-2 inhibitor celecoxib has therapeutic effects in major depression: Results of a double-blind, randomized, placebo controlled, add-on pilot study to reboxetine. *Molecular Psychiatry*, 11(7), 680–684.

Müller-Oerlinghausen, B., Retzow, A., Henn, F.A., *et al.* (2000). Valproate as an adjunct to neuroleptic medication for the treatment of acute episodes of mania: A prospective, randomized, double-blind, placebo-controlled, multicenter study. European Valproate Mania Study Group. *Journal of Clinical Psychopharmacology*, 20(2), 195–203.

Nelson, J.C., Mazure, C.M., Bowers, M.B. Jr. and Jatlow, P.I. (1991). A preliminary, open study of the combination of fluoxetine and desipramine for rapid treatment of major depression. *Archives of General Psychiatry*, 48(4), 303–307.

Nelson, J.C., Mazure, C.M., Jatlow, P.I., *et al.* (2004). Combining norepinephrine and serotonin reuptake inhibition mechanisms for treatment of depression: A double-blind, randomized study. *Biological Psychiatry*, 55(3), 296–300.

Nery, F.G., Monkul, E.S., Hatch, J.P., *et al.* (2008). Celecoxib as an adjunct in the treatment of depressive or mixed episodes of bipolar disorder: A double-blind, randomized, placebo-controlled study. *Human Psychopharmacology*, 23(2), 87–94.

Ninan, P., Hassman, H., Glass, S.J. and Sciamanna, A. (2004). Adjunctive modafinil at initiation of treatment with a selective serotonin reuptake inhibitor enhances the degree and onset of therapeutic effects in patients with major depressive disorder and fatigue. *Journal of Clinical Psychiatry*, 65(3), 414–420.

Nolen, W.A., Haffmans, P.M., Bouvy, P.F. and Duivenvoorden, H.J. (1993). Hypnotics as concurrent medication in depression. A placebo-controlled, double-blind comparison of flunitrazepam and lormetazepam in patients with major depression, treated with a (tri)cyclic antidepressant. *Journal of Affective Disorders*, 28(3), 179–188.

Normann, C., Hummel, B., Scharer, L.O., *et al.* (2002). Lamotrigine as adjunct to paroxetine in acute depression: A placebo-controlled, double-blind study. *Journal of Clinical Psychiatry*, 63(4), 337–344.

O'Hara, H., O'Hara, J., Valle-Jones, J.C., *et al.* (1978). Maprotiline and fluphenazine/nortriptyline in depression. *Practitioner*, 221(1323), 419–423.

Ota, K.Y., Turek, I., Berman, S.A. and Kurland, A.A. (1970). A comparative study of fluphenazine-amitriptyline combination and amitriptyline alone in the treatment of depressed psychiatric patients. *Current Therapeutic Research, Clinical and Experimental*, 12(9), 585–593.

Papakostas, G.I., Alpert, J.E. and Fava, M. (2003). SAMe in the treatment of depression: A comprehensive review of the literature. *Current Psychiatry Reports*, 5(6), 460–466.

Papakostas, G.I., Clain, A., Ameral, V.E., *et al.* (in press). Fluoxetine-clonazepam cotherapy for anxious depression: An exploratory, post-hoc analysis of a randomized, double blind study. *International Clinical Psychopharmacology*.

Papakostas, G.I., Cooper-Kazaz, R., Appelhof, B.C., *et al.* (2009). Simultaneous initiation (coinitiation) of pharmacotherapy with triiodothyronine and a selective serotonin reuptake inhibitor for major depressive disorder: A quantitative synthesis of double-blind studies. *International Clinical Psychopharmacology*, 24(1), 19–25.

Parker, G., Brotchie, H. and Parker, K. (2005). Is combination olanzapine and antidepressant medication associated with a more rapid response trajectory than antidepressant alone? *American Journal of Psychiatry*, 162(4), 796–798.

Pelton, G.H., Harper, O.L., Tabert, M.H., Sackeim, H.A., Scarmeas, N., Roose, S.P. and Devanand, D.P. (2008) Randomized double-blind placebo-controlled donepezil augmentation in antidepressant-treated elderly patients with depression and cognitive impairment: A pilot study. *International Journal of Geriatric Psychiatry*, 23(7), 670–676.

Perez, V., Gilaberte, I., Faries, D., *et al.* (1997). Randomised, double-blind, placebo-controlled trial of pindolol in combination with fluoxetine antidepressant treatment. *The Lancet*, 349(9065), 1594–1597.

Petersen, T., Dording, C., Neault, N.B., *et al.* (2002). A survey of prescribing practices in the treatment of depression. *Progress in Neuropsychopharmacology and Biological Psychiatry*, 26(1), 177–187.

Petersen, T., Papakostas, G.I., Posternak, M.A., *et al.* (2005). Empirical testing of two models for staging antidepressant treatment resistance. *Journal of Clinical Psychopharmacology*, 25(4), 336–341.

Pollack, B. (1962). Imipramine-promazine therapy for depression. *American Journal of Psychiatry*, 118, 842–845.

Pope, H.G. Jr., McElroy, S.L., Keck, P.E. Jr. and Hudson, J.I. (1991). Valproate in the treatment of acute mania. A placebo-controlled study. *Archives of General Psychiatry*, 48(1), 62–68.

Posternak, M.A., Novak, S.P., Stern, R.A., *et al.* (2008). A pilot effectiveness study: placebo-controlled trial of adjunctive L-triiodothyronine (T3) used to accelerate and potentiate the antidepressant response. *International Journal of Neuropsychopharmacology*, 11, 15–25.

Postolache, T.T., Rosenthal, R.N., Hellerstein, D.J., *et al.* (1999). Early augmentation of sertraline with methylphenidate. *Journal of Clinical Psychiatry*, 60(2), 123–124.

Potkin, S.G., Keck, P.E. Jr., Segal, S., *et al.* (2005). Ziprasidone in acute bipolar mania: A 21-day randomized, double-blind, placebo-controlled replication trial. *Journal of Clinical Psychopharmacology*, 25(4), 301–310.

Prange, A.J. Jr., Wilson, I.C., Knox, A., McClane, *et al.* (1970). Enhancement of imipramine by thyroid stimulating hormone: Clinical and theoretical implications. *American Journal of Psychiatry*, 127(2), 191–199.

Prange, A.J. Jr., Wilson, I.C., Rabon, A.M. and Lipton, M.A. (1969). Enhancement of imipramine antidepressant activity by thyroid hormone. *American Journal of Psychiatry*, 126(4), 457–469.

Prange, A.J., Wilson, I.C. and Alltop, L.B. (1972). Estrogen may well affect response to antidepressant. *Journal of the American Medical Association*, 219(2), 143–144.

Rabiner, E.A., Bhagwagar, Z., Gunn, R.N., *et al.* (2001). Pindolol augmentation of selective serotonin reuptake inhibitors: PET evidence that the dose used in clinical trials is too low. *American Journal of Psychiatry*, 158(12), 2080–2082.

Rasgon, N.L., Dunkin, J., Fairbanks, L., *et al.* (2007). Estrogen and response to sertraline in postmenopausal women with major depressive disorder: A pilot study. *Journal of Psychiatric Research*, 41(3–4), 338–343.

Ravn, J. (1961). The combined treatment of endogenous depression with imipramine (tofranil) and chlorprothixene (truxal), with special reference to ambulant therapy. *Acta Psychiatrica Scandinavica, Supplementum*, 162, 168–178.

Resler, G., Lavie, R., Campos, J., *et al.* (2008). Effect of folic acid combined with fluoxetine in patients with major depression on plasma homocysteine and vitamin B(12), and serotonin levels in lymphocytes. *Neuroimmunomodulation*, 15(3), 145–152.

Rickels, K., Csanalosi, I., Werblowsky, J., *et al.* (1982). Amitriptyline-perphenazine and doxepin in depressed outpatients: A controlled double-blind study. *Journal of Clinical Psychiatry*, 43(10), 419–422.

Rickels, K., Gordon, P.E., Jenkins, W.B., *et al.* (1970). Drug treatment of depressive illness. *Diseases of the Nervous System*, 31, 30–42.

Rickels, K., Hutchison, J.C., Weise, C.C., *et al.* (1972). Doxepin and amitriptyline-perphenazine in mixed anxious-depressed neurotic outpatients: A collaborative controlled study. *Psychopharmacologia*, 23(4), 305–318.

Rickels, K., Jenkins, B.W., Zamostien, B., *et al.* (1967). Pharmacotherapy in neurotic depression. Differential population responses. *Journal of Nervous and Mental Disease*, 145(6), 475–485.

Sachs, G., Chengappa, K.N., Suppes, T., *et al.* (2004). Quetiapine with lithium or divalproex for the treatment of bipolar mania: A randomized, double-blind, placebo-controlled study. *Bipolar Disorders*, 6(3), 213–223.

Sachs, G.S., Grossman, F., Ghaemi, S.N., *et al.* (2002). Combination of a mood stabilizer with risperidone or haloperidol for treatment of acute mania: A double-blind, placebo-controlled comparison of efficacy and safety. *American Journal of Psychiatry*, 159(7), 1146–1154.

Sachs, G., Sanchez, R., Marcus, R., *et al.* (2006). Aripiprazole in the treatment of acute manic or mixed episodes in patients with bipolar I disorder: A 3-week placebo-controlled study. *Journal of Psychopharmacology*, 20(4), 536–546.

Sanacora, G., Berman, R.M., Cappiello, A., *et al.* (2004). Addition of the alpha2-antagonist yohimbine to fluoxetine: Effects on rate of antidepressant response. *Neuropsychopharmacology*, 29(6), 1166–1171.

Schneider, L.S., Small, G.W., Hamilton, S.H., *et al.* (1997). Estrogen replacement and response to fluoxetine in a multicenter geriatric depression trial. Fluoxetine Collaborative Study Group. *American Journal of Geriatric Psychiatry*, 5(2), 97–106.

Shahal, B., Piel, E., Mecz, L., *et al.* (1996). Lack of advantage for imipramine combined with lithium versus imipramine alone in the treatment of major depression — a double-blind controlled study. *Biological Psychiatry*, 40(11), 1181–1183.

Shaw, D.M., Macsweeney, D.A., Hewland, R. and Johnson, A.L. (1975). Tricyclic antidepressants and tryptophan in unipolar depression. *Psychological Medicine*, 5(3), 276–278.

Shubin, H. and Mandel, S. (1967). Amitriptyline + perphenazine, an effective tranquilizer-antidepressant combination. *Psychosomatics*, 8(2), 79–81.

Sinclair, J.M., Walsh, M.R., Valle-Jones, J.C. and Schiff, A.A. (1975). Treatment of anxiety/depressive conditions in the elderly: A double-blind comparative study of Motival and amitriptyline. *Age and Ageing*, 4(4), 226–231.

Siwek, M., Dudek, D., Paul, I.A., *et al.* (2009). Zinc supplementation augments efficacy of imipramine in treatment resistant patients: A double blind, placebo-controlled study. *Journal of Affective Disorders*, 118(1–3), 187–195.

Smith, E. Incas, J. (1965). Combined amitriptyline and perphenazine (etrafon) in the treatment of severe emotional disorders. *Journal of the National Medical Association*, 57(4), 284–286.

Smith, M. (1973). Clinical response to amitriptyline and chlordiazepoxide-amitriptyline (Limbitrol) in anxiety-depressive states. A double-blind study. *Psychosomatics*, 14(3), 168–175.

Smith, L.A., Cornelius, V., Warnock, A., *et al.* (2007). Pharmacological interventions for acute bipolar mania: A systematic review of randomized placebo-controlled trials.*Bipolar Disorders*, 9(6), 551–560.

Smith, W.T., Londborg, P.D., Glaudin, V. and Painter, J.R. (1998). Short-term augmentation of fluoxetine with clonazepam in the treatment of depression: A double-blind study. *American Journal of Psychiatry*, 155(10), 1339–1345.

Smulevich, A.B., Khanna, S., Eerdekens, M., *et al.* (2005). Acute and continuation risperidone monotherapy in bipolar mania: A 3 week placebo-controlled trial followed by a 9-week double-blind trial of risperidone and haloperidol. *European Neuropsychopharmacology*, 15(1), 75–84.

Stewart, J.W., McGrath, P.J., Deliyannides, R.A. and Quitkin, F.M. (2009). Does dual antidepressant therapy as initial treatment hasten and increase remission from depression? *Journal of Psychiatric Practice*, 15(5), 337–345.

Sussex Clinical Trials Group. (1985). Separate and combined anxiolytic and anti-depressant treatment of mixed anxiety/depression. *Acta Psychiatrica Scandinavica*, 72, 81–88.

Taragano, F.E., Allegri, R., Vicario, A., *et al.* (2001). A double blind, randomized clinical trial assessing the efficacy and safety of augmenting standard antidepressant therapy with nimodipine in the treatment of 'vascular depression'. *International Journal of Geriatric Psychiatry*, 16(3), 254–260.

Taylor, M.J., Carney, S.M., Goodwin, G.M. and Geddes, J.R. (2004). Folate for depressive disorders: Systematic review and meta-analysis of randomized controlled trials. *Journal of Psychopharmacology*, 18(2), 251–256.

Thase, M.E., Macfadden, W., Weisler, R.H., *et al.* (2006). Efficacy of quetiapine monotherapy in bipolar I and II depression: A double-blind, placebo-controlled study (the BOLDER II study). *Journal of Clinical Psychopharmacology*, 26(6), 600–609.

Thomson, J., Rankin, H., Ashcroft, G.W., *et al.* (1982). The treatment of depression in general practice: A comparison of L-tryptophan, amitriptyline, and a combination of L-tryptophan and amitriptyline with placebo. *Psychological Medicine*, 12(4), 741–751.

Tohen, M., Bowden, C.L., Smulevich, A.B., *et al.* (2008). Olanzapine plus carbamazepine v. carbamazepine alone in treating manic episodes. *British Journal of Psychiatry*, 192, 135–143.

Tohen, M., Chengappa, K.N., Suppes, T., *et al.* (2002). Efficacy of olanzapine in combination with valproate or lithium in the treatment of mania in patients partially nonresponsive to valproate or lithium monotherapy. *Archives of General Psychiatry*, 59(1), 62–69.

Tohen, M., Jacobs, T.G., Grundy, S.L., *et al.* (2000). Efficacy of olanzapine in acute bipolar mania: A double-blind, placebo controlled study. The Olanzipine HGGW Study Group. *Archives of General Psychiatry*, 57(9), 841–849.

Tohen, M., Kryzhanovskaya, L., Carlson, G., *et al.* (2007). Olanzapine versus placebo in the treatment of adolescents with bipolar mania. *American Journal of Psychiatry*, 164(10), 1547–1556.

Tohen, M., Sanger, T.M., McElroy, S.L., *et al.* (1999). Olanzapine versus placebo in the treatment of acute mania. Olanzapine HGEH Study Group. *American Journal of Psychiatry*, 156(5), 702–709.

Tohen, M., Vieta, E., Calabrese, J., *et al.* (2003). Efficacy of olanzapine and olanzapine-fluoxetine combination in the treatment of bipolar I depression. *Archives of General Psychiatry*, 60(11), 1079–1088.

Tome, M.B., Isaac, M.T., Harte, R. and Holland, C. (1997). Paroxetine and pindolol: A randomized trial of serotonergic autoreceptor blockade in the reduction of antidepressant latency. *International Clinical Psychopharmacology*, 12(2), 81–89.

Tsai, J., Tourkodimitris, S. and Bose, A. (2008). Low-dose combination of bupropion and escitalopram is an effective treatment combination for adult outpatients. APA Annual Meeting.

Uchida, H., Takeuchi, H., Suzuki, T., *et al.* (2005). Combined treatment with sulpiride and paroxetine for accelerated response in patients with major depressive disorder. *Journal of Clinical Psychopharmacology*, 25(6), 545–551.

Valle-Jones, J.C., Craven, J.R, Wallis, T.D. and Schiff, A.A. (1983). Mixed anxiety/depressive illness in general practice. A therapeutic comparison of nomifensine with fluphenazine/nortriptyline. *Acta Psychiatrica Scandinavica*, 68(6) 494–500.

Vann, D. (1959). Promazine-iproniazid: A brief report. *American Journal of Psychiatry*, 115(9), 824–825.

Vieta, E., Calabrese, J.R., Goikolea, J.M., *et al.* (2007). Quetiapine monotherapy in the treatment of patients with bipolar I or II depression and a rapid-cycling disease course: A randomized, double-blind, placebo-controlled study. *Bipolar Disorders*, 9(4), 413–425.

Wells, B.G., Evans, R.L., Ereshefsky, L., *et al.* (1988). Clinical outcome and adverse effect profile associated with concurrent administration of alprazolam and imipramine. *Journal of Clinical Psychiatry*, 49(10), 394–399.

Wheatley, D. (1972). Potentiation of amitriptyline by thyroid hormone. *Archives of General Psychiatry*, 26(3), 229–233.

Wilson, I.C., Prange, A.J. Jr., McClane, T.K., *et al.* (1970). Thyroid-hormone enhancement of imipramine in nonretarded depressions. *New England Journal of Medicine*, 282(19), 1063–1067.

Yatham, L.N., Paulsson, B., Mullen, J. and Vågerö, A.M. (2004). Quetiapine versus placebo in combination with lithium or divalproex for the treatment of bipolar mania. *Journal of Clinical Psychopharmacology*, 24(6), 599–606.

Young, A.H., Carlsson, A, Olausson, B., *et al.* (2008). A double-blind, placebo-controlled study with acute and continuation phase of quetiapine and lithium in adults with bipolar depression (Embolden I). Annual Meeting of the Association of European Psychiatrists (AEP).

Young, J.P., Lader, M.H. and Hughes, W.C. (1979). Controlled trial of trimipramine, monoamine oxidase inhibitors, and combined treatment in depressed outpatients. *British Medical Journal*, 2(6201), 1315–1317.

Zanardi, R., Artigas, F., Franchini, L., *et al.* (1997). How long should pindolol be associated with paroxetine to improve the antidepressant response? *Journal of Clinical Psychopharmacology*, 17(6), 446–450.

Chapter 6

Abraham, G., Milev, R. and Stuart Lawson, J. (2006). T3 augmentation of SSRI resistant depression. *Journal of Affective Disorders*, 91(2–3), 211–215.

Adson, D.E., Kushner, M.G., Eiben, K.M. and Schulz, C. (2004). Preliminary experience with adjunctive quetiapine in patients receiving selective serotonin reuptake inhibitors. *Depression and Anxiety*, 19, 121–126.

Adson, D.E., Kushner, M.G. and Fahnhorst, T.A. (2005). Treatment of residual anxiety symptoms with adjunctive aripiprazole in depressed patients taking selective serotonin reuptake inhibitors. *Journal of Affective Disorders*, 86(1), 99–104.

Agid, O. and Lerer, B. (2003). Algorithm-based treatment of major depression in an outpatient clinic: Clinical correlates of response to a specific serotonin reuptake inhibitor and to triiodothyronine augmentation. *International Journal of Neuropsychopharmacology*, 6(1), 41–49.

Alpert, J.E., Mischoulon, D., Rubenstein, G.E., *et al.* (2002). Folinic acid (Leucovorin) as an adjunctive treatment for SSRI-refractory depression. *Annals of Clinical Psychiatry*, 14(1), 33–38.

Alpert, J.E., Papakostas, G., Mischoulon, D., *et al.* (2004). S-adenosyl-L-methionine (SAMe) as an adjunct for resistant major depressive disorder: An open trial following partial or nonresponse to selective serotonin reuptake inhibitors or venlafaxine. *Journal of Clinical Psychopharmacology*, 24(6), 661–664.

Altamura, A.C., Dell'Osso, B., Buoli, M., *et al.* (2008). Short-term intravenous citalopram augmentation in partial/nonresponders with major depression: A randomized placebo-controlled study. *International Clinical Psychopharmacology*,23(4), 198–202.

Altamura, A.C., Dell'Osso, B., Buoli, M., *et al.* (2008). Intravenous augmentative citalopram versus clomipramine in partial/nonresponders depressed patients: A short-term, low dose, randomized, placebo controlled study. *Journal of Clinical Psychopharmacology*, 28(4), 406–410.

Amiaz, R., Stein, O., Dannon, P.N., *et al.* (1999). Resolution of treatment-refractory depression with naltrexone augmentation of paroxetine — a case report. *Psychopharmacology*, 143(4), 433–444.

Amsterdam, J.D., Garcia-Espana, F. and Rosenzweig, M. (1997). Clomipramine augmentation in treatment-resistant depression. *Depression and Anxiety*, 5(2), 84–90.

Anderson, I.M., Sarsfield, A. and Haddad, P.M. (2009). Efficacy, safety and tolerability of quetiapine augmentation in treatment resistant depression: An open-label, pilot study. *Journal of Affective Disorders*, 117(1–2), 116–119.

Appelberg, B.G., Syvalahti, E.K., Koskinen, T.E., *et al.* (2001). Patients with severe depression may benefit from buspirone augmentation of selective serotonin reuptake inhibitors: Results from a placebo-controlled, randomized, double-blind, placebo wash-in study. *Journal of Clinical Psychiatry*, 62(6), 448–452.

Aronson, R., Offman, H.J., Joffe, R.T. and Naylor, C.D. (1996). Triiodothyronine augmentation in the treatment of refractory depression. A meta-analysis. *Archives of General Psychiatry*, 53(9), 842–828.

Artigas, F., Perez, V. and Alvarez, E. (1994). Pindolol induces a rapid improvement of depressed patients treated with serotonin reuptake inhibitors. *Archives of General Psychiatry*, 51(3), 248–251.

Ashton, A.K. (2004). Modafinil augmentation of phenelzine for residual fatigue in dysthymia. *American Journal of Psychiatry*, 161(9), 1716–1717.

Bader, G.M., Hawley, J.M. and Short, D.D. (1998). Venlafaxine augmentation with methylphenidate for treatment-refractory depression: A case report. *Journal of Clinical Psychopharmacology*, 18(3), 255–256.

Bakish, D., Hooper, C.L., Thornton, M.D., *et al.* (1997). Fast onset: An open study of the treatment of major depressive disorder with nefazodone and pindolol combination therapy. *International Clinical Psychopharmacology*, 12(2), 91–97.

Banki, C.M. (1977). Cerebrospinal fluid amine metabolites after combined amitriptyline-triiodothyronine treatment of depressed women. *European Journal of Clinical Pharmacology*, 11(4), 311–315.

Barbee, J.G. (2003). Topiramate in the treatment of severe bulimia nervosa with comorbid mood disorders: A case series. *International Journal of Eating Disorders*, 33(4), 468–472.

Barbee, J.G., Conrad, E.J. and Jamhour, N.J. (2004b). Aripiprazole augmentation in treatment-resistant depression. *Annals of Clinical Psychiatry*, 16(4), 189–194.

Barbee, J.G., Conrad, E.J. and Jamhour, N.J. (2004a). The effectiveness of olanzapine, risperidone, quetiapine, and ziprasidone as augmentation agents in treatment-resistant major depressive disorder. *Journal of Clinical Psychiatry*, 65(7), 975–981.

Barbee, J.G. and Jamhour, N.J. (2002). Lamotrigine as an augmentation agent in treatment-resistant depression. *Journal of Clinical Psychiatry*, 63(8), 737–741.

Barbee, J.G., Jamhour, N.J., Stewart, J.W., *et al.* (2007). Lamotrigine as an antidepressant augmentation in treatment refractory unipolar depression. Presented at the 160th Annual Meeting of the American Psychiatric Association. San Diego, California.

Barbosa, L., Berk, M. and Vorster, M. (2003). A double-blind, randomized, placebo-controlled trial of augmentation with lamotrigine or placebo in patients concomitantly treated with fluoxetine for resistant major depressive episodes. *Journal of Clinical Psychiatry*, 64(4), 403–407.

Bauer, M., Baur, H., Berghofer, A., *et al*. (2002). Effects of supraphysiological thyroxine administration in healthy controls and patients with depressive disorders. *Journal of Affective Disorders*, 68(2–3), 285–294.

Bauer, M., Bschor, T., Kunz, D., *et al.* (2000). Double-blind, placebo-controlled trial of the use of lithium to augment antidepressant medication in continuation treatment of unipolar major depression. *American Journal of Psychiatry*, 157(9), 1429–1435.

Bauer, M. and Dopfmer, S. (1999). Lithium augmentation in treatment-resistant depression: Meta-analysis of placebo-controlled studies. *Journal of Clinical Psychopharmacology*, 19(5), 427–434.

Bauer, M., Forsthoff, A., Baethge, C., *et al.* (2003). Lithium augmentation therapy in refractory depression-update 2002. *European Archives of Psychiatry and Clinical Neuroscience*, 253(3), 132–139.

Bauer, M., Hellweg, R., Graf, K.J. and Baumgartner, A. (1998). Treatment of refractory depression with high-dose thyroxine. *Neuropsychopharmacology*, 18(6), 444–455.

Bauer, M., Pretorius, H.W., Constant, E.L., *et al.* (2009). Extended-release quetiapine as adjunct to an antidepressant in patients with major depressive disorder: Results of a randomized, placebo-controlled, double-blind study. *Journal of Clinical Psychiatry*, 70(4), 540–549.

Bauman, P., Nil, R., Souche, A., *et al.* (1996). A double-blind, placebo-controlled study of citalopram with and without lithium in the treatment of therapy-resistant depressive patients: A clinical, pharmacokinetic, and pharmacogenetic invesigation. *Journal of Clinical Psychopharmacology*, 16(4), 307–314.

Baune, B.T., Caliskan, S. and Todder, D. (2007). Effects of adjunctive antidepressant therapy with quetiapine on clinical outcome, quality of sleep and daytime motor activity in patients with treatment-resistant depression. *Human Psychopharmacology*, 22(1), 1–9.

Bell, I.R., Edman, J.S., Morrow, F.D., *et al*. (1992). Brief communication. Vitamin B1, B2, and B6 augmentation of tricyclic antidepressant treatment in geriatric depression with cognitive dysfunction. *Journal of the American College of Nutrition*, 11(2), 159–163.

Bellino, S., Paradiso, E., Bogetto, F. (2008). Efficacy and tolerability of aripiprazole augmentation in sertraline-resistant patients with borderline personality disorder. *Psychiatry Research*, 161(2), 206–212.

Berigan, T.R. (2004). Atomoxetine used adjunctively with selective serotonin reuptake inhibitors to treat depression. *Primary Care Companion of the Journal of Clinical Psychiatry*, 6(2), 93–94.

Berigan, T.R. (2001). Augmentation with modafinil to achieve remission in depression: A case report. *Primary Care Companion of the Journal of Clinical Psychiatry*, 3(1), 32.

Berigan, T.R. and Zeff, K.N. (2000). Thyroid augmentation of mirtazapine: A case report. *Primary Care Companion of the Journal of Clinical Psychiatry*, 2(1), 27–28.

Berk, M., Copolov, D.L., Dean, O., *et al.* (2008). N-Acetyl cysteine for depressive symptoms in bipolar disorder-A double-blind randomized placebo-controlled trial. *Biological Psychiatry*, 64(6), 468–475.

Berlanga, C. (1988). Potentiating effect of estrogen in a patient with treatment-resistant depression. *Journal of Clinical Psychiatry*, 49(12), 504.

Berlanga, C. and Ortega-Soto, H.A. (1995). A 3-year follow-up of a group of treatment-resistant depressed patients with a MAOI/tricyclic combination. *Journal of Affective Disorders*, 34(3), 187–192.

Berman, R.M., Fava, M., Thase, M.E., *et al.* (2009). Aripiprazole augmentation in major depressive disorder: A double-blind, placebo-controlled study in patients with inadequate response to antidepressants. *CNS Spectrums*, 14(4), 197–206.

Berman, R.M., Marcus, R.N., Swanink, R., *et al.* (2007). The efficacy of aripiprazole as adjunctive therapy in major depressive disorder: A multicenter, randomized, double-blind, placebo-controlled study. *Journal of Clinical Psychiatry*, 68(6), 843–853.

Bertschy, G., Ragama-Pardos, E., Ait-Ameur, A., *et al.* (2003). Lithium augmentation in venlafaxine non-responders: An open study. *European Psychiatry*, 18(6), 314–317.

Bertschy, G., Ragama-Pardos, E., Muscionico, M., *et al.* (2005). Trazodone addition for insomnia in venlafaxine-treated, depressed inpatients: A semi-naturalistic study. *Pharmacology Research*, 51(1), 79–84.

Birkenhager, T.K., van den Broek, W.W., Moleman, P. and Bruijn, J.A. (2006). Outcome of a 4-step treatment algorithm for depressed inpatients. *Journal of Clinical Psychiatry*, 67(8), 1266–1271.

Birkenhager, T.K., Vegt, M. and Nolen, W.A. (1997). An open study of triiodothyronine augmentation of tricyclic antidepressants in inpatients with refractory depression. *Pharmacopsychiatry*, 30(1), 23–26.

Blier, P. and Bergeron, R. (1995). Effectiveness of pindolol with selected antidepressant drugs in the treatment of major depression. *Journal of Clinical Psychopharmacology*, 15(3), 217–222.

Bodkin, J.A., Lasser, R.A., Wines, J.D. Jr., *et al.* (1997). Combining serotonin reuptake inhibitors and bupropion in partial responders to antidepressant monotherapy. *Journal of Clinical Psychiatry*, 58(4), 137–145.

Bondolfi, G., Chautems, C., Rochat, B., *et al.* (1996). Non-response to citalopram in depressive patients: Pharmacokinetic and clinical consequences of a fluvoxamine augmentation. *Psychopharmacology*, 128(4), 421–425.

Bondolfi, G., Lissner, C., Kosel, M., *et al.* (2000). Fluoxetine augmentation in citalopram non-responders: Pharmacokinetic and clinical consequences. *International Journal of Neuropsychopharmacology*, 3(1), 55–60.

Bouckoms, A. and Mangini, L. (1993). Pergolide: An antidepressant adjuvant for mood disorders? *Psychopharmacology Bulletin*, 29(2), 207–211.

Bouwer, C., Claassen, J., Dinan, T.G. and Nemeroff, C.B. (2000). Prednisone augmentation in treatment-resistant depression with fatigue and hypocortisolaemia: A case series. *Depression and Anxiety*, 12(1), 44–50.

Browne, J.L., Rice, J.L., Evans, D.L. and Prange, A.J. (1990a). Triiodothyronine augmentation of the antidepressant effect of the nontricyclic antidepressant trazodone. *Journal of Nervous and Mental Disease*, 178(9), 598–599.

Browne, M., Lapierre, Y.D., Hrdina, P.D. and Horn, E. (1990b). Lithium as an adjunct in the treatment of major depression. *International Clinical Psychopharmacology*, 5, 103–110.

Buhagiar, K. and Cassar, J. (2007). Methylphenidate augmentation of fluvoxamine for treatment-resistant depression: A case report and review literature. *Turk Psikiyatri Dergisi*, 18(2), 179–183.

Camprubi, M.E. and Puri, B.K. (1995). The treatment of refractory depression using paroxetine with lithium augmentation. *Progress in Neuropsychopharmacology and Biological Psychiatry*, 19(3), 515–517.

Carta, M.G., Zairo, F., Mellino, G. and Hardoy, M.C. (2007). Add-on quetiapine in the treatment of major depressive disorder in elderly patients with cerebrovascular damage. *Clinical Practice in Epidemiology and Mental Health*, 3, 28.

Cassano, P., Lattanzi, L., Fava, M., *et al.* (2005). Ropinirole in treatment-resistant depression: A 16-week pilot study. *Canadian Journal of Psychiatry*, 50(6), 357–360.

Cassano, P., Lattanzi, L., Soldani, F., *et al.* (2004). Pramipexole in treatment-resistant depression: An extended follow-up. *Depression and Anxiety*, 20(3), 131–138.

Cappiello, A., McDougle, C.J., Malison, R.T., *et al.* (1995). Yohimbine augmentation of fluvoxamine in refractory depression: A single-blind study. *Biological Psychiatry*, 38(11), 765–767.

Carpenter, L.L., Leon, Z., Yasmin, S. and Price, L.H. (2002b). Do obese depressed patients respond to topiramate? A retrospective chart review. *Journal of Affective Disorders*, 69(1–3), 251.

Carpenter, L.L., Milosavljevic, N., Schecter, J.M., (2005). Augmentation with open-label atomoxetine for partial or nonresponse to antidepressants. *Journal of Clinical Psychiatry*, 66(10), 1234–1238.

Carpenter, L.L., Yasmin, S. and Price, L.H. (2002a). A double-blind, placebo-controlled study of antidepressant augmentation with mirtazapine. *Biological Psychiatry*, 51(2), 183–188.

Charney, D.S., Price, L.H. and Heninger, G.R. (1986). Desipramine-yohimbine combination treatment of refractory depression. Implications for the beta-adrenergic receptor hypothesis of antidepressant action. *Archives of General Psychiatry*, 43(12), 1155–1161.

Ciusani, E., Zullino, D.F., Eap, C.B., *et al.* (2004). Combination therapy with venlafaxine and carbamazepine in depressive patients not responding to venlafaxine: Pharmacokinetic and clinical aspects. *Journal of Psychopharmacology*, 18(4), 559–566.

Clayton, A.H. and Kaltsounis-Puckett, J. (2002). Combination therapy in the treatment of major depressive disorder complicated by fibromyalgia and menopause. *Psychosomatics*, 43(6), 491–493.

Cooke, R.G. (1990). T3 augmentation of a tricyclic antidepressant in a patient receiving T4 maintenance therapy. *American Journal of Psychiatry*, 147(2), 255.

Cooke, R.G., Joffe, R.T. and Levitt, A.J. (1992). T3 augmentation of antidepressant treatment in T4-replaced thyroid patients. *Journal of Clinical Psychiatry*, 53(1), 16–18.

Coppen, A., Whybrow, P.C., Noguera, R., *et al.* (1972). The comparative antidepressant value of L-tryptophan and imipramine with and without attempted potentiation by liothyronine. *Archives of General Psychiatry*, 26(3), 234–241.

Corrigan, F.M. (1992). Sodium valproate augmentation of fluoxetine or fluvoxamine effects. *Biological Psychiatry*, 31(11), 1178–1179.

Corya, S.A., Andersen, S.W., Detke, H.C., *et al.* (2003). Long-term antidepressant efficacy and safety of olanzapine/fluoxetine combination: A 76-week open-label study. *Journal of Clinical Psychiatry*, 64(11), 1349–1356.

Corya, S.A., Williamson, D., Sanger, T.M., *et al.* (2006). A randomized, double-blind comparison of olanzapine/fluoxetine combination, olanzapine, fluoxetine, and venlafaxine in treatment-resistant depression. *Depression and Anxiety*, 23(6), 364–372.

Cullen, M., Mitchell, P., Brodaty, H., *et al.* (1991). Carbamazepine for treatment-resistant melancholia. *Journal of Clinical Psychiatry*, 52(11), 472–476.

Dallal, A., Fontaine, R., Ontiveros, A. and Elie, R. (1990). Lithium carbonate augmentation of desipramine in refractory depression. *Canadian Journal of Psychiatry*, 35(7), 608–611.

Dalton, E.J., Rotondi, D., Levitan, R.D., *et al.* (2000). Use of slow-release melatonin in treatment-resistant depression. *Journal of Psychiatry and Neuroscience*, 25(1), 48–52.

De la Fuente, J.M. and Mendlewicz, J. (1992). Carbamazepine addition in tricyclic antidepressant-resistant unipolar depression. *Biological Psychiatry*, 32(4), 369–374.

De Montigny, C., Cournoyer, G., Morissette, R., *et al.* (1983). Lithium carbonate addition in tricyclic antidepressant-resistant unipolar depression. Correlations with the neurobiologic actions of tricyclic antidepressant drugs and lithium ion on the serotonin system. *Archives of General Psychiatry*, 40(12), 1327–1334.

De Montigny, C., Elie, R. and Caille, G. (1985). Rapid response to the addition of lithium in iprindole-resistant unipolar depression: A pilot study. *American Journal of Psychiatry*. 1985, 142(2), 220–223.

De Montigny, C., Grunberg, F., Mayer, A. and Descenes, JP. (1981). Lithium induces rapid relief of depression in tricyclic antidepressant drug non-responders. *British Journal of Psychiatry*, 138, 252–256.

DeBattista, C., Dighramji, K., Menza, M., *et al.* (2003b). Adjunct modafinil for the short-term treatment of fatigue and sleepiness in patients with major depressive disorder: A preliminary double-blind, placebo-controlled study. *Journal of Clinical Psychiatry*, 64(9), 1057–1064.

DeBattista, C., Lembke, A., Solvason, H.B., *et al.* (2004). A prospective trial of modafinil as an adjunctive treatment of major depression. *Journal of Clinical Psychopharmacology*, 24(1), 87–90.

DeBattista, C., Solvason, H.B., Poirier, J., *et al.* (2003a). A prospective trial of bupropion SR augmentation of partial and non-responders to serotonergic antidepressants. *Journal of Clinical Psychopharmacology*, 23(1), 27–30.

Delgado, P.L., Price, L.H., Charney, D.S. and Heninger, G.R. (1988). Efficacy of fluvoxamine in treatment-refractory depression. *Journal of Affective Disorders*, 15(1), 55–60.

Deicken, R.F. (1987). Combined alprazolam and phenelzine treatment of refractory depression with panic attacks. *Biological Psychiatry*, 22(6), 762–766.

Detweiler, M.B. and Trinkle, D.B. (2003). Fluoxetine augmentation with olanzapine for treatment of chronic resistant depression in an elderly patient: A case report. *Journal of Clinical Psychiatry*, 64(7), 851–852.

Dietrich, D.E., Bode, L., Spannhuth, C.W., *et al.* (2000). Amantadine in depressive patients with Borna disease virus (BDV) infection: An open trial. *Bipolar Disorders*, 2(1), 65–70.

Dietrich, D.E. and Emrich, H.M. (1998). The use of anticonvulsants to augment antidepressant medication. *Journal of Clinical Psychiatry*, 59(Suppl 5), 51–58.

Dimitriou, E.C. and Dimitriou, C.E. (1998). Buspirone augmentation of antidepressant therapy. *Journal of Clinical Psychopharmacology*, 18(6), 465–469.

Dinan, T.G. (1993). Lithium augmentation in sertraline-resistant depression: A preliminary dose-response study. *Acta Psychiatrica Scandinavica*, 88(4), 300.

Dinan, T.G. and Barry, S. (1989). A comparison of electroconvulsive therapy with a combined lithium and tricyclic combination among depressed tricyclic nonresponders. *Acta Psychiatrica Scandinavica*, 80(1), 97–100.

Dinan, T.G., Lavelle, E., Cooney, J., *et al.* (1997). Dexamethasone augmentation in treatment-resistant depression. *Acta Psychiatrica Scandinavica*, 95(1), 58–61.

Doree, J.P., Des Rosiers, J., Lew, V., *et al.* (2007). Quetiapine augmentation of treatment-resistant depression: A comparison with lithium. *Current Medical and Research Opinion*, 23(2), 333–341.

Dunbar, G., Kuchibhalta, R. and Kumar, R. (2007). Mecamylamine as an augmentation treatment for depressed patients who were nonresponders to citalopram. *European Neuropsychopharmacology*, 17(s4), S348.

Dunner, D.L., Amsterdam, J.D., Shelton, R.C., *et al.* (2007). Efficacy and tolerability of adjunctive ziprasidone in treatment-resistant depression: A randomized, open-label, pilot study. *Journal of Clinical Psychiatry*, 68(7), 1071–1077.

Earle, B.V. (1970). Thyroid hormone and tricyclic antidepressants in resistant depressions. *American Journal of Psychiatry*, 126(11), 1667–1669.

Elgamal, S. and MacQueen, G. (2008). Galantamine as an adjunctive treatment in major depression. *Journal of Clinical Psychopharmacology*, 28(3), 357–359.

El-Khalili, N., Joyce, M., Atkinson, S., *et al.* (2008). Adjunctive extended release quetiapine fumarate (quetiapine XR) in patients with major depressive disorder and inadequate response. *American Psychiatric Association Annual Meeting*.

Eller, T., Vasar, V., Shlik, J. and Maron, E. (2009). Effects of bupropion augmentation on pro-inflammatory cytokines in escitalopram-resistant patients with major depressive disorder. *Journal of Psychopharmacology*, 23(7), 854–858.

Even, C., Friedman, S., Dardennes, R. and Guelfi, J.D. (2004). Modafinil as an alternative to light therapy for winter depression. *European Psychiatry*, 19(1), 66.

Fanelli, J. and Montgomery, C. (1996). Use of the analgesic tramadol in antidepressant potentiation. *Psychopharmacology Bulletin*, 32, 442.

Fatemi, S.H., Emamian, E.S. and Kist, D.A. (1999). Venlafaxine and bupropion combination therapy in a case of treatment-resistant depression. *Annals of Pharmacotherapy*, 33(6), 701–703.

Fava, M., Alpert, J., Nierenberg, A., *et al.* (2002). Double-blind study of high-dose fluoxetine versus lithium or desipramine augmentation of fluoxetine in partial responders and nonresponders to fluoxetine. *Journal of Clinical Psychopharmacology*, 22(4), 379–387.

Fava, M., Thase, M.E. and DeBattista, C. (2005). A multicenter, placebo-controled study of modafinil augmentation in partial responders to selective serotonin reuptake inhibitors with persistent fatigue and hypersomnia. *Journal of Clinical Psychiatry*, 66(1), 85–93.

Fava, M., Thase, M.E., DeBattista, C., *et al.* (2007). Modafinil augmentation of selective serotonin reuptake inhibitor therapy in MDD partial responders with persistent fatigue and sleepiness. *Annals of Clinical Psychiatry*, 19(3), 153–159.

Fava, M., Rosenbaum, J.F., McGrath, P.J., *et al.* (1994). Lithium and tricyclic augmentation of fluoxetine treatment for resistant major depression: A double-blind, controlled study. *American Journal of Psychiatry*, 151(9), 1372–1374.

Fawcett, J., Kravitz, H.M., Zajecka, J.M. and Schaff, M.R. (1991). CNS stimulant potentiation of monoamine oxidase inhibitors in treatment-refractory depression. *Journal of Clinical Psychopharmacology*, 11(2), 127–132.

Fe-Bornstein, M., Watt, S.D. and Gitlin, M.C. (2002). Improvement in the level of psychosocial functioning in chronic pain patients with the use of risperidone. *Pain Medicine*, 3(2), 128–131.

Feighner, J.P., Herbstein, J. and Damlouji, N. (1985). Combined MAOI, TCA, and direct stimulant therapy of treatment-resistant depression. *Journal of Clinical Psychiatry*, 46(6), 206–209.

Feinberg, S.S. (2004). Combining stimulants with monoamine oxidase inhibitors: A review of uses and one possible additional indication. *Journal of Clinical Psychiatry*, 65(11), 1520–1524.

Feldmesser-Reiss, E.E. (1958). The application of triiodothyronine in the treatment of mental disorders. *Journal of Nervous and Mental Disease*, 127(6), 540–545.

Ferreri, M., Lavergne, F., Berlin, L., *et al.* (2001). Benefits from mianserin augmentation of fluoxetine in patients with major depression non-responders to fluoxetine alone. *Acta Psychiatrica Scandinavica*, 103(1), 66–72.

Finch, E.J.L. and Katona, C.L.E. (1989). Lithium augmentation in the treatment of refractory depression in old age. *International Journal of Geriatric Psychiatry*, 4, 41–46.

Fischer, P., Tauscher, J., Kufferle, B. and Kasper, S. (1998). Weak antidepressant response after buspirone augmentation of serotonin reuptake inhibitors in refractory severe depression. *International Clinical Psychopharmacology*, 13(2), 83–86.

Flach, F.F., Celian, C.I. and Rawson, R.W. (1958). Treatment of psychiatric disorders with triiodothyronine. *American Journal of Psychiatry*, 114(9), 841–842.

Flint, A.J. and Rifat, S.L. (1994). A prospective study of lithium augmentation in antidepressant-resistant geriatric depression. *Journal of Clinical Psychopharmacology*, 14(5), 353–355.

Flint, A.J. and Rifat, S.L. (1996). The effect of sequential antidepressant treatment on geriatric depression. *Journal of Affective Disorders*, 36(3–4), 95–105.

Fontaine, R., Ontiveros, R., Elie, R. and Vezina, M. (1991). Lithium carbonate augmentation of desipramine and fluoxetine in refractory depression. *Biological Psychiatry*, 29, 946–948.

Frye, M.A., Grunze, H., Suppes, T., *et al.* (2007). A placebo-controlled evaluation of adjunctive modafinil in the treatment of bipolar depression. *American Journal of Psychiatry*, 164(8), 1242–1249.

Gabriel, A. (2006). Lamotrigine adjunctive treatment in resistant unipolar depression: An open, descriptive study. *Depression and Anxiety*, 23(8), 485–488.

Garbutt, J.C., Mayo, J.P. Jr., Gillette, G.M., *et al.* (1986). Lithium potentiation of tricyclic antidepressants following lack of T3 potentiation. *American Journal of Psychiatry*, 143(8), 1038–1039.

George, T.P., Sacco, K.A., Vessicchio, J.C., *et al.* (2008). Nicotinic antagonist augmentation of selective serotonin reuptake inhibitor-refractory major depressive disorder: A preliminary study. *Journal of Clinical Psychopharmacology*, 28(3), 340–344.

Gitlin, M.J., Suri, R., Altshuler, L., *et al.* (2002). Bupropion-sustained release as a treatment for SSRI-induced sexual side effects. *Journal of Sex and Marital Therapy*, 28(2), 131–138.

Gitlin, M.J., Weiner, H., Fairbanks, L., *et al.* (1987). Failure of T3 to potentiate tricyclic antidepressant response. *Journal of Affective Disorders*, 13(3), 267–272.

Goforth, H.W. and Carroll, B.T. (2007). Aripiprazole augmentation of tranylcypromine in treatment-resistant major depression. *Journal of Clinical Psychopharmacology*, 27(2), 216–217.

Goldberg, J.F., Burdick, K.E. and Endick, C.J. (2004). Preliminary randomized, double-blind, placebo-controlled trial of pramipexole added to mood stabilizers for treatment-resistant bipolar depression. *American Journal of Psychiatry*, 161(3), 564–566.

Gomez Gomez, J.M. and Teixido Perramon, C. (2000). Combined treatment with venlafaxine and tricyclic antidepressants in depressed patients who had partial response to clomipramine or imipramine: Initial findings. *Journal of Clinical Psychiatry*, 61(4), 285–289.

Goodwin, F.K., Prange, A.J. Jr., Post, R.M., *et al.* (1982). Potentiation of antidepressant effects by L-triiodothyronine in tricyclic nonresponders. *American Journal of Psychiatry*, 139(1), 34–38.

Grigoriadis, S., Kennedy, S.H., Srinivisan, J., *et al.* (2005). Antidepressant augmentation with raloxifene. *Journal of Clinical Psychopharmacology*, 25(1), 96–98.

Gupta, S., Vincent, J.L. and Frank, B. (2006). Pramipexole: Augmentation in the treatment of depressive symptoms. *CNS Spectrum*, 11(3), 172–175.

Gutierrez, R.L., McKertcher, R., Galea, J. and Jamison, K.L. (2005). Lamotrigine augmentation strategy for patients with treatment-resistant depression. *CNS Spectrum*, 10(10), 800–805.

Hantouche, E.G., Akiskal, H.S., Lancrenon, S. and Chetenet-Duchene, L. (2005). Mood stabilizer augmentation in apparently "unipolar" MDD: Predictors of response in the naturalistic French national EPIDEP study. *Journal of Affective Disorders*, 84(2–3), 243–249.

Hawley, C.J., Quick, S.J., Ratnam, S., *et al.* (1996). Safety and tolerability of combined treatment with moclobemide and SSRIs: A systematic study of 50 patients. *International Clinical Psychopharmacology*, 11(3), 187–191.

Hawley, C.J., Roberts, A.G. and Baldwin, D.S. (1994). Tolerability of combined treatment with lithium and fluoxetine: 14 cases treated under open conditions. *International Clinical Psychopharmacology*, 9(1), 31–33.

Hawley, C.J., Sivakumaran, T., Ochoki, M. and Bevan, J. (2000). Coadministration therapy with reboxetine and serotonin specific reuptake inhibitors in twenty-four patients with major depression. *European Neuropsychopharmacology*, 10(3), S231.

Hellerstein, D.J. (2004). Aripiprazole as an adjunctive treatment for refractory major depression. *Progress in Neuropsychopharmacology and Biological Psychiatry*, 28(8), 1347–1348.

Hellerstein, D.J., Batchelder, S., Hyler, S., *et al.* (2008). Aripiprazole as an adjunctive treatment for refractory unipolar depression. *Progress in Neuropsychopharmacologgy and Biological Psychiatry*, 32(3), 744–750.

Heninger, G.R., Charney, D.S. and Sternberg, D.E. (1983). Lithium carbonate augmentation of antidepressant treatment. *Archives of General Psychiatry*, 40, 1335–1342.

Heresco-Levy, U., Javitt, D.C., Gelfin, Y., *et al.* (2006). Controlled trial of D-cycloserine adjuvant therapy for treatment-resistant major depressive disorder. *Journal of Affective Disorders*, 93(1–3), 239–243.

Hoencamp, E., Haffmans, P.M., Dijken, W.A., *et al.* (1994). Brofaromine versus lithium addition to maprotiline. A double-blind study in maprotiline refractory depressed outpatients. *Journal of Affective Disorders*, 30(3), 219–227.

Hoencamp, E., Haffmans, J., Dijken, W.A. and Huijbrechts, I. (2000). Lithium augmentation of venlafaxine: An open-label trial. *Journal of Clinical Psychopharmacology*, 20(5), 538–543.

Holder, G., Brand, S., Hatzinger, M. and Holsboer-Trachsler, E. (2002). Reduction of daytime sleepiness in a depressive patient during adjunct treatment with modafinil. *Journal of Psychiatric Research*, 36(1), 49–52.

Hornig-Rohan, M. and Amsterdam, J.D. (2002). Venlafaxine versus stimulant therapy in patients with dual diagnosis ADD and depression. *Progress in Neuropsychopharmacology and Biological Psychiatry*, 26(3), 585–589.

Howland, R.H. (1991). Lithium augmentation of fluoxetine in the treatment of OCD and major depression: A case report. *Canadian Journal of Psychiatry*, 36(2), 154–155.

Inoue, T., Tsuchiya, K., Miura, J., *et al.* (1996). Bromocriptine treatment of tricyclic and heterocyclic antidepressant-resistant depression. *Biological Psychiatry*, 40(2), 151–153.

Iosifescu, D.V., Nierenberg, A.A., Mischoulon, D., *et al.* (2005). An open study of triiodothyronine augmentation of selective serotonin reuptake inhibitors in treatment-resistant major depressive disorder. *Journal of Clinical Psychiatry*, 66(8), 1038–1042.

Izumi, T., Inoue, T., Kitagawa, N., *et al.* (2000). Open pergolide treatment of tricyclic and heterocyclic antidepressant-resistant depression. *Journal of Affective Disorders*, 61(1–2), 127–132.

Jackson, W.C., Manning, J.S., Connor, P.D. and Deardorff, O.G. (2004). Retrospective study of olanzapine in depressive and anxious states in primary care. *Primary Care Companion of the Journal of Clinical Psychiatry*, 6(5), 199–202.

Jaracz, J., Chlopocka-Wozniak, M. and Rybakowski, J.K. (2004). Reboxetine added to SSRI accelerates the improvement in depressed patients who failed to respond to SSRI alone. *European Neuropsychopharmacology*, 14s1, S200.

Joffe, R.T. (1992). Triiodothyronine potentiation of fluoxetine in depressed patients. *Canadian Journal of Psychiatry*, 37(1), 48–50.

Joffe, R.T. (1988). Triiodothyronine potentiation of the antidepressant effect of phenelzine. *Journal of Clinical Psychiatry*, 49(10), 409–410.

Joffe, R.T. and Schuller, D.R. (1993). An open study of buspirone augmentation of serotonin reuptake inhibitors in refractory depression. *Journal of Clinical Psychiatry*, 54(7), 269–271.

Joffe, R.T. and Singer, W. (1990). A comparison of triiodothyronine and thyroxine in the potentiation of tricyclic antidepressants. *Psychiatry Research*, 32(3), 241–251.

Joffe, R.T., Singer, W., Levitt, A.J. and McDonald C. (1993). A placebo-controlled comparison of lithium and triiodothyronine augmentation of tricyclic antidepressants in unipolar refractory depression. *Archives of General Psychiatry*, 50, 387–393.

Joffe, R.T., Sokolov, S.T. and Levitt, A.J. (2006). Lithium and triiodothyronine augmentation of antidepressants. *Canadian Journal of Psychiatry*, 51(12), 791–793.

Kan, C.K. and Ho, T.P. (2001). Triiodothyronine augmentation for the treatment of depression in substance misusers unresponsive to tricyclic antidepressants. *Hong Kong Medical Journal*, 7(3), 299–302.

Kantor, D., McNevin, S., Leichner, P., *et al.* (1986). The benefit of lithium carbonate adjunct in refractory depression-fact or fiction? *Canadian Journal of Psychiatry*, 31, 416–418.

Kaplan, M. (2000). Atypical antipsychotics for treatment of mixed depression and anxiety. *Journal of Clinical Psychiatry*, 61(5), 388–389.

Katona, C.L., Abou-Saleh, M.T., Harrison, D.A., *et al.* (1995). Placebo-controlled trial of lithium augmentation of fluoxetine and lofepramine. *British Journal of Psychiatry*, 166, 80–86.

Keitner, G.I., Garlow, S.J., Ryan, C.E., *et al.* (2009). Risperidone augmentation for patients with difficult-to-treat major depression. *Journal of Psychiatric Research*, 43(3), 205–214.

Kelly, T.F. and Lieberman, D.Z. (2009). Long term augmentation with T(3) in refractory major depression. *Journal of Affective Disorders*, 115(1–2), 230–233.

Ketter, T.A., Post, R.M., Parekh, P.I. and Worthington, K. (1995). Addition of monoamine oxidase inhibitors to carbamazepine: Preliminary evidence of safety and antidepressant efficacy in treatment-resistant depression. *Journal of Clinical Psychiatry*, 56(10), 471–475.

Khullar, A., Chokka, P., Fullerton, D., *et al.* (2006). Quetiapine as treatment of non-psychotic unipolar depression with residual symptoms: Double blind, randomized, placebo controlled study. Presented at the 159th Annual Meeting of the American Psychiatric Association. Toronto, Canada.

Kok, R.M., Vink, D., Heeren, T.J. and Nolen, W.A. (2007). Lithium augmentation compared with phenelzine in treatment-resistant depression in the elderly: An open, randomized, controlled trial. *Journal of Clinical Psychiatry*, 68(8), 1177–1185.

Konig, F. and Wolfersdorf, M. (1997). Combination therapy using moclobemide with tricyclic and tetracyclic antidepressants to treat therapy-resistant depression. *Pharmacopsychiatry*, 30(3), 93.

Kudoh, A., Ishihara, H. and Matsuki, A. (1998). Effect of carbamazepine on pain scores of unipolar depressed patients with chronic pain: A trial of off-on-off-on design. *Clinical Journal of Pain*, 14(1), 61–65.

Kushnir, S.L. (1986). Lithium-antidepressant combinations in the treatment of depressed, physically ill geriatric patients. *American Journal of Psychiatry*, 143(3), 378–379.

Lafferman, J., Solomon, K. and Ruskin, P. (1988). Lithium augmentation for treatment-resistant depression in the elderly. *Journal of Geriatric Psychiatry and Neurology*, 1(1), 49–52.

Lam, R.W., Hossie, H., Solomons, K. and Yatham, L.N. (2004). Citalopram and bupropion-SR combining versus switching in patients with treatment-resistant depression. *Journal of Clinical Psychiatry*, 65(3), 337–340.

Landen, M., Bjorling, G., Agren, H. and Fahlen, T. (1998). A randomized, double-blind, placebo-controlled trial of buspirone in combination with an SSRI in patients with treatment-refractory depression. *Journal of Clinical Psychiatry*, 59(12), 664–668.

Lattanzi, L., Dell'Osso, L., Cassano, P., *et al.* (2002). Pramipexole in treatment-resistant depression: A 16-week naturalistic study. *Bipolar Disorders*, 4(5), 307–314.

Levine, J., Gonsalves, M., Babur, I., *et al.* (1993). Inositiol 6g daily may be effective in depression but not in schizophrenia. *Human Psychopharmacology*, 8, 49–53.

Levitt, A.J., Chaput, Y., Lam, R., *et al.* (2004). Risperidone versus olanzapine as add-on treatment in resistant depression. *International Journal of Neuropsychopharmacology*, 7(s2), s1–s503.

Levitt, A.J., Joffe, R.T., Kamil, R. and McIntyre, R. (1999). Do depressed subjects who have failed both fluoxetine and a tricyclic antidepressant respond to the combination? *Journal of Clinical Psychiatry*, 60(9), 613–616.

Licht, R.W. and Qvitzau, S. (2002). Treatment strategies in patients with major depression not responding to first-line sertraline treatment. A randomised study of extended duration of treatment, dose increase or mianserin augmentation. *Psychopharmacology*, 161(2), 143–151.

Linet, L.S. (1989). Treatment of a refractory depression with a combination of fluoxetine and *d*-amphetamine. *American Journal of Psychiatry*, 146(6), 803–804.

Lojko, D. and Rybakowski, J.K. (2007). l-thyroxine augmentation of serotonergic antidepressants in female patients with refractory depression. *Journal of Affective Disorders*, 103(1–3), 253–256.

Lopez-Munoz, F., Alamo, C., Rubio, G., *et al.* (2007). Reboxetine combination in treatment-resistant depression to selective serotonin reuptake inhibitors. *Pharmacopsychiatry*, 40(1), 14–19.

Lopez-Munoz, F., Rubio, G., Alamo, C., *et al.* (2006). Reboxetine addition in patients with mirtazapine-resistant depression: A case series. *Clinical Neuropharmacology*, 29(4), 192–196.

Louie, A.K. and Meltzer, H.Y. (1984). Lithium potentiation of antidepressant treatment. *Journal of Clinical Psychopharmacology*, 4(6), 316–321.

Lundt, L. (2004). Modafinil treatment in patients with seasonal affective disorder/winter depression: An open-label pilot study. *Journal of Affective Disorders*, 81(2), 173–178.

Maes, M., Libbrecht, I., van Hunsel, F., *et al.* (1999). Pindolol and mianserin augment the antidepressant activity of fluoxetine in hospitalized major depressed patients, including those with treatment resistance. *Journal of Clinical Psychopharmacology*, 19(2), 177–182.

Maes, M., Vandoolaeghe, E. and Desnyder, R. (1996). Efficacy of treatment with trazodone in combination with pindolol or fluoxetine in major depression. *Journal of Affective Disorders*, 41(3), 201–210.

Mago, R., Patkar, A.A., Evenden, M., *et al.* (2004). An open-label, rater-blinded study of aripiprazole as an augmentation agent in patients with treatment-resistant depression. Presented at the 44th Annual Meeting of the New Clinical Drug Evaluation Unit (NCDEU) of the National Institute of Mental Health. Scottsdale, Arizona.

Mahmoud, R.A., Pandina, G.J., Turkoz, I., *et al.* (2007). Risperidone for treatment-refractory major depressive disorder: A randomized trial. *Annals of Internal Medicine*, 147(9), 593–602.

Malison, R.T., Price, L.H., Nestler, E.J., *et al.* (1997). Efficacy of papaverine addition for treatment-refractory major depression. *American Journal of Psychiatry*, 154(4), 579–580.

Maltese, T.M. (1999). Adjunctive lamotrigine treatment for major depression. *American Journal of Psychiatry*, 156(11), 1833.

Manning, J.S. and Connor, P.D. (1994). Antidepressant augmentation with lithium. *Journal of Family Practice*, 39(4), 379–383.

Marcus, R.N., McQuade, R.D., Carson, W.H., *et al.* (2008). The efficacy and safety of aripiprazole as adjunctive therapy in major depressive disorder: A second multicenter, randomized, double-blind, placebo-controlled study. *Journal of Clinical Psychopharmacology*, 28(2), 156–165.

Markowitz, J.S. and Patrick, K.S. (1998). Venlafaxine-tramadol similarities. *Medical Hypotheses*, 51(2), 167–168.

Markovitz, P.J. and Wagner, S. (2003). An open-label trial of modafinil augmentation in patients with partial response to antidepressant therapy. *Journal of Clinical Psychopharmacology*, 23(2), 207–209.

Maron, E., Eller, T., Vasar, V. and Nutt, D.J. (2009). Effects of bupropion augmentation in escitalopram-resistant patients with major depressive disorder: An open-label, naturalistic study. *Journal of Clinical Psychiatry*, 70(7), 1054–1056.

Masand, P.S., Anand, V.S. and Tanquary, J.F. (1998). Psychostimulant augmentation of second generation antidepressants: A case series. *Depression and Anxiety*, 7(2), 89–91.

Mattingly, G.W., Ilivicky, H.J., Canale, J.P. and Anderson, R.H. (2006). Quetiapine augmentation for treatment-resistant depression. Presented at the 159th Annual Meeting of the American Psychiatric Association, Toronto, Canada.

Maurer, I., Volz, H.P. and Sauer, H. (1999). Gabapentin leads to remission of somatoform pain disorder with major depression. *Pharmacopsychiatry*, 32(6), 255.

McGrath, P.J., Stewart, J.W., Fava, M., *et al.* (2006). Tranylcypromine versus venlafaxine plus mirtazapine following three failed antidepressant medication trials for depression: A STAR*D report. *American Journal of Psychiatry*, 163(9), 1531–1541.

McIntyre, A., Gendron, A. and McIntyre, A. (2007). Quetiapine adjunct to selective serotonin reuptake inhibitors or venlafaxine in patients with major depression, comorbid anxiety, and residual depressive symptoms: A randomized, placebo-controlled pilot study. *Depression and Anxiety*, 24(7), 487–494.

McLeod, M.N., Gaynes, B.N. and Golden, R.N. (1999). Chromium potentiation of antidepressant pharmacotherapy for dysthymic disorder in 5 patients. *Journal of Clinical Psychiatry*, 60(4), 237–240.

Mendlewicz, J., Kriwin, P., Oswald, P., *et al.* (2006). Shortened onset of action of antidepressants in major depression using acetylsalicylic acid augmentation: A pilot open-label study. *International Clinical Psychopharmacology*, 21(4), 227–231.

Menza, M.A., Kaufman, K.R. and Castellanos, A. (2000). Modafinil augmentation of antidepressant treatment in depression. *Journal of Clinical Psychiatry*, 61(5), 378–381.

Mischoulon, D., Fava, M. and Rosenbaum, JF. (1999). Strategies for augmentation of SSRI treatment: A survey of an academic psychopharmacology practice. *Harvard Review of Psychiatry*, 6(6), 322–326.

Michelson, D., Adler, L.A., Amsterdam, J.D., *et al.* (2007). Addition of atomoxetine for depression incompletely responsive to sertraline: A randomized, double-blind, placebo-controlled study. *Journal of Clinical Psychiatry*, 68, 582–587.

Moeller, O., Hetzel, G. and Arolt, V. (2004). Quetiapine in the treatment of agitation in major depressive disorder. *European Neuropsychopharmacology*. 2004, 14(s1), S176.

Montes, J.M., Ferrando, L. and Saiz-Ruiz, J. (2004). Remission in major depression with two antidepressant mechanisms: Results from a naturalistic study. *Journal of Affective Disorders*, 79(1–3), 229–234.

Morgan, M.L., Cook, I.A., Rapkin, A.J. and Leuchter, A.F. (2005). Estrogen augmentation of antidepressants in perimenopausal depression: A pilot study. *Journal of Clinical Psychiatry*, 66(6), 774–780.

Morgan, M.L., Cook, I.A., Rapkin, A.J. and Leuchter, A.F. (2007). Neurophysiologic changes during estrogen augmentation in perimenopausal depression. *Maturitas*, 56(1), 54–60.

Morishita, S. and Aoki, S. (2002). Clonazepam augmentation of antidepressants: Does it distinguish unipolar from bipolar depression? *Journal of Affective Disorders*, 71(1–3), 217–220.

Morishita, S. and Aoki, S. (1999). Clonazepam in the treatment of prolonged depression. *Journal of Affective Disorders*, 53(3), 275–278.

Morishita, S. and Arita, S. (2007). Possible predictors of response to clonazepam augmentation therapy in patients with protracted depression. *Human Psychopharmacology*, 22, 27–31.

Mountjoy, C.Q., Price, J.S, Weller, M., *et al.* (1974). A double-blind crossover sequential trial of oral thyrotrophin-releasing hormone in depression. *The Lancet*, 1(7864), 958–960.

Nasr, S. (2004). Modafinil as adjunctive therapy in depressed outpatients. *Annals of Clinical Psychiatry*, 16(3), 133–138.

Nelson, J.C. and Byck, R. (1982). Rapid response to lithium in phenelzine non-responders. *British Journal of Psychiatry*, 141, 85–86.

Nelson, J.C., Mazure, C.M., Jatlow, P.I., *et al.* (2004). Combining norepinephrine and serotonin reuptake inhibition mechanisms for treatment of depression: A double-blind, randomized study. *Biological Psychiatry*, 55(3), 296–300.

Nelson, J.C. and Papakostas, G.I. (2009). Atypical antipsychotic augmentation in major depressive disorder: A meta analysis of placebo-controlled randomized trials. *American Journal of Psychiatry*, 166(9), 980–991.

Nemets, B., Mishory, A., Levine, J. and Belmaker, R.H. (1999). Inositol addition does not improve depression in SSRI treatment failures. *Journal of Neural Transmission*, 106(7–8), 795–798.

Nemets, B., Stahl, Z. and Belmaker, R.H. (2002). Addition of omega-3 fatty acid to maintenance medication treatment for recurrent unipolar depressive disorder. *American Journal of Psychiatry*, 159(3), 477–479.

Nierenberg, A.A., Cole, J.O. and Glass, L. (1992). Possible trazodone potentiation of fluoxetine: A case series. *Journal of Clinical Psychiatry*, 53(3), 83–85.

Nierenberg, A.A., Farabaugh, A.H., Alpert, J.E., *et al.* (2000). Timing of onset of antidepressant response with fluoxetine treatment. *American Journal of Psychiatry*, 157(9), 1423–1428.

Nierenberg, A.A., Fava, M., Trivedi, M.H., *et al.* (2006). A comparison of lithium and T(3) augmentation following two failed medication treatments for depression: A STAR*D report. *American Journal of Psychiatry*, 163(9), 1519–1530.

Nierenberg, A.A., Papakostas, G.I., Petersen, T., *et al.* (2003). Lithium augmentation of nortriptyline for subjects resistant to multiple antidepressants. *Journal of Clinical Psychopharmacology*, 23(1), 92–95.

O'Connor, M. and Silver, H. (1998). Adding risperidone to selective serotonin reuptake inhibitor improves chronic depression. *Journal of Clinical Psychopharmacology*, 18(1), 89–91.

Olver, J.S., Ignatidis, S., Maruff, P., *et al.* (2008). Quetiapine augmentation in depressed patients with partial response to antidepressants. *Human Psychopharmacology*, 23(8), 653–660.

Orengo, C.A., Fullerton, L. and Kunik, M.E. (2005). Safety and efficacy of testosterone gel 1% augmentation in depressed men with partial response to antidepressant therapy. *Journal of Geriatric Psychiatry and Neurology*, 18(1), 20–24.

Ostroff, R.B. and Nelson, C.J. (1999). Risperidone augmentation of selective serotonin reuptake inhibitors in major depression. *Journal of Clinical Psychiatry*, 60, 256–259.

Otani, K., Yasui, N., Kaneko, S., *et al.* (1996). Carbamazepine augmentation therapy in three patients with trazodone-resistant unipolar depression. *International Clinical Psychopharmacology*, 11(1), 55–57.

Pae, C.U., Patkar, A.A., Jun, T.Y., *et al.* (2007). Aripiprazole augmentation for treatment of patients with inadequate antidepressants response. *Depression and Anxiety*, 24(7), 522–526.

Papakostas, G.I., Alpert, J.E. and Fava, M. (2003). SAMe in the treatment of depression: A comprehensive review of the literature. *Current Psychiatry Reports*, 5(6), 460–466.

Papakostas, G.I., Petersen, T.J., Kinrys, G., *et al.* (2005). Aripiprazole augmentation of selective serotonin reuptake inhibitors for treatment-resistant major depressive disorder. *Journal of Clinical Psychiatry*, 66(10), 1326–1330.

Papakostas, G.I., Petersen, T.J., Nierenberg, A.A., *et al.* (2004). Ziprasidone augmentation of selective serotonin reuptake inhibitors (SSRIs) for SSRI-resistant major depressive disorder. *Journal of Clinical Psychiatry*, 65(2), 217–221.

Papakostas, G.I., Shelton, R.C., Smith, J. and Fava, M. (2007). Augmentation of antidepressants with atypical antipsychotic medications for treatment-resistant major depressive disorder: A meta-analysis. *Journal of Clinical Psychiatry*, 68(6), 826–831.

Papakostas, G.I., Worthington, J.J. 3rd, Iosifescu, D.V., *et al.* (2006). The combination of duloxetine and bupropion for treatment-resistant major depressive disorder. *Depression and Anxiety*, 23(3), 178–181.

Parker, G. (2002). Olanzapine augmentation in the treatment of melancholia: The trajectory of improvement in rapid responders. *International Clinical Psychopharmacology*, 17(2), 87–89.

Pasquini, M., Picardi, A., Speca, A., *et al.* (2007). Combining an SSRI with an anticonvulsant in depressed patients with dysphoric mood: An open study. *Clinical Practice and Epidemiology in Mental Health*, 3, 3.

Patkar, A.A., Masand, P.S., Pae, C.U., *et al.* (2006b). A randomized, double-blind, placebo-controlled trial of augmentation with an extended release formulation of methylphenidate in outpatients with treatment-resistant depression. *Journal of Clinical Psychopharmacology*, 26(6), 653–656.

Patkar, A.A., Peindl, K., Mago, R., *et al.* (2006a). An open-label, rater-blinded, augmentation study of aripiprazole in treatment-resistant depression. *Primary Care Companion of the Journal of Clinical Psychiatry*, 8(2), 82–87.

Peet, M. and Horrobin, D.F. (2002). A dose-ranging study of the effects of ethyl-eicosapentaenoate in patients with ongoing depression despite apparently adequate treatment with standard drugs. *Archives of General Psychiatry*, 59(10), 913–919.

Perez, V., Soler, J., Puigdemont, D., *et al.* (1999). A double-blind, randomized, placebo-controlled trial of pindolol augmentation in depressive patients resistant to serotonin reuptake inhibitors. Grup de Recerca en Trastorns Afectius. *Archives of General Psychiatry*, 56(4), 375–379.

Perry, E.B., Berman, R.M., Sancora, G., *et al.* (2004). Pindolol augmentation in depressed patients resistant to selective serotonin reuptake inhibitors: A double-blind, randomized, controlled trial. *Journal of Clinical Psychiatry*, 65(2), 238–243.

Pestality, P., Rihmer, Z. and Kiss, H.G. (2003). Moclobemide-amitriptyline combination therapy in treatment-resistant depression. *European Neuropsychopharmacology*, 13(4), S275.

Philip, N.S., Carpenter, L.L., Tyrka, A.R., *et al.* (2009). Varenecline augmentation in depressed smokers: An 8-week, open-label study. *Journal of Clinical Psychiatry*, 70(7), 1026–1031.

Pitchot, W. and Ansseau, M. (2001). Addition of olanzapine for treatment-resistant depression. *American Journal of Psychiatry*, 158(10), 1737.

Pollack, M.H. and Hammerness, P. (1993). Adjunctive yohimbine for treatment in refractory depression. *Biological Psychiatry*, 33(3), 220–221.

Pope, H.G. Jr., Cohane, G.H., Kanayama, G., *et al.* (2003). Testosterone gel supplementation for men with refractory depression: A randomized, placebo-controlled trial. *American Journal of Psychiatry*, 160(1), 105–111.

Preskorn, S.H., Baker, B., Kolluri, S., *et al.* (2008). An innovative design to establish proof of concept of the antidepressant effects of the NR2B subunit selective N-methyl-D-aspartate antagonist, CP-101,606, in patients with treatment-refractory major depressive disorder. *Journal of Clinical Psychopharmacology*, 28(6), 631–637.

Price, C.S. and Taylor, F.B. (2005). A retrospective chart review of the effects of modafinil on depression as monotherapy and as adjunctive therapy. *Depression and Anxiety*, 21(4), 149–153.

Price, L.H., Charney, D.S., Delgado, P.L. and Heninger, G.R. (1990). Fenfluramine augmentation in tricyclic-refractory depression. *Journal of Clinical Psychopharmacology*, 10(5), 312–317.

Price, L.H., Charney, D.S. and Heninger, G.R. (1987). Reserpine augmentation of desipramine in refractory depression: Clinical and neurobiological effects. *Psychopharmacology*, 92(4), 431–437.

Price, L.H., Charney, D.S. and Heninger, G.R. (1986). Variability of response to lithium augmentation in refractory depression. *American Journal of Psychiatry*, 143, 1387–1392.

Rabkin, J.G., Rabkin, R. and Wagner, G. (1994). Effects of fluoxetine on mood and immune status in depressed patients with HIV illness. *Journal of Clinical Psychiatry*, 55(3), 92–97.

Raffa, R.B., Friderichs, E., Reimann, W., *et al.* (1992). Opioid and nonopioid components independently contribute to the mechanism of action of tramadol, an 'atypical' opioid analgesic. *Journal of Pharmacology and Experimental Therapeutics*, 260(1), 275–285.

Rampello, L., Alvano, A., Chiechio, S., *et al.* (2004). Evaluation of the prophylactic efficacy of amitriptyline and citalopram, alone or in combination, in patients with comorbidity of depression, migraine, and tension-type headache. *Neuropsychobiology*, 50(4), 322–328.

Rapaport, M., Wilcox, C., Heiser, J., *et al.* (2002). Reboxetine augmentation of fluoxetine for patients with major depressive disorder: An 8-week open-label study. *European Neuropsychopharmacology*, 12(3), S205.

Rasgon, N.L., Altshuler, L.L., Fairbanks, L.A., *et al.* (2002). Estrogen replacement therapy in the treatment of major depressive disorder in perimenopausal women. *Journal of Clinical Psychiatry*, 63(Suppl 7), 45–48.

Rasmussen, N.A., Schroder, P., Olsen, L.R., *et al.* (2005). Modafinil augmentation in depressed patients with partial response to antidepressants: A pilot study on self-reported symptoms covered by the Major Depression Inventory (MDI) and the Symptom Checklist (SCL-92). *Nordic Journal of Psychiatry*, 59(3), 173–178.

Ravindran, A.V., Kennedy, S.H., O'Donovan, C., *et al.* (2008). Osmotic-release oral system methylphenidate augmentation of antidepressant monotherapy in major depressive disorder: Results of a double-blind, randomized, placebo-controlled trial. *Journal of Clinical Psychiatry*, 69(1), 87–94.

Reeves, H., Batra, S., May, R.S., *et al.* (2008). Efficacy of risperidone augmentation to antidepressants in the management of suicidality in major depressive disorder: A randomized, double-blind, placebo-controlled pilot study. *Journal of Clinical Psychiatry*, 69(8), 1228–1235.

Ries, R.K. and Wittkowsky, A.K. (1986). Synergistic action of alprazolam with tranylcypromine in drug-resistant atypical depression with panic attacks. *Biological Psychiatry*, 21(5–6), 522–526.

Rocca, P, Marchiaro, L., Rasetti, R., *et al.* (2002). A comparison of paroxetine versus paroxetine plus amisulpride in the treatment of dysthymic disorder: Efficacy and psychosocial outcomes. *Psychiatry Research*, 112(2), 145–152.

Rocha, F.L. and Hara, C. (2003). Lamotrigine augmentation in unipolar depression. *International Clinical Psychopharmacology*, 18(2), 97–99.

Rogoz, Z., Dziedzicka-Wasylewska, M., Daniel, W.A., *et al.* (2004b). Effects of joint administration of imipramine and amantadine in patients with drug-resistant unipolar depression. *Polish Journal of Pharmacology*, 56(6), 735–742.

Rogoz, Z., Skuza, G., Wojcikowski, J., *et al.* (2004a). Effect of metyrapone supplementation on imipramine therapy in patients with treatment-resistant unipolar depression. *Polish Journal of Pharmacology*, 56(6), 849–855.

Roitman, S., Green, T., Osher, Y., *et al.* (2007). Creatine monohydrate in resistant depression: A preliminary study. *Bipolar Disorders*, 9(7), 754–758.

Rubio, G., San, L., Lopez-Munoz, F. and Alamo, C. (2004). Reboxetine adjunct for partial or nonresponders to antidepressant treatment. *Journal of Affective Disorders*, 81, 67–72.

Rudas, S., Schmitz, M., Pichler, P. and Baumgartner, A. (1999). Treatment of refractory chronic depression and dysthymia with high-dose thyroxine. *Biological Psychiatry*, 45(2), 229–233.

Rybakowski, J.K., Suwalska, A. and Chlopocka-Wozniak, M. (1999). Potentiation of antidepressants with lithium or carbamazepine in treatment-resistant depression. *Neuropsychobiology*, 40(3), 134–139.

Sagud, M., Mihaljevic-Peles, A., Muck-Seler, D., *et al.* (2006). Quetiapine augmentation in treatment-resistant depression: A naturalistic study. *Psychopharmacology*, 187(4), 511–514.

Sanacora, G., Kendell, S.F., Levin, Y., *et al.* (2007). Preliminary evidence of riluzole efficacy in antidepressant-treated patients with residual depressive symptoms. *Biological Psychiatry*, 61(6), 822–825.

Santos, M.A., Rocha, F.L. and Hara, C. (2008). Efficacy and safety of antidepressant augmentation with lamotrigine in patients with treatment-resistant depression: A randomized, placebo-controlled, double-blind study. *Journal of Clinical Psychiatry*. 10(3): 187–190.

Sato, Y., Yasui-Furukori, N., Nakagami, T., *et al.* (2009). Augmentation of antidepressants with perospirone for treatment-resistant major depressive disorder. *Progress in Neuropsychopharmacology and Biological Psychiatry*, 33(3), 416–418.

Schindler, F. and Anghelescu, I.G. (2007). Lithium versus lamotrigine augmentation in treatment resistant unipolar depression: A randomized, open-label study. *International Clinical Psychopharmacology*, 22(3), 179–182.

Schmauss, M., Laakmann, G. and Dieterle, D. (1998). Effects of alpha 2-receptor blockade in addition to tricyclic antidepressants in therapy-resistant depression. *Journal of Clinical Psychopharmacology*, 8(2), 108–111.

Schmauss, M., Kapfhammer, H.P., Meyr, P. and Hoff, P. (1988). Combined MAO-inhibitor and tri- (tetra) cyclic antidepressant treatment in therapy resistant depression. *Progress in Neuropsychopharmacology and Biological Psychiatry*, 12(4), 523–532.

Schopf, J., Baumann, P., Lemarchand, T. and Rey, M. (1989). Treatment of endogenous depressions resistant to tricyclic antidepressants or related drugs by lithium addition. Results of a placebo-controlled double-blind study. *Pharmacopsychiatry*, 22, 183–187.

Schrader, G.D. and Levien, H.E. (1985). Response to sequential administration of clomipramine and lithium carbonate in treatment-resistant depression. *British Journal of Psychiatry*, 147, 573–575.

Schwarcz, G., Halaris, A., Baxter, L., *et al.* (1984). Normal thyroid function in desipramine nonresponders converted to responders by the addition of L-triiodothyronine. *American Journal of Psychiatry*, 141(12), 1614–1616.

Schwartz, T.L., Azhar, N., Cole, K., *et al.* (2004). An open-label study of adjunctive modafinil in patients with sedation related to serotonergic antidepressant therapy. *Journal of Clinical Psychiatry*, 65(9), 1223–1227.

Schwartz, T.L., Leso, L., Beale, M., *et al.* (2002). Modafinil in the treatment of depression with severe comorbid medical illness. *Psychosomatics*, 43(4), 336–337.

Schwartz, T.L., Nasra, G.S., Chilton, M., *et al.* (2007). Aripiprazole augmentation of selective serotonin reuptake inhibitors or serotonin norepinephrine reuptake inhibitors in the treatment of major depressive disorder. *Primary Psychiatry*, 14(1), 67–69.

Seidman, S.N. and Rabkin, J.G. (1998). Testosterone replacement therapy for hypogonadal men with SSRI-refractory depression. *Journal of Affective Disorders*, 48(2–3), 157–161.

Sekine, Y., Iyo, M., Tanaka, K., *et al.* (2000). Effective adjunctive use of low-dose methylphenidate with mianserin for major depression with silent cerebral infarction: A case report. *Journal of Clinical Psychopharmacology*, 20(5), 584–585.

Sharpley, A.L., Attenburrow, M.E., Hafizi, S. and Cowen, P.J. (2005). Olanzapine increases slow wave sleep and sleep continuity in SSRI-resistant depressed patients. *Journal of Clinical Psychiatry*, 66(4), 450–454.

Shapira, B., Oppenheim, G., Zohar, J., *et al.* (1985). Lack of efficacy of estrogen supplementation to imipramine in resistant female depressives. *Biological Psychiatry*, 20(5), 576–579.

Shapira, B., Nemets, B., Trachtenberg, A. and Belmaker, R.H. (2006). Phenytoin as an augmentation for SSRI failures: A small controlled study. *Journal of Affective Disorders*, 96(1–2), 123–126.

Shelton, R.C. and Addington, S. (2005). Risperidone versus bupropion combined with SSRIs in treatment-resistant unipolar major depression. *Neuropsychopharmacology*. 30(s1), s238.

Shelton, R.C., Tollefson, G.D., Tohen, M., *et al.* (2001). A novel augmentation strategy for treating resistant major depression. *American Journal of Psychiatry*, 158(1), 131–134.

Shelton, R.C., Williamson, D.J., Corya, S.A., *et al.* (2005). Olanzapine/ fluoxetine combination for treatment-resistant depression: A controlled study of SSRI and nortriptyline resistance. *Journal of Clinical Psychiatry*, 66(10), 1289–1297.

Shingo, N., Hisashi, H., Kazuhiro, S., *et al.* (2004). Augmentation effect of cabergoline to milnacipran in a case with refractory depression. *International Clinical Psychopharmacology*, 19(3), 186–187.

Showraki, M. (2007). Pregabalin in the treatment of depression. *Journal of Psychopharmacology*, 21(8), 883–884.

Simon, J.S. and Nemeroff, C.B. (2005). Aripiprazole augmentation of antidepressants for the treatment of partially responding and nonresponding patients with major depressive disorder. *Journal of Clinical Psychiatry*, 66(10), 1216–1220.

Sloan Manning, J., Haykal, R.F., Connor, P.D., *et al.* (2005). Sustained remission with lamotrigine augmentation or monotherapy in female resistant depressives with mixed cyclothymic-dysthymic temperament. *Journal of Affective Disorders*, 84(2–3), 259–266.

Sluzewska, A., Sobieska, M. and Rybakowski, J.K. (1997). Changes in acute-phase proteins during lithium potentiation of antidepressants in refractory depression. *Neuropsychobiology*, 35(3), 123–127.

Sokolski, K.N. (2008). Adjunctive aripiprazole for bupropion-resistant major depression. *Annals of Pharmacotherapy*, 42(9), 1348–1349.

Sokolski, K.N. and Brown, B.J. (2006). Quetiapine for insomnia associated with refractory depression exacerbated by phenelzine. *Annals of Pharmacotherapy*, 40(3), 567–570.

Sokolski, K.N., Conney, J.C., Brown, B.J. and DeMet, E.M. (2004). Once-daily high-dose pindolol for SSRi-refractory depression. *Psychiatry Research*, 125, 81–86.

Sovner, R. (1990). Amphetamine and tranylcypromine in treatment-resistant depression. *Biological Psychiatry*, 28(11), 1011–1012.

Sporn, J., Ghaemi, S.N., Sambur, M.R., *et al.* (2000). Pramipexole augmentation in the treatment of unipolar and bipolar depression: A retrospective chart review. *Annals of Clinical Psychiatry*, 12(3), 137–140.

Stabl, M., Kasas, A., Blajev, B., *et al.* (1995). A double-blind comparison of moclobemide and thioridazine versus moclobemide and placebo in the treatment of refractory, severe depression. *Journal of Clinical Psychopharmacology*, 15(4 Suppl 2), 41S–45S.

Steinacher, L., Vandel, P., Zullino, D.F., *et al.* (2002). Carbamazepine augmentation in depressive patients non-responding to citalopram: A pharmacokinetic and clinical pilot study. *European Neuropsychopharmacology*, 12(3), 255–260.

Steiner, M., Radwan, M., Elizur, A., *et al.* (1978). Failure of l-triiodothyronine (T3) to potentiate tricyclic antidepressant response. *Current Therapeutic Research*, 23(5), 655–659.

Stein, G. and Bernadt, M. (1993). Lithium augmentation therapy in tricyclic-resistant depression. A controlled trial using lithium in low and normal doses. *British Journal of Psychiatry*, 162, 634–640.

Stoll, A.L. and Haura, G. (2000). Tranylcypromine plus risperidone for treatment-refractory major depression. *Journal of Clinical Psychopharmacology*, 20(4), 495–496.

Stoll, A.L., Pillay, S.S., Diamond, L., *et al.* (1996). Methylphenidate augmentation of serotonin selective reuptake inhibitors: A case series. *Journal of Clinical Psychiatry*, 57(2), 72–76.

Stoll, A.L. and Rueter, S. (1999). Treatment augmentation with opiates in severe and refractory major depression. *American Journal of Psychiatry*, 156(12), 2017.

Stryjer, R., Strous, R.D., Shaked, G., *et al.* (2003). Amantadine as augmentation therapy in the management of treatment-resistant depression. *International Clinical Psychopharmacology*, 18(2), 93–96.

Su, K.P., Huang, S.Y., Chiu, C.C. and Shen, W.W. (2003). Omega-3 fatty acids in major depressive disorder. A preliminary double-blind, placebo-controlled trial. *European Neuropsychopharmacology*, 13(4), 267–271.

Sumiyoshi, A., Miki, K., Kamimura, M. and Yamada, K. (2008). Tandospirone augmentation therapy is useful in depressed patients with inadequate response to SSRIs or SNRIs. *European Neuropsychopharmacology*, 18(s4), s332.

Takahashi, H., Kamata, M., Yoshida, K., *et al.* (2008). Augmentation with olanzapine in TCA-refractory depression with melancholic features: A consecutive case series. *Human Psychopharmacology*, 23(3), 217–220.

Takahashi, H., Kamata, M., Yoshida, K., *et al.* (2005). Remarkable effect of milnacipran, a serotonin-noradrenalin reuptake inhibitor (SNRI), on depressive symptoms in patients with Parkinson's disease who have insufficient response to selective serotonin reuptake inhibitors (SSRIs): Two case reports. *Progress in Neuropsychopharmacology and Biological Psychiatry*, 29(2), 351–353.

Takahashi, H., Yoshida, K., Higuchi, H., *et al.* (2003). Addition of a dopamine agonist, cabergoline, to a serotonin-noradrenalin reuptake inhibitor, milnacipran as a therapeutic option in the treatment of refractory depression: Two case reports. *Clinical Neuropharmacology*, 26(5), 230–232.

Tani, K., Takei, N., Kawai, M., *et al.* (2004). Augmentation of milnacipran by risperidone in treatment for major depression. *International Journal of Neuropsychopharmacology*, 7(1), 55–58.

Targum, S.D., Greenberg, R.D., Harmon, R.L., *et al.* (1984). Thyroid hormone and the TRH stimulation test in refractory depression. *Journal of Clinical Psychiatry*, 45(8), 345–346.

Targum, S.D., Hassman, H., Bastani, B. and Bari, M. (2004). Quetiapine reduces persistent anxiety in patients with major depressive disorder. Presented at the 44th Annual Meeting of the New Clinical Drug Evaluation Unit (NCDEU) of the National Institute of Mental Health. Scottsdale, Arizona.

Tavormina, G., Corea, S. and Citron, A. (2002). Reboxetine utilization as an add-on therapy to SSRI in treatment-resistant depression. *European Neuropsychopharmacology*, 12(3), S178.

Taylor, F.B. and Prather, M.R. (2003). The efficacy of nefazodone augmentation for treatment-resistant depression with anxiety symptoms or anxiety disorder. *Depression and Anxiety*, 18(2), 83–88.

Thase, M.E., Corya, S.A., Osuntokun, O., *et al.* (2007). A randomized, double-blind comparison of olanzapine/fluoxetine combination, olanzapine, and fluoxetine in treatment-resistant major depressive disorder. *Journal of Clinical Psychiatry*, 68(2), 224–236.

Thase, M.E., Fava, M., DeBattista, C., *et al.* (2006). Modafinil augmentation of SSRI therapy in patients with major depressive disorder and excessive sleepiness and fatigue: A 12-week, open-label, extension study. *CNS Spectrums*, 11(2), 93–102.

Thase, M.E., Kupfer, D.J., Frank, E. and Jarrett, D.B. (1989b). Treatment of imipramine-resistant recurrent depression: An open clinical trial of lithium augmentation. *Journal of Clinical Psychiatry*, 50(11), 413–417.

Thase, M.E., Kupfer, D.J. and Jarrett, D.B. (1989a). Treatment of imipramine-resistant recurrent depression: I. An open clinical trial of adjunctive L-triiodothyronine. *Journal of Clinical Psychiatry*, 50(10), 385–388.

Trivedi, M.H., Fava, M., Wisniewski, S.R., *et al.* (2006). Medication augmentation after the failure of SSRIs for depression. *New England Journal of Medicine*, 354(12), 1243–1252.

Tsutsui, S., Yamazaki, Y., Namba, T. and Tsushima, M. (1979). Combined therapy of T3, and antidepressants in depression. *Journal of International Medical Research*, 7(2), 138–146.

van Marwijk, H.W., Bekker, F.M., Nolen, W.A., *et al.* (1990). Lithium augmentation in geriatric depression. *Journal of Affective Disorders*, 20(4), 217–223.

Varga, E., Sugerman, A.A. and Apter, J. (1982). The effect of codeine on involutional and senile depression. *Annals of the New York Academy of Sciences*, 398, 103–105.

Viner, M.W., Chen, Y., Bakshi, I. and Kamper, P. (2003). Low-dose risperidone augmentation of antidepressants in nonpsychotic depressive disorders with suicidal ideation. *Journal of Clinical Psychopharm*acology, 23(1), 104–106.

Weilburg, J.B., Rosenbaum, J.F., Biederman, J., *et al.* (1989). Fluoxetine added to non-MAOI antidepressants converts nonresponders to responders: A preliminary report. *Journal of Clinical Psychiatry*, 50(12), 447–449.

Whyte, E.M., Basinski, J., Farhi, P., *et al.* (2004). Geriatric depression treatment in nonresponders to selective serotonin reuptake inhibitors. *Journal of Clinical Psychiatry*, 65(12), 1634–1641.

Worthington, J.J. 3rd, Kinrys, G., Wygant, L.E. and Pollack, M.H. (2005). Aripiprazole as an augmentor of selective serotonin reuptake inhibitors in depression and anxiety disorder patients. *International Clinical Psychopharmacology*, 20(1), 9–11.

Xiong, G.L., Christopher, E.J. and Goebel, J. (2005). Modafinil as an alternative to methylphenidate as augmentation for depression treatment. *Psychosomatics*, 46(6), 578–579.

Yasmin, S., Carpenter, L.L., Leon, Z., *et al.* (2001). Adjunctive gabapentin in treatment-resistant depression: A retrospective chart review. *Journal of Affective Disorders*, 63(1–3), 243–247.

Zajecka, J.M., Jeffries, H. and Fawcett, J. (1995). The efficacy of fluoxetine combined with heterocyclic antidepressant in treatment-resistant depression: A retrospective analysis. *Journal of Clinical Psychiatry*, 56, 338–343.

Zarate, C.A. Jr., Payne, J.L., Singh, J., *et al.* (2004). Pramipexole for bipolar II depression: A placebo-controlled proof of concept study. *Biological Psychiatry*, 56(1), 54–60.

Zarate, C.A Jr., Singh, J.B., Carlson, P.J., *et al.* (2006). A randomized trial of an N-methyl-D-aspartate antagonist in treatment-resistant major depression. *Archives of General Psychiatry*, 63(8), 856–864.

Zetin, M. (1984). Combined use of trazodone and phenelzine in depression: Case report. *Journal of Clinical Psychiatry*, 45(4), 182–183.

Zheng, L., Jing, C., Xia, L. and Jun, C. (2007). Efficacy and tolerability of quetiapine combined with antidepressants in patients with treatment-resistant depression. *European Neuropsychopharmacology*, 17(s4), S471.

Zimmer, B., Rosen, J., Thornton, J.E., *et al.* (1991). Adjunctive lithium carbonate in nortriptyline-resistant elderly depressed patients. *Journal of Clinical Psychopharmacology*, 11(4), 254–256.

Zohar, J., Shapira, B., Oppenheim, G., *et al.* (1985). Addition of estrogen to imipramine in female-resistant depressives. *Psychopharmacology Bulletin*, 21(3), 705–706.

Zullino, D., Preisig, M. and Baumann, P. (2001). Lithium augmentation in venlafaxine-refractory depression. *Journal of Clinical Psychopharmacology*, 21(2), 242–243.

Zusky, P.M., Biederman, J., Rosenbaum, J.F., *et al.* (1988). Adjunct low dose lithium carbonate in treatment-resistant depression: A placebo controlled study. *Journal of Clinical Psychopharmacology*, 8, 120–124.

Chapter 7

Amsterdam, J.D. and Berwish, N.J. (1989). High dose tranylcypromine therapy for refractory depression. *Pharmacopsychiatry*, 22(1), 21–25.

Amsterdam, J.D., Maislin, G. and Potter, L. (1994). Fluoxetine efficacy in treatment resistant depression. *Progress in Neuropsychopharmacology and Biological Psychiatry*, 18(2), 243–261.

Amsterdam, J.D. and Shults, J. (2005). MAOI efficacy and safety in advanced stage treatment resistant depression-A retrospective study. *Journal of Affective Disorders*, 89(1–3), 183–188.

Baldomero, E.B., Ubago, J.G., Cercos, C.L., *et al.* (2005). Venlafaxine extended release versus conventional antidepressants in the remission of depressive disorders after previous antidepressant failure: ARGOS study. *Depression and Anxiety*, 22, 68–76.

Beasley, C.M. Jr., Sayler, M.E., Cunningham, G.E., *et al.* (1990). Fluoxetine in tricyclic refractory major depressive disorder. *Journal of Affective Disorders*, 20(3), 193–200.

Benkert, O., Szegedi, A., Wetzel, H., *et al.* (1997). Dose escalation vs. continued doses of paroxetine and maprotiline: A prospective study in depressed out-patients with inadequate treatment response. *Acta Psychiatrica Scandinavica*, 95(4), 288–296.

Birkenhager, T.K., van den Broek, W.W., Mulder, P.G., *et al.* (2004). Comparison of two-phase treatment with imipramine or fluvoxamine, both followed by lithium addition, in inpatients with major depressive disorder. *American Journal of Psychiatry*, 161(11), 2060–2065.

Brent, D., Emslie, G., Clarke, G., *et al.* (2008). Switching to another SSRI or to venlafaxine with or without cognitive behavioral therapy for adolescents with SSRI-resistant depression: The TORDIA randomized controlled trial. *Journal of the American Medical Association*, 299(8), 901–913.

Cantrell, R., Gillespie, W. and Altshuler, L. (1999). Fluoxetine and sertraline dosages in major depression. *Depression and Anxiety*, 9(2), 78–82.

Cole, J.O., Schatzberg, A.F., Sniffin, C., *et al.* (1981). Trazodone in treatment-resistant depression: An open-label study. *Journal of Clinical Psychopharmacology*, 1(s6), 49–54.

de Montigny, C., Silverstone, P.H., Debonnel, G., *et al.* (1999). Venlafaxine in treatment-resistant major depression: A Canadian multicenter, open-label trial. *Journal of Clinical Psychopharmacology*, 19(5), 401–406.

Dornseif, B.E., Dunlop, S.R., Potvin, J.H. and Wernicke, J.F. (1989). Effect of dose escalation after low-dose fluoxetine therapy. *Psychopharmacology Bulletin*, 25(1), 71–79.

Fava, M., Alpert, J., Nierenberg, A., *et al.* (2002). Double-blind study of high-dose fluoxetine versus lithium or desipramine augmentation of fluoxetine in partial responders and nonresponders to fluoxetine. *Journal of Clinical Psychopharmacology*, 22(4), 379–387.

Fava, M., Dunner, D.L., Greist, J.H., *et al.* (2001). Efficacy and safety of mirtazapine in major depressive disorder patients after SSRI treatment failure: An open-label trial. *Journal of Clinical Psychiatry*, 62(6), 413–420.

Fava, M., McGrath, P.J., Sheu, W.P. & Reboxetine Study Group. (2003b). Switching to reboxetine: An efficacy and safety study in patients with major depressive disorder unresponsive to fluoxetine. *Journal of Clinical Psychopharmacology*, 23(4), 365–369.

Fava, M., Papakostas, G.I., Petersen, T., *et al.* (2003a). Switching to bupropion in fluoxetine-resistant major depressive disorder. *Annals of Clinical Psychiatry*, 15(1), 17–22.

Fava, M., Rosenbaum, J.F., Cohen, L., *et al.* (1992). High-dose fluoxetine in the treatment of depressed patients not responsive to a standard dose of fluoxetine. *Journal of Affective Disorders*, 25(4), 229–234.

Fava, M., Rosenbaum, J.F., McGrath, P.J., *et al.* (1994). Lithium and tricyclic augmentation of fluoxetine treatment for resistant major depression: A double-blind, controlled study. *American Journal of Psychiatry*, 151(9), 1372–1374.

Fava, M., Rush, A.J., Wisniewski, S.R., *et al.* (2006). A comparison of mirtazapine and nortriptyline following two consecutive failed medication treatments for depressed outpatients: A STAR*D report. *American Journal of Psychiatry*, 163(7), 1161–1172.

Ferreri, M., Lavergne, F., Berlin, I., *et al.* (2001). Benefits from mianserin augmentation of fluoxetine in patients with major depression nonresponders to fluoxetine alone. *Acta Psychiatrica Scandinavica*, 103(1), 66–72.

Flint, A.J. and Rifat, S.L. (1996). The effect of sequential antidepressant treatment on geriatric depression. *Journal of Affective Disorders*, 36(3–4), 95–105.

Fredman, S.J., Fava, M., Kienke, A.S., *et al.* (2000). Partial response, nonresponse, and relapse with selective serotonin reuptake inhibitors in major depression: A survey of current "next-step" practices. *Journal of Clinical Psychiatry*, 61(6), 403–408.

George, T., Theodoros, M.T., Chiu, E., *et al.* (1999). An open study of sertraline in patients with major depression who failed to respond to moclobemide. *Australian and New Zealand Journal of Psychiatry*, 33(6), 889–895.

Georgotas, A., Friedman, E., McCarthy, M., *et al.* (1983). Resistant geriatric depressions and therapeutic response to monoamine oxidase inhibitors. *Biological Psychiatry*, 18(2), 195–205.

Gervasoni, N., Aubry, J.M., Gex-Fabry, M., *et al.* (2009). Is there a place for tricyclic antidepressants and subsequent augmentation strategies in obtaining remission for patients with treatment resistant depression? *Pharmacology Research*, 59(3), 202–206.

Heiligenstein, J.H., Hoog, S.L., Wagner, K.D., *et al.* (2006). Fluoxetine 40–60 mg versus fluoxetine 20 mg in the treatment of children and adolescents with a less-than-complete response to nine-week treatment with fluoxetine 10–20 mg: A pilot study. *Journal of Child and Adolescent Psychopharmacology*, 16(1–2), 207–217.

Hoencamp, E., Haffmans, P.M., Dijken, W.A., *et al.* (1994). Brofaromine versus lithium addition to maprotiline. A double-blind study in maprotiline refractory depressed outpatients. *Journal of Affective Disorders*, 30(3), 219–227.

Joffe, R.T., Levitt, A.J., Sokolov, S.T. and Young, L.T. (1996). Response to an open trial of a second SSRI in major depression. *Journal of Clinical Psychiatry*, 57(3), 114–115.

Kaplan, E.M. (2002). Efficacy of venlafaxine in patients with major depressive disorder who have unsustained or no response to selective serotonin reuptake inhibitors: An open-label, uncontrolled study. *Clinical Therapeutics*, 24(7), 1194–2000.

Karp, J.F., Whyte, E.M., Lenze, E.J., *et al.* (2008). Rescue pharmacotherapy with duloxetine for selective serotonin reuptake inhibitor nonresponders in late-life depression: Outcome and tolerability. *Journal of Clinical Psychiatry*, 69(3), 457–463.

Kornstein, S.G., Dunner, D.L., Meyers, A.L., *et al.* (2008). A randomized, double-blind study of increasing or maintaining duloxetine dose in patients without remission of major depressive disorder after initial duloxetine therapy. *Journal of Clinical Psychiatry*, 69(9), 1383–1392.

Lam, R.W., Hossie, H., Solomons, K. and Yatham, L.N. (2004). Citalopram and bupropion-SR combining versus switching in patients with treatment-resistant depression. *Journal of Clinical Psychiatry*, 65(3), 337–340.

Lenox-Smith, A.J. and Jiang, Q. (2008). Venlafaxine extended release versus citalopram in patients with depression unresponsive to a selective serotonin reuptake inhibitor. *International Clinical Psychopharmacology*, 23(3), 113–119.

Licht, R.W. and Qvitzau, S. (2002). Treatment strategies in patients with major depression not responding to first-line sertraline treatment. A randomised study of extended duration of treatment, dose increase or mianserin augmentation. *Psychopharmacology*, 161(2), 143–151.

Mazeh, D., Shahal, B., Aviv, A., *et al.* (2007). A randomized, single-blind, comparison of venlafaxine with paroxetine in elderly patients suffering from resistant depression.*International Clinical Psychopharmacology*, 22(6), 371–375.

Mbaya, P. (2002). Safety and efficacy of high dose of venlafaxine XL in treatment resistant major depression. *Human Psychopharmacology*, 17(7), 335–339.

McGrath, P.J., Stewart, J.W., Fava, M., *et al.* (2006). Tranylcypromine versus venlafaxine plus mirtazapine following three failed antidepressant medication trials for depression: A STAR*D report. *American Journal of Psychiatry*, 163(9), 1531–1541.

McGrath, P.J., Stewart, J.W., Harrison, W. and Quitkin, F.M. (1987). Treatment of tricyclic refractory depression with a monoamine oxidase inhibitor antidepressant. *Psychopharmacology Bulletin*, 23(1), 169–172.

McGrath, P.J., Stewart, J.W., Nunes, E.V., *et al.* (1993). A double-blind crossover trial of imipramine and phenelzine for outpatients with treatment-refractory depression. *American Journal of Psychiatry*, 150(1), 118–123.

Mischoulon, D., Opitz, G., Kelly, K., *et al.* (2004). A preliminary open study of the tolerability and effectiveness of nefazodone in major depressive disorder: Comparing patients who recently discontinued an SSRI with those on no recent antidepressant treatment. *Depression and Anxiety*, 19(1), 43–50.

Mitchell, P.B., Schweitzer, I., Burrows, G., *et al.* (2000). Efficacy of venlafaxine and predictors of response in a prospective open-label study of patients with treatment-resistant major depression. *Journal of Clinical Psychopharmacology*, 20(4), 483–487.

Montes, J.M., Ferrando, L. and Saiz-Ruiz, J. (2004). Remission in major depression with two antidepressant mechanisms: Results from a naturalistic study. *Journal of Affective Disorders*, 79(1–3), 229–234.

Nierenberg, A.A., Farabaugh, A.H., Alpert, J.E., *et al.* (2000). Timing of onset of antidepressant response with fluoxetine treatment. *American Journal of Psychiatry*, 157(9), 1423–1428.

Nierenberg, A.A., Feighner, J.P., Rudolph, R., *et al.* (1994). Venlafaxine for treatment-resistant unipolar depression. *Journal of Clinical Psychopharmacology*, 14(6), 419–423.

Nierenberg, A.A., Papakostas, G.I., Petersen, T., *et al.* (2003). Nortriptyline for treatment-resistant depression. *Journal of Clinical Psychiatry*, 64(1), 35–39.

Nolen, W.A., Haffmans, P.M., Bouvy, P.F. and Duivenvoorden, H.J. (1993). Monoamine oxidase inhibitors in resistant major depression. A double-blind comparison of brofaromine and tranylcypromine in patients resistant to tricyclic antidepressants. *Journal of Affective Disorders*, 28(3), 189–197.

Nolen, W.A., van de Putte, J.J., Dijken, W.A. and Kamp, J.S. (1985). L-5HTP in depression resistant to re-uptake inhibitors. An open comparative study with tranylcypromine. *British Journal of Psychiatry*, 147, 16–22.

Nolen, W.A., van de Putte, J.J., Dijken, W.A., *et al.* (1988). Treatment strategy in depression. II. MAO inhibitors in depression resistant to cyclic antidepressants: Two controlled crossover studies with tranylcypromine versus L-5-hydroxytryptophan and nomifensine. *Acta Psychiatrica Scandinavica*, 78(6), 676–683.

Papakostas, G.I., Petersen, T., Worthington, J.J., *et al.* (2003). A pilot, open study of sertraline in outpatients with treatment-resistant depression (TRD) or with a history of TRD who responded but later relapsed. *International Clinical Psychopharmacology*, 18(5), 293–296.

Papakostas, G.I., Fava, M. and Thase, M.E. (2008). Treatment of SSRI-resistant depression: A meta-analysis comparing within- versus across-class switches. Biological Psychiatry, 63(7), 699–704.

Perahia, D.G.S., Quail, D., Desaiah, D., *et al.* (2008). Switching to duloxetine from selective serotonin reuptake inhibitor antidepressants: A multicenter trial comparing 2 switching techniques. *Journal of Clinical Psychiatry*, 69(1), 95–105.

Peselow, E.D., Filippi, A.M., Goodnick, P., *et al.* (1989). The short- and long-term efficacy of paroxetine HCl: B. Data from a double-blind crossover study and from a year-long term trial vs. imipramine and placebo. *Psychopharmacology Bulletin*, 25(2), 272–276.

Petersen, T., Dording, C., Neault, N.B., *et al.* (2002). A survey of prescribing practices in the treatment of depression. *Progress in Neuropsychopharmacology and Biological Psychiatry*, 26(1), 177–187.

Poirier, M.F. and Boyer, P. (1999). Venlafaxine and paroxetine in treatment-resistant depression. Double-blind, randomised comparison. *British Journal of Psychiatry*, 175, 12–16.

Raynaert-Dupuis, G., Zdanowicz, N., Leyman, S., *et al.* (2002). Efficacy and tolerance of venlafaxine in depressed patients switched from prior antidepressant treatment. *Primary Care Psychiatry*, 8(2), 63–68.

Ruhé, H.G., Booij, J., Weert, H.C., *et al.* (2009). Evidence why paroxetine dose escalation is not effective in major depressive disorder: A randomized controlled trial with assessment of serotonin transporter occupancy. *Neuropsychopharmacology*, 34(4), 999–1010.

Rush, A.J., Trivedi, M.H., Wisniewski, S.R., *et al.* (2006). Bupropion-SR, sertraline, or venlafaxine-XR after failure of SSRIs for depression. *New England Journal of Medicine*, 354(12), 1231–1242.

Sajatovic, M., DiGiovanni, S., Fuller, M., *et al.* (1999). Nefazodone therapy in patients with treatment-resistant or treatment-intolerant depression and high psychiatric comorbidity. *Clinical Therapeutics*, 21(4), 733–740.

Saiz-Ruiz, J., Ibanez, A., Diaz-Marsa, M., *et al.* (2002). Efficacy of venlafaxine in major depression resistant to selective serotonin reuptake inhibitors. *Progress in Neuropsychopharmacology and Biological Psychiatry*, 26(6), 1129–1134.

Schweizer, E., Rickels, K., Amsterdam, J.D., *et al.* (1990). What constitutes an adequate antidepressant trial for fluoxetine? *Journal of Clinical Psychiatry*, 51(1), 8–11.

Smith, W.T., Londborg, P.D., Glaudin, V. and Painter, J.R. (1998). Short-term augmentation of fluoxetine with clonazepam in the treatment of depression: A double-blind study. *American Journal of Psychiatry*, 155(10), 1339–1345.

Thase, M.E., Blomgren, S.L., Birkett, M.A., *et al.* (1997). Fluoxetine treatment of patients with major depressive disorder who failed initial treatment with sertraline. *Journal of Clinical Psychiatry*, 58(1), 16–21.

Thase, M.E., Feighner, J.P. and Lydiard, R.B. (2001a). Citalopram treatment of fluoxetine nonresponders. *Journal of Clinical Psychiatry*, 62(9), 683–687.

Thase, M.E., Frank, E., Mallinger, A.G., *et al.* (1992). Treatment of imipramine-resistant recurrent depression, III: Efficacy of monoamine oxidase inhibitors. *Journal of Clinical Psychiatry*, 53(1), 5–11.

Thase, M.E., Kremer, C. and Rodrigues, H. (2001b). Mirtazapine versus sertraline after SSRI non-response. Presented at the 41st Annual Meeting of the New Clinical Drug Evaluation Unit of the National Institute of Mental Health. Boca Raton, Florida.

Thase, M.E., Rush, A.J., Howland, R.H., *et al.* (2002). Double-blind switch study of imipramine or sertraline treatment of antidepressant-resistant chronic depression. *Archives of General Psychiatry*, 59(3), 233–239.

Thase, M.E., Shelton, R.C. and Khan, A. (2006). Treatment with venlafaxine extended release after SSRI nonresponse or intolerance: A randomized comparison of standard- and higher-dosing strategies. *Journal of Clinical Psychopharmacology*, 26(3), 250–258.

Volz, H.P., Faltus, F., Magyar, I. and Moller, H.J. (1994). Brofaromine in treatment-resistant depressed patients — a comparative trial versus tranylcypromine. *Journal of Affective Disorders*, 30(3), 209–217.

Walker, P.W., Cole, J.O., Gardner, E.A., *et al.* (1993). Improvement in fluoxetine-associated sexual dysfunction in patients switched to bupropion. *Journal of Clinical Psychiatry*, 54(12), 459–465.

Weintraub, D. (2001). Nortriptyline in geriatric depression resistant to serotonin reuptake inhibitors: Case series. *Journal of Geriatric Psychiatry and Neurology*, 14(1), 28–32.

Whyte, E.M., Basinski, J., Farhi, P., *et al.* (2004). Geriatric depression treatment in nonresponders to selective serotonin reuptake inhibitors. *Journal of Clinical Psychiatry*, 65(12), 1634–1641.

Wohlreich, M.M., Mallinckrodt, C.H., Prakash, A., *et al.* (2006). Duloxetine for the treatment of major depressive disorder: Safety and tolerability associated with dose escalation. *Depression and Anxiety*, 24(1), 41–52.

Wohlreich, M.M., Mallinckrodt, C.H., Watkin, J.G., *et al.* (2005a). Immediate switching of antidepressant therapy: Results from a clinical trial of duloxetine. *Annals of Clinical Psychiatry*, 17(4), 259–268.

Wohlreich, M.M., Martinez, J.M., Mallinckrodt, C.H., *et al.* (2005b). An open-label study of duloxetine for the treatment of major depressive disorder: Comparison of switching versus initiating treatment approaches. *Journal of Clinical Psychopharmacology*, 25(6), 552–560.

Zarate, C.A., Kando, J.C., Tohen, M., *et al.* (1996). Does intolerance or lack of response with fluoxetine predict the same will happen with sertraline? *Journal of Clinical Psychiatry*, 57(2), 67–71.

Chapter 8

Abbass, A.A. (2006). Intensive short-term dynamic psychotherapy of treatment-resistant depression: A pilot study. *Depression and Anxiety*, 23(7), 449–452.

Allen, J.J., Schnyer, R.N., Chambers, A.S., *et al.* (2006). Acupuncture for depression: A randomized controlled trial. *Journal of Clinical Psychiatry*, 67(11), 1665–1673.

Antonuccio, D.O., Akins, W.T., Chatham, P.M., *et al.* (1984). An exploratory study: The psychoeducational group treatment of drug-refractory unipolar depression. *Journal of Behavior Therapy and Experimental Psychiatry*, 15(4), 309–313.

Astin, J.A., Berman, B.M., Bausell, B., *et al.* (2003). The efficacy of mindfulness meditation plus Qigong movement therapy in the treatment of fibromyalgia: A randomized controlled trial. *Journal of Rheumatology*, 30(10), 2257–2262.

Avery, D.H., Holtzheimer, P.E. 3rd, Fawaz, W., *et al.* (2006). A controlled study of repetitive transcranial magnetic stimulation in medication-resistant major depression. *Biological Psychiatry*, 59(2) 187–194.

Bares, M., Kopecek, M., Novak, T., *et al.* (2009). Low frequency (1-Hz), right prefrontal repetitive transcranial magnetic stimulation (rTMS) compared with venlafaxine ER in the treatment of resistant depression: A double-blind, single-centre, randomized study. *Journal of Affective Disorders*, 118(1–3), 94–100.

Barker, W.A., Scott, J. and Eccleston, D. (1987). The Newcastle chronic depression study: Results of a treatment regimen. *International Clinical Psychopharmacology*, 2, 261–272.

Berman, R.M., Narasimhan, M., Sanacora, G., *et al.* (2000). A randomized clinical trial of repetitive transcranial magnetic stimulation in the treatment of major depression. *Biological Psychiatry*, 47(4), 332–337.

Boggio, P.S., Rigonatti, S.P., Ribeiro, R.B., *et al.* (2008). A randomized, double-blind clinical trial on the efficacy of cortical direct current stimulation for the treatment of major depression. *International Journal of Neuropsychopharmacology*, 11(2), 249–254.

Brent, D., Emslie, G., Clarke, G., *et al.* (2008). Switching to another SSRI or to venlafaxine with or without cognitive behavioral therapy for adolescents with SSRI-resistant depression: The TORDIA randomized controlled trial. *Journal of the American Medical Association*, 299(8), 901–913.

Bristow, M. (1995). Group cognitive therapy in chronic depression: Results from two intervention studies. *Behavioural and Cognitive Psychotherapy*, 23, 373–380.

Cooper, M. (1994). Cognitive behavioral therapy in an in-patient with chronic difficulties: A case report. *Behavioural and Cognitive Psychotherapy*, 22, 171–176.

Cuijpers, P., Dekker, J., Hollon, S.D. and Andersson, G. (2009). Adding psychotherapy to pharmacotherapy in the treatment of depressive disorders in adults: A meta-analysis. *Journal of Clinical Psychiatry*, 70(9), 1219–1229.

Davidson, J., McLeod, M., Law-Yone, B. and Linnoila, M. (1978). A comparison of electroconvulsive therapy and combined phenelzine-amitriptyline in refractory depression. *Archives of General Psychiatry*, 35(5), 639–642.

De Jong, R., Treiber, R. and Henrich, G. (1986). Effectiveness of two psychological treatments for inpatients with severe and chronic depressions. *Cognitive Therapy and Research*, 10, 645–663.

Dennehy, E.B., Schnyer, R., Bernstein, I.H., *et al.* (2009). The safety, acceptability, and effectiveness of acupuncture as an adjunctive treatment for acute symptoms in bipolar disorder. *Journal of Clinical Psychiatry*, 70(6), 897–905.

DeRubeis, R.J., Gelfand, L.A., Tang, T.Z. and Simons, A.D. (1989). Medications versus cognitive behavior therapy for severely depressed outpatients: Mega-analysis of four randomized comparisons. *American Journal of Psychiatry*, 156(7), 1007–1013.

Dinan, T.G. and Barry, S. (1989). A comparison of electroconvulsive therapy with a combined lithium and tricyclic combination among depressed tricyclic nonresponders. *Acta Psychiatrica Scandinavica*, 80(1), 97–100.

Dunn, A.L., Trivedi, M.H., Kampert, J.B., *et al.* (2005). Exercise treatment for depression: Efficacy and dose response. *American Journal of Preventive Medicine*, 28(1), 1–8.

Eschweiler, G.W., Vonthein, R., Bode, R., *et al.* (2007). Clinical efficacy and cognitive side effects of bifrontal versus right unilateral electroconvulsive therapy (ECT): A short-term randomised controlled trial in pharmaco-resistant major depression, *Journal of Affective Disorders*, 101(1–3), 149–157.

Fava, G.A., Savron, G., Grandi, S. and Rafanelli, C. (1997). Cognitive-behavioral management of drug-resistant major depressive disorder. *Journal of Clinical Psychiatry*, 58(6), 278–282.

Fennell, M.J. and Teasdale, J.D. (1982). Cognitive therapy with chronic, drug-refractory depressed outpatients: A note of caution. *Cognitive Therapy and Research*, 6, 455–460.

Fitzgerald, P.B., Brown, T.L., Marston, N.A., *et al.* (2003). Transcranial magnetic stimulation in the treatment of depression: A double-blind, placebo-controlled trial. *Archives of General Psychiatry*, 60(10), 1002–1008.

Fitzgerald, P.B., Hoy, K., McQueen, S., *et al.* (2009). A randomized trial of rTMS targeted with MRI based neuro-navigation in treatment-resistant depression. *Neuropsychopharmacology*, 34(5), 1255–1262.

Folkerts, H.W., Michael, N., Tolle, R., *et al.* (1997). Electroconvulsive therapy vs. paroxetine in treatment-resistant depression — a randomized study. *Acta Psychiatrica Scandinavica*, 96(5), 334–342.

George, M.S., Nahas, Z., Molloy, M., *et al.* (2000). A controlled trial of daily left prefrontal cortex TMS for treating depression. *Biological Psychiatry*, 8(10), 962–970.

George, M.S., Rush, A.J., Marangell, L.B., *et al.* (2005). A one-year comparison of vagus nerve stimulation with treatment as usual for treatment-resistant depression. *Biological Psychiatry*, 58(5), 364–373.

Golden, R.N., Gaynes, B.N., Ekstrom, R.D., *et al.* (2005). The efficacy of light therapy in the treatment of mood disorders: A review and meta-analysis of the evidence. *American Journal of Psychiatry*, 162(4), 656–662.

Grunhaus, L., Schreiber, S., Dolberg, O.T., *et al.* (2003). A randomized controlled comparison of electroconvulsive therapy and repetitive transcranial magnetic stimulation in severe and resistant nonpsychotic major depression. *Biological Psychiatry*, 53(4), 324–331.

Harpin, R., Liberman, R.P., Marks, I., *et al.* (1982). Cognitive behaviour therapy for chronically depressed patients: A controlled pilot study. *Journal of Nervous and Mental Disorders*, 170, 295–301.

Janakiramaiah, N., Gangadhar, B.N., Naga Venkatesha Murthy, P.J., *et al.* (2000). Antidepressant efficacy of Sudarshan Kriya Yoga (SKY) in melancholia: A randomized comparison with electroconvulsive therapy (ECT) and imipramine. *Journal of Affective Disorders*, 57(1–3), 255–259.

Jorge, R.E., Robinson, R.G., Tateno, A., *et al.* (2004). Repetitive transcranial magnetic stimulation as treatment of poststroke depression: A preliminary study. *Biological Psychiatry*, 55(4), 398–405.

Kauffmann, C.D., Cheema, M.A. and Miller, B.E. (2004). Slow right prefrontal transcranial magnetic stimulation as a treatment for medication-resistant depression: A double-blind, placebo-controlled study. *Depression and Anxiety*, 19(1), 59–62.

Kellner, C.H., Knapp, R.G., Petrides, G., *et al.* (2006). Continuation electroconvulsive therapy vs. pharmacotherapy for relapse prevention in major depression: A multisite study from the Consortium for Research in Electroconvulsive Therapy (CORE). *Archives of General Psychiatry*, 63(12), 1337–1344.

Lauritzen, L., Odgaard, K., Clemmesen, L., *et al.* (1996). Relapse prevention by means of paroxetine in ECT-treated patients with major depression: A comparison with imipramine and placebo in medium-term continuation therapy. *Acta Psychiatrica Scandinavica*, 94(4), 241–251.

Leykin, Y., Amsterdam, J.D., DeRubeis, R.J., *et al.* (2007). Progressive resistance to a selective serotonin reuptake inhibitor but not to cognitive therapy in the treatment of major depression. *Journal of Consulting and Clinical Psychology*, 75(2), 267–276.

Loo, C.K., Mitchell, P.B., Croker, V.M., *et al.* (2003). Double-blind controlled investigation of bilateral prefrontal transcranial magnetic stimulation for the treatment of resistant major depression. *Psychological Medicine*, 33(1), 33–40.

Loo, C.K. and Mitchell, P.B. (2005). A review of the efficacy of transcranial magnetic stimulation (TMS) treatment for depression, and current and future strategies to optimize efficacy. *Journal of Affective Disorders*, 88(3), 255–267.

Loo, C., Mitchell, P., Sachdev, P., *et al.* (1999). Double-blind controlled investigation of transcranial magnetic stimulation for the treatment of resistant major depression. *American Journal of Psychiatry*, 156(6), 946–948.

Malone, D.A. Jr., Dougherty, D.D., Rezai, A.R., *et al.* (2009). Deep brain stimulation of the ventral capsule/ventral striatum for treatment-resistant depression. *Biological Psychiatry*, 65(4), 267–275.

Manes, F., Jorge, R., Morcuende, M., *et al.* (2001). A controlled study of repetitive transcranial magnetic stimulation as a treatment of depression in the elderly. *International Psychogeriatrics*, 13(2), 225–231.

Mayberg, H.S., Lozano, A.M., Voon, V., *et al.* (2005). Deep brain stimulation for treatment-resistant depression. *Neuron*, 45(5), 651–660.

Miller, I.W., Bishop, S.B., Norman, W.H. and Keitner, G.I. (1985). Cognitive behavioral therapy and pharmacotherapy with chronic, drug-refractory depressed inpatients: A note of optimism. *Behavioural Psychotherapy*, 13, 320–327.

Miniussi, C., Bonato, C., Bignotti, S., *et al.* (2005). Repetitive transcranial magnetic stimulation (rTMS) at high and low frequency: An efficacious therapy for major drug-resistant depression? *Clinical Neurophysiology*, 116(5), 1062–1071.

Mirabel-Sarron, C., Morell, C. and Samuel-Lajeunesse, B. (1993). Beck's cognitive therapy for patients with pharmacotherapy-resistant chronic depression. *Annales Médico-Psychologiques*, 151, 697–701.

Nahas, Z., Marangell, L.B., Husain, M.M., *et al.* (2005). Two-year outcome of vagus nerve stimulation (VNS) for treatment of major depressive episodes. *Journal of Clinical Psychiatry*, 66(9), 1097–1104.

Neumeister, A., Goessler, R., Lucht, M., *et al.* (1996). Bright light therapy stabilizes the antidepressant effect of partial sleep deprivation. *Biological Psychiatry*, 39(1), 16–21.

O'reardon, J.P., Solvason, H.B., Janicak, P.G., *et al.* (2007). Efficacy and safety of transcranial magnetic stimulation in the acute treatment of major depression: A multisite randomized controlled trial. *Biological Psychiatry*, 62(11), 1208–1216.

Padberg, F., Zwanzger, P., Keck, M.E., *et al.* (2002). Repetitive transcranial magnetic stimulation (rTMS) in major depression: Relation between efficacy and stimulation intensity. *Neuropsychopharmacology*, 27(4), 638–645.

Padberg, F., Zwanzger, P., Thoma, H., *et al.* (1999). Repetitive transcranial magnetic stimulation (rTMS) in pharmacotherapy-refractory major depression: Comparative study of fast, slow and sham rTMS. *Psychiatry Research*, 88(3), 163–171.

Pampallona, S., Bollini, P., Tibaldi, G., *et al.* (2004). Combined pharmacotherapy and psychological treatment for depression: A systematic review. *Archives of General Psychiatry*, 61(7), 714–719.

Pascual-Leone, A., Rubio, B., Pallardo, F. and Catala, M.D. (1996). Rapid-rate transcranial magnetic stimulation of left dorsolateral prefrontal cortex in drug-resistant depression. *The Lancet*, 348(9022), 233–227.

Rush, A.J., George, M.S., Sackeim, H.A., *et al.* (2000). Vagus nerve stimulation (VNS) for treatment-resistant depressions: A multicenter study. *Biological Psychiatry*, 47(4), 276–286.

Rush, A.J., Marangell, L.B., Sackeim, H.A., *et al.* (2005a). Vagus nerve stimulation for treatment-resistant depression: A randomized, controlled acute phase trial. *Biological Psychiatry*, 58(5), 347–354.

Rush, A.J., Sackeim, H.A., Marangell, L.B., *et al.* (2005b). Effects of 12 months of vagus nerve stimulation in treatment-resistant depression: A naturalistic study. *Biological Psychiatry*, 58(5), 355–363.

Sackeim, H.A., Dillingham, E.M., Prudic, J., *et al.* (2009). Effect of concomitant pharmacotherapy on electroconvulsive therapy outcomes: Short-term efficacy and adverse effects. *Archives of General Psychiatry*, 66(7), 729–737.

Sackeim, H.A., Haskett, R.F., Mulsant, B.H., *et al.* (2001a). Continuation pharmacotherapy in the prevention of relapse following electroconvulsive therapy: A randomized controlled trial. *Journal of the American Medical Association*, 285(10), 1299–1307.

Sackeim, H.A., Rush, A.J., George, M.S., *et al.* (2001b). Vagus nerve stimulation (VNS) for treatment-resistant depression: Efficacy, side effects, and predictors of outcome. *Neuropsychopharmacology*, 25(5), 713–728.

Schatzberg, A.F., Rush, A.J., Arnow, B.A., *et al.* (2005). Chronic depression: Medication (nefazodone) or psychotherapy (CBASP) is effective when the other is not. *Archives of General Psychiatry*, 62(5), 513–520.

Scott, J. (1992). Chronic depression: Can cognitive therapy succeed when other treatments fail? *Behavioural Psychotherapy*, 20, 25–36.

Seager, C.P. and Bird, R.L. (1962). Imipramine with electrical treatment in depression — a controlled trial. *Journal of Mental Science*, 108, 704–707.

Sephton, S.E., Salmon, P., Weissbecker, I., *et al.* (2007). Mindfulness meditation alleviates depressive symptoms in women with fibromyalgia: Results of a randomized clinical trial. *Arthritis and Rheumatism*, 57(1), 77–85.

Sharma, V.K., Das, S., Mondal, S., *et al.* (2006). Effect of Sahaj Yoga on neurocognitive functions in patients suffering from major depression. *Indian Journal of Physiology and Pharmacology*, 50(4), 375–383.

Steiner, M., Radwan, M., Elizur, A., *et al.* (1978). Failure of l-triiodothyronine to potentiate tricyclic antidepressant response. *Current Therapeutic Research*, 23(5), 655–659.

Thase, M.E., Friedman, E.S., Biggs, M.M., *et al.* (2007). Cognitive therapy versus medication in augmentation and switch strategies as second-step treatments: A STAR*D report. *American Journal of Psychiatry*, 164(5), 739–752.

Thase, M.E., Greenhouse, J.B., Frank, E., *et al.* (1997). Treatment of major depression with psychotherapy or psychotherapy-pharmacotherapy combinations. *Archives of General Psychiatry*, 54(11), 1009–1015.

Thase, M.E. and Howland, R.H. (1994). Refractory depression: Relevance of psychosocial factors and therapies. *Psychiatric Annals*, 24, 232–240.

Trivedi, M.H., Greer, T.L., Grannemann, B.D., *et al.* (2006). Exercise as an augmentation strategy for treatment of major depression. *Journal of Psychiatric Practice*, 12(4), 205–213.

U.K. E.C.T. Review Group. (2003). Efficacy and safety of electroconvulsive therapy in depressive disorders: A systematic review and meta-analysis. *The Lancet*, 361(9360), 799–808.

van den Broek, W.W., Birkenhager, T.K., Mulder, P.G., *et al.* (2006). Imipramine is effective in preventing relapse in electroconvulsive therapy-responsive depressed inpatients with prior pharmacotherapy treatment failure: A randomized, placebo-controlled trial. *Journal of Clinical Psychiatry*, 67(2), 263–268.

Zhang, W.J., Yang, X.B. and Zhong, B.L. (2009). Combination of acupuncture and fluoxetine for depression: A randomized, double-blind, sham-controlled trial. *J Alternative and Complementary Medicine*, 15(8), 837–844.

Introduction to Part III

Kocsis, J.H., Schatzberg, A., Rush, A.J., *et al.* (2002). Psychosocial outcomes following long-term, double-blind treatment of chronic depression with sertraline versus placebo. *Archives of General Psychiatry*, 59(8), 723–728.

Lavori, P.W., Keller, M.B. and Klerman, G.L. (1984). Relapse in affective disorders: A reanalysis of the literature using life table methods. *Journal of Psychiatric Research*, 18(1), 13–25.

Solomon, D.A., Keller, M.B., Leon, A.C., *et al.* (2000). Multiple recurrences of major depressive disorder. *American Journal of Psychiatry*, 157(2), 229–233.

Chapter 9

Alexopoulos, G.S., Meyers, B.S., Young, R.C., *et al.* (2000). Executive dysfunction and long-term outcomes of geriatric depression. *Archives of General Psychiatry*, 57(3), 285–290.

Amsterdam, J.D. and Bodkin, J.A. (2006). Selegiline transdermal system in the prevention of relapse of major depressive disorder: A 52-week, double-blind, placebo-substitution, parallel-group clinical trial. *Journal of Clinical Psychopharmacology*, 26(6), 579–586.

Amsterdam, J., Brunswick, D.J. and Gilbertini, M. (2004). Sustained efficacy of gepirone-IR in major depressive disorder: A double-blind placebo substitution trial. *Journal of Psychiatric Research*, 38(3), 259–265.

Anton, S.F., Robinson, D.S., Roberts, D.L., *et al.* (1994). Long-term treatment of depression with nefazodone. *Psychopharmacology Bulletin*, 30(2), 165–169.

Bauer, M., Bschor, T., Kunz, D., *et al.* (2000). Double-blind, placebo-controlled trial of the use of lithium to augment antidepressant medication in continuation treatment of unipolar major depression. *American Journal of Psychiatry*, 157(9), 1429–1435.

Bialos, D., Giller, E., Jatlow, P., *et al.* (1982). Recurrence of depression after discontinuation of long-term amitriptyline treatment. *American Journal of Psychiatry*, 139(3), 325–329.

Bjork, K. (1983). The efficacy of zimeldine in preventing depressive episodes in recurrent major depressive disorders — a double-blind placebo-controlled study. *Acta Psychiatrica Scandinavica Supplementum*, 308, 182–189.

Claghorn, J.L. and Feighner, J.P. (1993). A double-blind comparison of paroxetine with imipramine in the long-term treatment of depression. *Journal of Clinical Psychopharmacology*, 13(6 Suppl 2), 23S–27S.

Cohen, B.M. and Baldessarini, R.J. (1985). Tolerance to therapeutic effects of antidepressants. *American Journal of Psychiatry*, 142(4), 489–490.

Cook, B.L., Helms, P.M., Smith, R.E. and Tsai, M. (1986). Unipolar depression in the elderly. Reoccurrence on discontinuation of tricyclic antidepressants. *Journal of Affective Disorders*, 10(2), 91–94.

Coppen, A., Ghose, K., Montgomery, S., *et al.* (1978). Continuation therapy with amitriptyline in depression. *British Journal of Psychiatry*, 133, 28–33.

Dalery, J., Dagens-Lafont, V. and De Bodinat, C. (2001). Efficacy of tianeptine vs placebo in the long-term treatment (16.5 months) of unipolar major recurrent depression. *Human Psychopharmacology*, 16(S1), S39–S47.

Davidson, J. and Raft, D. (1984). Use of phenelzine in continuation therapy. *Neuropsychobiology*, 11(3), 191–194.

Doogan, D.P. and Caillard, V. (1992). Sertraline in the prevention of depression. *British Journal of Psychiatry*, 160, 217–222.

Emslie, G.J., Heiligenstein, J.H., Hoog, S.L., *et al.* (2004). Fluoxetine treatment for prevention of relapse of depression in children and adolescents: A double-blind, placebo-controlled study. *Journal of the American Academy of Child and Adolescent Psychiatry*, 43(11), 1397–1405.

Emslie, G.J., Kennard, B.D., Mayes, T.L., *et al.* (2008). Fluoxetine versus placebo in preventing relapse of major depression in children and adolescents. *American Journal of Psychiatry*, 165(4), 459–467.

Faravelli, C., Ambonetti, A., Pallanti, S. and Pazzagli, A. (1986). Depressive relapses and incomplete recovery from index episode. *American Journal of Psychiatry*, 143(7), 888–891.

Fava, M., Detke, M.J., Balestrieri, M., *et al.* (2006). Management of depression relapse: Re-initiation of duloxetine treatment or dose increase. *Journal of Psychiatric Research*, 40(4), 328–336.

Fava, M., Rappe, S.M., Pava, J.A., *et al.* (1995). Relapse in patients on long-term fluoxetine treatment: Response to increased fluoxetine dose. *Journal of Clinical Psychiatry*, 56(2), 52–55.

Fava, M., Schmidt, M.E., Zhang, S., *et al.* (2002). Treatment approaches to major depressive disorder relapse. Part 2: Reinitiation of antidepressant treatment. *Psychotherapy and Psychosomatics*, 71(4), 195–199.

Feiger, A.D., Bielski, R.J., Bremner, J., *et al.* (1999). Double-blind, placebo-substitution study of nefazodone in the prevention of relapse during continuation treatment of outpatients with major depression. *International Clinical Psychopharmacology*, 14(1), 19–28.

Ferreri, M., Colonna, L. and Leger, J.M. (1997). Efficacy of amineptine in the prevention of relapse in unipolar depression. *International Clinical Psychopharmacology*, 12(Suppl 3), S39–45.

Fieve, R.R., Dunner, D.L., Kumbarachi, T. and Stallone, F. (1975). Lithium carbonate in affective disorders. IV. A double-blind study of prophylaxis in unipolar recurrent depression. *Archives of General Psychiatry*, 32(12), 1541–1544.

Flint, A.J. and Rifat, S.L. (2001). Nonresponse to first-line pharmacotherapy may predict relapse and recurrence of remitted geriatric depression. *Depression and Anxiety*, 13(3), 125–131.

Franchini, L., Gasperini, M., Perez, J., *et al.* (1998). Dose-response efficacy of paroxetine in preventing depressive recurrences: A randomized, double-blind study. *Journal of Clinical Psychiatry*, 59(5), 229–232.

Franchini, L., Rossini, D., Bongiorno, F., *et al.* (2000). Will a second prophylactic treatment with a higher dosage of the same antidepressant either prevent or delay new depressive episodes? *Psychiatry Research*, 96(1), 81–85.

Frank, E., Kupfer, D.J., Perel, J.M., *et al.* (1990). Three-year outcomes for maintenance therapies in recurrent depression. *Archives of General Psychiatry*, 47(12), 1093–1099.

Frank, E., Kupfer, D.J., Perel, J.M., *et al.* (1993). Comparison of full-dose versus half-dose pharmacotherapy in the maintenance treatment of recurrent depression. *Journal of Affective Disorders*, 27(3), 139–145.

Geddes, J.R., Carney, S.M., Davies, C., *et al.* (2003). Relapse prevention with antidepressant drug treatment in depressive disorders: A systematic review. *The Lancet*, 361(9358), 653–661.

Gelenberg, A.J., Trivedi, M.H., Rush, A.J., *et al.* (2003). Randomized, placebo-controlled trial of nefazodone maintenance treatment in preventing recurrence in chronic depression. *Biological Psychiatry*, 54(8), 806–817.

Gilaberte, I., Montejo, A.L., de la Gandara, J., *et al.* (2001). Fluoxetine in the prevention of depressive recurrences: A double-blind study. *Journal of Clinical Psychopharmacology*, 21(4), 417–424.

Goodwin, G.M., Emsley, R., Rembry, S., *et al.* (2009). Agomelatine prevents relapse in patients with major depressive disorder without evidence of a discontinuation syndrome: A 24-week randomized, double-blind, placebo-controlled trial. *Journal of Clinical Psychiatry*, 70(8), 1128–1137.

Gorwood, P., Weiller, E., Lemming, O. and Katona, C. (2007). Escitalopram prevents relapse in older patients with major depressive disorder. *American Journal of Geriatric Psychiatry*, 15(7), 581–593.

Hardy, B.G., Shulman, K.I. and Zucchero, C. (1997). Gradual discontinuation of lithium augmentation in elderly patients with unipolar depression. *Journal of Clinical Psychopharmacology*, 17(1), 22–26.

Harrison, W., Rabkin, J., Stewart, J.W., *et al.* (1986). Phenelzine for chronic depression: A study of continuation treatment. *Journal of Clinical Psychiatry*, 47(7), 346–349.

Hochstrasser, B., Isaksen, P.M., Koponen, H., *et al.* (2001). Prophylactic effect of citalopram in unipolar, recurrent depression: Placebo-controlled study of maintenance therapy. *British Journal of Psychiatry*, 178, 304–310.

Kamijima, K., Burt, T., Cohen, G., *et al.* (2006). A placebo-controlled, randomized withdrawal study of sertraline for major depressive disorder in Japan. *International Clinical Psychopharmacology*, 21(1), 1–9.

Kanai, T., Takeuchi, H., Furukawa, T.A., *et al.* (2003). Time to recurrence after recovery from major depressive episodes and its predictors. *Psychological Medicine*, 33(5), 839–845.

Keller, M.B., Kocsis, J.H., Thase, M.E., *et al.* (1998). Maintenance phase efficacy of sertraline for chronic depression: A randomized controlled trial. *Journal of the American Medical Association*, 280(19), 1665–1672.

Keller, M.B., Ruwe, F.J., Janssens, C.J., *et al.* (2005). Relapse prevention with gepirone ER in outpatients with major depression. *Journal of Clinical Psychopharmacology*, 25(1), 79–84.

Keller, M.B., Trivedi, M.H., Thase, M.E., *et al.* (2007a). The prevention of recurrent episodes of depression with venlafaxine for two years (PREVENT) study: Outcomes from the 2-year and combined maintenance phases. *Journal of Clinical Psychiatry*, 68(8), 1246–1256.

Keller, M.B., Trivedi, M.H., Thase, M.E., *et al.* (2007b). The prevention of recurrent episodes of depression with venlafaxine for two years (PREVENT) study: Outcomes from the acute and continuation phases. *Biological Psychiatry*, 62(12):1371–1379.

Kishimoto, A., Mizukawa, R., Matsuzaki, F., *et al.* (1994). Prophylactic effect of mianserin on recurrent depression. *Acta Psychiatrica Scandinavica*, 89(1), 46–51.

Klerman, G.L., Dimascio, A., Weissman, M., *et al.* (1974). Treatment of depression by drugs and psychotherapy. *American Journal of Psychiatry*, 131(2), 186–191.

Klysner, R., Bent-Hansen, J., Hansen, H.L., *et al.* (2002). Efficacy of citalopram in the prevention of recurrent depression in elderly patients: Placebo-controlled study of maintenance therapy. *British Journal of Psychiatry*, 181, 29–35.

Kocsis, J.H., Friedman, R.A., Markowitz, J.C., *et al.* (1996). Maintenance therapy for chronic depression. A controlled clinical trial of desipramine. *Archives of General Psychiatry*, 53(9), 769–774.

Kocsis, J.H., Thase, M.E., Trivedi, M.H., *et al.* (2007). Prevention of recurrent episodes of depression with venlafaxine ER in a 1-year maintenance phase from the PREVENT Study. *Journal of Clinical Psychiatry*, 68(7), 1014–1023.

Koran, L.M., Gelenberg, A.J., Kornstein, S.G., *et al.* (2001). Sertraline versus imipramine to prevent relapse in chronic depression. *Journal of Affective Disorders*, 65(1), 27–36.

Kornstein, S.G., Bose, A., Li, D., *et al.* (2006). Escitalopram Maintenance treatment for prevention of recurrent depression: A randomized, placebo-controlled trial. *Journal of Clinical Psychiatry*, 67(11), 1767–1775.

Kupfer, D.J., Frank, E., Perel, J.M., *et al.* (1992). Five-year outcome for maintenance therapies in recurrent depression. *Archives of General Psychiatry*, 49(10), 769–773.

Lepine, J.P., Caillard, V., Bisserbe, J.C., *et al.* (2004). A randomized, placebo-controlled trial of sertraline for prophylactic treatment of highly recurrent major depressive disorder. *American Journal of Psychiatry*, 161(5), 836–842.

Lonnqvist, J., Sihvo, S., Syvalahti, E., *et al.* (1995). Moclobemide and fluoxetine in the prevention of relapses following acute treatment of depression. *Acta Psychiatrica Scandinavica*, 91(3), 189–194.

Mann, J.J. (1983). Loss of antidepressant effect with long-term monoamine oxidase inhibitor treatment without loss of monoamine oxidase inhibition. *Journal of Clinical Psychopharmacology*, 3(6), 363–366.

McGrath, P.J., Fava, M., Nierenberg, A.A., *et al.* (2002). Bupropion SR for relapses of MDD during or after fluoxetine treatment. Presented at the 42th Annual Meeting of the New Clinical Drug Evaluation Unit of the National Institute of Mental Health. Boca Raton, Florida.

McGrath, P.J., Quitkin, F.M. and Klein, D.F. (1995). Bromocriptine treatment of relapses seen during selective serotonin re-uptake inhibitor treatment of depression. *Journal of Clinical Psychopharmacology*, 15(4), 289–291.

McGrath, P.J., Stewart, J.W., Petkova, E., *et al.* (2000). Predictors of relapse during fluoxetine continuation or maintenance treatment of major depression. *Journal of Clinical Psychiatry*, 61(7), 518–524.

McGrath, P.J., Stewart, J.W., Quitkin, F.M., *et al.* (2006). Predictors of relapse in a prospective study of fluoxetine treatment of major depression. *American Journal of Psychiatry*, 163(9), 1542–1548.

Mindham, R.H., Howland, C. and Shepherd, M. (1973). An evaluation of continuation therapy with tricyclic antidepressants in depressive illness. *Psychological Medicine*, 3(1), 5–17.

Mindham, R.H., Howland, C. and Shepherd, M. (1972). Continuation therapy with tricyclic antidepressants in depressive illness. *The Lancet*, 2(7782), 854–855.

Montgomery, S.A., Dufour, H., Brion, S., *et al.* (1988). The prophylactic efficacy of fluoxetine in unipolar depression. *British Journal of Psychiatry Supplementum*, 3, 69–76.

Montgomery, S.A. and Dunbar, G. (1993). Paroxetine is better than placebo in relapse prevention and the prophylaxis of recurrent depression. *International Clinical Psychopharmacology*, 8(3), 189–195.

Montgomery, S.A., Entsuah, R., Hackett, D., *et al.* (2004). Venlafaxine versus placebo in the preventitive treatment of recurrent major depression. *Journal of Clinical Psychiatry*, 65(3), 328–336.

Montgomery, S.A. and Rasmussen, J.G. (1992). Citalopram 20 mg, citalopram 40 mg and placebo in the prevention of relapse of major depression. *International Clinical Psychopharmacology*, 6 (Suppl 5), 71–73.

Montgomery, S.A., Rasmussen, J.G. andTanghoj, P. (1993). A 24-week study of 20 mg citalopram, 40 mg citalopram, and placebo in the prevention of relapse of major depression. *International Clinical Psychopharmacology*, 8(3), 181–188.

Montgomery, S.A., Reimitz, P.E. and Zivkov, M. (1998). Mirtazapine versus amitriptyline in the long-term treatment of depression: A double-blind placebo-controlled study. *International Clinical Psychopharmacology*, 13(2), 63–73.

Nemeroff, C.B., Evans, D.L., Gyulai, L., *et al.* (2001). Double-blind, placebo-controlled comparison of imipramine and paroxetine in the treatment of bipolar depression. *American Journal of Psychiatry*, 158(6), 906–912.

Nierenberg, A.A. and DeCecco, L.M. (2001). Definitions of antidepressant treatment response, remission, nonresponse, partial response, and other relevant outcomes: A focus on treatment-resistant depression. *Journal of Clinical Psychiatry*, 62(Suppl 16), 5–9.

Nierenberg, A.A., Price, L.H., Charney, D.S. and Heninger, G.R. (1990). After lithium augmentation: A retrospective follow-up of patients with antidepressant-refractory depression. *Journal of Affective Disorders*, 18(3), 167–175.

Nierenberg, A.A., Quitkin, F.M., Kremer, C., *et al.* (2004). Placebo-controlled continuation treatment with mirtazapine: Acute pattern of response predicts relapse. Neuropsychopharmacology. Placebo-controlled continuation treatment with mirtazapine: Acute pattern of response predicts relapse. *Neuropsychopharmacology*, 29(5), 1012–1018.

Papakostas, G.I., Perlis, R.H., Seifert, C. and Fava, M. (2007a). Antidepressant dose reduction and the risk of relapse in major depressive disorder. *Psychotherapy and Psychosomatics*, 76(5), 266–270.

Papakostas, G.I., Petersen, T., Sklarsky, K.G., *et al.* (2007b). Timing of clinical improvement and symptom resolution in the treatment of major depressive disorder. *Psychiatry Research*, 149(1–3), 195–200.

Papakostas, G.I., Petersen, T., Worthington, J.J., *et al.* (2003). A pilot, open study of sertraline in outpatients with treatment-resistant depression (TRD) or with a history of TRD who responded but later relapsed. *International Clinical Psychopharmacology*, 18(5), 293–296.

Paykel, E.S., Ramana, R., Cooper, Z., *et al.* (1995). Residual symptoms after partial remission: An important outcome in depression. *Psychological Medicine*, 25(6), 1171–1180.

Perahia, D.G., Gilaberte, I., Wang, F., *et al.* (2006). Duloxetine in the prevention of relapse of major depressive disorder: Double-blind placebo-controlled study. *British Journal of Psychiatry*, 188, 346–353.

Perahia, D.G., Maina, G., Thase, M.E., *et al.* (2009). Duloxetine in the prevention of depressive recurrences: A randomized, double-blind, placebo-controlled trial. *Journal of Clinical Psychiatry*, 70(5), 706–716.

Petersen, T., Pava, J.A., Buchin, J., *et al.* (in press). The role of cognitive-behavioral therapy and fluoxetine in prevention of recurrence of major depressive disorder. *Cognitive Therapy and Research*.

Prien, R.F. and Kupfer, D.J. (1986). Continuation drug therapy for major depressive episodes: How long should it be maintained? *American Journal of Psychiatry*, 143(1), 18–23.

Prien, R.F., Kupfer, D.J., Mansky, P.A., *et al.* (1984). Drug therapy in the prevention of recurrences in unipolar and bipolar affective disorders. Report of the NIMH Collaborative Study Group comparing lithium carbonate, imipramine, and a lithium carbonate-imipramine combination. *Archives of General Psychiatry*, 41(11), 1096–1104.

Rapaport, M.H., Bose, A. and Zheng, H. (2004). Escitalopram continuation treatment prevents relapse of depressive episodes. *Journal of Clinical Psychiatry*, 65(1), 44–49.

Rapaport, M.H., Gharabawi, G.M., Canuso, C.M., *et al.* (2006). Effects of risperidone augmentation in patients with treatment-resistant depression: Results of open-label treatment followed by double-blind continuation. *Neuropsychopharmacology*, 31(11), 2505–2513.

Rasmussen, K.G., Mueller, M., Rummans, T.A., *et al.* (2009). Is baseline medication resistance associated with potential relapse after successful remission of a depressive episode with ECT? Data from the consortium for research on electroconvulsive therapy (CORE). *Journal of Clinical Psychiatry*, 70(2), 232–237.

Reimherr, F.W., Amsterdam, J.D., Quitkin, F.M., *et al.* (1998). Optimal length of continuation therapy in depression: A prospective assessment during long-term fluoxetine treatment. *American Journal of Psychiatry*, 155(9), 1247–1253.

Remillard, A.J., Blackshaw, S.L. and Dangor, A. (1994). Differential responses to a single antidepressant in recurrent episodes of major depression. *Hospital and Community Psychiatry*, 45(4), 359–361.

Reynolds, C.F. 3rd, Dew, M.A., Pollock, B.G., *et al.* (2006). Maintenance treatment of major depression in old age. *New England Journal of Medicine*, 354(11), 1130–1138.

Reynolds, C.F. 3rd, Frank E., Perel, J.M., *et al.* (1999). Nortriptyline and interpersonal psychotherapy as maintenance therapies for recurrent major depression: A randomized controlled trial in patients older than 59 years. *Journal of the American Medical Association*, 281(1), 39–45.

Reynolds, C.F. 3rd, Frank, E., Perel, J.M., *et al.* (1996). High relapse rate after discontinuation of adjunctive medication for elderly patients with recurrent major depression. *American Journal of Psychiatry*, 153(11), 1418–1422.

Rickels, K., Montgomery, S.A., Guelfi, J.D., *et al.* (2007). A multicenter, randomized, double-blind, placebo-controlled, parallel-group study of desvenlafaxine succinate for prevention of depressive relapse in adult outpatients with major depressive disorder. Presented at the 160th

Annual Meeting of the American Psychiatric Association. San Diego, California.

Robert, P. and Montgomery, S.A. (1995). Citalopram in doses of 20–60 mg is effective in depression relapse prevention: A placebo-controlled 6 month study. *International Clinical Psychopharmacology*, 10(Suppl 1), 29–35.

Robinson, D.S., Lerfald, S.C., Bennett, B., *et al*. (1991). Continuation and maintenance treatment of major depression with the monoamine oxidase inhibitor phenelzine: A double-blind placebo-controlled discontinuation study. *Psychopharmacology Bulletin*, 27(1), 31–39.

Rouillon, F., Phillips, R., Serruirier, D., *et al*. (1991b). Rechutes de depression unipolaire et efficacite de la Maprotiline. *Encephale*, 15, 527–534.

Rouillon, F., Serrurier, D., Miller, H.D. and Gerard, M.J. (1991a) Prophylactic efficacy of maprotiline on unipolar depression relapse. *Journal of Clinical Psychiatry*, 52(10), 423–431.

Rouillon, F., Warner, B., Pezous, N. and Bisserbe, J.C. (2000). Milnacipran efficacy in the prevention of recurrent depression: A 12-month placebo-controlled study. Milnacipran recurrence prevention study group. *International Clinical Psychopharmacology*, 15(3), 133–140.

Rush, A.J., Trivedi, M.H., Wisniewski, S.R., *et al*. (2006). Acute and longer-term outcomes in depressed outpatients requiring one or several treatment steps: A STAR*D report. *American Journal of Psychiatry*, 163(11), 1905–1917.

Schmidt, M.E., Fava, M., Robinson, J.M. and Judge, R. (2000) The efficacy and safety of a new enteric-coated formulation of fluoxetine given once weekly during the continuation treatment of major depressive disorder. *Journal of Clinical Psychiatry*, 61(11), 851–857.

Schmidt, M.E., Fava, M., Zhang, S., *et al*. (2002). Treatment approaches to major depressive disorder relapse. Part 1: Dose increase. *Psychotherapy and Psychosomatics*, 71(4), 190–194.

Simons, A.D., Murphy, G.E., Levine, J.L. and Wetzel, R.D. (1986). Cognitive therapy and pharmacotherapy for depression. Sustained improvement over one year. *Archives of General Psychiatry*, 43(1), 43–48.

Souza, F.G., Mander, A.J. and Goodwin, G.M. (1990). The efficacy of lithium in prophylaxis of unipolar depression Evidence from its discontinuation. *British Journal of Psychiatry*, 157, 718–722.

Stein, M.K., Rickels, K. and Weise, C.C. (1980). Maintenance therapy with amitriptyline: A controlled trial. *American Journal of Psychiatry*, 137(3), 370–371.

Stewart, J.W., Quitkin, F.M., McGrath, P.J., *et al*. (1998). Use of pattern analysis to predict differential relapse of remitted patients with major depression during 1 year of treatment with fluoxetine or placebo. *Archives of General Psychiatry*, 55(4), 334–343.

Stewart, J.W., Tricamo, E., McGrath, P.J. and Quitkin, F.M. (1997). Prophylactic efficacy of phenelzine and imipramine in chronic atypical depression: Likelihood of recurrence on discontinuation after 6 months' remission. *American Journal of Psychiatry*, 154(1), 31–36.

Terra, J.L. and Montgomery, S.A. (1998). Fluvoxamine prevents recurrence of depression: Results of a long-term, double-blind, placebo-controlled study. *International Clinical Psychopharmacology*, 13(2), 55–62.

Thase, M.E., Nierenberg, A.A., Keller, M.B., *et al.* (2001). Efficacy of mirtazapine for prevention of depressive relapse: A placebo-controlled double-blind trial of recently remitted high-risk patients. *Journal of Clinical Psychiatry*, 62(10), 782–788.

Versiani, M., Mehilane, L., Gaszner, P. and Arnaud-Castiglioni, R. (1999). Reboxetine, a unique selective NRI, prevents relapse and recurrence in long-term treatment of major depressive disorder. *Journal of Clinical Psychiatry*, 60(6), 400–406.

Weihs, K.L., Houser, T.L., Batey, S.R., *et al.* (2002). Continuation phase treatment with bupropion SR effectively decreases the risk for relapse of depression. *Biological Psychiatry*, 51(9), 753–761.

Zetin, M., Aden, G. and Moldawsky, R. (1983). Tolerance to amoxapine antidepressant effects. *Clinical Therapeutics*, 5(6), 638–643.

Chapter 10

Adson, D.E., Kushner, M.G. and Fahnhorst, T.A. (2005). Treatment of residual anxiety symptoms with adjunctive aripiprazole in depressed patients taking selective serotonin reuptake inhibitors. *Journal of Affective Disorders*, 86(1), 99–104.

Aizenberg, D., Zemishlany, Z. and Weizman, A. (1995). Cyproheptadine treatment of sexual dysfunction induced by serotonin reuptake inhibitors. *Clinical Neuropharmacology*, 18(4), 320–324.

Alevizos, B., Vaidakis, N. and Alevizos, E. (2005). Increased libido with the combined use of venlafaxine and mirtazapine. *Journal of Clinical Psychopharmacology*, 25(2), 194–196.

Alvarez-Jimenez, M., Gonzalez-Blanch, C., Vazquez-Barquero, J.L., *et al.* (2006). Attenuation of antipsychotic-induced weight gain with early behavioral intervention in drug-naive first-episode psychosis patients: A randomized controlled trial. *Journal of Clinical Psychiatry*, 67(8), 1253–1260.

Amsterdam, J.D., Hornig-Rohan, M. and Maislin, G. (1994). Efficacy of alprazolam in reducing fluoxetine-induced jitteriness in patients with major depression. *Journal of Clinical Psychiatry*, 55(9), 394–400.

Anghelescu, I., Klawe, C. and Benkert, O. (2000). Orlistat in the treatment of psychopharmacologically induced weight gain. *Journal of Clinical Psychopharmacology*, 20(6), 716–717.

Anghelescu, I. and Urbanek, C. (2005). Tadalafil in a patient with treatment-resistant depression and antidepressant polypharmacy. *Journal of Clinical Psychopharmacology*, 25(2), 191–192.

Arnott, S., Nutt, D. (1994). Successful treatment of fluvoxamine-induced anorgasmia by cyproheptadine. *British Journal of Psychiatry*, 164(6), 838–839.

Ashton, A.K. (2004). Modafinil augmentation of phenelzine for residual fatigue in dysthymia. *American Journal of Psychiatry*, 161(9), 1716–1717.

Ashton, A.K. (1999). Sildenafil treatment of paroxetine-induced anorgasmia in a woman. *American Journal of Psychiatry*, 156(5), 800.

Ashton, A.K., Ahrens, K., Gupta, S. and Masand, P.S. (2000). Antidepressant-induced sexual dysfunction and Ginkgo Biloba. *American Journal of Psychiatry*, 157(5), 836–837.

Ashton, A.K. and Bennett, R.G. (1999). Sildenafil treatment of serotonin reuptake inhibitor-induced sexual dysfunction. *Journal of Clinical Psychiatry*, 60(3), 194–195.

Ashton, A.K. and Rosen, R.C. (1998). Bupropion as an antidote for serotonin reuptake inhibitor-induced sexual dysfunction. *Journal of Clinical Psychiatry*, 59(3), 112–115.

Asnis, G.M., Chakraburtty, A., DuBoff, E.A., *et al.* (1999). Zolpidem for persistent insomnia in SSRI-treated depressed patients. *Journal of Clinical Psychiatry*, 60(10), 668–676.

Bagheri, H., Picault, P., Schmitt, L., *et al.* (1994). Pharmacokinetic study of yohimbine and its pharmacodynamic effects on salivary secretion in patients treated with tricyclic antidepressants. *British Journal of Clinical Pharmacology*, 37(1), 93–96.

Bagheri, H., Schmitt, L., Berlan, M. and Montastruc, J.L. (1997). A comparative study of the effects of yohimbine and anetholtrithione on salivary secretion in depressed patients treated with psychotropic drugs. *European Journal of Clinical Pharmacology*, 52(5), 339–342.

Bagheri, H., Schmitt, L., Berlan, M. and Montastruc, J.L. (1992). Effect of 3 weeks treatment with yohimbine on salivary secretion in healthy volunteers and in depressed patients treated with tricyclic antidepressants. *British Journal of Clinical Pharmacology*, 34(6), 555–558.

Bahk, W.M., Lee, K.U., Chae, J.H., *et al.* (2004). Open label study of the effect of amantadine on weight gain induced by olanzapine. *Psychiatry and Clinical Neurosciences*, 58(2), 163–167.

Baldwin, D.S., Hutchinson, J., Donaldson, K., *et al.* (2008). Selective serotonin re-uptake inhibitor treatment-emergent sexual dysfunction: Randomized double-blind placebo-controlled parallel-group fixed-dose study of a potential adjuvant compound, VML-670. *Journal of Psychopharmacology*, 22(1), 55–63.

Balogh, S., Hendricks, S.E. and Kang, J. (1992). Treatment of fluoxetine-induced anorgasmia with amantadine. *Journal of Clinical Psychiatry*, 53(6), 212–213.

Balon, R. (1993). Fluoxetine-induced sexual dysfunction and yohimbine. *Journal of Clinical Psychiatry*, 54(4), 161–162.

Balon, R. (1998). Fluvoxamine-induced erectile dysfunction responding to sildenafil. *Journal of Sex and Marital Therapy*, 24(4), 313–317.

Balon, R. (1996). Intermittent amantadine for fluoxetine-induced anorgasmia. *Journal of Sex and Marital Therapy*, 22(4), 290–292.

Balon, R. (1999). Sildenafil and sexual dysfunction associated with antidepressants. *Journal of Sex and Marital Therapy*, 25(4), 259–264.

Baptista, T., Martinez, J., Lacruz, A., *et al.* (2006). Metformin for prevention of weight gain and insulin resistance with olanzapine: A double-blind placebo-controlled trial. *Canadian Journal of Psychiatry*, 51(3), 192–196.

Baptista, T., Rangel, N., Fernandez, V., *et al.* (2007). Metformin as an adjunctive treatment to control body weight and metabolic dysfunction during olanzapine administration: A multicentric, double-blind, placebo-controlled trial. *Schizophrenia Research*, 93(1–3), 99–108.

Bartlik, B.D., Kaplan, P. and Kaplan, H.S. (1995). Psychostimulants apparently reverse sexual dysfunction secondary to selective serotonin reuptake inhibitors. *Journal of Sex and Marital Therapy*, 21(4), 264–271.

Berigan, T.R. (2001). Augmentation with modafinil to achieve remission in depression: A case report. *Primary Care Companion of the Journal of Clinical Psychiatry*, 3(1), 32.

Bertschy, G., Ragama-Pardos, E., Muscionico, M., *et al.* (2005). Trazodone addition for insomnia in venlafaxine-treated, depressed inpatients: A semi-naturalistic study. *Pharmacology Research*, 51(1), 79–84.

Bostwick, J.M. and Jaffee, M.S. (1999). Buspirone as an antidote to SSRI-induced bruxism in 4 cases. *Journal of Clinical Psychiatry*, 60(12), 857–860.

Brown, W.A. and Harrison, W. (1995). Are patients who are intolerant to one serotonin selective reuptake inhibitor intolerant to another? *Journal of Clinical Psychiatry*, 56(1), 30–34.

Brubaker, R.V. (2002). Fluoxetine-induced sexual dysfunction reversed by loratadine. *Journal of Clinical Psychiatry*, 63(6), 534.

Calabrese, J.R., Londborg, P.D., Shelton, M.D. and Thase, M.E. (2003). Citalopram treatment of fluoxetine-intolerant depressed patients. *Journal of Clinical Psychiatry*, 64(5), 562–567.

Calcedo Ordonez, A., Arosamene, X., Otero Perez, F.J., *et al.* (1992). Clomipramine/bentazepam combination in the treatment of major depressive disorders. *Human Psychopharmacology*, 7, 115–122.

Caldis, E.V. and Gair, R.D. (2004). Mirtazapine for treatment of nausea induced by selective serotonin reuptake inhibitors. *Canadian Journal of Psychiatry*, 49(10), 707.

Carpenter, L., Leon, Z., Yasmin, S. and Price, L.H. (2002). Do obese patients respond to topiramate? A retrospective chart review. *Journal of Affective Disorders*, 69, 251–255.

Cavazzoni, P., Tanaka, Y., Roychowdhury, S.M., *et al.* (2003). Nizatidine for prevention of weight gain with olanzapine: A double-blind placebo-controlled trial. *European Neuropsychopharmacology*, 13(2), 81–85.

Chen, J.J., Swope, D.M. (2005). A case of complex movement disorder induced by fluoxetine with management of dystonia by botulinum toxin type A. *Journal of Clinical Psychiatry*, 66(2), 267–268.

Chengappa, K.N., Kambhampati, R.K., Perkins, K., *et al.* (2001). Bupropion sustained release as a smoking cessation treatment in remitted depressed patients maintained on treatment with selective serotonin reuptake inhibitor antidepressants. *Journal of Clinical Psychiatry*, 62(7), 503–508.

Clayton, A.H., Pradko, J.F., Croft, H.A., *et al.* (2002). Prevalence of sexual dysfunction among newer antidepressants. *Journal of Clinical Psychiatry*, 63(4), 357–366.

Clayton, A.H., Warnock, J.K., Kornstein, S.G., *et al.* (2004). A placebo-controlled trial of bupropion SR as an antidote for selective serotonin reuptake inhibitor-induced sexual dysfunction. *Journal of Clinical Psychiatry*, 65(1), 62–67.

Cohen, A.J. (1992). Fluoxetine-induced yawning and anorgasmia reversed by cyproheptadine treatment. *Journal of Clinical Psychiatry*, 53(5), 174.

Cohen, A.J. and Bartlik, B. (1998). Ginkgo biloba for antidepressant-induced sexual dysfunction. *Journal of Sex and Marital Therapy*, 24(2), 139–143.

Cohn, J.B. (1983). Triazolam treatment of insomnia in depressed patients taking tricyclics. *Journal of Clinical Psychiatry*, 44(11), 401–406.

Dalton, E.J., Rotondi, D., Levitan, R.D., Kennedy, S.H. and Brown, G.M. (2000). Use of slow-release melatonin in treatment-resistant depression. *Journal of Psychiatry and Neuroscience*, 25(1), 48–52.

Damis, M., Patel, Y. and Simpson, G.M. (1999). Sildenafil in the treatment of SSRI-induced sexual dysfunction: A pilot study. *Primary Care Companion to Journal of Clinical Psychiatry*, 1(6), 184–187.

DeBattista, C., Dighramji, K., Menza, M., *et al.* (2003). Adjunct modafinil for the short-term treatment of fatigue and sleepiness in patients with major depressive disorder: A preliminary double-blind, placebo-controlled study. *Journal of Clinical Psychiatry*, 9, 1057–1064.

DeBattista, C., Lembke, A., Solvason, H.B., *et al.* (2004). A prospective trial of modafinil as an adjunctive treatment of major depression. *Journal of Clinical Psychopharmacology*, 24(1), 87–90.

Debattista, C., Solomon, A., Arnow, B., *et al.* (2005b). The efficacy of divalproex sodium in the treatment of agitation associated with major depression. *Journal of Clinical Psychopharmacology*, 25(5), 476–479.

DeBattista, C., Solvason, B., Poirier, J., *et al.* (2005a). A placebo-controlled, randomized, double-blind study of adjunctive bupropion sustained release in the treatment of SSRI-induced sexual dysfunction. *Journal of Clinical Psychiatry*, 66(7), 844–848.

Deberdt, W., Winokur, A., Cavazzoni, P.A., *et al.* (2005). Amantadine for weight gain associated with olanzapine treatment. *European Neuropsychopharmacology*, 15(1), 13–21.

Demyttenaere, K. and Huygens, R. (2002). Painful ejaculation and urinary hesitancy in association with antidepressant therapy: Relief with tamsulosin. *European Neuropsychopharmacology*, 12(4), 337–341.

Demyttenaere, K., Huygens, R. and Van Buggenhout, R. (2001). Tamsulosin as an effective treatment for reboxetine-associated urinary hesitancy. *International Clinical Psychopharmacology*, 16(6), 353–355.

deVries, M.W. and Peeters, F.P. (1997). Melatonin as a therapeutic agent in the treatment of sleep disturbance in depression. *Journal of Nervous and Mental Disease*, 185(3), 201–202.

Delva, N.J., Horgan, S.A. and Hawken, E.R. (2000). Valproate prophylaxis for migraine induced by selective serotonin reuptake inhibitors. *Headache*, 40(3), 248–251.

DeVane, C.L. (2003). Immediate-release versus controlled-release formulations: Pharmacokinetics of newer antidepressants in relation to nausea. *Journal of Clinical Psychiatry*, 64(Suppl 18), 14–19.

Dobkin, R.D., Menza, M., Marin, H., *et al.* (2006). Bupropion improves sexual functioning in depressed minority women: An open-label switch study. *Journal of Clinical Psychopharmacology*, 26(1), 21–26.

Dolberg, O.T., Hirschmann, S. and Grunhaus, L. (1998). Melatonin for the treatment of sleep disturbances in major depressive disorder. *American Journal of Psychiatry*, 155(8), 1119–1121.

Dolberg, O.T., Klag, E., Gross, Y. and Schreiber, S. (2002). Relief of serotonin selective reuptake inhibitor induced sexual dysfunction with low-dose mianserin in patients with traumatic brain injury. *Psychopharmacology*, 161(4), 404–407.

Dominguez, R.A., Jacobson, A.F., Goldstein, B.J. and Steinbrook, R.M. (1984). Comparison of triazolam and placebo in the treatment of insomnia in depressed patients. *Current Therapeutic Research*, 36(5), 856–865.

Dording, C.M., Fisher, L., Papakostas, G., *et al.* (2008). A double-blind, randomized, pilot dose-finding study of maca root (*L. Meyenii*) for the management of SSRI-induced sexual dysfunction. *CNS Neuroscience and Therapeutics*, 14(3), 182–191.

Dording, C.M., Mischoulon, D., Petersen, T.J., *et al.* (2002). The pharmacologic management of SSRI-induced side effects: A survey of psychiatrists. *Annals of Clinical Psychiatry*, 14(3), 143–147.

Dunlop, B.W., Crits-Christoph, P., Evans, D.L., *et al.* (2007). Coadministration of modafinil and a selective serotonin reuptake inhibitor from the initiation of treatment of major depressive disorder with fatigue and sleepiness: A double-blind, placebo controlled study. *Journal of Clinical Psychopharmacology*, 27(6), 614–619.

Elgamal, S. and Macqueen, G. (2008). Galantamine as an adjunctive treatment in major depression. *Journal of Clinical Psychopharmacology*, 28(3), 357–359.

Ellison, J.M. and DeLuca, P. (1998). Fluoxetine-induced genital anesthesia relieved by Ginkgo biloba extract. *Journal of Clinical Psychiatry*, 59(4), 199–200.

Ellison, J.M. and Stanziani, P. (1993). SSRI-associated nocturnal bruxism in four patients. *Journal of Clinical Psychiatry*, 54(11), 432–434.

Even, C., Friedman, S., Dardennes, R. and Guelfi, J.D. (2004). Modafinil as an alternative to light therapy for winter depression. *European Psychiatry*, 19(1), 66.

Fava, M., Asnis, G., Shrivastava, R., *et al.* (2008). Zolpidem extended-release, co-administered with escitalopram, improves insomnia in patients with comorbid insomnia and major depressive disorder. APA 2008.

Fava, M., McCall, W.V., Krystal, A., *et al.* (2006b). Eszopiclone co-administered with fluoxetine in patients with insomnia coexisting with major depressive disorder. *Biological Psychiatry*, 59(11), 1052–1060.

Fava, M., Nurnberg, H.G., Seidman, S.N., *et al.* (2006a). Efficacy and safety of sildenafil in men with serotonergic antidepressant-associated erectile dysfunction: Results from a randomized, double-blind, placebo-controlled trial. *Journal of Clinical Psychiatry*, 67(2), 240–246.

Fava, M., Rankin, M.A., Alpert, J.E., *et al.* (1998). An open trial of oral sildenafil in antidepressant-induced sexual dysfunction. *Psychotherapy and Psychosomatics*, 67(6), 328–331.

Fava, M., Thase, M.E. and DeBattista, C. (2005). A multicenter, placebo-controlled study of modafinil augmentation in partial responders to selective serotonin reuptake inhibitors with persistent fatigue and hypersomnia. *Journal of Clinical Psychiatry*, 66(1), 85–93.

Fawcett, J., Edwards, J.H., Kravitz, H.M. and Jeffriess, H. (1987). Alprazolam: An antidepressant? Alprazolam, desipramine, and an alprazolam-desipramine combination in the treatment of adult depressed outpatients. *Journal of Clinical Psychopharmacology*, 7(5), 295–310.

Fleischhacker, W.W. (1991). Propanolol for fluoxetine-induced akathisia. *Biological Psychiatry*, 30(5), 531–532.

Floris, M., Lejeune, J. and Deberdt, W. (2001). Effect of amantadine on weight gain during olanzapine treatment. *European Neuropsychopharmacology*, 11(2), 181–182.

Gadde, K.M., Zhang, W. and Foust, M.S. (2006). Bupropion treatment of olanzapine-associated weight gain: An open-label, prospective trial. *Journal of Clinical Psychopharmacology*, 26(4), 409–413.

Gitlin, M.J., Suri, R., Altshuler, L., *et al.* (2002). Bupropion-sustained release as a treatment for SSRI-induced sexual side effects. *Journal of Sex and Marital Therapy*, 28(2), 131–138.

Gracious, B.L., Krysiak, T.E. and Youngstrom, E.A. (2002). Amantadine treatment of psychotropic-induced weight gain in children and adolescents: Case series. *Journal of Child and Adolescent Psychopharmacology*, 12(3), 249–257.

Green, T.R. (1997). Bupropion for SSRI-induced fatigue. *Journal of Clinical Psychiatry*, 58(4), 174.

Gross, M.D. (1982). Reversal by bethanechol of sexual dysfunction caused by anticholinergic antidepressants. *American Journal of Psychiatry*, 139(9), 1193–1194.

Gupta, S., Droney, T., Masand, P. and Ashton, A.K. (1999a). SSRI-induced sexual dysfunction treated with sildenafil. *Depression and Anxiety*, 9(4), 180–192.

Gupta, S., Masand, P., Ashton, A.K. and Berry, S.L. (1999b). Phenelzine-induced sexual dysfunction treated with sildenafil. *Journal of Sex and Marital Therapy*, 25(2), 131–135.

Hemmeter, U., Annen, B., Bischof, R., *et al.* (2001). Polysomnographic effects of adjuvant ginkgo biloba therapy in patients with major depression medicated with trimipramine. *Pharmacopsychiatry*, 34(2), 50–59.

Henderson, D.C., Copeland, P.M., Daley, T.B., *et al.* (2005). A double-blind, placebo-controlled trial of sibutramine for olanzapine-associated weight gain. *American Journal of Psychiatry*, 162(5), 954–962.

Holder, G., Brand, S., Hatzinger, M. and Holsboer-Trachsler, E. (2002). Reduction of daytime sleepiness in a depressive patient during adjunct treatment with modafinil. *Journal of Psychiatric Research*, 36(1), 49–52.

Hollander, E. and McCarley, A. (1992). Yohimbine treatment of sexual side effects induced by serotonin reuptake blockers. *Journal of Clinical Psychiatry*, 53(6), 207–209.

Hyatt, M. and Messer, M. (1986). Yohimbine and imipramine-induced orthostatia. *American Journal of Psychiatry*, 143(3), 389–390.

Jacobsen, F.M. (1992). Fluoxetine-induced sexual dysfunction and an open trial of yohimbine. *Journal of Clinical Psychiatry*, 53(4), 119–122.

Jacobsen, F.M. (1990). Low-dose trazodone as a hypnotic in patients treated with MAOIs and other psychotropics: A pilot study. *Journal of Clinical Psychiatry*, 51(7), 298–302.

Jacobsen, F.M. and Comas-Díaz, L. (1999). Donepezil for psychotropic-induced memory loss. *Journal of Clinical Psychiatry*, 60(10), 698–704.

Jaffee, M.S. and Bostwick, J.M. (2000). Buspirone as an antidote to venlafaxine-induced bruxism. *Psychosomatics*, 41(6), 535–536.

Jespersen, S., Berk, M., Wyk, C.V., *et al.* (2004). A pilot randomized, double-blind, placebo-controlled study of granisetron in the treatment of sexual dysfunction in women associated with antidepressant use. *International Clinical Psychopharmacology*, 19(3), 161–164.

Ji, J.L., Liu, W.J., Zhang, N., *et al.* (2007). Effects of paroxetine with or without zolpidem on depression with insomnia: A multi-center randomized comparative study. *Zhonghua Yi Xue Za Zhi*, 87(23), 1585–1589.

Johnna, R.L. (1996). Relatively low doses of cisapride in the treatment of nausea in patients treated with venlafaxine for treatment-refractory depression. *Journal of Clinical Psychopharmacology*, 16(1), 35–37.

Kang, B.J., Lee, S.J., Kim, M.D. and Cho, M.J. (2002). A placebo-controlled, double-blind trial of *Ginkgo biloba* for antidepressant-induced sexual dysfunction. *Human Psychopharmacology*, 17(6), 279–284.

Kasper, S. (2002). Managing reboxetine-associated urinary hesitancy in a patient with major depressive disorder: A case study. *Psychopharmacology*, 159(4), 445–446.

Kasper, S. and Wolf, R. (2002). Successful treatment of reboxetine-induced urinary hesitancy with tamsulosin. *European Neuropsychopharmacology*, 12(2), 119–122.

Keller, A.A., Hamer, R. and Rosen, R.C. (1997). Serotonin reuptake inhibitor-induced sexual dysfunction and its treatment: A large-scale retrospective study of 596 psychiatric outpatients. *Journal of Sex and Marital Therapy*, 23(3), 165–175.

Kim, J.H., Yim, S.J. and Nam, J.H. (2006). A 12-week, randomized, open-label, parallel-group trial of topiramate in limiting weight gain during olanzapine treatment in patients with schizophrenia. *Schizophrenia Research*, 82(1), 115–117.

Klein, D.J., Cottingham, E.M., Sorter, M., *et al.* (2006). A randomized, double-blind, placebo-controlled trial of metformin treatment of weight gain associated with initiation of atypical antipsychotic therapy in children and adolescents. *American Journal of Psychiatry*, 163(12), 2072–2079.

Kwon, J.S., Choi, J.S., Bahk, W.M., *et al.* (2006). Weight management program for treatment-emergent weight gain in olanzapine-treated patients with schizophrenia or schizoaffective disorder: A 12-week randomized controlled clinical trial. *Journal of Clinical Psychiatry*, 67(4), 547–553.

Labbate, L.A., Grimes, J.B., Hines, A. and Pollack, M.H. (1997). Bupropion treatment of serotonin reuptake antidepressant-associated sexual dysfunction. *Annals of Clinical Psychiatry*, 9(4), 241–245.

Labbate, L.A. and Pollack, M.H. (1994). Treatment of fluoxetine-induced sexual dysfunction with bupropion: A case report. *Annals of Clinical Psychiatry*, 6(1), 13–15.

Lacomblez, L., Bensimon, G., Isnard, F., *et al.* (1989). Effect of yohimbine on blood pressure in patients with depression and orthostatic hypotension induced by clomipramine. *Clinical Pharmacology and Therapeutics*, 45(3), 241–251.

Lara, D.R., Busnello, E.D. and Souza, D.O. (2001). Ondansetron rather than metoclopramide for bupropion-induced nausea. *Canadian Journal of Psychiatry*, 46(4), 371.

Lauerma, H. (1996). Successful treatment of citalopram-induced anorgasmia by cyproheptadine. *Acta Psychiatrica Scandinavica*, 93(1), 69–70.

Lecrubier, Y., Puech, A.J. and Des Lauriers, A. (1981). Favourable effects of yohimbine on clomipramine-induced orthostatic hypotension: A double-blind study. *British Journal of Clinical Pharmacology*, 12(1), 90–93.

Lipinski, J.F. Jr., Mallya, G., Zimmerman, P. and Pope, H.G. Jr. (1989). Fluoxetine-induced akathisia: Clinical and theoretical implications. *Journal of Clinical Psychiatry*, 50(9), 339–342.

Levy, E., Agbokou, C., Ferreri, F., *et al.* (2007). Topiramate-induced weight loss in schizophrenia: A retrospective case series study. *Canadian Journal of Pharmacology*, 14(2), 234–239.

Londborg, P.D., Smith, W.T., Glaudin, V. and Painter, J.R. (2000). Short-term cotherapy with clonazepam and fluoxetine: Anxiety, sleep disturbance and core symptoms of depression. *Journal of Affective Disorders*, 61(1–2), 73–79.

Lundt, L. (2004). Modafinil treatment in patients with seasonal affective disorder/winter depression: An open-label pilot study. *Journal of Affective Disorders*, 81(2), 173–178.

Manber, R., Edinger, J.D., Gress, J.L., *et al.* (2008). Cognitive behavioral therapy for insomnia enhances depression outcome in patients with comorbid major depressive disorder and insomnia. *Sleep*, 31(4), 489–495.

Markovitz, P.J. and Wagner, S. (2003). An open-label trial of modafinil augmentation in patients with partial response to antidepressant therapy. *Journal of Clinical Psychopharmacology*, 23(2), 207–209.

Masand, P.S., Anand, V.S. and Tanquary, J.F. (1998). Psychostimulant augmentation of second generation antidepressants: A case series. *Depression and Anxiety*, 7(2), 89–91.

Masand, P.S., Ashton, A.K., Gupta, S. and Frank, B. (2001). Sustained-release bupropion for selective serotonin reuptake inhibitor-induced sexual dysfunction: A randomized, double-blind, placebo-controlled, parallel-group study. *American Journal of Psychiatry*, 158(5), 805–807.

Maskall, D.D. and Lam, R.W. (1993). Midodrine for TCA-induced orthostatic hypotension. *Journal of Psychiatry and Neuroscience*, 18(5), 276–277.

McCormick, S., Olin, J. and Brotman, A.W. (1990). Reversal of fluoxetine-induced anorgasmia by cyproheptadine in two patients. *Journal of Clinical Psychiatry*, 51(9), 383–384.

Menza, M.A., Kaufman, K.R. and Castellanos, A. (2000). Modafinil augmentation of antidepressant treatment in depression. *Journal of Clinical Psychiatry*, 61(5), 378–381.

Meston, C.M. (2004). A randomized, placebo-controlled, crossover study of ephedrine for SSRI-induced female sexual dysfunction. *Journal of Sex and Marital Therapy*, 30(2), 57–68.

Metz, A. and Shader, R.I. (1990). Adverse interactions encountered when using trazodone to treat insomnia associated with fluoxetine. *International Clinical Psychopharmacology*, 5(3), 191–194.

Michael, A. and O'Donnell, E.A. (2000). Fluoxetine-induced sexual dysfunction reversed by trazodone. *Canadian Journal of Psychiatry*, 45(9), 847–848.

Michael, A., Tubbe, P.A. and Praseedom, A. (1999). Sertraline-induced anorgasmia reversed by nefazodone. *British Journal of Psychiatry*, 175, 491.

Michelson, D., Bancroft, J., Targum, S., *et al.* (2000). Female sexual dysfunction associated with antidepressant administration: A randomized, placebo-controlled study of pharmacologic intervention. *American Journal of Psychiatry*, 157(2), 239–243.

Michelson, D., Kociban, K., Tamura, R. and Morrison, M.F. (2002). Mirtazapine, yohimbine or olanzapine augmentation therapy for serotonin reuptake-associated female sexual dysfunction: A randomized, placebo controlled trial. *Journal of Psychiatric Research*, 36(3), 147–152.

Milano, W., Grillo, F., Del Mastro, A., *et al.* (2007). Appropriate intervention strategies for weight gain induced by olanzapine: A randomized controlled study. *Advances in Therapy*, 24(1), 123–134.

Nasr, S. (2004). Modafinil as adjunctive therapy in depressed outpatients. *Annals of Clinical Psychiatry*, 16(3), 133–138.

Nelson, E.B., Keck, P.E. Jr. and McElroy, S.L. (1997). Resolution of fluoxetine-induced sexual dysfunction with the 5-HT3 antagonist granisetron. *Journal of Clinical Psychiatry*, 58(11), 496–497.

Nelson, E.B., Shah, V.N., Welge, J.A. and Keck, P.E. Jr. (2001). A placebo-controlled, crossover trial of granisetron in SRI-induced sexual dysfunction. *Journal of Clinical Psychiatry*, 62(6), 469–473.

Nickel, M.K., Nickel, C., Muehlbacher, M., *et al.* (2005). Influence of topiramate on olanzapine-related adiposity in women: A random, double-blind, placebo-controlled study. *Journal of Clinical Psychopharmacology*, 25(3), 211–217.

Nierenberg, A.A., Adler, L.A., Peselow, E., *et al.* (1994). Trazodone for antidepressant-associated insomnia. *American Journal of Psychiatry*, 151(7), 1069–1072.

Nierenberg, A.A. and Keck, P.E. Jr. (1989). Management of monoamine oxidase inhibitor-associated insomnia with trazodone. *Journal of Clinical Psychopharmacology*, 9(1), 42–45.

Nurnberg, H.G., Fava, M., Gelenberg, A.J., *et al.* (2007). Open-label sildenafil treatment of partial and non-responders to double-blind treatment in men with antidepressant-associated sexual dysfunction. *International Journal of Impotence Research*, 19(2), 167–175.

Nurnberg, H.G., Hensley, P.L., Gelenberg, A.J., *et al.* (2003). Treatment of antidepressant-associated sexual dysfunction with sildenafil: A randomized controlled trial. *Journal of the American Medical Association*, 289(1), 56–64.

Nurnberg, H.G., Hensley, P.L., Heiman, J.R., *et al.* (2008). Sildenafil treatment of women with antidepressant-associated sexual dysfunction: A randomized controlled trial. *Journal of the American Medical Association*, 300(4), 395–404.

Nurnberg, H.G., Hensley, P.L., Lauriello, J., *et al.* (1999a). Sildenafil for women patients with antidepressant-induced sexual dysfunction. *Psychiatric Services*, 50(8), 1076–1078.

Nurnberg, H.G., Lauriello, J., Hensley, P.L, *et al.* (1999b). Sildenafil for sexual dysfunction in women taking antidepressants. *American Journal of Psychiatry*, 156(10), 1664.

Nurnberg, H.G., Lauriello, J., Hensley, P.L., *et al.* (1999c). Sildenafil for iatrogenic serotonergic antidepressant medication-induced sexual dysfunction in 4 patients. *Journal of Clinical Psychiatry*, 60(1), 33–35.

Orr, G., Weiser, M., Pollack, M., *et al.* (2006). Effectiveness of sildenafil in treating erectile dysfunction in PTSD patients: A double-blind, placebo-controlled crossover study. *Journal of Clinical Psychopharmacology*, 26(4), 426–430.

Oulis, P., Kouzoupis, A.V., Koulouris, G., *et al.* (2008). Acute pregabalin reversal of citalopram induced sexual dysfunction in generalized anxiety disorder. *Journal of Clinical Psychopharmacology*, 28(3), 332–363.

Pae, C.U., Marks, D.M., Masand, P.S., *et al.* (2009). Methylphenidate extended release (OROS MPH) for the treatment of antidepressant-related sexual dysfunction in patients with treatment-resistant depression: Results from a 4-week, double-blind, placebo-controlled trial. *Clinical Neuropharmacology*, 32(2), 85–88.

Papakostas, G.I., Petersen, T.J., Burns, A.M. and Fava, M. (2006). Adjunctive atomoxetine for residual fatigue in major depressive disorder. *Journal of Psychiatric Research*, 40(4), 370–373.

Pavlovic, Z.M. (2004). Buspirone to improve compliance in venlafaxine-induced movement disorder. *International Journal of Neuropsychopharmacology*, 7(4), 523–524.

Pierre, J.M. and Guze, B.H. (2000). Benztropine for venlafaxine-induced night sweats. *Journal of Clinical Psychopharmacology*, 20(2), 269.

Price, D. (1998). Sildenafil (Viagra): Efficacy in the treatment of erectile dysfunction in depressed patients treated with common concomitant conditions. *Journal of Impotence Research*, 10, 584.

Price, J. and Grunhaus, L.J. (1990). Treatment of clomipramine-induced anorgasmia with yohimbine: A case report. *Journal of Clinical Psychiatry*, 51(1), 32–33.

Posternak, M.A. and Zimmerman, M. (2002). The effectiveness of switching antidepressants during remission: A case series of depressed patients who experienced intolerable side effects. *Journal of Affective Disorders*, 69(1–3), 237–240.

Poyurovsky, M., Tal, V., Maayan, R., *et al.* (2004). The effect of famotidine addition on olanzapine-induced weight gain in first-episode schizophrenia patients: A double-blind placebo-controlled pilot study. *European Neuropsychopharmacology*, 14(4), 332–336.

Ravindran, A.V., Kennedy, S.H., O'Donovan, C., *et al.* (2008). Osmotic-release oral system methylphenidate augmentation of antidepressant monotherapy in major depressive disorder: Results of a double-blind, randomized, placebo-controlled trial. *Journal of Clinical Psychiatry*, 69(1), 87–94.

Reynolds, R.D. (1997). Sertraline-induced anorgasmia treated with intermittent nefazodone. *Journal of Clinical Psychiatry*, 58(2), 89.

Rickels, K., Hutchison, J.C., Weise, C.C., *et al.* (1972). Doxepin and amitriptyline-perphenazine in mixed anxious-depressed neurotic outpatients: A collaborative controlled study. *Psychopharmacologia*, 23(4), 305–318.

Rickels, K., Jenkins, B.W., Zamostien, B., *et al.* (1967). Pharmacotherapy in neurotic depression. Differential population responses. *Journal of Nervous and Mental Disease*, 145(6), 475–485.

Rispail, Y., Schmitt, L., Berlan, M., *et al.* (1990). Yohimbine increases salivary secretion in depressed patients treated with tricyclic antidepressants. *European Journal of Clinical Pharmacology*, 39(4), 425–426.

Romanelli, F., Adler, D.A. and Bungay, K.M. (1996). Possible paroxetine-induced bruxism. *Annals of Pharmacotherapy*, 30(11), 1246–1248.

Rosenberg, K.P. (1999). Sildenafil citrate for SSRI-induced sexual side effects. *American Journal of Psychiatry*, 156(1), 157.

Sacchetti, E., Guarneri, L. and Bravi, D. (2000). H(2) antagonist nizatidine may control olanzapine-associated weight gain in schizophrenic patients. *Biological Psychiatry*, 48(2), 167–168.

Schaller, J.L. and Behar, D. (1999). Sildenafil citrate for SSRI-induced sexual side effects. *American Journal of Psychiatry*, 156(1), 156–157.

Schaefer, D.M., Ruggiero, L.D., Iyengar, M.K. and Lipschitz, A. (2004). Tolerability of controlled release paroxetine in patients with previously intolerant SSRI/SNRI therapy. Presented at the 44th Annual Meeting of the New Clinical Drug Evaluation Unit of the National Institute of Mental Health. Scottsdale, Arizona.

Schonfeldt-Lecuona, C., Connemann, B.J., Wolf, R.C., *et al.* (2006). Bupropion augmentation in the treatment of chronic fatigue syndrome with coexistent major depression episode. *Pharmacopsychiatry*, 39(4), 152–154.

Schwartz, T.L., Azhar, N., Cole, K., *et al.* (2004a). An open-label study of adjunctive modafinil in patients with sedation related to serotonergic antidepressant therapy. *Journal of Clinical Psychiatry*, 65(9), 1223–1227.

Schwartz, T.L. and Beale, M. (2003). Psychotropic induced weight gain alleviated with orlistat: A case-series. *Psychopharmacology Bulletin*, 37(1), 5–8.

Schwartz, T.L., Jindal, S., Simionescu, M., *et al.* (2004b). Effectiveness of orlistat versus diet and exercise for weight gain associated with antidepressant use: A pilot study. *Journal of Clinical Psychopharmacology*, 24(5), 555–556.

Schwartz, T.L., Leso, L., Beale, M., *et al.* (2002). Modafinil in the treatment of depression with severe comorbid medical illness. *Psychosomatics*, 43(4), 336–337.

Scocco, P., Longo, R. and Caon, F. (2006). Weight change in treatment with olanzapine and a psychoeducational approach. *Eating Behaviors*, 7(2), 115–124.

Seibyl, J.P., Krystal, J.H., Price, L.H. and Charney, D.S. (1989). Use of yohimbine to counteract nortriptyline-induced orthostatic hypotension. *Journal of Clinical Psychopharmacology*, 9(1), 67–68.

Seidman, S.N., Pesce, V.C. and Roose, S.P. (2003). High-dose sildenafil citrate for selective serotonin reuptake inhibitor-associated ejaculatory delay: Open clinical trial. *Journal of Clinical Psychiatry*, 64(6), 721–725.

Seidman, S.N., Roose, S.P., Menza, M.A., *et al.* (2001). Treatment of erectile dysfunction in men with depressive symptoms: Results of a placebo-controlled trial with sildenafil citrate. *American Journal of Psychiatry*, 158(10), 1623–1630.

Shrivastava, R.K., Shrivastava, S., Overweg, N. and Schmitt, M. (1995). Amantadine in the treatment of sexual dysfunction associated with selective serotonin reuptake inhibitors. *Journal of Clinical Psychopharmacology*, 15(1), 83–84.

Sokolski, K.N. and Brown, B.J. (2006). Quetiapine for insomnia associated with refractory depression exacerbated by phenelzine. *Annals of Pharmacotherapy*, 40(3), 567–570.

Sovner, R. (1984). Treatment of tricyclic antidepressant-induced orgasmic inhibition with cyproheptadine. *Journal of Clinical Psychopharmacology*, 4(3), 169.

Sporn, J., Ghaemi, S.N., Sambur, M.R., *et al.* (2000). Pramipexole augmentation in the treatment of unipolar and bipolar depression: A retrospective chart review. *Annals of Clinical Psychiatry*, 12(3), 137–140.

Steele, T.E. and Howell, E.F. (1986). Cyproheptadine for imipramine-induced anorgasmia. *Journal of Clinical Psychopharmacology*, 6(5), 326–327.

Stryjer, R., Spivak, B., Strous, R.D., *et al.* (2009). Trazodone for the treatment of sexual dysfunction induced by serotonin reuptake inhibitors: A preliminary open-label study. *Clinical Neuropharmacology*, 32(2), 82–84.

Thase, M.E., Blomgren, S.L., Birkett, M.A., *et al.* (1997). Fluoxetine treatment of patients with major depressive disorder who failed initial treatment with sertraline. *Journal of Clinical Psychiatry*, 58(1), 16–21.

Thase, M.E., Ferguson, J.M., Lydiard, R.B. and Wilcox, C.S. (2002). Citalopram treatment of paroxetine-intolerant depressed patients. *Depression and Anxiety*, 16(3), 128–133.

Tignol, J., Furlan, P.M., Gomez-Beneyto, M., *et al.* (2004). Efficacy of sildenafil citrate (Viagra) for the treatment of erectile dysfunction in men in remission from depression. *International Clinical Psychopharmacology*, 19(4), 191–199.

Tramontina, S., Zeni, C.P., Pheula, G. and Rohde, L.A. (2007). Topiramate in adolescents with juvenile bipolar disorder presenting weight gain due to atypical antipsychotics or mood stabilizers: An open clinical trial. *Journal of Child and Adolescent Psychopharmacology*, 17(1), 129–134.

Ueda, N., Yoshimura, R., Shinkai, K., *et al.* (2001). Characteristics of fluvoxamine-induced nausea.*Psychiatry Research*, 104(3), 259–264.

Van Ameringen, M., Mancini, C., Pipe, B., *et al.* (2002). Topiramate treatment for SSRI-induced weight gain in anxiety disorders. *Journal of Clinical Psychiatry*, 63(11), 981–984.

Walker, P.W., Cole, J.O., Gardner, E.A., *et al.* (1993). Improvement in fluoxetine-associated sexual dysfunction in patients switched to bupropion. *Journal of Clinical Psychiatry*, 54(12), 459–465.

Wang, P.W., Yang, Y.S., Chandler, R.A., *et al.* (2008). Adjunctive zonisamide for weight loss in euthymic bipolar disorder patients: A pilot study. *Journal of Psychiatric Research*, 42(6), 451–457.

Wheatley, D. (2004). Triple-blind, placebo-controlled trial of Ginkgo biloba in sexual dysfunction due to antidepressant drugs. *Human Psychopharmacology*, 19(8), 545–548.

Wohlreich, M.M., Martinez, J.M., Mallinckrodt, C.H., *et al.* (2005). An open-label study of duloxetine for the treatment of major depressive disorder: Comparison of switching versus initiating treatment approaches. *Journal of Clinical Psychopharmacology*, 25(6), 552–560.

Worthington, J.J. 3rd., Simon, N.M., Korbly, N.B., *et al.* (2002). Ropinirole for antidepressant-induced sexual dysfunction. *International Clinical Psychopharmacology*, 17(6), 307–310.

Wu, R.R., Zhao, J.P., Guo, X.F., *et al.* (2008). Metformin addition attenuates olanzapine-induced weight gain in drug-naive first-episode schizophrenia patients: A double-blind, placebo-controlled study. *American Journal of Psychiatry*, 165, 352–358.

Yamada, K., Kanba, S., Yagi, G. and Asai, M. (1999). Herbal medicine in the treatment of fluvoxamine-induced nausea and dyspepsia. *Psychiatry and Clinical Neurosciences*, 53(6), 681.

Yamada, K., Yagi, G. and Kanba, S. (2003). Effectiveness of Gorei-san (TJ-17) for treatment of SSRI-induced nausea and dyspepsia: Preliminary observations. *Clinical Neuropharmacology*, 26(3), 112–114.

Zarate, C.A., Kando, J.C., Tohen, M., *et al.* (1996). Does intolerance or lack of response with fluoxetine predict the same will happen with sertraline? *Journal of Clinical Psychiatry*, 57(2), 67–71.

Zimmermann, U., Rechlin, T., Plaskacewicz, G.J., *et al.* (1997). Effect of naltrexone on weight gain and food craving induced by tricyclic antidepressants and lithium: An open study. *Biological Psychiatry*, 41(6), 747–749.

Chapter 11

Abadie, P., Rioux, P., Scatton, B., *et al.* (1996). Central benzodiazepine receptor occupancy by zolpidem in the human brain as assessed by positron emission tomography. *European Journal of Pharmacology*, 295(1), 35–44.

Ablon, S.L. and Goodwin, F.K. (1974). High frequency of dysphoric reactions to tetrahydrocannabinol among depressed patients. *American Journal of Psychiatry*, 131(4), 448–453.

Anand, A., Bukhari, L., Jennings, S.A., *et al.* (2005). A preliminary open-label study of zonisamide treatment for bipolar depression in 10 patients. *Journal of Clinical Psychiatry*, 66(2), 195–198.

Ansseau, M., Ansoms, C., Beckers, G., *et al.* (1984). Double-blind clinical study comparing alprazolam and doxepin in primary unipolar depression. *Journal of Affective Disorders*, 7(3–4), 287–296.

Ansseau, M., Devoitille, J.M., Papart, P., *et al.* (1991). Comparison of adinazolam, amitriptyline, and diazepam in endogenous depressive inpatients exhibiting DST nonsuppression or abnormal contingent negative variation. *Journal of Clinical Psychopharmacology*, 11(3), 160–165.

Armbruster, K.F., Rahn, A.C., Ing, T.S., *et al.* (1974). Amantadine toxicity in a patient with renal insufficiency. *Nephron*, 13(2), 183–186.

Arnold, L.M., Goldenberg, D.L., Stanford, S.B., *et al.* (2007). Gabapentin in the treatment of fibromyalgia: A randomized, double-blind, placebo-controlled, multicenter trial. *Arthritis and Rheumatism*, 56(4), 1336–1344.

Arnold, L.M., Russell, I.J., Diri, E.W., *et al.* (2008). A 14-week, randomized, double-blinded, placebo-controlled monotherapy trial of pregabalin in patients with fibromyalgia. *Journal of Pain*, 9(9), 792–805.

Atack, J.R. (2003). Anxioselective compounds acting at the GABA(A) receptor benzodiazepine binding site. Current Drug Targets. *CNS and Neurological Disorders*, 2(4), 213–232.

Avenet, P., Leonardon, J., Besnard, F., *et al.* (1997). Antagonist properties of eliprodil and other NMDA receptor antagonists at rat NR1A/NR2A and NR1A/NR2B receptors expressed in Xenopus oocytes. *Neuroscience Letters*, 223(2), 133–136.

Barnard, E.A., Skolnick, P., Olsen, R.W., *et al.* (1998). International Union of Pharmacology. XV. Subtypes of gamma-aminobutyric acid A receptors: Classification on the basis of subunit structure and receptor function. *Pharmacology Reviews*, 50(2), 291–313.

Banerji, J.R., Brantingham, P., McEwan, G.D., *et al.* (1989). A comparison of alprazolam with amitriptyline in the treatment of patients with neurotic or reactive depression. A report of a randomised, double blind study by a General Practitioner Working Party. *Irish Journal of Medical Science*, 158(5), 110–113.

Bech, P. (2007). Dose-response relationship of pregabalin in patients with generalized anxiety disorder. A pooled analysis of four placebo-controlled trials. *Pharmacopsychiatry*, 40(4), 163–168.

Bellino, S., Paradiso, E. and Bogetto, F. (2005). Oxcarbazepine in the treatment of borderline personality disorder: A pilot study. *Journal of Clinical Psychiatry*, 66(9), 1111–1115.

Bergink, V. and Westenberg, H.G. (2005). Metabotropic glutamate II receptor agonists in panic disorder: A double blind clinical trial with LY354740. *International Clinical Psychopharmacology*, 20(6), 291–293.

Bergstrom, M., Fasth, K.J., Kilpatrick, G., *et al.* (2000). Brain uptake and receptor binding of two [11C]labelled selective high affinity NK1-antagonists, GR203040 and GR205171 — PET studies in rhesus monkey. *Neuropharmacology*, 39(4), 664–670.

Berman, R.M., Cappiello, A., Anand, A., *et al.* (2000). Antidepressant effects of ketamine in depressed patients. *Biological Psychiatry*, 47(4), 351–354.

Biancosino, B., Facchi, A., Marmai, L. and Grassi, L. (2002). Gabapentin treatment of impulsive-aggressive behaviour. *Canadian Journal of Psychiatry*, 47(5), 483–484.

Bodkin, J.A., Zornberg, G.L., Lukas, S.E. and Cole, J.O. (1995). Buprenorphine treatment of refractory depression. *Journal of Clinical Psychopharmacology*, 15(1), 49–57.

Borison, R.L. (1979). Amantadine-induced psychosis in a geriatric patient with renal disease. *American Journal of Psychiatry*, 136(1) 111–112.

Bray, G.A., Hollander, P., Klein, S., *et al.* (2003). A 6-month randomized, placebo-controlled, dose-ranging trial of topiramate for weight loss in obesity. *Obesity Research*, 11(6), 722–733.

Breier, A., Adler, C.M., Weisenfeld, N., *et al.* (1998). Effects of NMDA antagonism on striatal dopamine release in healthy subjects: Application of a novel PET approach. *Synapse*, 29(2), 142–147.

Bremner, J.D., Mletzko, T., Welter, S., *et al.* (2004). Treatment of posttraumatic stress disorder with phenytoin: An open-label pilot study. *Journal of Clinical Psychiatry*, 65(11), 1559–1564.

Bryans, J.S. and Wustrow, D.J. (1999). 3-substituted GABA analogs with central nervous system activity: A review. *Medicinal Research Reviews*, 19(2), 149–177.

Callaway, E. (1996). Buprenorphine for depression: The un-adoptable orphan. *Biological Psychiatry*, 39(12), 989–990.

Carta, M.G., Hardoy, M.C., Hardoy, M.J., *et al.* (2003). The clinical use of gabapentin in bipolar spectrum disorders. *Journal of Affective Disorders*, 75(1), 83–91.

Ceskova, E., Svestka, J., Nahunek, K. and Obrovska, V. (1989). Double blind comparison of alprazolam with dosulepine in endogenous depression. *Activitas Nervosa Superior*, 31(4), 290–291.

Chambers, M.S., Atack, J.R., Broughton, H.B., *et al.* (2003). Identification of a novel, selective GABA(A) alpha5 receptor inverse agonist which enhances cognition. *Journal of Medicinal Chemistry*, 46(11), 2227–2240.

Chen, Y., Sharples, T.J., Phillips, K.G., *et al.* (2003). The nicotinic alpha4 beta2 receptor selective agonist, TC-2559, increases dopamine neuronal activity in the ventral tegmental area of rat midbrain slices. *Neuropharmacology*, 45(3), 334–344.

Chouinard, G. (2004). Issues in the clinical use of benzodiazepines: Potency, withdrawal, and rebound. *Journal of Clinical Psychiatry*, 65(Suppl 5), 7–12.

Claudino, A.M., de Oliveira, I.R., Appolinario, J.C., *et al.* (2007). Double-blind, randomized, placebo-controlled trial of topiramate plus cognitive-behavior therapy in binge-eating disorder. *Journal of Clinical Psychiatry*, 68(9), 1324–1332.

Coccaro, E.F. and Kavoussi, R.J. (1997). Fluoxetine and impulsive aggressive behavior in personality-disordered subjects. *Archives of General Psychiatry*, 54(12), 1081–1088.

Cohen, B.M. and Zubenko, G.S. (1988). Captopril in the treatment of recurrent major depression. *Journal of Clinical Psychopharmacology*, 8(2), 143–144.

Cohen, C., Bergis, O.E., Galli, F., *et al.* (2003). SSR591813, a novel selective and partial alpha4beta2 nicotinic receptor agonist with potential as an aid to smoking cessation. *Journal of Pharmacology and Experimental Therapeutics*, 306(1), 407–420.

Cohen, M.R., Cohen, R.M., Pickar, D., *et al.* (1984). High dose naloxone in depression. *Biological Psychiatry*, 19(6), 825–832.

Covi, L., Lipman, R.S., McNair, D.M. and Czerlinsky, T. (1979). Symptomatic volunteers in multicenter drug trials. *Progress in Neuropsychopharmacology*, 3(5–6), 521–533.

Cowdry, R.W. and Gardner, D.L. (1988). Pharmacotherapy of borderline personality disorder. Alprazolam, carbamazepine, trifluoperazine, and tranylcypromine. *Archives of General Psychiatry*, 45(2), 111–119.

Cox, L.S., Patten, C.A., Krahn, L.E., *et al.* (2003). The effect of nicotine patch therapy on depression in nonsmokers: A preliminary study. *Journal of Addictive Disorders*, 22(4), 75–85.

Crane, G.E. (1959). Cycloserine as an antidepressant agent. *American Journal of Psychiatry*, 115, 1025–1026.

Crane, G.E. (1961). The psychotropic effects of cycloserine. *Comprehensive Psychiatry*, 2, 51–59.

Crofford, L.J., Mease, P.J., Simpson, S.L., *et al.* (2008). Fibromyalgia relapse evaluation and efficacy for durability of meaningful relief (FREEDOM):

A 6-month, double-blind, placebo-controlled trial with pregabalin. *Pain*, 136(3), 419–431.

Crofford, L.J., Rowbotham, M.C., Mease, P.J., *et al.* (2005). Pregabalin for the treatment of fibromyalgia syndrome: Results of a randomized, double-blind, placebo-controlled trial. *Arthritis and Rheumatism*, 52(4), 1264–1273.

Czuczwar, S.J. and Patsalos, P.N. (2001). The new generation of GABA enhancers. Potential in the treatment of epilepsy. *CNS Drugs*, 15(5), 339–350.

Dani, J.A. (2001). Overview of nicotinic receptors and their roles in the central nervous system. *Biological Psychiatry*, 49(3), 166–174.

Davies, J.A. (1995). Mechanisms of action of antiepileptic drugs. *Seizure*, 4(4), 267–271.

Davis, L.L., Bartolucci, A. and Petty, F. (2005). Divalproex in the treatment of bipolar depression: A placebo-controlled study. *Journal of Affective Disorders*, 85(3), 259–266.

Davis, L.L., Kabel, D., Patel, D., *et al.* (1996). Valproate as an antidepressant in major depressive disorder. *Psychopharmacology Bulletin*, 32(4), 647–652.

de Wit, H., Metz, J., Wagner, N. and Cooper, M. (1991). Effects of diazepam on cerebral metabolism and mood in normal volunteers. *Neuropsychopharmacology*, 5(1), 33–41.

Deep, P., Dagher, A., Sadikot, A., *et al.* (1999). Stimulation of dopa decarboxylase activity in striatum of healthy human brain secondary to NMDA receptor antagonism with a low dose of amantadine. *Synapse*, 34(4), 313–318.

Deicken, R.F. (1986). Captopril treatment of depression. *Biological Psychiatry*, 21(14), 1425–1428.

Delbello, M.P., Findling, R.L., Kushner, S., *et al.* (2005). A pilot controlled trial of topiramate for mania in children and adolescents with bipolar disorder. *Journal of the American Academy of Child and Adolescent Psychiatry*, 44(6), 539–547.

Dewey, S.L., Chaurasia, C.S., Chen, C.E., *et al.* (1997). GABAergic attenuation of cocaine-induced dopamine release and locomotor activity. *Synapse*, 25(4), 393–398.

Dewey, S.L., Smith, G.S., Logan, J., *et al.* (1992). GABAergic inhibition of endogenous dopamine release measured *in vivo* with 11C-raclopride and positron emission tomography. *Journal of Neuroscience*, 12(10), 3773–3780.

Dietrich, D.E., Bode, L., Spannhuth, C.W., *et al.* (2000). Amantadine in depressive patients with Borna disease virus (BDV) infection: An open trial. *Bipolar Disorders*, 2(1), 65–70.

Doble, A. (1996). The pharmacology and mechanism of action of riluzole. *Neurology*, 47(6 Suppl 4), S233–241.

Domino, E.F., Minoshima, S., Guthrie, S.K., *et al.* (2000a). Effects of nicotine on regional cerebral glucose metabolism in awake resting tobacco smokers. *Neuroscience*, 101(2), 277–282.

Domino, E.F., Minoshima, S., Guthrie, S., *et al.* (2000b). Nicotine effects on regional cerebral blood flow in awake, resting tobacco smokers. *Synapse*, 38(3) 313–321.

Dunayevich, E., Erickson, J., Levine, L., *et al.* (2008). Efficacy and tolerability of an mGlu2/3 agonist in the treatment of generalized anxiety disorder. *Neuropsychopharmacology*, 33(7), 1603–1610.

Eden Evins, A., Demopulos, C., Nierenberg, A., *et al.* (2006). A double-blind, placebo-controlled trial of adjunctive donepezil in treatment-resistant mania. *Bipolar Disorders*, 8(1), 75–80.

Emrich, H.M., Vogt, P. and Herz, A. (1982a). Possible antidepressive effects of opioids: Action of buprenorphine. *Annals of the New York Academy of Sciences*, 398, 108–112.

Emrich, H.M., Vogt, P., Herz, A. and Kissling, W. (1982b). Antidepressant effects of buprenorphine. *The Lancet*, 2(8300), 709.

Eriksson, B., Nagy, A., Starmark, J.E. and Thelander, U. (1987). Alprazolam compared to amitriptyline in the treatment of major depression. *Acta Psychiatrica Scandinavica*, 75(6), 656–663.

Ernst, C.L. and Goldberg, J.F. (2003). Antidepressant properties of anticonvulsant drugs for bipolar disorder. *Journal of Clinical Psychopharmacology*, 23(2), 182–192.

Ernst, M., Matochik, J.A., Heishman, S.J., *et al.* (2001). Effect of nicotine on brain activation during performance of a working memory task. *Proceedings of the National Academy of Sciences of the United States of America*, 98(8) 4728–4733.

Extein, I., Pickar, D., Gold, M.S., *et al.* (1981). Methadone and morphine in depression. *Psychopharmacology Bulletin*, 17(1), 29–33.

Fahn, S., Craddock, G. and Kumin, G. (1971). Acute toxic psychosis from suicidal overdosage of amantadine. *Archives of Neurology*, 25(1), 45–48.

Faravelli, C., Albanesi, G. and Sessarego, A. (1988). Viqualine in resistant depression: A double-blind, placebo-controlled trial. *Neuropsychobiology*, 20(2), 78–81.

Fava, M., Alpert, J., Nierenberg, A.A., *et al.* (1996). Fluoxetine treatment of anger attacks: A replication study. *Annals of Clinical Psychiatry*, 8(1), 7–10.

Fava, M., Nierenberg, A.A., Quitkin, F.M., *et al.* (1997). A preliminary study on the efficacy of sertraline and imipramine on anger attacks in atypical depression and dysthymia. *Psychopharmacology Bulletin*, 33(1), 101–103.

Fava, M., Rosenbaum, J.F., McCarthy, M., *et al.* (1991). Anger attacks in depressed outpatients and their response to fluoxetine. *Psychopharmacology Bulletin*, 27(3), 275–279.

Fava, M., Rosenbaum, J.F., Pava, J.A., *et al.* (1993). Anger attacks in unipolar depression, Part 1: Clinical correlates and response to fluoxetine treatment. *American Journal of Psychiatry*, 150(8), 1158–1163.

Fawcett, J., Edwards, J.H., Kravitz, H.M. and Jeffriess, H. (1987). Alprazolam: An antidepressant? Alprazolam, desipramine, and an alprazolam-desipramine combination in the treatment of adult depressed outpatients. *Journal of Clinical Psychopharmacology*, 7(5), 295–310.

Feighner, J.P., Aden, G.C., Fabre, L.F., *et al.* (1983b). Comparison of alprazolam, imipramine, and placebo in the treatment of depression. *Journal of the American Medical Association*, 249(22), 3057–3064.

Feighner, J.P., Brauzer, B., Gelenberg, A.J., *et al.* (1979). A placebo-controlled multicenter trial of Limbitrol versus its components (amitriptyline and chlordiazepoxide) in the symptomatic treatment of depressive illness. *Psychopharmacology*, 61(2), 217–225.

Feighner, J.P., Meredith, C.H., Frost, N.R., *et al.* (1983a). A double-blind comparison of alprazolam vs. imipramine and placebo in the treatment of major depressive disorder. *Acta Psychiatrica Scandinavica*, 68(4), 223–233.

Feltner, D.E., Crockatt, J.G., Dubovsky, S.J., *et al.* (2003). A randomized, double-blind, placebo-controlled, fixed-dose, multicenter study of pregabalin in patients with generalized anxiety disorder. *Journal of Clinical Psychopharmacology*, 23(3), 240–249.

Feltner, D., Wittchen, H.U., Kavoussi, R., *et al.* (2008) Long-term efficacy of pregabalin in generalized anxiety disorder. *International Clinical Psychopharmacology*, 23(1), 18–28.

Ferguson, J., McDonald, S., Bel, J., *et al.* (2003). Evaluation of the antidepressant effect of memantine in patients with major depressive disorder. Presented at the 42nd Annual Meeting of the American College of Neuropsychopharmacology. San Juan, Puerto Rico.

Ferszt, R., Kuhl, K.P., Bode, L., *et al.* (1999). Amantadine revisited: An open trial of amantadinesulfate treatment in chronically depressed patients with Borna disease virus infection. *Pharmacopsychiatry*, 32(4), 142–147.

Fhager, B., Meiri, I.M., Sjogren, M. and Edman, A. (2003). Treatment of aggressive behavior in dementia with the anticonvulsant topiramate: A retrospective pilot study. *International Psychogeriatrics*, 15(3), 307–309.

Fink, M., Simeon, J., Itil, T.M. and Freedman, A.M. (1970). Clinical antidepressant activity of cyclazocine — a narcotic antagonist. *Clinical Pharmacology and Therapeutics*, 11(1), 41–48.

Foster, H.G., Hillbrand, M., Chi, C.C. (1989). Efficacy of carbamazepine in assaultive patients with frontal lobe dysfunction. *Progress in Neuropsychopharmacology and Biological Psychiatry*, 13(6), 865–874.

French, J.A. (1999). Vigabatrin. *Epilepsia*, 40(Suppl 5), S11–16.

Friedman, H., Greenblatt, D.J., Peters, G.R., *et al.* (1992). Pharmacokinetics and pharmacodynamics of oral diazepam: Effect of dose, plasma concentration, and time. *Clinical Pharmacology and Therapeutics*, 52(2), 139–150.

Furey, M.L., Drevets, W.C. (2006). Antidepressant efficacy of the antimuscarinic drug scopolamine: A randomized, placebo-controlled clinical trial. *Archives of General Psychiatry*, 63(10), 1121–1129.

Fujita, M., Woods, S.W., Verhoeff, N.P., *et al.* (1999). Changes of benzodiazepine receptors during chronic benzodiazepine administration in humans. *European Journal of Pharmacology*, 368(2–3), 161–172.

Gardner, D.L., Cowdry, R.W. (1986). Positive effects of carbamazepine on behavioral dyscontrol in borderline personality disorder. *American Journal of Psychiatry*, 143(4), 519–522.

Germain, L. and Chouinard, G. (1989). Captopril treatment of major depression with serial measurements of blood cortisol concentrations. *Biological Psychiatry*, 25(4), 489–493.

Germain, L. and Chouinard, G. (1988). Treatment of recurrent unipolar major depression with captopril. *Biological Psychiatry*, 23(6), 637–641.

Gerner, R.H., Catlin, D.H., Gorelick, D.A., *et al.* (1980). beta-Endorphin. Intravenous infusion causes behavioral change in psychiatric inpatients. *Archives of General Psychiatry*, 37(6), 642–647.

Ghaemi, S.N., Gilmer, W.S., Goldberg, J.F., *et al.* (2007). Divalproex in the treatment of acute bipolar depression: A preliminary double-blind, randomized, placebo-controlled pilot study. *Journal of Clinical Psychiatry*, 68(12): 1840–1844.

Ghaemi, S.N., Zablotsky, B., Filkowski, M.M., *et al.* (2006). An open prospective study of zonisamide in acute bipolar depression. *Journal of Clinical Psychopharmacology*, 26(4), 385–388.

Ghatan, P.H., Ingvar, M., Eriksson, L., *et al.* (1998). Cerebral effects of nicotine during cognition in smokers and non-smokers. *Psychopharmacology*, 136(2), 179–189.

Giakas, W.J., Seibyl, J.P. and Mazure, C.M. (1990). Valproate in the treatment of temper outbursts. *Journal of Clinical Psychiatry*, 51(12), 525.

Gillin, J.C., Buchsbaum, M.S., Valladares-Neto, D.C., *et al.* (1996). Effects of zolpidem on local cerebral glucose metabolism during non-REM sleep in normal volunteers: A positron emission tomography study. *Neuropsychopharmacology*, 15(3), 302–313.

Glassman, A.H., Covey, L.S., Stetner, F. and Rivelli S. (2001). Smoking cessation and the course of major depression: A follow-up study. *The Lancet*, 357(9272), 1929–1932.

Gleason, R.P. and Schneider, L.S. (1990). Carbamazepine treatment of agitation in Alzheimer's outpatients refractory to neuroleptics. *Journal of Clinical Psychiatry*, 51(3), 115–118.

Glover, E.D. and Rath, J.M. (2007). Varenicline: Progress in smoking cessation treatment. *Expert Opinion in Pharmacotherapy*, 8(11), 1757–1767.

Goldberg, S.C., Ettigi, P., Schulz, P.M., *et al.* (1986). Alprazolam versus imipramine in depressed out-patients with neurovegetative signs. *Journal of Affective Disorders*, 11(2), 139–145.

Goldenberg, G., Kahaner, K., Basavaraju, N. and Rangu, S. (1998). Gabapentin for disruptive behaviour in an elderly demented patient. *Drugs and Aging*, 13(2), 183–184.

Greenblatt, D.J. and Wright, C.E. (1993). Clinical pharmacokinetics of alprazolam. Therapeutic implications. *Clinical Pharmacokinetics*, 24(6), 453–471.

Guay, D.R. (1994). Amantadine and rimantadine prophylaxis of influenza A in nursing homes. A tolerability perspective. *Drugs and Aging*, 5(1), 8–19.

Gupta, S., Frank, B.L. and Masand, P.S. (2000). Gabapentin in the treatment of aggression associated with conduct disorder. *Primary Care Companion of the Journal of Clinical Psychiatry*, 2(2), 60–61.

Hamilton, M. (1959). The assessment of anxiety states by rating. *British Journal of Medical Psychology*, 32(1), 50–55.

Hamouz, W., Pinder, R.M. and Stulemeijer, S.M. (1980). A double-blind group comparative trial of mianserin and diazepam in depressed outpatients. *Pharmakopsychiatrie Neuro-Psychopharmakologie*, 13(2), 79–83.

Hargreaves, R. (2002). Imaging substance P receptors (NK1) in the living human brain using positron emission tomography. *Journal of Clinical Psychiatry*, 63(Suppl 11), 18–24.

Haro, R. and Drucker-Colin, R. (2004a). A two-year study on the effects of nicotine and its withdrawal on mood and sleep. *Pharmacopsychiatry*, 37(5), 221–227.

Haro, R. and Drucker-Colin, R. (2004b). Effects of long-term administration of nicotine and fluoxetine on sleep in depressed patients. *Archives of Medical Research*, 35(6) 499–506.

Harper, R.W. and Knothe, B.U. (1973). Coloured Lilliputian hallucinations with amantadine. *Medical Journal of Australia*, 1(9), 444–445.

Hartvig, P., Valtysson, J., Antoni, G., *et al.* (1994). Brain kinetics of (R)- and (S)-[N-methyl-11C]ketamine in the rhesus monkey studied by positron emission tomography (PET). *Nuclear Medicine and Biology*, 21(7), 927–934.

Harwood, A.J., Agam, G. (2003). Search for a common mechanism of mood stabilizers. *Biochemistry and Pharmacology*, 66(2), 179–119.

Hashimoto, K., Shimizu, E. and Iyo, M. (2004). Critical role of brain-derived neurotrophic factor in mood disorders. Brain Research. *Brain Research Reviews*, 45(2), 104–114.

Hawkins, J.W., Tinklenberg, J.R., Sheikh, J.I., *et al.* (2000). A retrospective chart review of gabapentin for the treatment of aggressive and agitated behavior in patients with dementias. *American Journal of Geriatric Psychiatry*, 8(3), 221–225.

Hayashi, T., Su, T.P. (2004). Sigma-1 receptor ligands: Potential in the treatment of neuropsychiatric disorders. *CNS Drugs*, 18(5), 269–284.

Hedges, D.W., Reimherr, F.W., Hoopes, S.P., *et al.* (2003). Treatment of bulimia nervosa with topiramate in a randomized, double-blind, placebo-controlled trial, part 2: Improvement in psychiatric measures. *Journal of Clinical Psychiatry*, 64(12), 1449–1454.

Herrmann, N. (1998). Valproic acid treatment of agitation in dementia. *Canadian Journal of Psychiatry*, 43(1), 69–72.

Hertzberg, M.A., Butterfield, M.I., Feldman, M.E., *et al.* (1999). A preliminary study of lamotrigine for the treatment of posttraumatic stress disorder. *Biological Psychiatry*, 45(9), 1226–1229.

Hollander, E., Allen, A., Lopez, R.P., *et al.* (2001). A preliminary double-blind, placebo-controlled trial of divalproex sodium in borderline personality disorder. *Journal of Clinical Psychiatry*, 62(3), 199–203.

Hollander, E., Tracy, K.A., Swann, A.C., *et al.* (2003). Divalproex in the treatment of impulsive aggression: Efficacy in cluster B personality disorders. *Neuropsychopharmacology*, 28(6), 1186–1197.

Hoopes, S.P., Reimherr, F.W., Hedges, D.W., *et al.* (2003). Treatment of bulimia nervosa with topiramate in a randomized, double-blind, placebo-controlled trial, part 1: Improvement in binge and purge measures. *Journal of Clinical Psychiatry*, 64(11), 1335–1341.

Horne, M. and Lindley, S.E. (1995). Divalproex sodium in the treatment of aggressive behavior and dysphoria in patients with organic brain syndromes. *Journal of Clinical Psychiatry*, 56(9), 430–431.

Hubain, P.P., Castro, P., Mesters, P., *et al.* (1990). Alprazolam and amitriptyline in the treatment of major depressive disorder: A double-blind clinical and sleep EEG study. *Journal of Affective Disorders*, 18(1), 67–73.

Hunter, J.W., Owen, S., Eksi, A. and Scott, J.F. (1967). A controlled cross-over study of trimipramine and amylobarbitone. *British Journal of Psychiatry*, 113(499), 667–670.

Imlah, N.W. (1985). An evaluation of alprazolam in the treatment of reactive or neurotic (secondary) depression. *British Journal of Psychiatry*, 146, 515–519.

Innis, R.B., al-Tikriti, M.S., Zoghbi, S.S., *et al.* (1991). SPECT imaging of the benzodiazepine receptor: Feasibility of *in vivo* potency measurements from stepwise displacement curves. *Journal of Nuclear Medicine*, 32(9), 1754–1761.

Ishizuka, H., Sawada, Y., Ito, K., *et al.* (1989). Nonlinear relationship between benzodiazepine receptor occupancy and glucose metabolic response in the conscious mouse brain *in vivo*. *Journal of Pharmacology and Experimental Therapeutics*, 251(1), 362–367.

Janowsky, D.S., Kraus, J.E., Barnhill, J., *et al.* (2003). Effects of topiramate on aggressive, self-injurious, and disruptive/destructive behaviors in the intellectually disabled: An open-label retrospective study. *Journal of Clinical Psychopharmacology*, 23(5), 500–504.

Jarvis, B. and Figgitt, D.P. (2003). Memantine. *Drugs and Aging*, 20(6), 465–476.

Johns, M.W. (1977). Self-poisoning with barbiturates in England and Wales during 1959–1974. *British Medical Journal*, 1(6069), 1128–1130.

Johnson, D.A. (1979). A double-blind comparison of flupenthixol, nortriptyline and diazepam in neurotic depression. *Acta Psychiatrica Scandinavica*, 59(1), 1–8.

Kavoussi, R.J. and Coccaro, E.F. (1998). Divalproex sodium for impulsive aggressive behavior in patients with personality disorder. *Journal of Clinical Psychiatry*, 59(12), 676–680.

Kavoussi, R.J., Liu, J. and Coccaro, E.F. (1994). An open trial of sertraline in personality disordered patients with impulsive aggression. *Journal of Clinical Psychiatry*, 55(4), 137–141.

Kaufman, K.R., Kugler, S.L. and Sachdeo, R.C. (2002). Tiagabine in the management of postencephalitic epilepsy and impulse control disorder. *Epilepsy and Behavior*, 3(2), 190–194.

Kegeles, L.S., Abi-Dargham, A., Zea-Ponce, Y., *et al.* (2000). Modulation of amphetamine-induced striatal dopamine release by ketamine in humans: Implications for schizophrenia. *Biological Psychiatry*, 48(7), 627–640.

Keller, M., Montgomery, S., Ball, W., *et al.* (2006). Lack of efficacy of the substance P (neurokinin(1) receptor) antagonist aprepitant in the treatment of major depressive disorder. *Biological Psychiatry*, 59(3), 216–223.

Kinrys, G., Vasconcelos e Sa, D. and Nery, F. (2007b). Adjunctive zonisamide for treatment refractory anxiety. *International Journal of Clinical Practice*, 61(6), 1050–1053.

Kinrys G, Worthington, J.J., Wygant, L., *et al.* (2007a). Levetiracetam as adjunctive therapy for refractory anxiety disorders. *Journal of Clinical Psychiatry*, 68(7), 1010–1013.

Kinrys, G., Wygant, L.E., Pardo, T.B. and Melo, M. (2006). Levetiracetam for treatment-refractory posttraumatic stress disorder. *Journal of Clinical Psychiatry*, 67(2), 211–214.

Kishimoto, A., Kamata, K., Sugihara, T., *et al.* (1988). Treatment of depression with clonazepam. *Acta Psychiatrica Scandinavica*, 77(1), 81–86.

Kline, N.S., Li, C.H., Lehmann, H.E., *et al.* (1977). Beta-endorphin–induced changes in schizophrenic and depressed patients. *Archives of General Psychiatry*, 34(9), 1111–1113.

Kotin, J., Post, R.M. and Goodwin, F.K. (1973). 9-Tetrahydrocannabinol in depressed patients. *Archives of General Psychiatry*, 28(3), 345–348.

Kramer, M.S. (2001). Substance P (NK1) receptor antagonists (SPAs) in patients with major depression. Presented at the 40th Annual Annual Meeting of the American College of Neuropsychopharmacology. Waikoloa, Hawaii.

Kramer, M.S., Cutler, N., Feighner, J., *et al.* (1998). Distinct mechanism for antidepressant activity by blockade of central substance P receptors. *Science*, 281(5383), 1640–1645.

Kramer, M.S., Winokur, A., Kelsey, J., *et al.* (2004). Demonstration of the efficacy and safety of a novel substance P (NK1) receptor antagonist in major depression. *Neuropsychopharmacology*, 29(2), 385–392.

Krishnan, R. (2002). Clinical experience with substance P receptor (NK1) antagonists in depression. *Journal of Clinical Psychiatry*, 63(Suppl 11), 25–29.

Kunik, M.E., Puryear, L., Orengo, C.A., *et al.* (1998). The efficacy and tolerability of divalproex sodium in elderly demented patients with behavioral disturbances. *International Journal of Geriatric Psychiatry*, 13(1), 29–34.

Kushner, S.F., Khan, A., Lane, R. and Olson, W.H. (2006). Topiramate monotherapy in the management of acute mania: Results of four double-blind placebo-controlled trials. *Bipolar Disorders*, 8(1), 15–27.

Laakman, G., Faltermaier-Temizel, M., Bossert-Zaudig, S., *et al.* (1995). Treatment of depressive outpatients with lorazepam, alprazolam, amytriptyline and placebo. *Psychopharmacology*, 120(1), 109–115.

Lader, M. and Scotto, J.C. (1998). A multicentre double-blind comparison of hydroxyzine, buspirone and placebo in patients with generalized anxiety disorder. *Psychopharmacology*, 139(4), 402–406.

Lapierre, Y.D., Browne, M., Oyewumi, K. and Sarantidis, D. (1994). Alprazolam and amitriptyline in the treatment of moderate depression. *International Clinical Psychopharmacology*, 9(1), 41–45.

Laws, D., Ashford, J.J. and Anstee, J.A. (1990). A multicentre double-blind comparative trial of fluvoxamine versus lorazepam in mixed anxiety and depression treated in general practice. *Acta Psychiatrica Scandinavica*, 81(2), 185–189.

Leaderbetter, R., Pande, A., Slomkowski, A. and Smith, F. (1999). Igmesine: A novel antidepressant. *Biological Psychiatry*, 8(s1), 76S.

Lee, D.O., Steingard, R.J., Cesena, M., *et al.* (1996). Behavioral side effects of gabapentin in children. *Epilepsia*, 37(1), 87–90.

Lehmann, H.E., Ananth, J.V., Geagea, K.C. and Ban, T.A. (1971). Treatment of depression with dexedrine and demerol. *Current Therapeutic Research, Clinical and Experimental*, 13(1), 42–49.

Lemoine, P., Boulenger, J.P., Caillard, V., *et al.* (1991). Compared efficacy of prazepam and clomipramine in major depression with anxiety: A multicenter controlled study. *Pharmacopsychiatry*, 24(5), 175–179.

Lenox, R.H., Shipley, J.E., Peyser, J.M., *et al.* (1984). Double-blind comparison of alprazolam versus imipramine in the inpatient treatment of major depressive illness. *Psychopharmacology Bulletin*, 20(1), 79–82.

Leon, A.C., Shear, M.K., Portera, L. and Klerman, G.L. (1993). Effect size as a measure of symptom-specific drug change in clinical trials. *Psychopharmacology Bulletin*, 29(2), 163–167.

Levin, E.D., Bettegowda, C., Blosser, J. and Gordon, J. (1999). AR-R17779, and alpha7 nicotinic agonist, improves learning and memory in rats. *Behavioural Pharmacology*, 10(6–7), 675–680.

Levin, E.D. and Rezvani, A.H. (2002). Nicotinic treatment for cognitive dysfunction. Current drug targets. *CNS and Neurological Disorders*, 1(4), 423–431.

Lindley, S.E., Carlson, E.B. and Hill, K. (2007). A randomized, double-blind, placebo-controlled trial of augmentation topiramate for chronic combat-related posttraumatic stress disorder. *Journal of Clinical Psychopharmacology*, 27(6), 677–681.

Lingford-Hughes, A., Hume, S.P., Feeney, A., *et al.* (2002). Imaging the GABA-benzodiazepine receptor subtype containing the alpha5-subunit *in vivo* with [11C]Ro15 4513 positron emission tomography. *Journal of Cerebral Blood Flow and Metabolism*, 22(7), 878–889.

Lipman, R.S., Covi, L., Rickels, K., *et al.* (1986). Imipramine and chlordiazepoxide in depressive and anxiety disorders. I. Efficacy in depressed outpatients. *Archives of General Psychiatry*, 43(1), 68–77.

Lipton, S.A. and Rosenberg, P.A. (1994). Excitatory amino acids as a final common pathway for neurologic disorders. *New England Journal of Medicine*, 330(9), 613–622.

Lloyd, K.G., Zivkovic, B., Sanger, D., *et al.* (1987). Fengabine, a novel antidepressant GABAergic agent. I. Activity in models for antidepressant drugs and psychopharmacological profile. *Journal of Pharmacology and Experimental Therapeutics*, 241(1), 245–250.

Loew, T.H., Nickel, M.K., Muehlbacher, M., *et al.* (2006). Topiramate treatment for women with borderline personality disorder: A double-blind, placebo-controlled study. *Journal of Clinical Psychopharmacology*, 26(1), 61–66.

Lott, A.D., McElroy, S.L. and Keys, M.A. (1995). Valproate in the treatment of behavioral agitation in elderly patients with dementia. *Journal of Neuropsychiatry and Clinical Neurosciences*, 7(3), 314–319.

Low, R.A. Jr. and Brandes, M. (1999). Gabapentin for the management of agitation. *Journal of Clinical Psychopharmacology*, 19(5), 482–483.

Luchins, D.J. (1983). Carbamazepine for the violent psychiatric patient. *The Lancet*, 1(8327), 766.

Luchins, D.J. (1984). Carbamazepine in violent non-epileptic schizophrenics. *Psychopharmacology Bulletin*, 20(3), 569–571.

Lynch, D.R and Guttmann, R.P. (2002). Excitotoxicity: Perspectives based on N-methyl-D-aspartate receptor subtypes. *Journal of Pharmacology and Experimental Therapeutics*, 300(3), 717–723.

Macchio, G.J., Ito, V. and Sahgal, V. (1993). Amantadine-induced coma. *Archives of Physical and Medicine Rehabilitation*, 74(10), 1119–1120.

Maeda, J., Suhara, T., Kawabe, K., *et al.* (2003). Visualization of alpha5 subunit of GABAA/benzodiazepine receptor by 11C Ro15–4513 using positron emission tomography. *Synapse*, 47(3), 200–208.

Magni, G., Garreau, M., Orofiamma, B. and Palminteri, R. (1989). Fengabine, a new GABAmimetic agent in the treatment of depressive disorders: An overview of six double-blind studies versus tricyclics. *Neuropsychobiology*, 20(3), 126–131.

Markowitz, J.S. and Patrick, K.S. (1998). Venlafaxine-tramadol similarities. *Medical Hypotheses*, 51(2), 167–168.

Martins, J.K. (1966). Combined amitriptyline-perphenazine (Etrafon) compared with chlordiazepoxide hydrochloride: A double-blind, crossover study. *Current Therapeutic Research, Clinical and Experimental*, 8(1), 17–22.

Mattes, J.A. (1990). Comparative effectiveness of carbamazepine and propranolol for rage outbursts. *Journal of Neuropsychiatry and Clinical Neurosciences*, 2(2), 159–164.

Mattes, J.A. (2008). Levetiracetam in patients with impulsive aggression: A double-blind, placebo-controlled trial. *Journal of Clinical Psychiatry*, 69(2), 310–315.

McClernon, F.J., Hiott, F.B. and Westman, E.C., (2006). Transdermal nicotine attenuates depression symptoms in nonsmokers: A double-blind, placebo-controlled trial. *Psychopharmacology*, 189(1), 125–133.

McElroy, S.L., Arnold, L.M., Shapira, N.A., *et al.* (2003). Topiramate in the treatment of binge eating disorder associated with obesity: A randomized, placebo-controlled trial. *American Journal of Psychiatry*, 160(2), 255–261.

McElroy, S.L., Hudson, J.I., Capece, J.A., *et al.* (2007). Topiramate for the treatment of binge eating disorder associated with obesity: A placebo-controlled study. *Biological Psychiatry*, 61(9), 1039–1048.

McElroy, S.L., Kotwal, R., Guerdjikova, A.I., *et al.* (2006). Zonisamide in the treatment of binge eating disorder with obesity: A randomized controlled trial. *Journal of Clinical Psychiatry*, 67(12), 1897–1906.

McElroy, S.L., Shapira, N.A., Arnold, L.M., *et al.* (2004). Topiramate in the long-term treatment of binge-eating disorder associated with obesity. *Journal of Clinical Psychiatry*, 65(11), 1463–1469.

McElroy, S.L., Suppes, T., Keck, P.E. Jr., *et al.* (2005). Open-label adjunctive zonisamide in the treatment of bipolar disorders: A prospective trial. *Journal of Clinical Psychiatry*, 66(5), 617–624.

McIntyre, R.S., Mancini, D.A., McCann, S., *et al.* (2002). Topiramate versus bupropion SR when added to mood stabilizer therapy for the depressive phase of bipolar disorder: A preliminary single-blind study. *Bipolar Disorders*, 4(3), 207–213.

McKay, P.F., Foster, K.L., Mason, D., *et al.* (2004). A high affinity ligand for GABAA-receptor containing alpha5 subunit antagonizes ethanol's neurobehavioral effects in Long-Evans rats. *Psychopharmacology*, 172(4), 455–462.

McLeod, M., Pralong, D., Copolov, D. and Dean, B. (2002). The heterogeneity of central benzodiazepine receptor subtypes in the human hippocampal formation, frontal cortex and cerebellum using [3H]flumazenil and zolpidem. *Brain Research. Molecular Brain Research*, 104(2), 203–209.

Mease, P.J., Russell, I.J., Arnold, L.M., *et al.* (2008). A randomized, double-blind, placebo-controlled, phase III trial of pregabalin in the treatment of patients with fibromyalgia. *Journal of Rheumatology*, 35(3), 502–514.

Mehta, A.K. and Ticku, M.K. (1999). An update on GABAA receptors. *Brain Research. Brain Research Reviews*, 29(2–3), 196–217.

Melander, A., Henricson, K., Stenberg, P., *et al.* (1991). Anxiolytic-hypnotic drugs: Relationships between prescribing, abuse and suicide. *European Journal of Clinical Pharmacology*, 41(6), 525–529.

Meldrum, B.S. (1996). Update on the mechanism of action of antiepileptic drugs. *Epilepsia*, 37(Suppl 6), S4–11.

Mellow, A.M., Solano-Lopez, C. and Davis, S. (1993). Sodium valproate in the treatment of behavioral disturbance in dementia. *Journal of Geriatric Psychiatry and Neurology*, 6(4), 205–209.

Mendels, J. and Schless, A.P. (1986). Comparative efficacy of alprazolam, imipramine, and placebo administered once a day in treating depressed patients. *Journal of Clinical Psychiatry*, 47(7), 357–361.

Mendelson, W.B. and Rich, C.L. (1993). Sedatives and suicide: The San Diego study. *Acta Psychiatrica Scandinavica*, 88(5), 337–341.

Miller, D.K., Sumithran, S.P., Dwoskin, L.P. (2002). Bupropion inhibits nicotine-evoked [(3)H]overflow from rat striatal slices preloaded with [(3)H]dopamine and from rat hippocampal slices preloaded with [(3)H]norepinephrine. *Journal of Pharmacology and Experimental Therapeutics*, 302(3), 1113–1122.

Miller, L.J. (2001). Gabapentin for treatment of behavioral and psychological symptoms of dementia. *Annals of Pharmacotherapy*, 35(4), 427–431.

Mishory, A., Yaroslavsky, Y., Bersudsky, Y. and Belmaker, R.H. (2000). Phenytoin as an antimanic anticonvulsant: A controlled study. *American Journal of Psychiatry*, 157(3), 463–465.

Monk, J.P. and Brogden, R.N. (1990). Mexiletine. A review of its pharmacodynamic and pharmacokinetic properties, and therapeutic use in the treatment of arrhythmias. *Drugs*, 40(3), 374–411.

Montgomery, S., Chatamra, K., Pauer, L., *et al.* (2008). Efficacy and safety of pregabalin in elderly people with generalised anxiety disorder. *British Journal of Psychiatry*, 193(5), 389–394.

Montgomery, B.A., Cullinan, T.R. and Bayley, A.J. (1970). A double-blind comparative trial of doxepin hydrochloride and chlordiazepoxide in anxiety and depression in general practice. *British Journal of Clinical Practice*, 24(5), 207–209.

Montgomery, S.A., Tobias, K., Zornberg, G.L., *et al.* (2006). Efficacy and safety of pregabalin in the treatment of generalized anxiety disorder: A 6-week, multicenter, randomized, double-blind, placebo-controlled comparison of pregabalin and venlafaxine. *Journal of Clinical Psychiatry*, 67(5), 771–782.

Möller, H.J., Volz, H.P., Reimann, I.W. and Stoll, K.D. (2001). Opipramol for the treatment of generalized anxiety disorder: A placebo-controlled trial including an alprazolam-treated group. *Journal of Clinical Psychopharmacology*, 21(1), 59–65.

Neppe, V.M. (1983). Carbamazepine as adjunctive treatment in nonepileptic chronic inpatients with EEG temporal lobe abnormalities. *Journal of Clinical Psychiatry*, 44(9), 326–331.

Nickel, C., Lahmann, C., Tritt, K., *et al.* (2005a). Topiramate in treatment of depressive and anger symptoms in female depressive patients: A randomized, double-blind, placebo-controlled study. *Journal of Affective Disorders*, 87(2–3), 243–252.

Nickel, C., Tritt, K., Muehlbacher, M., *et al.* (2005b). Topiramate treatment in bulimia nervosa patients: A randomized, double-blind, placebo-controlled trial. *International Journal of Eating Disorders*, 38(4), 295–300.

Nickel, M.K., Nickel, C., Kaplan, P., *et al.* (2005). Treatment of aggression with topiramate in male borderline patients: A double-blind, placebo-controlled study. *Biological Psychiatry*, 57(5), 495–499.

Nickel, M.K, Nickel, C., Mitterlehner, F.O., *et al.* (2004). Topiramate treatment of aggression in female borderline personality disorder patients: A double-blind, placebo-controlled study. *Journal of Clinical Psychiatry*, 65(11), 1515–1519.

Nielsen, N.P., Cesana, B., Zizolfi, S., *et al.* (1990). Therapeutic effects of fengabine, a new GABAergic agent, in depressed outpatients: A double-blind study versus clomipramine. *Acta Psychiatrica Scandinavica*, 82(5), 366–371.

Obata, T. and Yamamura, H.I. (1988). Modulation of GABA-stimulated chloride influx into membrane vesicles from rat cerebral cortex by triazolobenzodiazepines. *Life Sciences*, 42(6), 659–665.

Olver, I.N. (2004). Aprepitant in antiemetic combinations to prevent chemotherapy-induced nausea and vomiting. *International Journal of Clinical Practice*, 58(2), 201–206.

Oommen, K.J. and Mathews, S. (1999). Zonisamide: A new antiepileptic drug. *Clinical Neuropharmacology*, 22(4), 192–200.

Overall, J.E., Biggs, J., Jacobs, M. and Holden, K. (1987). Comparison of alprazolam and imipramine for treatment of outpatient depression. *Journal of Clinical Psychiatry*, 48(1), 15–19.

Pande, A.C., Crockatt, J.G., Feltner, D.E., *et al.* (2003). Pregabalin in generalized anxiety disorder: A placebo-controlled trial. *American Journal of Psychiatry*, 160(3), 533–540.

Pande, A.C., Crockatt, J.G., Janney, C.A., *et al.* (2000a). Gabapentin in bipolar disorder: A placebo-controlled trial of adjunctive therapy. Gabapentin Bipolar Disorder Study Group. *Bipolar Disorder*, 2(3 Pt 2), 249–255.

Pande, A.C., Davidson, J.R., Jefferson, J.W., *et al.* (1999). Treatment of social phobia with gabapentin: A placebo-controlled study. *Journal of Clinical Psychopharmacology*, 19(4), 341–348.

Pande, A.C., Feltner, D.E., Jefferson, J.W., *et al.* (2004). Efficacy of the novel anxiolytic pregabalin in social anxiety disorder: A placebo-controlled, multicenter study. *Journal of Clinical Psychopharmacology*, 24(2), 141–149.

Pande, A.C., Pollack, M.H., Crockatt, J., *et al.* (2000b). Placebo-controlled study of gabapentin treatment of panic disorder. *Journal of Clinical Psychopharmacology*, 20(4), 467–471.

Papakostas, G.I. and Zarate, C.A. Jr. (2007). Novel augmentation strategies for treatment-resistant major depressive disorder. *Primary Psychiatry*, 14(1), 59–65.

Parker, C.S. and Wrigley, F. (1950). Synthetic cannabis preparations in psychiatry: Synhexyl. *Journal of Mental Science*, 96, 276–279.

Parsons, C.G., Panchenko, V.A., Pinchenko, V.O., *et al.* (1996). Comparative patch-clamp studies with freshly dissociated rat hippocampal and striatal neurons on the NMDA receptor antagonistic effects of amantadine and memantine. *European Journal of Neuroscience*, 8(3), 446–454.

Paterson, D. and Nordberg, A. (2000). Neuronal nicotinic receptors in the human brain. *Progress in Neurobiology*, 61(1), 75–111.

Perucca, E. (2002). Pharmacological and therapeutic properties of valproate: A summary after 35 years of clinical experience. *CNS Drugs*, 16(10), 695–714.

Petty, F., Trivedi, M.H., Fulton, M. and Rush, A.J. (1995). Benzodiazepines as antidepressants: Does GABA play a role in depression? *Biological Psychiatry*, 38(9), 578–591.

Phillips, M.L., Drevets, W.C., Rauch, S.L. and Lane, R. (2003a). Neurobiology of emotion perception I: The neural basis of normal emotion perception. *Biological Psychiatry*, 54(5), 504–514.

Phillips, M.L., Drevets, W.C., Rauch, S.L. and Lane, R. (2003b). Neurobiology of emotion perception II: Implications for major psychiatric disorders. *Biological Psychiatry*, 54(5), 515–528.

Pickar, D., Davis, G.C., Schulz, S.C., *et al.* (1981). Behavioral and biological effects of acute beta-endorphin injection in schizophrenic and depressed patients. *American Journal of Psychiatry*, 138(2), 160–166.

Pimentel, L. and Hughes, B. (1991). Amantadine toxicity presenting with complex ventricular ectopy and hallucinations. *Pediatric Emergency Care*, 7(2), 89–92.

Pinninti, N.R. and Mahajan, D.S. (2001). Gabapentin-associated aggression. *Journal of Neuropsychiatry and Clinical Neurosciences*, 13(3), 424.

Pohl, R.B., Feltner, D.E., Fieve, R.R. and Pande A.C. (2005). Efficacy of pregabalin in the treatment of generalized anxiety disorder: Double-blind, placebo-controlled comparison of BID versus TID dosing. *Journal of Clinical Psychopharmacology*, 25(2), 151–158.

Pollack, M.H., Roy-Byrne, P.P., Van Ameringen, M., *et al.* (2005). The selective GABA reuptake inhibitor tiagabine for the treatment of generalized anxiety disorder: Results of a placebo-controlled study. Journal of Clinical Psychiatry, 66(11), 1401–1408.

Pollack, M.H., Tiller, J., Xie, F. and Trivedi, M.H. (2008). Tiagabine in adult patients with generalized anxiety disorder: Results from 3 randomized, double-blind, placebo-controlled, parallel-group studies. *Journal of Clinical Psychopharmacology*, 28(3), 308–316.

Pond, D.A. (1948). Psychological effects in depressive patients of the marihuana homologye synhexyl. *Journal of Neurology, Neurosurgery, and Psychiatry*, 11, 271–279.

Porter, A.C. and Felder, C.C. (2001). The endocannabinoid nervous system: Unique opportunities for therapeutic intervention. *Pharmacology and Therapeutics*, 90(1), 45–60.

Post, R.M., Altshuler, L.L., Frye, M.A., *et al.* (2005). Preliminary observations on the effectiveness of levetiracetam in the open adjunctive treatment of refractory bipolar disorder. *Journal of Clinical Psychiatry*, 66(3), 370–374.

Post, R.M., Ketter, T.A., Joffe, R.T. and Kramlinger, K.L. (1991). Lack of beneficial effects of l-baclofen in affective disorder. *International Clinical Psychopharmacology*, 6(4), 197–207.

Puryear, L.J., Kunik, M.E. and Workman, R. (1995). Jr. Tolerability of divalproex sodium in elderly psychiatric patients with mixed diagnoses. *Journal of Geriatric Psychiatry and Neurology*, 8(4), 234–237.

Quirk, J.C., Nisenbaum, E.S. (2002). LY404187: A novel positive allosteric modulator of AMPA receptors. *CNS Drug Reviews*, 8(3), 255–282.

Raffa, R.B., Friderichs, E., Reimann, W., *et al.* (1992). Opioid and nonopioid components independently contribute to the mechanism of action of tramadol, an 'atypical' opioid analgesic. *Journal of Pharmacology and Experimental Therapeutics*, 260(1), 275–285.

Raskin, A., Schulterbrandt, J.G., Reatig, N., *et al.* (1974). Depression subtypes and response to phenelzine, diazepam, and a placebo. Results of a nine hospital collaborative study. *Archives of General Psychiatry*, 30(1), 66–75.

Regan, W.M. and Gordon, S.M. (1997). Gabapentin for behavioral agitation in Alzheimer's disease. *Journal of Clinical Psychopharmacology*, 17(1), 59–60.

Reife, R., Pledger, G. and Wu, S.C. (2000). Topiramate as add-on therapy: Pooled analysis of randomized controlled trials in adults. *Epilepsia*, 41(Suppl 1), S66–71.

Remick, R.A., Fleming, J.A., Buchanan, R.A., *et al.* (1985). A comparison of the safety and efficacy of alprazolam and desipramine in moderately severe depression. *Canadian Journal of Psychiatry*, 30(8), 597–601.

Remick, R.A., Keller, F.D., Buchanan, R.A., *et al.* (1988). A comparison of the efficacy and safety of alprazolam and desipramine in depressed outpatients. *Canadian Journal of Psychiatry*, 33(7), 590–594.

Richards, H.H., Midha, R.N. and Miller, S. (1982). A double-blind study of trazodone and mianserin in the treatment of depression in general practice. *Journal of International Medical Research*, 10(3), 147–156.

Rice, M.E. and Cragg, S.J. (2004). Nicotine amplifies reward-related dopamine signals in striatum. *Nature Neuroscience*, 7(6), 583–584.

Rickels, K., Chung, H.R., Csanalosi, I.B., *et al.* (1987). Alprazolam, diazepam, imipramine, and placebo in outpatients with major depression. *Archives of General Psychiatry*, 44(10), 862–866.

Rickels, K., Chung, H.R., Feldman, H.S., *et al.* (1973). Amitriptyline, diazepam, and phenobarbital sodium in depressed outpatients. *Journal of Nervous and Mental Disorders*, 157(6), 442–351.

Rickels, K., Feighner, J.P. and Smith, W.T. (1985). Alprazolam, amitriptyline, doxepin, and placebo in the treatment of depression. *Archives of General Psychiatry*, 42(2), 134–141.

Rickels, K., Gordon, P.E., Jenkins, B.W., *et al.* (1970). Drug treatment in depressive illness. *Diseases of the Nervous System*, 31(1) 30–42.

Rickels, K., London, J., Fox, I., *et al.* (1991). Adinazolam, diazepam, imipramine, and placebo in major depressive disorder: A controlled study. *Pharmacopsychiatry*, 24(4), 127–131.

Rickels, K., Pollack, M.H., Feltner, D.E., *et al.* (2005). Pregabalin for treatment of generalized anxiety disorder: A 4-week, multicenter, double-blind, placebo-controlled trial of pregabalin and alprazolam. *Archives of General Psychiatry*, 62(9), 1022–1030.

Rickels, K., Schweizer, E., Case, W.G. and Greenblatt, D.J. (1990). Long-term therapeutic use of benzodiazepines. I. Effects of abrupt discontinuation. *Archives of General Psychiatry*, 47(10), 899–907.

Rigo, J.M., Hans, G., Nguyen, L., *et al.* (2002). The anti-epileptic drug levetiracetam reverses the inhibition by negative allosteric modulators of neuronal GABA- and glycine-gated currents. *British Journal of Pharmacology*, 136(5), 659–672.

Rose, J.E., Behm, F.M., Westman, E.C., *et al.* (2003). PET studies of the influences of nicotine on neural systems in cigarette smokers. *American Journal of Psychiatry*, 160(2), 323–333.

Rosenthal, M. (2003). Tiagabine for the treatment of generalized anxiety disorder: A randomized, open-label, clinical trial with paroxetine as a positive control. *Journal of Clinical Psychiatry*, 64(10), 1245–1249.

Roth, T., Wright, K.P. Jr. and Walsh, J. (2006). Effect of tiagabine on sleep in elderly subjects with primary insomnia: A randomized, double-blind, placebo-controlled study. *Sleep*, 29(3), 335–341.

Roy-Byrne, P., Fleishaker, J., Arnett, C., *et al.* (1993). Effects of acute and chronic alprazolam treatment on cerebral blood flow, memory, sedation, and plasma catecholamines. *Neuropsychopharmacology*, 8(2), 161–169.

Roy Chengappa, K.N., Schwarzman, L.K., Hulihan, J.F., *et al.* (2006). Adjunctive topiramate therapy in patients receiving a mood stabilizer for bipolar I disorder: A randomized, placebo-controlled trial. *Journal of Clinical Psychiatry*, 67(11), 1698–1706.

Rush, A.J., Erman, M.K., Schlesser, M.A., *et al.* (1985). Alprazolam vs amitriptyline in depressions with reduced REM latencies. *Archives of General Psychiatry*, 42(12), 1154–1159.

Rush, R., Kuryatov, A., Nelson, M.E. and Lindstrom, J. (2002). First and second transmembrane segments of alpha3, alpha4, beta2, and beta4 nicotinic acetylcholine receptor subunits influence the efficacy and potency of nicotine. *Molecular Pharmacology*, 61(6), 1416–1422.

Russell, G.F., Niaz, U., Wakeling, A. and Slade, P.D. (1978). Comparative double-blind trial of mianserin hydrochloride (Organon GB94) and diazepam in patients with depressive illness. *British Journal of Clinical Pharmacology*, 5(Suppl 1), 57S–65S.

Ryback, R. and Ryback, L. (1995). Gabapentin for behavioral dyscontrol. *American Journal of Psychiatry*, 152(9), 1399.

Salminen, O., Murphy, K.L., McIntosh, J.M., *et al.* (2004). Subunit composition and pharmacology of two classes of striatal presynaptic nicotinic acetylcholine receptors mediating dopamine release in mice. *Molecular Pharmacology*, 65(6), 1526–1535.

Salin-Pascual, R.J. (2002). Relationship between mood improvement and sleep changes with acute nicotine administration in non-smoking major depressed patients. *Revista de Investigación Clínica*, 54(1), 36–40.

Salin-Pascual, R.J., de la Fuente, J.R., Galicia-Polo, L. and Drucker-Colin, R. (1995). Effects of transderman nicotine on mood and sleep in nonsmoking major depressed patients. *Psychopharmacology*, 121(4), 476–479.

Salin-Pascual, R.J. and Drucker-Colin, R. (1998). A novel effect of nicotine on mood and sleep in major depression. *Neuroreport*, 9(1), 57–60.

Salin-Pascual, R.J., Rosas, M., Jimenez-Genchi, A., *et al.* (1996). Antidepressant effect of transdermal nicotine patches in nonsmoking patients with major depression. *Journal of Clinical Psychiatry*, 57(9), 387–389.

Salloum, I.M., Cornelius, J.R., Thase, M.E., *et al.* (1998). Naltrexone utility in depressed alcoholics. *Psychopharmacology Bulletin*, 34(1), 111–115.

Salzman, C., Wolfson, A.N., Schatzberg, A., *et al.* (1995). Effect of fluoxetine on anger in symptomatic volunteers with borderline personality disorder. *Journal of Clinical Psychopharmacology*, 15(1), 23–29.

Samochocki, M., Hoffle, A., Fehrenbacher, A., *et al.* (2003). Galantamine is an allosterically potentiating ligand of neuronal nicotinic but not of muscarinic acetylcholine receptors. *Journal of Pharmacology and Experimental Therapeutics*, 305(3), 1024–1036.

Sanna, E., Busonero, F., Talani, G., *et al.* (2002). Comparison of the effects of zaleplon, zolpidem, and triazolam at various GABA(A) receptor subtypes. *European Journal of Pharmacology*, 451(2), 103–110.

Sapolsky, R.M. (2000). The possibility of neurotoxicity in the hippocampus in major depression: A primer on neuron death. *Biological Psychiatry*, 48(8), 755–765.

Sattler, R. and Tymianski, M. (2001). Molecular mechanisms of glutamate receptor-mediated excitotoxic neuronal cell death. *Molecular Neurobiology*, 24(1–3), 107–129.

Scatton, B. (1993). The NMDA receptor complex. *Fundamental and Clinical Pharmacology*, 7(8), 389–400.

Schaffer, A. and Levitt, A.J. (2005). Double-blind, placebo-controlled pilot study of mexiletine for acute mania or hypomania. *Journal of Clinical Psychopharmacology*, 25(5), 507–508.

Schoepp, D.D., Wright, R.A., Levine, L.R., *et al.* (2003). LY354740, an mGlu2/3 receptor agonist as a novel approach to treat anxiety/stress. *Stress*, 6(3), 189–197.

Schweizer, E., Rickels, K., Case, W.G. and Greenblatt, D.J. (1990). Long-term therapeutic use of benzodiazepines. II. Effects of gradual taper. *Archives of General Psychiatry*, 47(10), 908–915.

Shapira, N.A., Verduin, M.L. and DeGraw, J.D. (2001). Treatment of refractory major depression with tramadol monotherapy. *Journal of Clinical Psychiatry*, 62(3), 205–206.

Sharples, C.G., Kaiser, S., Soliakov, L., *et al.* (2000). UB-165: A novel nicotinic agonist with subtype selectivity implicates the alpha4beta2* subtype in the modulation of dopamine release from rat striatal synaptosomes. *Journal of Neuroscience*, 20(8), 2783–2791.

Sheldon, L.J., Ancill, R.J. and Holliday, S.G. (1998). Gabapentin in geriatric psychiatry patients. *Canadian Journal of Psychiatry*, 43(4), 422–423.

Shinotoh, H., Iyo, M., Yamada, T., *et al.* (1989). Detection of benzodiazepine receptor occupancy in the human brain by positron emission tomography. *Psychopharmacology*, 99(2), 202–207.

Shytle, R.D., Silver, A.A., Lukas, R.J., *et al.* (2002a). Nicotinic acetylcholine receptors as targets for antidepressants. *Molecular Psychiatry*, 7(6), 525–535.

Shytle, R.D., Silver, A.A., Sheehan, K.H., *et al.* (2002b). Neuronal nicotinic receptor inhibition for treating mood disorders: Preliminary controlled evidence with mecamylamine. *Depression & Anxiety*, 16, 89–92.

Siafaka-Kapadai, A., Patiris, M., Bowden, C. and Javors, M. (1998). Incorporation of [3H]valproic acid into lipids in GT1-7 neurons. *Biochemistry and Pharmacology*, 56(2), 207–212.

Sieghart, W. (1995). Structure and pharmacology of gamma-aminobutyric acidA receptor subtypes. *Pharmacology Reviews*, 47(2), 181–234.

Singh, A.N., Nair, N.P., Suranyi-Cadotte, B., *et al.* (1988). A double blind comparison of alprazolam and amitriptyline hydrochloride in the treatment of nonpsychotic depression. *Canadian Journal of Psychiatry*, 33(3), 218–222.

Simon, N.M., Worthington, J.J., Doyle, A.C, *et al.* (2004). An open-label study of levetiracetam for the treatment of social anxiety disorder. *Journal of Clinical Psychiatry*, 65(9), 1219–1222.

Sival, R.C., Haffmans, P.M., Jansen, P.A., *et al.* (2002). Sodium valproate in the treatment of aggressive behavior in patients with dementia — a randomized placebo controlled clinical trial. *International Journal of Geriatric Psychiatry*, 17(6), 579–585.

Sival, R.C., Duivenvoorden, H.J., Jansen, P.A., *et al.* (2004). Sodium valproate in aggressive behaviour in dementia: A twelve-week open label follow-up study. *International Journal of Geriatric Psychiatry*, 19(4), 305–312.

Smith, G.S., Schloesser, R., Brodie, J.D., *et al.* (1998). Glutamate modulation of dopamine measured *in vivo* with positron emission tomography (PET) and 11C-raclopride in normal human subjects. *Neuropsychopharmacology*, 18(1), 18–25.

Snoey, E.R. and Bessen, H.A. (1990). Acute psychosis after amantadine overdose. *Annals of Emergency Medicine*, 19(6), 668–670.

Stahl, S.M. and Grady, M.M. (2003). Differences in mechanism of action between current and future antidepressants. *Journal of Clinical Psychiatry*, 64(Suppl 13), 13–17.

Stapleton, J.M., Gilson, S.F., Wong, D.F., *et al.* (2003). Intravenous nicotine reduces cerebral glucose metabolism: A preliminary study. *Neuropsychopharmacology*, 28(4), 765–772.

Steece-Collier, K., Chambers, L.K., Jaw-Tsai, S.S., *et al.* (2000). Antiparkinsonian actions of CP-101,606, an antagonist of NR2B subunit-containing N-methyl-d-aspartate receptors. *Experimental Neurology*, 163(1), 239–243.

Stein, D.J., Baldwin, D.S., Baldinetti, F. and Mandel, F. (2008). Efficacy of pregabalin in depressive symptoms associated with generalized anxiety disorder: A pooled analysis of 6 studies. *European Neuropsychopharmacology*, 18(6), 422–430.

Stein, D.J., Simeon, D., Frenkel, M., *et al.* (1995). An open trial of valproate in borderline personality disorder. *Journal of Clinical Psychiatry*, 56(11), 506–510.

Sternfeld, F., Carling, R.W., Jelley, R.A., *et al.* (2004). Selective, orally active gamma-aminobutyric acidA alpha5 receptor inverse agonists as cognition enhancers. *Journal of Medicinal Chemistry*, 47(9), 2176.

Stockings, G.T. (1947). A new euphoriant for depressive mental states. *British Medical Journal*, 1, 918–922.

Strong, D.K., Eisenstat, D.D., Bryson, S.M., *et al.* (1991). Amantadine neurotoxicity in a pediatric patient with renal insufficiency. DICP, 25(11), 1175–1177.

Tallian, K.B., Nahata, M.C., Lo, W. and Tsao, C.Y. (1996). Gabapentin associated with aggressive behavior in pediatric patients with seizures. *Epilepsia*, 37(5), 501–502.

Tariot, P.N., Farlow, M.R., Grossberg, G.T., *et al.* (2004). Memantine treatment in patients with moderate to severe Alzheimer disease already receiving donepezil: A randomized controlled trial. *Journal of the American Medical Association*, 291(3), 317–324.

Terenius, L., Wahlstrom, A. and Agren, H. (1977). Naloxone (Narcan) treatment in depression: Clinical observations and effects on CSF endorphins and monoamine metabolites. *Psychopharmacology*, 54(1), 31–33.

Tiller, J., Schweitzer, I., Maguire, K. and Davies, B. (1989b). A sequential double-blind controlled study of moclobemide and diazepam in patients with atypical depression. *Journal of Affective Disorders*, 16(2–3), 181–187.

Tiller, J.W., Schweitzer, I., Maguire, K.P. and Davis, B. (1989a). Is diazepam an antidepressant? *British Journal of Psychiatry*, 155, 483–489.

Trinh, N.H., Hoblyn, J., Mohanty, S. and Yaffe, K. (2003). Efficacy of cholinesterase inhibitors in the treatment of neuropsychiatric symptoms and functional impairment in Alzheimer disease: A meta-analysis. *Journal of the American Medical Association*, 289(2), 210–216.

Tucker, P., Trautman, R.P., Wyatt, D.B., *et al.* (2007). Efficacy and safety of topiramate monotherapy in civilian posttraumatic stress disorder: A randomized, double-blind, placebo-controlled study. *Journal of Clinical Psychiatry*, 68(2), 201–206.

Tyrer, P., Seivewright, N., Murphy, S., *et al.* (1988). The Nottingham study of neurotic disorder: Comparison of drug and psychological treatments. *The Lancet*, 2(8605), 235–240.

Vale, S., Espejel, M.A. and Dominguez, J.C. (1971). Amantadine in depression. *The Lancet*, 2(7721), 437.

van der Stelt, M. and Di Marzo, V. (2003). The endocannabinoid system in the basal ganglia and in the mesolimbic reward system: Implications for neurological and psychiatric disorders. *European Journal of Pharmacology*, 480(1–3), 133–150.

Van Kampen, M., Selbach, K., Schneider, R., *et al.* (2004). AR-R 17779 improves social recognition in rats by activation of nicotinic alpha7 receptors. *Psychopharmacology*, 172(4), 375–383.

Varga, E., Sugerman, A.A. and Apter, J. (1982). The effect of codeine on involutional and senile depression. *Annals of the New York Academy of Sciences*, 398, 103–105.

Verner, J.V. (1969). Comparison of imipramine and chlordiazepoxide in the treatment of the depressed and anxious patient. *Journal of the Florida Medical Association*, 56(1), 15–21.

Vieta, E., Manuel Goikolea, J., Martínez-Arán, A., *et al.* (2006). A double-blind, randomized, placebo-controlled, prophylaxis study of adjunctive gabapentin for bipolar disorder. *Journal of Clinical Psychiatry*, 67(3), 473–477.

Videbaek, C., Friberg, L., Holm, S., *et al.* (1993). Benzodiazepine receptor equilibrium constants for flumazenil and midazolam determined in humans with the single photon emission computer tomography tracer [123I]iomazenil. *European Journal of Pharmacology*, 249(1), 43–51.

Volkow, N.D., Wang, G.J., Fowler, J.S., *et al.* (1998). Enhanced sensitivity to benzodiazepines in active cocaine-abusing subjects: A PET study. *American Journal of Psychiatry*, 155(2), 200–206.

Volkow, N.D., Wang, G.J., Hitzemann, R., *et al.* (1995). Depression of thalamic metabolism by lorazepam is associated with sleepiness. *Neuropsychopharmacology*, 12(2), 123–132.

Vollenweider, F.X., Vontobel, P., Oye, I., *et al.* (2000). Effects of (S)-ketamine on striatal dopamine: A [11C]raclopride PET study of a model psychosis in humans. *Journal of Psychiatric Research*, 34(1), 35–43.

Vuckovic, A., Cohen, B.M. and Zubenko, G.S. (1991). The use of captopril in treatment-resistant depression: An open trial. *Journal of Clinical Psychopharmacology*, 11(6), 395–396.

Wagner, K.D., Kowatch, R.A., Emslie, G.J., *et al.* (2006). A double-blind, randomized, placebo-controlled trial of oxcarbazepine in the treatment of bipolar disorder in children and adolescents. *American Journal of Psychiatry*, 163(7), 1179–1186.

Walsh, S.L. and Eissenberg, T. (2003). The clinical pharmacology of buprenorphine: Extrapolating from the laboratory to the clinic. *Drug and Alcohol Dependence*, 70(Suppl 2), S13–27.

Walsh, J.K., Randazzo, A.C., Frankowski, S., *et al.* (2005). Dose-response effects of tiagabine on the sleep of older adults. *Sleep*, 28(6), 673–676.

Walsh, J.K., Zammit, G., Schweitzer, P.K., *et al.* (2006). Tiagabine enhances slow wave sleep and sleep maintenance in primary insomnia. *Sleep Medicine*, 7(2), 155–161.

Wang, G.J., Volkow, N.D., Franceschi, D., *et al.* (2000). Regional brain metabolism during alcohol intoxication. *Alcoholism, Clinical and Experimental Research*, 24(6), 822–829.

Waterhouse, R.N. (2003). Imaging the PCP site of the NMDA ion channel. *Nuclear Medicine and Biology*, 30(8), 869–878.

Weisler, R.H., Kalali, A.H., Ketter, T.A.; SPD417 Study Group. (2004). A multicenter, randomized, double-blind, placebo-controlled trial of extended-release carbamazepine capsules as monotherapy for bipolar disorder patients with manic or mixed episodes. *Journal of Clinical Psychiatry*, 65(4), 478–484.

Weisler, R.H., Keck, P.E. Jr., Swann, A.C., *et al.* (2005). Extended-release carbamazepine capsules as monotherapy for acute mania in bipolar disorder: A multicenter, randomized, double-blind, placebo-controlled trial. *Journal of Clinical Psychiatry*, 66(3), 323–330.

Weissman, M.M., Prusoff, B., Sholomskas, A.J. and Greenwald, S. (1992). A double-blind clinical trial of alprazolam, imipramine, or placebo in the depressed elderly. *Journal of Clinical Psychopharmacology*, 12(3), 175–182.

Wheatley, D. (1969). A comparative trial of imipramine and phenobarbital in depressed patients seen in general practice. *Journal of Nervous and Mental Disorders*, 148(5), 542–549.

Wilcox, J.A. (1995). Divalproex sodium as a treatment for borderline personality disorder. *Annals of Clinical Psychiatry*, 7(1), 33–37.

Wilcox, J. (1985). Psychoactive properties of amantadine. *Journal of Psychoactive Drugs*, 17(1), 51–53.

Wolf, S.M., Shinnar, S., Kang, H., *et al.* (1995). Gabapentin toxicity in children manifesting as behavioral changes. *Epilepsia*, 36(12), 1203–1205.

Woods, T.M., Eichner, S.F. and Franks, A.S. (2004). Weight gain mitigation with topiramate in mood disorders. *Annals of Pharmacotherapy*, 38(5), 887–891.

Woods, J.H., Katz, J.L. and Winger, G. (1992). Benzodiazepines: Use, abuse, and consequences. *Pharmacology Reviews*, 44(2), 151–347.

Zarate, C.A. Jr., Payne, J.L., Quiroz, J., *et al.* (2004). An open-label trial of riluzole in patients with treatment-resistant major depression. *American Journal of Psychiatry*, 161(1), 171–174.

Zarate, C.A. Jr., Singh, J.B., Quiroz, J.A., *et al.* (2006). A double-blind, placebo-controlled study of memantine in the treatment of major depression. *American Journal of Psychiatry*, 163(1), 153–155.

Zawertailo, L.A., Busto, U.E., Kaplan, H.L., *et al.* (2003). Comparative abuse liability and pharmacological effects of meprobamate, triazolam, and butabarbital. *Journal of Clinical Psychopharmacology*, 23(3), 269–280.

Zhang, W., Connor, K.M. and Davidson, J.R. (2005). Levetiracetam in social phobia: A placebo controlled pilot study. *Journal of Psychopharmacology*, 19(5), 551–553.

Zhang, Z.J., Tan, Q.R., Tong, Y., *et al.* (2008). The effectiveness of carbamazepine in unipolar depression: A double-blind, randomized, placebo-controlled study. *Journal of Affective Disorders*, 109(1–2), 91–97.

Zubenko, G.S. and Nixon, R.A. (1984). Mood-elevating effect of captopril in depressed patients. *American Journal of Psychiatry*, 141(1), 110–111.

Zubieta, J., Lombardi, U., Minoshima, S., *et al.* (2001). Regional cerebral blood flow effects of nicotine in overnight abstinent smokers. *Biological Psychiatry*, 49(11), 906–913.

Chapter 12

Adams, J.B., Pyke, R.E., Costa, J., *et al.* (1995). A double-blind, placebo-controlled study of a CCK-B receptor antagonist, CI-988, in patients with generalized anxiety disorder. *Journal of Clinical Psychopharmacology*, 15(6), 428–434.

Ahokas, A., Aito, M. and Rimon, R. (2000). Positive treatment effect of estradiol in postpartum psychosis: A pilot study. *Journal of Clinical Psychiatry*, 61, 166–169.

Ahokas, A., Kaukoranta, J., Wahlbeck, K. and Aito, M. (2001). Estrogen deficiency in severe postpartum depression: Successful treatment with sublingual physiologic 17beta-estradiol: A preliminary study. *Journal of Clinical Psychiatry*, 62, 332–336.

Allolio, B., Callies, F. and Arlt, W. (1999). Dehydroepiandrosterone substitution in women. *Journal of Endocrinological Investigation*, 22, 29–31.

Altschule, M.D. and Tillotson, K.J. (1948). The use of testosterone in the treatment of depressions. *New England Journal of Medicine*, 239, 1036–1038.

Anand, A., Malison, R., McDougle, C.J. and Price, L.H. (1995). Antiglucocorticoid treatment of refractory depression with ketoconazole: A case report. *Biological Psychiatry*, 37, 338–340.

Andersch, B. and Hahn, L. (1985). Progesterone treatment of premenstrual tension — A double blind study. *Journal of Psychosomatic Research*, 29, 489–493.

Andreen, L., Bixo, M., Nyberg, S., *et al.* (2003). Progesterone effects during sequential hormone replacement therapy. *European Journal of Endocrinology*, 148, 571–577.

Arana, G.W. and Forbes, R.A. (1991). Dexamethasone for the treatment of depression: A preliminary report. *Journal of Clinical Psychiatry*, 52, 304–306.

Arana, G.W., Santos, A.B., Laraia, M.T., *et al.* (1995). Dexamethasone for the treatment of depression: A randomized, placebo-controlled, double-blind trial. *American Journal of Psychiatry*, 152, 265–267.

Arwert, L.I., Deijen, J.B. and Drent, M.L. (2003). Effects of an oral mixture containing glycine, glutamine and niacin on memory, GH and IGF-I secretion in middle-aged and elderly subjects. *Nutritional Neuroscience*, 6(5), 269–275.

Attardi, B.J., Burgenson, J., Hild, S.A. and Reel, J.R. (2004). *In vitro* antiprogestational/antiglucocorticoid activity and progestin and glucocorticoid receptor binding of the putative metabolites and synthetic derivatives of CDB-2914, CDB-4124, and mifepristone. *Journal of Steroid Biochemistry and Molecular Biology*, 88(3), 277–288.

Bech, P., Raabaek Olsen, L., Jarlov, N., *et al.* (1999). A case of sequential anti-stress medication in a patient with major depression resistant to amine-reuptake inhibitors. *Acta Psychiatrica Scandinavica*, 100, 76–78.

Belanoff, J.K., Flores, B.H., Kalezhan, M., *et al.* (2001). Rapid reversal of psychotic depression using mifepristone. *Journal of Clinical Psychopharmacology*, 21, 516–521.

Belanoff, J.K., Rothschild, A.J., Cassidy, F., *et al.* (2002). An open label trial of C-1073(mifepristone) for psychotic major depression. *Biological Psychiatry*, 52, 386–392.

Bellipanni, G., Bianchi, P., Pierpaoli, W., *et al.* (2001). Effects of melatonin in perimenopausal and menopausal women: A randomized and placebo controlled study. *Experimental Gerontology*, 36, 297–310.

Benedict, C., Hallschmid, M., Hatke, A., *et al.* (2004). Intranasal insulin improves memory in humans. *Psychoneuroendocrinology*, 29(10), 1326–1334.

Benkert, O., Martschke, D. and Gordon, A. (1974). Comparison of T.R.H., L.H.-R.H., and placebo in depression. *The Lancet*, 2(7889), 1146.

Binneman, B., Feltner, D., Kolluri, S., *et al.* (2008). A 6-week randomized, placebo-controlled trial of CP-316,311 (a selective CRH1 antagonist) in the treatment of major depression. *American Journal of Psychiatry*, 165(5), 617–620.

Brown, E.S., Bobadilla, L. and Rush, A.J. (2001). Ketoconazole in bipolar patients with depressive symptoms: A case series and literature review. *Bipolar Disorders*, 3, 23–29.

Campbell, S. and Whitehead, M. (1977). Oestrogen therapy and the menopausal syndrome. *Clinical Obstetrics and Gynaecology*, 4, 31–47.

Carman, J.S., Post, R.M., Buswell, R. and Goodwin, F.K. (1976). Negative effects of melatonin on depression. *American Journal of Psychiatry*, 133, 1181–1186.

Carranza-Lira, S. and Valentino-Figueroa, M.L. (1999). Estrogen therapy for depression in postmenopausal women. *International Journal of Gynaecology and Obstetrics*, 65, 35–38.

Cavallini, G., Caracciolo, S., Vitali, G., *et al.* (2004). Carnitine versus androgen administration in the treatment of sexual dysfunction, depressed mood, and fatigue associated with male aging. *Urology*, 63, 641–646.

Chu, J.W., Matthias, D.F., Belanoff, J., *et al.* (2001). Successful long-term treatment of refractory Cushing's disease with high-dose mifepristone (RU 486). *Journal of Clinical Endocrinology and Metabolism*, 86, 3568–3573.

Citera, G., Arias, M.A., Maldonado-Cocco, J.A., *et al.* (2000). The effect of melatonin in patients with fibromyalgia: A pilot study. *Clinical Rheumatology*, 19, 9–13.

Civic, D., Scholes, D., Ichikawa, L., *et al.* (2000). Depressive symptoms in users and non-users of depot medroxyprogesterone acetate. *Contraception*, 61, 385–390.

Cohen, L.S., Soares, C.N., Poitras, J.R., *et al.* (2003). Short-term use of estradiol for depression in perimenopausal and postmenopausal women: A preliminary report. *American Journal of Psychiatry*, 160, 1519–1522.

Coope, J. (1981). Is oestrogen therapy effective in the treatment of menopausal depression? *Journal of the Royal College of General Practitioners*, 31, 134–140.

Corney, R.H., Stanton, R. and Newell, R. (1990). Comparison of progesterone, placebo and behavioral psychotherapy in the treatment of premenstrual syndrome. *Journal of Psychosomatic Obstetrics and Gynaecology*, 11, 211–220.

Craft, S., Asthana, S., Newcomer, J.W., *et al.* (1999). Enhancement of memory in Alzheimer disease with insulin and somatostatin, but not glucose. *Archives of General Psychiatry*, 56(12), 1135–1140.

Craft, S., Newcomer, J., Kanne, S., *et al.* (1996). Memory improvement following induced hyperinsulinemia in Alzheimer's disease. *Neurobiology of Aging*, 17(1), 123–130.

Danziger, L. and Blank, H.R. (1942). Androgen therapy of agitated depressions in male. *Medical Annals of the District of Columbia*, 11, 181–183.

Danziger, L., Schroeder, H.T. and Unger, A.A. (1944). Androgen therapy for involutional melancholia. *Archives of Neurology and Psychiatry*, 51, 457–461.

Debattista, C., Belanoff, J., Glass, S., *et al.* (2006). Mifepristone versus placebo in the treatment of psychosis in patients with psychotic major depression. *Biological Psychiatry*, 60(12), 1343–1349.

DeBattista, C., Posener, J.A., Kalehzan, B.M. and Schatzberg, A.F. (2000). Acute antidepressant effects of intravenous hydrocortisone and CRH in depressed patients: A double-blind, placebo-controlled study. *American Journal of Psychiatry*, 157, 1334–1337.

Dennerstein, L., Spencer-Gardner, C., Gotts, G., *et al.* (1985). Progesterone and the premenstrual syndrome: A double blind crossover trial. *British Medical Journal (Clinical Research Edition)*, 290, 1617–1621.

Ditkoff, E.C, Crary, W.G., Cristo, M. and Lobo, R.A. (1991). Estrogen improves psychological function in asymptomatic postmenopausal women. *Obstetrics and Gynecology*, 78, 991–995.

Doggrell, R.A. (2003). Does the melanin-concentrating hormone antagonist SNAP-7941 deserve 3As? *Expert Opinion on Investigational Drugs*, 12, 1035–1038.

Dubocovich, M.L., Rivera-Bermudez, M.A., Gerdin, M.J. and Masana, M.I. (2003). Molecular pharmacology, regulation and function of mammalian melatonin receptors. *Frontiers in Bioscience*, 8, 1093–1108.

Ehrensing, R.H. and Kastin, A.J. (1978). Dose-related biphasic effect of prolyl-leucyl-glycinamide (MIF-I) in depression. *American Journal of Psychiatry*, 135(5), 562–566.

Ehrensing, R.H. and Kastin, A.J. (1974). Melanocyte-stimulating hormone-release inhibiting hormone as an antidepressant. A pilot study. *Archives of General Psychiatry*, 30(1), 63–65.

Ehrensing, R.H., Kastin, A.J., Schalch, D.S., *et al.* (1974). Affective state and thyrotropin and prolactin responses after repeated injections of thyrotropin-releasing hormone in depressed patients. *American Journal of Psychiatry*, 131(6), 714–718.

Ehrensing, R.H., Kastin, A.J., Wurzlow, G.F., *et al.* (1994). Improvement in major depression after low subcutaneous doses of MIF-1. *Journal of Affective Disorders*, 31(4), 227–233.

Erman, M., Seiden, D., Zammit, G., *et al.* (2006). An efficacy, safety, and dose-response study of Ramelteon in patients with chronic primary insomnia. *Sleep Medicine*, 7(1), 17–24.

Fraser, I., Wang, Y. (1998). New delivery systems for hormone replacement therapy. In J. Studd (Ed.), *The Management of Menopause-Annual Review*. 1st ed., pp. 101–110. London, UK: Parthenon.

Freeman, E., Rickels, K., Sondheimer, S.J. and Polansky, M. (1990). Ineffectiveness of progesterone suppository treatment for premenstrual syndrome. *Journal of the American Medical Association*, 264, 349–353.

Freeman, E.W., Rickels, K., Sondheimer, S.J. and Polansky, M. (1995). A double-blind trial of oral progesterone, alprazolam, and placebo in treatment of severe premenstrual syndrome. *Journal of the American Medical Association*, 274, 51–57.

Freeman, E.W., Sondheimer, S.J., Rickels, K. and Albert, J. (1993). Gonadotropin-releasing hormone agonist in treatment of premenstrual symptoms with and without comorbidity of depression: A pilot study. *Journal of Clinical Psychiatry*, 54, 192–195.

Freeman, M.P. and Freeman, S.A. (2003). Treatment of leuprolide-induced depression with intramuscular testosterone: A case report. *Journal of Clinical Psychiatry*, 64, 341–343.

George, G.C., Utian, W.H., Beaumont, P.J. and Beardwood, C.J. (1973). Effect of exogenous oestrogens on minor psychiatric symptoms in postmenopausal women. *South African Medical Journal*, 47, 2387–2388.

Ghadirian, A.M., Engelsmann, F., Dhar, V., *et al.* (1995). The psychotropic effects of inhibitors of steroid biosynthesis in depressed patients refractory to treatment. *Biological Psychiatry*, 37, 369–375.

Giusti, M., Meineri, I., Malagamba, D., *et al.* (1998). Impact of recombinant human growth hormone treatment on psychological profiles in hypopituitary patients with adult-onset growth hormone deficiency. *European Journal of Clinical Investigation*, 28, 13–19.

Gold, P.W., Weingartner, H., Ballenger, J.C., *et al.* (1979). Effects of 1-desamo-8-D-arginine vasopressin on behaviour and cognition in primary affective disorder. *The Lancet*, 2, 992–994.

Goodwin, G.M., Muir, W.J., Seckl, J.R., *et al.* (1992). The effects of cortisol infusion upon hormone secretion from the anterior pituitary and subjective mood in depressive illness and in controls. *Journal of Affective Disorders*, 26, 73–83.

Griebel, G., Simiand, J., Stemmelin, J., *et al.* (2003). The vasopressin V1b receptor as a therapeutic target in stress-related disorders. *Current Drug Targets. CNS and Neurological Disorders*, 2, 191–200.

Grinspoon, S., Corcoran, C., Stanley, T., *et al.* (2000). Effects of hypogonadism and testosterone administration on depression indices in HIV-infected men. *Journal of Clinical Endocrinology and Metabolism*, 85, 60–65.

Gregoire, A.J., Kumar, R., Everitt, B., *et al.* (1996). Transdermal oestrogen for treatment of severe postnatal depression. *The Lancet*, 347, 930–933.

Grunhaus, L., Hirschman, S., Dolberg, O.T., *et al.* (2001). Coadministration of melatonin and fluoxetine does not improve the 3-month outcome following ECT. *Journal of Electroconvulsive Therapy*, 17, 124–128.

Gupta, N., O'Brien, R., Jacobsen, L.J., *et al.* (2001). Mood changes in adolescents using depot-medroxyprogesterone acetate for contraception: A prospective study. *Journal of Pediatric and Adolescent Gynecology*, 14, 71–76.

Halbreich, U. and Kahn, L.S. (2001). Role of estrogen in the aetiology and treatment of mood disorders. *CNS Drugs*, 15, 797–817.

Haren, M.T., Wittert, G.A., Chapman, I.M., *et al.* (2005). Effect of oral testosterone undecanoate on visuospatial cognition, mood and quality of life in elderly men with low-normal gonadal status. *Maturitas*, 50(2), 124–133.

Herranz, R. (2003). Cholecystokinin antagonists: Pharmacological and therapeutic potential. *Medicinal Research Reviews*, 23(5), 559–605.

Heinrichs, S.C., De Souza, E.B., Schulteis, G., *et al.* (2002). Brain penetrance, receptor occupancy and antistress *in vivo* efficacy of a small molecule corticotropin releasing factor type I receptor selective antagonist. *Neuropsychopharmacology*, 27(2), 194–202.

Hollister, L.E., Berger, P., Ogle, F.L., *et al.* (1974). Protirelin (TRH) in depression. *Archives of General Psychiatry*, 31(4), 468–470.

Itil, T.M., Michael, S.T., Shapiro, D.M. and Itil, K.Z. (1984). The effects of mesterolone, a male sex hormone in depressed patients (a double blind controlled study). *Methods and Findings in Experimental and Clinical Pharmacology*, 6, 331–337.

Itil, T.M., Patterson, C.D., Polvan, N., *et al.* (1975). Clinical and CNS effects of oral and I.V. Thyrotropin-releasing hormone in depressed patients. *Diseases of the Nervous System*, 36(9), 529–536.

Karlberg, B.E., Kjellman, B.F. and Kagedal, B. (1978). Treatment of endogenous depression with oral thyrotropin-releasing hormone and amitriptyline. *Acta Psychiatrica Scandinavica*, 58(5), 389–400.

Kastin, A.J., Ehrensing, R.H., Schalch, D.S. and Anderson, M.S. (1972). Improvement in mental depression with decreased thyrotropin response after administration of thyrotropin-releasing hormone. *The Lancet*, 2(7780), 740–742.

Kern, W., Peters, A., Fruehwald-Schultes, B., *et al.* (2001). Improving influence of insulin on cognitive functions in humans. *Neuroendocrinology*, 74(4), 270–280.

Kiely, W.F., Adrian, A.D., Lee, J.H. and Nicoloff, J.T. (1976). Therapeutic failure of oral thyrotropin-releasing hormone in depression. *Psychosomatic Medicine*, 38(4), 233–241.

Kramer, M.S., Cutler, N.R., Ballenger, J.C., *et al.* (1995). A placebo-controlled trial of L-365,260, a CCKB antagonist, in panic disorder. *Biological Psychiatry*, 37(7), 462–466.

Kunzel, H.E., Zobel, A.W., Nickel, T., *et al.* (2003). Treatment of depression with the CRH-1-receptor antagonist R121919: Endocrine changes and side effects. *Journal of Psychiatric Research*, 37, 525–533.

Leppamaki, S., Partonen, T., Vakkuri, O., *et al.* (2003). Effect of controlled-release melatonin on sleep quality, mood, and quality of life in subjects with seasonal or weather-associated changes in mood and behaviour. *European Neuropsychopharmacology*, 13, 137–145.

Levy, M.I., DeNigris, Y. and Davis, K.L. (1982). Rapid antidepressant activity of melanocyte-inhibiting factor: A clinical trial. *Biological Psychiatry*, 17(2), 259–263.

Lewy, A.J., Bauer, V.K., Cutler, N.L. and Sack, R.L. (1998). Melatonin treatment of winter depression: A pilot study. *Psychiatry Research*, 77, 57–61.

Lloyd, R.L., Pekary, A.E., Sattin, A. and Amundson, T. (2001). Antidepressant effects of thyrotropin-releasing hormone analogues using a rodent model of depression. *Pharmacology, Biochemistry, and Behavior*, 70(1), 15–22.

Maddocks, S., Hahn, P., Moller, F. and Reid, R.L. (1986). A double-blind placebo-controlled trial of progesterone vaginal suppositories in the treatment of premenstrual syndrome. *American Journal of Obstetrics and Gynecology*, 154, 573–581.

Magill, P.J. (1995). Investigation of the efficacy of progesterone pessaries in the relief of symptoms of premenstrual syndrome. progesterone Study Group. *British Journal of General Practice*, 45, 589–593.

Malison, R.T., Anand, A., Pelton, G.H., *et al.* (1999). Limited efficacy of ketoconazole in treatment-refractory major depression. *Journal of Clinical Psychopharmacology*, 19, 466–470.

Malkin, C.J., Pugh, P.J., Morris, P.D., *et al.* (2004). Testosterone replacement in hypogonadal men with angina improves ischaemic threshold and quality of life. *Heart*, 90(8), 871–876.

Mattes, J.A., Pettinati, H.M., Nilsen, S.M., *et al.* (1989). Vasopressin for ECT-induced memory impairment: A placebo-controlled comparison. *Psychopharmacology Bulletin*, 25, 80–84.

Mattes, J.A., Pettinati, H.M., Stephens, S., *et al.* (1990). A placebo-controlled evaluation of vasopressin for ECT-induced memory impairment. *Biological Psychiatry*, 27, 289–303.

Morrison, M.F., Kallan, M.J., Ten Have, T., *et al.* (2004). Lack of efficacy of estradiol for depression in postmenopausal women: A randomized, controlled trial. *Biological Psychiatry*, 55, 406–412.

Murphy, B.E. (1991). Treatment of major depression with steroid suppressive drugs. *Journal of Steroid Biochemistry and Molecular Biology*, 39, 239–244.

Murphy, B.E., Dhar, V., Ghadirian, A.M., *et al.* (1991). Response to steroid suppression in major depression resistant to antidepressant therapy. *Journal of Clinical Psychopharmacology*, 11, 121–126.

Murphy, B.E., Filipini, D. and Ghadirian, A.M. (1993). Possible use of glucocorticoid receptor antagonists in the treatment of major depression: Preliminary results using RU 486. *Journal of Psychiatry and Neuroscience*, 18, 209–213.

Murphy, B.E., Ghadirian, A.M. and Dhar, V. (1998). Neuroendocrine responses to inhibitors of steroid biosynthesis in patients with major depression resistant to antidepressant therapy. *Canadian Journal of Psychiatry*, 43, 279–286.

O'Dwyer, A.M., Lightman, S.L., Marks, M.N. and Checkley, S.A. (1995). Treatment of major depression with metyrapone and hydrocortisone. *Journal of Affective Disorders*, 33, 123–128.

Okun, M.S., Walter, B.L., McDonald, W.M., *et al.* (2002). Beneficial effects of testosterone replacement for the nonmotor symptoms of Parkinson disease. *Archives of Neurology*, 59, 1750–1753.

Pande, A.C., Greiner, M., Adams, J.B., *et al.* (1999). Placebo-controlled trial of the CCK-B antagonist, CI-988, in panic disorder. *Biological Psychiatry*, 46(6), 860–862.

Perry, P.J., Yates, W.R., Williams, R.D., *et al.* (2002). Testosterone therapy in late-life major depression in males. *Journal of Clinical Psychiatry*, 63, 1096–1101.

Prange, A.J. Jr., Lara, P.P., Wilson, I.C., *et al.* (1972). Effects of thyrotropin-releasing hormone in depression. *The Lancet*, 2(7785), 999–1002.

Rabkin, J.G., McElhiney, M.C., Rabkin, R., *et al.* (2006). Placebo-controlled trial of dehydroepiandrosterone (DHEA) for treatment of nonmajor depression in patients with HIV/AIDS. *American Journal of Psychiatry*, 163(1), 59–66.

Rabkin, J. and Wagner, G. (1995). Testosterone Replacement Therapy: A recent innovation in the treatment of AIDS. *SIDAhora*, 1, 51–52.

Rabkin, J.G., Wagner, G.J., McElhiney, M.C., *et al.* (2004). Testosterone versus fluoxetine for depression and fatigue in HIV/AIDS: A placebo-controlled trial. *Journal of Clinical Psychopharmacology*, 24(4), 379–385.

Rabkin, J.G., Wagner, G.J. and Rabkin, R. (2000). A double-blind, placebo-controlled trial of testosterone therapy for HIV-positive men with hypogonadal symptoms. *Archives of General Psychiatry*, 57, 141–147.

Rabkin, J.G., Wagner, G.J. and Rabkin, R. (1999). Testosterone therapy for human immunodeficiency virus-positive men with and without hypogonadism. *Journal of Clinical Psychopharmacology*, 19, 19–27.

Ramachandran, C. and Fleisher, D. (2000). Transdermal delivery of drugs for the treatment of bone diseases. *Advanced Drug Delivery Reviews*, 42, 197–223.

Rapkin, A.J., Chang, L.C. and Reading, A.E. (1987). Premenstrual Syndrome: A double-blind placebo controlled study of treatment with progesterone vaginal suppositories. *Journal of Obstetrics and Gynecology*, 135, 209–215.

Rasgon, N.L., Altshuler, L.L. and Fairbanks, L. (2001). Estrogen-replacement therapy for depression. *American Journal of Psychiatry*, 158, 1738.

Rasgon, N.L., Altshuler, L.L., Fairbanks, L.A., *et al.* (2002). Estrogen replacement therapy in the treatment of major depressive disorder in perimenopausal women. *Journal of Clinical Psychiatry*, 63(Suppl 7), 45–48.

Raven, P.W., O'Dwyer, A.M., Taylor, N.F. and Checkley, S.A. (1996). The relationship between the effects of metyrapone treatment on depressed mood and urinary steroid profiles. *Psychoneuroendocrinology*, 21, 277–286.

Rubinow, D.R., Schmidt, P.J. and Roca, C.A. (1998). Estrogen-serotonin interactions: Implications for affective regulation. *Biological Psychiatry*, 44, 839–850.

Saletu, B., Brandstatter, N., Metka, M., *et al.* (1995). Double-blind, placebo-controlled, hormonal, syndromal and EEG mapping studies with transdermal oestradiol therapy in menopausal depression. *Psychopharmacology*, 122, 321–329.

Schmidt, P.J., Daly, R.C., Bloch, M., *et al.* (2005). Dehydroepiandrosterone monotherapy in midlife-onset major and minor depression. *Archives of General Psychiatry*, 62(2), 154–162.

Schmidt, P.J., Nieman, L., Danaceau, M.A., *et al.* (2000). Estrogen replacement in perimenopause-related depression: A preliminary report. *American Journal of Obstetrics and Gynecology*, 183, 414–220.

Schmidt, P.J., Roca, C.A., Bloch, M. and Rubinow, D.R. (1997). The perimenopause and affective disorders. *Seminars in Reproductive Endocrinology*, 15(1), 91–100.

Schneider, M.A., Brotherton, P.L. and Hailes, J. (1977). The effect of exogenous oestrogens on depression in menopausal women. *Medical Journal of Australia*, 2, 162–163.

Seidman, S.N., Orr, G., Raviv, G., *et al.* (2009). Effects of testosterone replacement in middle-aged men with dysthymia: A randomized, placebo-controlled clinical trial. *Journal of Clinical Psychopharmacology*, 29(3), 216–221.

Seidman, S.N. and Roose, S.P. (2006). The sexual effects of testosterone replacement in depressed men: Randomized, placebo-controlled clinical trial. *Journal of Sex and Marital Therapy*, 32(3), 267–273.

Seidman, S.N., Spatz, E., Rizzo, C. and Roose, S.P. (2001). Testosterone replacement therapy for hypogonadal men with major depressive disorder: A randomized, placebo-controlled clinical trial. *Journal of Clinical Psychiatry*, 62, 406–412.

Shifren, J.L., Braunstein, G.D., Simon, J.A., *et al.* (2000). Transdermal testosterone treatment in women with impaired sexual function after oophorectomy. *New England Journal of Medicine*, 343, 682–688.

Shores, M.M., Kivlahan, D.R., Sadak, T.I., *et al.* (2009). A randomized, double-blind, placebo-controlled study of testosterone treatment in hypogonadal older men with subthreshold depression (dysthymia or minor depression). *Journal of Clinical Psychiatry*, 70(7), 1009–1016.

Smith, R.N., Studd, J.W., Zamblera, D. and Holland, E.F. (1995). A randomised comparison over 8 months of 100 micrograms and 200 micrograms twice weekly doses of transdermal oestradiol in the treatment of severe premenstrual syndrome. *British Journal of Obstetrics and Gynaecology*, 102, 475–484.

Soares, C.N. (2003). Sex, hormones and depression: The impact of sex steroids on mood across the reproductive life cycle. Presented at the 156th Annual Meeting of the American Psychiatric Association. San Francisco, California.

Soares, C.N., Almeida, O.P., Joffe, H. and Cohen, L.S. (2001). Efficacy of estradiol for the treatment of depressive disorders in perimenopausal women: A double-blind, randomized, placebo-controlled trial. *Archives of General Psychiatry*, 58, 529–534.

Soares, C.N., Musolino, N.R., Cunha Neto, M., *et al.* (1999). Impact of recombinant human growth hormone (RH-GH) treatment on psychiatric, neuropsychological and clinical profiles of GH deficient adults. A placebo-controlled trial. *Arquivos de Neuro-psiquiatria*, 57, 182–189.

Souetre, E., Salvati, E., Belugou, J.L., *et al.* (1987). 5-Methoxypsoralen increases the plasma melatonin levels in humans. *Journal of Investigative Dermatology*, 89, 152–155.

Souetre, E., Salvati, E., Belugou, J.L., *et al.* (1988). Antidepressant effect of 5-methoxypsoralen: A preliminary report. *Psychopharmacology*, 95, 430–431.

Sovner, R. and Fogelman, S. (1996). Ketoconazole therapy for atypical depression. *Journal of Clinical Psychiatry*, 57, 227–228.

Strickler, R.C., Borth, R., Cecutti, A., *et al.* (1977). The role of oestrogen replacement in the climacteric syndrome. *Psychological Medicine*, 7, 631–639.

Sramek, J.J., Kramer, M.S., Reines, S.A. and Cutler, N.R. (1994). Pilot study of a CCKB antagonist in patients with panic disorder: Preliminary findings. *Anxiety*, 1(3), 141–143.

Sun, Y., Lu, X. and Gershengorn, M.C. (2003). Thyrotropin-releasing hormone receptors — similarities and differences. *Journal of Molecular Endocrinology*, 30(2), 87–97.

Szuba, M.P., Amsterdam, J.D., Fernando, A.T. 3rd, *et al.* (2005). Rapid antidepressant response after nocturnal TRH administration in patients with bipolar type I and bipolar type II major depression. *Journal of Clinical Psychopharmacology*, 25(4), 325–330.

Takahashi, S., Kondo, H., Yoshimura, M. and Ochi, Y. (1973). Antidepressant effect of thyrotropin-releasing hormone (TRH) and the plasma thyrotropin levels in depression. *Folia Psychiatrica et Neurologica Japonica*, 27(4), 305–314.

Thakore, J.H. and Dinan, T.G. (1995). Cortisol synthesis inhibition: A new treatment strategy for the clinical and endocrine manifestations of depression. *Biological Psychiatry*, 37, 364–368.

Thompson, J. and Oswald, I. (1977). Effect of oestrogen on the sleep, mood, and anxiety of menopausal women. *British Medical Journal*, 2, 1317–1319.

Thompson, J.L., Butterfield, G.E., Gylfadottir, U.K., *et al.* (1998). Effects of human growth hormone, insulin-like growth factor I, and diet and exercise on body composition of obese postmenopausal women. *Journal of Clinical Endocrinology and Metabolism*, 83, 1477–1284.

Turek, I.S. and Rocha, J. (1974). Oral thyrotropin-releasing hormone (TRH) in depressive illness. *Journal of Clinical Pharmacology*, 14(11–12), 612–616.

van den Burg, W., van Praag, H.M., Bos, E.R., *et al.* (1976). TRH by slow, continuous infusion: An antidepressant? *Psychological Medicine*, 6(3), 393–397.

Van der Meer, Y.G., Benedek-Yaszmann, L.J. and Van Loenen, A.C. (1983). Effect of high-dose progesterone on the premenstrual syndrome: A double blind crossover trial. *Journal of Psychosomatic Obstetrics and Gynaecology*, 2, 220–222.

van der Velde, C.D. (1983). Rapid clinical effectiveness of MIF-I in the treatment of major depressive illness. *Peptides*, 4(3), 297–300.

Vanselow, W., Dennerstein, L., Greenwood, K.M. and de Lignieres, B. (1996). Effect of progesterone and its 5 alpha and 5 beta metabolites on symptoms of premenstrual syndrome according to route of administration. *Journal of Psychosomatic Obstetrics and Gynaecology*, 17, 29–38.

Vogel, H.P., Benkert, O., Illig, R., *et al.* (1977). Psychoendocrinological and therapeutic effects of TRH in depression. *Acta Psychiatrica Scandinavica*, 56(3), 223–232.

Wagner, G.J., Rabkin, J.G. and Rabkin, R. (1998). Testosterone as a treatment for fatigue in HIV+ men. *Gen Hosp Psychiatry*, 20, 209–213.

Westhoff, C., Wieland, D. and Tiezzi, L. (1995). Depression in users of depomedroxyprogesterone acetate. *Contraception*, 51, 351–354.

Wren, B.G., Champion, S.M., Willetts, K., *et al.* (2003). Transdermal progesterone and its effect on vasomotor symptoms, blood lipid levels, bone metabolic markers, moods, and quality of life for postmenopausal women. *Menopause*, 10, 13–18.

Wolkowitz, O.M. and Reus, V.I. (1999). Treatment of depression with antiglucocorticoid drugs. *Psychosomatic Medicine*, 61(5), 698–711.

Wolkowitz, O.M., Reus, V.I., Chan, T., *et al.* (1999b). Antiglucocorticoid treatment of depression: Double-blind ketoconazole. *Biological Psychiatry*, 45, 1070–1074.

Wolkowitz, O.M., Reus, V.I., Keebler, A., *et al.* (1999a). Double-blind treatment of major depression with dehydroepiandrosterone. *American Journal of Psychiatry*, 156, 646–649.

Wolkowitz, O.M., Reus, V.I., Manfredi, F., *et al.* (1993). Ketoconazole administration in hypercortisolemic depression. *American Journal of Psychiatry*, 150, 810–812.

Wolkowitz, O.M., Reus, V.I., Roberts, E., *et al.* (1997). Dehydroepiandrosterone (DHEA) treatment of depression. *Biological Psychiatry*, 41, 311–318.

Wirz-Justice, A., Graw, P., Krauchi, K., *et al.* (1990). Morning or night-time melatonin is ineffective in seasonal affective disorder. *Journal of Psychiatric Research*, 24, 129–137.

Young, A.H., Gallagher, P., Watson, S., *et al.* (2004). Improvements in neurocognitive function and mood following adjunctive treatment with mifepristone (RU-486) in bipolar disorder. *Neuropsychopharmacology*, 29(8), 1538–1545.

Zemlan, F.P., Mulchahey, J.J., Scharf, M.B., *et al.* (2005). The efficacy and safety of the melatonin agonist beta-methyl-6-chloromelatonin in primary insomnia: A randomized, placebo-controlled, crossover clinical trial. *Journal of Clinical Psychiatry*, 66(3), 384–390.

Zohar, J., Drummer, D., Edelstein, E.D., *et al.* (1985). Effect of lysine vasopressin in depressed patients on mood and 24-hour rhythm of growth hormone, cortisol, melatonin and prolactin. *Psychoneuroendocrinology*, 10, 273–279.

Chapter 13

Adams, P.W., Rose, D.P., Folkard, J., *et al.* (1973). Effect of pyridoxine hydrochloride (vitamin B 6) upon depression associated with oral contraception. *The Lancet*, 1(7809), 899–904.

Agnoli, A., Fazio, C. and Andreoli, V. (1975). Disturbi neuropsichiatrici e transmetilazioni. Effetti terapeutici della S adenosil-l-metionina. *La Clinica Terapeutica*, 75, 567–579.

Andreoli, V., Campedelli, A. and Maffei, F. (1977). La s-adenosil-l-metionina (SAMe) in geropsichiatria: Uno studio clinico controllato "in aperto" nelle sindromi depressive dell'eta' senile. *Giornale Di Gerontologia*, 25, 172–180.

Barberi, A. and Pusateri, C. (1978). Sugli effetti clinici della s-adenosil-l-metionina (SAMe) nelle sindromi depressive. *Minerva Psichiatrica*, 19, 235–243.

Bell, K.M., Plon, L., Bunney, W.E. Jr. and Potkin, (1988). S.G. S-adenosylmethionine treatment of depression: A controlled clinical trial. *American Journal of Psychiatry*, 145, 1110–1114.

Bell, M.B., Carreon, D., Plon, L., *et al.* (1990). Oral s-adenosylmethionine in the treatment of depression: A double-blind comparison with desipramine. Study Report Provided by BioResearch, Inc.

Bella, R., Biondi, R., Raffaele, R. and Pennisi, G. (1990). Effect of acetyl-L-carnitine on geriatric patients suffering from dysthymic disorders. *International Journal of Clinical Pharmacology Research*, 10(6), 355–360.

Berkowitz, H.L. (2005). Modafinil in poststroke depression. *Psychosomatics*, 46(1), 93.

Bertolino, A., Crippa, D., di Dio, S., *et al.* (1988). Rolipram versus imipramine in inpatients with major, "minor" or atypical depressive disorder: A double-blind double-dummy study aimed at testing a novel therapeutic approach. *International Clinical Psychopharmacology*, 3(3), 245–253.

Bjerkenstedt, L., Edman, G.V., Alken, R.G. and Mannel, M. (2005). Hypericum extract LI 160 and fluoxetine in mild to moderate depression. A randomized, placebo-controlled multi-center study in outpatients. *European Archives of Psychiatry and Clinical Neuroscience*, 255(1), 40–47.

Bladt, S. and Wagner, H. (1994). Inhibition of MAO by fractions and constituents of hypericum extract. *Journal of Geriatric Psychiatry and Neurology*, 7(Suppl 1), S57–59.

Bobon, D., Breulet, M., Gerard-Vandenhove, M.A., *et al.* (1988). Is phosphodiesterase inhibition a new mechanism of antidepressant action? A double blind double-dummy study between rolipram and desipramine in hospitalized major and/or endogenous depressives. *European Archives of Psychiatry and Neurological Sciences*, 238(1), 2–6.

Bottiglieri, T., Godfrey, P., Flynn, T., *et al.* (1990). Cerebrospinal fluid S-adenosylmethionine in depression and dementia: Effects of treatment with parenteral and oral S-adenosylmethionine. *Journal of Neurology, Neurosurgery and Psychiatry*, 53, 1096–1098.

Bressa, G.M. (1994). S-adenosyl-l-methionine (SAMe) as antidepressant: Meta-analysis of clinical studies. *Acta Neurologica Scandinavica Supplementum*, 154, 7–14.

Brody, S. (2002). High-dose ascorbic acid increases intercourse frequency and improves mood: A randomized controlled clinical trial. *Biological Psychiatry*, 52(4), 371–374.

Cagnacci, A., Arangino, S., Renzi, A., *et al.* (2003). Kava-Kava administration reduces anxiety in perimenopausal women. *Maturitas*, 44(2), 103–109.

Carney, M.W., Edeh, J., Bottiglieri, T., *et al.* (1986). Affective illness and s-adenosyl methionine: A preliminary report. *Clinical Neuropharmacology*, 9, 379–385.

Caruso, I., Fumagalli, M., Boccassini, L., *et al.* (1984). Antidepressant activity of S-adenosyl methionine. *The Lancet*, I, 904.

Castagna, A., Le Grazie, C. and Accordini, A. (1995). Cerebrospinal fluid S-adenosylmethionine (SAMe) and glutathione concentrations in HIV infection: Effect of parenteral treatment with SAMe. *Neurology*, 45(9), 1678–1683.

Cavallini, G., Caracciolo, S., Vitali, G., *et al.* (2004). Carnitine versus androgen administration in the treatment of sexual dysfunction, depressed mood, and fatigue associated with male aging. *Urology*, 63(4), 641–646.

Chatterjee, S.S., Bhattacharya, S.K., Wonnemann, M., *et al.* (1998). Hyperforin as a possible antidepressant component of hypericum extracts. *Life Sciences*, 63(6), 499–510.

Cocchi, P., Silenzi, M., Calabri, G. and Salvi, G. (1980). Antidepressant effect of vitamin C. *Pediatrics*, 65(4), 862–863.

Connor, K.M. and Davidson, J.R. (2002). A placebo-controlled study of Kava kava in generalized anxiety disorder. *International Clinical Psychopharmacology*, 17(4), 185–188.

Cott, J.M. (1997). *In vitro* receptor binding and enzyme inhibition by *Hypericum perforatum* extract. *Pharmacopsychiatry*, 30(Suppl 2), 108–112.

Curtius, H.C., Muldner, H. and Niederweiser, A. (1982). Tetrahydrobiopterin: Efficacy in endogenous depression and Parkinson's disease. *Journal of Neural Transmission*, 55, 301–318.

Curtius, H.C., Niederwieser, A., Levine, R.A., *et al.* (1983). Successful treatment of depression with tetrahydrobiopterin. *The Lancet*, 1(8325), 657–658.

Davidson, J.R., Abraham, K., Connor, K.M. and McLeod, M.N. (2003). Effectiveness of chromium in atypical depression: A placebo-controlled trial. *Biological Psychiatry*, 53(3), 261–264.

De Vanna, M. and Rigamonti, R. (1992). Oral S-adenosyl-L-Methionine in depression. *Current Therapeutic Research*, 52, 478–485.

Delle Chiaie, R., Pancheri, P. and Scapicchio, P. (2002). Efficacy and tolerability of oral and intramuscular S-adenosyl-L-methionine 1,4-butanedisulfonate (SAMe) in the treatment of major depression: Comparison with imipramine in 2 multicenter studies. *American Journal of Clinical Nutrition*, 76 Suppl, 1172S–1176S.

Di Rocco, A., Rogers, J.D., Brown, R., *et al.* (2000). S-Adenosyl-Methionine improves depression in patients with Parkinson's disease in an open-label clinical trial. *Movement Disorders*, 15(6), 1225–1229.

Docherty, J.P., Sack, D., Roffman, M., *et al.* (2004). Chromium picolinate: Atypical depression, carbohydrate craving and clinical response. Presented at the 44th Annual Meeting of the New Clinical Drug Evaluation Unit of the National Institute of Mental Health. Scottsdale, Arizona.

Donovan, J.L., Malcolm, R.J., Markowitz, J.S. and DeVane, C.L. (2003). Chiral analysis of d- and l-modafinil in human serum: Application to human pharmacokinetic studies. *Therapeutic Drug Monitoring*, 25(2), 197–202.

Doornbos, B., van Goor, S.A., Dijck-Brouwer, D.A., *et al.* (2009). Supplementation of a low dose of DHA and DHA+AA does not prevent peripartum depressive symptoms in a small population based sample. *Progress in Neuropsychopharmacology and Biological Psychiatry*, 33(1), 49–52.

Eckmann, F., Fichte, K., Meya, U. and Sastre-Y-Hernandez, M. (1988). Rolipram in major depression: Results of a double-blind comparative study with amitriptyline. *Current Therapeutic Research*, 43(2), 291–295.

Fava, M., Alpert, J., Nierenberg, A.A., *et al.* (2005). A double-blind, randomized trial of St John's wort, fluoxetine, and placebo in major depressive disorder. *Journal of Clinical Psychopharmacology*, 25(5), 441–447.

Fava, M., Gianelli, A., Rapisarda, V., *et al.* (1995). Rapidity of onset of the antidepressant effect of parenteral S-adenosyl-L-methionine. *Psychiatry Research*, 56, 295–297.

Fava, M., Rosenbaum, J.F., Birnbaum, R., *et al.* (1992). The thyrotropin response to thyrotropin-releasing hormone as a predictor of response to treatment in depressed outpatients. *Acta Psychiatrica Scandinavica*, 86(1), 42–45.

Fava, M., Rosenbaum, J.F., MacLaughlin, R., *et al.* (1990). Neuroendocrine effects of s-adenosyl-l-methionine, a novel putative antidepressant. *Journal of Psychiatric Research*, 24, 177–184.

Fazio, C., Andreoli, V., Agnoli, A., *et al.* (1973). Effetti terapeutici e meccanismo d'azione della S-adenosil-l-metionina (SAMe) nelle sindromi depressive. *Minerva Medica*, 64: 1515–1529.

Ferraro, L., Antonelli, T., Tanganelli, S., *et al.* (1999). The vigilance promoting drug modafinil increases extracellular glutamate levels in the medial preoptic area and the posterior hypothalamus of the conscious rat: Prevention by local GABAA receptor blockade. *Neuropsychopharmacology*, 20(4), 346–356.

Ferraro, L., Tanganelli, S., O'Connor, W.T., *et al.* (1996). The vigilance promoting drug modafinil increases dopamine release in the rat nucleus accumbens via the involvement of a local GABAergic mechanism. *European Journal of Pharmacology*, 306(1–3), 33–39.

Ferraro, L., Tanganelli, S., O'Connor, W.T., *et al.* (1996b). The vigilance promoting drug modafinil decreases GABA release in the medial preoptic area and in the posterior hypothalamus of the awake rat: Possible involvement of the serotonergic 5-HT3 receptor. *Neuroscience Letters*, 220(1), 5–8.

Fleischhacker, W.W., Hinterhuber, H., Bauer, H., *et al.* (1992). A multicenter double-blind study of three different doses of the new camp-phosphodiesterase inhibitor rolipram in patients with major depressive disorder. *Neuropsychobiology*, 26, 59–64.

Follesa, P., Cagetti, E., Porta, S., *et al.* (2000). Pivagabine-induced increases in the abundance of CRF mRNA in the cerebral cortex and hypothalamus of rats. *Brain Research. Molecular Brain Research*, 84(1–2), 52–57.

Freeman, M.P., Davis, M., Sinha, P., *et al.* (2008). Omega-3 fatty acids and supportive psychotherapy for perinatal depression: A randomized placebo-controlled study. *Journal of Affective Disorders*, 110(1–2), 142–148.

Freeman, M.P., Hibbeln, J.R., Wisner, K.L., *et al.* (2006). Randomized dose-ranging pilot trial of omega-3 fatty acids for postpartum depression. *Acta Psychiatrica Scandinavica*, 113(1), 31–35.

Garzya, G., Corallo, D., Fiore, A., *et al.* (1990). Evaluation of the effects of L-acetylcarnitine on senile patients suffering from depression. *Drugs Under Experimental and Clinical Research*, 16(2), 101–106.

Gastpar, M., Singer, A. and Zeller, K. (2006). Comparative efficacy and safety of a once-daily dosage of hypericum extract STW3-VI and citalopram in patients with moderate depression: A double-blind, randomised, multicentre, placebo-controlled study. *Pharmacopsychiatry*, 39(2), 66–75.

Gerra, G., Zaimovic, A., Giusti, F., *et al.* (2001). Pivagabine effects on neuroendocrine responses to experimentally-induced psychological stress in humans. *Behavioural Brain Research*, 122(1), 93–101.

Gigliotti, B., Multinu, A. and Lai, V.R. (1997). Role of pivagabine in the treatment of climacteric syndrome. *Arzneimittel-Forschung*, 47(11A), 1317–1321.

Gloth, F.M. 3rd, Alam, W. and Hollis, B. (1999). Vitamin D vs broad spectrum phototherapy in the treatment of seasonal affective disorder. *Journal of Nutrition, Health, and Aging*, 3(1), 5–7.

Gobbi, M., Moia, M., Pirona, L., *et al.* (2001). *In vitro* binding studies with two *Hypericum perforatum* extracts — hyperforin, hypericin and biapigenin — on 5-HT6, 5-HT7, GABA(A)/benzodiazepine, sigma, NPY-Y1/Y2 receptors and dopamine transporters. *Pharmacopsychiatry*, 34(Suppl 1), S45-48.

Gould, T.D., Einat, H., Bhat, R. and Manji, H.K. (2004). AR-A014418, a selective GSK-3 inhibitor, produces antidepressant-like effects in the forced swim test. *International Journal of Neuropsychopharmacology*, 7(4), 387–390.

Grenyer, B.F., Crowe, T., Meyer, B., *et al.* (2007). Fish oil supplementation in the treatment of major depression: A randomized double-blind placebo controlled trial. *Progress in Neuropsychopharmacology and Biological Psychiatry*, 31(7), 1393–1396.

Guarardi, G., Fava, M., Mazzi, F. and LaGreca, P. (1993). An open trial of methyltetrahydrofolate (MTHF) in elderly depressed patients. *Annals of Clinical Psychiatry*, 5, 101–106.

Guiot-Goffioul, F., Gerard-Vandenhove, M.A., Troisfontaines, B., *et al.* (1987). Preliminary results of a double-blind study between rolipram and desipramine in hospitalized patients with major depressive symptoms. *Acta Psychiatrica Belgica*, 87(2), 230–235.

Hamilton, M. (1960). A rating scale for depression. *Journal of Neurology, Neurosurgery, and Psychiatry*, 23, 56–62.

Hansgen, K.D., Vesper, J. and Ploch, M. (1994). Multicenter double-blind study examining the antidepressant effectiveness of the hypericum extract LI 160. *Journal of Geriatric Psychiatry and Neurology*, 7(Suppl 1), S15–18.

Harrer, G., Hubner, W.D. and Podzuweit, H. (1994). Effectiveness and tolerance of the hypericum extract LI 160 compared to maprotiline: A multicenter double-blind study. *Journal of Geriatric Psychiatry and Neurology*, 7(Suppl 1), S24–28.

Hartz, A.J., Bentler, S., Noyes, R., *et al.* (2004). Randomized controlled trial of Siberian ginseng for chronic fatigue. *Psychological Medicine*, 34(1), 51–61.

Hebenstreit, G.F., Fellerer, K., Fichte, K., *et al.* (1989). Rolipram in major depressive disorder: Results of a double-blind comparative study with imipramine. *Pharmacopsychiatry*, 22(4), 156–160.

Heron, D.S., Shinitzky, M., Hershkowitz, M. and Samuel, D. (1980). Lipid fluidity markedly modulates the binding of serotonin to mouse brain membranes. *Proceedings of the National Academy of Sciences of the United States of America*, 77, 7463–7467.

Holsboen, F., Benkert, O., Meier, L. and Kreuz-Kersting, A. (1985). Combined estradiol and vitamin B6 treatment in women with major depression. *American Journal of Psychiatry*, 142(5), 658.

Hongisto, V., Smeds, N., Brecht, S., *et al.* (2003). Lithium blocks the c-Jun stress response and protects neurons via its action on glycogen synthase kinase 3. *Molecular and Cellular Biology*, 23(17), 6027–6036.

Horowski, R. and Sastre-Y-Hernandez, M. (1985). Clinical effects of the neurotropic selective camp phosphodiesterase inhibitor rolipram in depressed patients: Global evaluation of the preliminary reports. *Current Therapeutic Research*, 38(1), 23–29.

Hubner, W.D., Lande, S. and Podzuweit, H. (1994). Hypericum treatment of mild depressions with somatic symptoms. *Journal of Geriatric Psychiatry and Neurology*, 7(Suppl 1), S12–14.

Hypericum Depression Trial Study Group. (2002). Effect of *Hypericum perforatum* (St John's wort) in major depressive disorder: A randomized controlled trial. *Journal of the American Medical Association*, 287(14), 1807–1814.

Ishizuka, T., Sakamoto, Y., Sakurai, T. and Yamatodani, A. (2003). Modafinil increases histamine release in the anterior hypothalamus of rats. *Neuroscience Letters*, 339(2), 143–146.

Janicak, P.G., Lipinski, J., Davis, J.M., *et al.* (1988). S-Adenosylmethionine in depression: A literature review and preliminary report. *Alabama Journal of Medical Sciences*, 25, 306–313.

Jazayeri, S., Tehrani-Doost, M., Keshavarz, S.A., *et al.* (2008). Comparison of therapeutic effects of omega-3 fatty acid eicosapentaenoic acid andfluoxetine, separately and in combination, in major depressive disorder. *Australian and New Zealand Journal of Psychiatry*, 42(3), 192–198.

Kagan, B.L., Sultzer, D.L., Rosenlicht, N. and Gerner, R.H. (1990). Oral S-adenosylmethionine in depression: A randomized, double-blind, placebo-controlled trial. *American Journal of Psychiatry*, 147, 591–595.

Kalb, R., Trautmann-Sponsel, R.D. and Kieser, M. (2001). Efficacy and tolerability of hypericum extract WS 5572 versus placebo in mildly to moderately depressed patients. A randomized double-blind multicenter clinical trial. *Pharmacopsychiatry*, 34(3), 96–103.

Kasper, S. (2001). *Hypericum perforatum* — a review of clinical studies. *Pharmacopsychiatry*, 34(Suppl 1), S51–55.

Kasper, S., Anghelescu, I.G., Szegedi, A., *et al.* (2006). Superior efficacy of St John's wort extract WS 5570 compared to placebo in patients with major depression: A randomized, double-blind, placebo-controlled, multicenter trial. *BMC Medicine*, 4, 14.

Kasper, S., Volz, H.P., Möller, H.J., *et al.* (2008). Continuation and longterm maintenance treatment with Hypericum extract WS((R)) 5570 after recovery from an acute episode of moderate depression — A double-blind, randomized, placebo controlled long-term trial. *European Neuropsychopharmacology*, 18(11), 803–813.

Kaufman, K.R., Menza, M.A. and Fitzsimmons, A. (2002). Modafinil monotherapy in depression. *European Psychiatry*, 17(3), 167–169.

Knuppel, L. and Linde, K. (2004). Adverse Effects of St. John's Wort: A systematic review. *Journal of Clinical Psychiatry*, 65(11), 1470–1479.

Kulkarni, J., Garland, K.A., Scaffidi, A., *et al.* (2006). A pilot study of hormone modulation as a new treatment for mania in women with bipolar affective disorder. *Psychoneuroendocrinology*, 31(4), 543–547.

Laakmann, G., Schule, C., Baghai, T. and Kieser, M. (1998). St. John's wort in mild to moderate depression: The relevance of hyperforin for the clinical efficacy. *Pharmacopsychiatry*, 31(Suppl 1), 54–59.

Lands, W.E.B. (1992). Biochemistry and physiology of n-3 fatty acids. *FASEB Journal*, 6, 2530–2536.

Leaf, A. and Weber, P.C. (1987). A new era for science in nutrition. *American Journal of Clinical Nutrition*, 45, 1048–1053.

Lecrubier, Y., Clerc, G., Didi, R. and Kieser, M. (2002). Efficacy of St. John's wort extract WS 5570 in major depression: A double-blind, placebo-controlled trial. *American Journal of Psychiatry*, 159(8), 1361–1366.

Lehrl, S. (2004). Clinical efficacy of kava extract WS 1490 in sleep disturbances associated with anxiety disorders. Results of a multicenter, randomized, placebo-controlled, double-blind clinical trial. *Journal of Affective Disorders*, 78(2), 101–110.

Levine, J., Barak, Y., Gonzalves, M., *et al.* (1995). Double-blind, controlled trial of inositol treatment of depression. *American Journal of Psychiatry*, 152(5), 792–794.

Lipinski, J.F., Cohen, B.M., Frankenburg, F., *et al.* (1984). Open trial of S-adenosylmethionine for treatment of depression. *American Journal of Psychiatry*, 141(3), 448–450.

Loehrer, F.M., Schwab, R., Angst, C.P., *et al.* (1997). Influence of oral S-adenosylmethionine on plasma 5-methyltetrahydrofolate, S-adenosylhomocysteine, homocysteine and methionine in healthy humans. *Journal of Pharmacology and Experimental Therapeutics*, 282(2), 845–850.

Lundt, L. (2004). Modafinil treatment in patients with seasonal affective disorder/winter depression: An open-label pilot study. *Journal of Affective Disorders*, 81(2), 173–178.

Mantero, M. and Pastorino, P. (1976). Sindromi depressive, malattie cutanee e transmetilazioni. Effetti terapeutici della s-adenosyl-l-metionina. *Gazzeta Medica Italiana*, 135, 707–716.

Marangell, L.B., Martinez, J.M., Zboyan, H.A., *et al.* (2003). A double-blind, placebo-controlled study of the omega-3 fatty acid docosahexaenoic acid in the treatment of major depression. *American Journal of Psychiatry*, 160(5), 996–998.

McLeod, M.N., Gaynes, B.N. and Golden, R.N. (1999). Chromium potentiation of antidepressant pharmacotherapy for dysthymic disorder in 5 patients. *Journal of Clinical Psychiatry*, 60(4), 237–240.

McLeod, M.N. and Golden, R.N. (2000). Chromium treatment of depression. *International Journal of Neuropsychopharmacology*, 3(4), 311–314.

Mischoulon, D., Best-Popescu, C., Laposata, M., *et al.* (2008). A double-blind dose-finding pilot study of docosahexaenoic acid (DHA) for major depressive disorder. *European Neuropsychopharmacology*, 18(9), 639–645.

Mischoulon, D., Papakostas, G.I., Dording, C.M., *et al.* (in press). A double-blind, placebo-controlled trial of ethyl-eicosapentanoic acid (EPA) monotherapy for major depressive disorder. *Journal of Clinical Psychiatry*,

Moreno, R.A., Teng, C.T., Almeida, K.M. and Tavares Junior, H. (2006). *Hypericum perforatum* versus fluoxetine in the treatment of mild to moderate depression: A randomized double-blind trial in a Brazilian sample. *Revista Brasileira de Psiquiatria*, 28(1), 29–32.

Muller, D., Pfeil, T. and von den Driesch, V. (2003). Treating depression comorbid with anxiety — results of an open, practice-oriented study with St John's wort WS 5572 and valerian extract in high doses. *Phytomedicine*, 10(Suppl 4), 25–30.

Muller, W.E., Singer, A., Wonnemann, M., *et al.* (1998). Hyperforin represents the neurotransmitter reuptake inhibiting constituent of hypericum extract. *Pharmacopsychiatry*, 31 (Suppl 1), 16–21.

Nahrstedt, A. and Butterweck, V. (1997). Biologically active and other chemical constituents of the herb of Hypericum perforatum L. *Pharmacopsychiatry*, 30(Suppl 2), 129–134.

Negri, L. (1997). Evaluation of the efficacy of pivagabine on insomnia associated with mood disorders. *Arzneimittel-Forschung*, 47(11A): 1322–1325.

Nemets, H., Nemets, B., Apter, A., *et al.* (2006). Omega-3 treatment of childhood depression: A controlled, double-blind pilot study. *American Journal of Psychiatry*, 163(6), 1098–1100.

Ochs, G., Penn, R.D., York, M., *et al.* (2000). A phase IvII trial of recombinant methionyl human brain derived neurotrophic factor administered by intrathecal infusion to patients with amyotrophic lateral sclerosis. *Amyotrophic Lateral Sclerosis and other Motor Neuron Disorders*, 1, 201–206.

Oren, D.A., Teicher, M.H., Schwartz, P.J., *et al.* (1994). A controlled trial of cyanocobalamin (vitamin B12) in the treatment of winter seasonal affective disorder. *Journal of Affective Disorders*, 32(3), 197–200.

Ori, C., Freo, U., Pizzolato, G. and Dam, M. (2002). Effects of acetyl-L-carnitine on regional cerebral glucose metabolism in awake rats. *Brain Research*, 951(2), 330–335.

Pancheri, P., Scapicchio, P. and Chiaie, R.D. (2002). A double-blind, randomized parallel-group, efficacy and safety study of intramuscular S-adenosyl-L-methionine 1,4-butanedisulphonate (SAMe) versus imipramine in patients with major depressive disorder. *International Journal of Neuropsychopharmacology*, 5(4), 287–294.

Papakostas, G.I. (2009). Evidence for S-adenosyl-l-methionine (SAM-e) for the treatment of major depressive disorder. *Journal of Clinical Psychiatry*, 70(s5), 18–23.

Papakostas, G.I., Alpert, J.E. and Fava, M. (2003). S-adenosyl-methionine in depression: A comprehensive review of the literature. *Current Psychiatry Reports*, 5(6), 460–466.

Passeri, M., Cucinotta, D., Abate, G., *et al.* (1993). Oral 5′-methyltetrahydrofolic acid in senile organic mental disorders with depression: Results of a double-blind multicenter study. *Aging* (*Milano*), 5(1), 63–71.

Passeri, M., Ventura, S., Abate, G. and Cucinola, D. (1991). Oral 5-methyltetrahydrofolate (MTHF) in depression associated with senile organic mental disorders. *European Journal of Clinical Investigation*, 21(2ptII), 24.

Pettegrew, J.W., Levine, J. and McClure, R.J. (2000). Acetyl-L-carnitine physical-chemical, metabolic, and therapeutic properties: Relevance for its mode of action in Alzheimer's disease and geriatric depression. *Molecular Psychiatry*, 5(6), 616–632.

Philipp, M., Kohnen, R. and Hiller, K.O. (1999). Hypericum extract versus imipramine or placebo in patients with moderate depression: Randomised multicentre study of treatment for eight weeks. *British Medical Journal*, 319(7224), 1534–1538.

Pittler, M.H. and Ernst, E. (2000). Efficacy of kava extract for treating anxiety: Systematic review and meta-analysis. *Journal of Clinical Psychopharmacology*, 20(1), 84–89.

Pinzello, A. and Andreoli, V. (1972). Le transmetilazioni SAM-dipendenti nelle sindromi depressive. Valutazione dell-effetto terapeutico della S-adenosilmetionina con la scala di Hamilton. *Quaderni di Terapia Sperimentale — Supplemento di Biochimica eBiologia Sperimentale*, X/2, 3–11.

Pizzolato, G., Cagnin, A., Mancia, D., *et al.* (1997). Randomised, double-blind, placebo-controlled study of pivagabine in neurasthenia. *Arzneimittel-Forschung*, 47(11A), 1329–1331.

Price, C.S. and Taylor, F.B. (2005). A retrospective chart review of the effects of modafinil on depression as monotherapy and as adjunctive therapy. *Depression and Anxiety*, 21(4), 149–153.

Rabkin, J.G., McElhiney, M.C., Rabkin, R. and Ferrando, S.J. (2004). Modafinil treatment for fatigue in HIV+ patients: A pilot study. *Journal of Clinical Psychiatry*, 65(12), 1688–1695.

Randlov, C., Mehlsen, J., Thomsen, C.F., *et al.* (2006). The efficacy of St. John's wort in patients with minor depressive symptoms or dysthymia — a double-blind placebo-controlled study. *Phytomedicine*, 13(4), 215–221.

Rayman, M., Thompson, A., Warren-Perry, M., *et al.* (2006). Impact of selenium on mood and quality of life: A randomized, controlled trial. *Biological Psychiatry*, 59(2), 147–154.

Rees, A.M., Austin, M.P. and Parker, G.B. (2008). Omega-3 fatty acids as a treatment for perinatal depression: Randomized double-blind placebo-controlled trial. *Australian and New Zealand Journal of Psychiatry*, 42(3), 199–205.

Renau, T.E. (2004). The potential of phosphodiesterase 4 inhibitors for the treatment of depression: Opportunities and challenges. *Current Opinion in Investigational Drugs*, 5(1), 34–39.

Ricny, J., Tucek, S. and Novakova, J. (1992). Acetylcarnitine, carnitine and glucose diminish the effect of muscarinic antagonist quinuclidinyl benzilate on striatal acetylcholine content. *Brain Research*, 576(2), 215–219.

Rogers, P.J., Appleton, K.M., Kessler, D., *et al.* (2008). No effect of n-3 long-chain polyunsaturated fatty acid (EPA and DHA) supplementation on depressed mood and cognitive function: A randomised controlled trial. *British Journal of Nutrition*, 99(2), 421–431.

Rosenbaum, J.F., Fava, M., Falk, W.E., *et al.* (1990). The antidepressant potential of oral S-adenosyl-l-methionine. *Acta Psychiatrica Scandinavica*, 81, 432–436.

Roz, N., Mazur, Y., Hirshfeld, A. and Rehavi, M. (2002). Inhibition of vesicular uptake of monoamines by hyperforin. *Life Sciences*, 71(19), 2227–2237.

Roz, N. and Rehavi, M. (2003). Hyperforin inhibits vesicular uptake of monoamines by dissipating pH gradient across synaptic vesicle membrane. *Life Sciences*, 73(4), 461–470.

Ryves, W.J. and Harwood, A.J. (2001). Lithium inhibits glycogen synthase kinase-3 by competition for magnesium. *Biochemical and Biophysical Research Communications*, 280(3), 720–725.

Salmaggi, P., Bressa, G.M., Nicchia, G., *et al.* (1993). Double-blind, placebo-controlled study of s-adenosyl-l-methionine in depressed postmenopausal women. *Psychotherapy and Psychosomatics*, 59, 34–40.

Salvadorini, F., Galeone, F., Saba, P., *et al.* (1980). Evaluation of s-adenosylmethionine (SAMe) effectiveness on depression. *Current Therapeutic Research*, 27, 908–918.

Sarris, J., Kavanagh, D.J., Byrne, G., *et al.* (2009). The Kava Anxiety Depression Spectrum Study (KADSS): A randomized, placebo controlled crossover trial using an aqueous extract of *Piper methysticum*. *Psychopharmacology*, 205(3), 399–407.

Sarris, J., Kavanagh, D.J., Deed, G. and Bone, K.M. (2009). St. John's wort and Kava in treating major depressive disorder with comorbid anxiety: A randomised double-blind placebo-controlled pilot trial. *Human Psychopharmacology*, 24(1), 41–48.

Schrader, E. (2000). Equivalence of St John's wort extract (Ze 117) and fluoxetine: A randomized, controlled study in mild-moderate depression. *International Clinical Psychopharmacology*, 15(2), 61.

Schrader, E., Meier, B. and Brattstrom, A. (1998). Hypericum treatment of mild-moderate depression in a placebo-controlled study. A prospective, double-blind, randomized, placebo-controlled, multicenre study. *Human Psychopharmacology*, 13, 163–169.

Scott, A.I., Perini, A.F., Shering, P.A. and Whalley, L.J. (1991). In-patient major depression: Is rolipram as effective as amitriptyline? *European Journal of Clinical Pharmacology*, 40(2), 127–129.

Serra, M., Concas, A., Mostallino, M.C., *et al.* (1999). Antagonism by pivagabine of stress-induced changes in GABAA receptor function and corticotropin-releasing factor concentrations in rat brain. *Psychoneuroendocrinology*, 24(3), 269–284.

Shelton, R.C. (2000). Intracellular mechanisms of antidepressant drug action. *Harvard Review of Psychiatry*, 8(4), 161–174.

Shelton, R.C., Keller, M.B., Gelenberg, A., *et al.* (2001). Effectiveness of St John's wort in major depression: A randomized controlled trial. *Journal of the American Medical Association*, 285(15), 1978–1986.

Simopoulos, A.P., Norman, H.A., Gillaspy, J.E. and Duke, J.A. (1992). Common purslane: A source of omega-3 fatty acids and antioxidants. *Journal of the American College of Nutrition*, 11, 374–382.

Simopoulos, A.P. and Salem, N. Jr. (1986). Purslane: A terrestrial source of omega-3 fatty acids. *New England Journal of Medicine*, 315, 833.

Sommer, H. and Harrer, G. (1994). Placebo-controlled double-blind study examining the effectiveness of an hypericum preparation in 105 mildly depressed patients. *Journal of Geriatric Psychiatry and Neurology*, 7(Suppl 1), S9–11.

Sperling, R.I., Benincaso, A.I., Knoell, C.T., *et al.* (1993). Dietary omega-3 polyunsaturated fatty acids inhibit phosphoinositide formation and chemotaxis in neutrophils. *Journal of Clinical Investigation*, 91, 651–660.

Stensby, M.E. (1969). Nutritional properties of fish oils. *World Review of Nutrition and Dietetics*, 11, 46–105.

Su, K.P., Huang, S.Y., Chiu, T.H., *et al.* (2008). Omega-3 fatty acids for major depressive disorder during pregnancy: Results from a randomized, double-blind, placebo-controlled trial. *Journal of Clinical Psychiatry*, 69(4), 644–651.

Sugden, S.G. and Bourgeois, J.A. (2004). Modafinil monotherapy in poststroke depression. *Psychosomatics*, 45(1), 80–81.

Szegedi, A., Kohnen, R., Dienel, A. and Kieser, M. (2005). Acute treatment of moderate to severe depression with hypericum extract WS 5570 (St John's wort): Randomised controlled double blind non-inferiority trial versus paroxetine. *British Medical Journal*, 330(7490), 503.

Takadera, T., Sakamoto, Y. and Ohyashiki, T. (2004). NMDA receptor 2B-selective antagonist ifenprodil-induced apoptosis was prevented by glycogen synthase kinase-3 inhibitors in cultured rat cortical neurons. *Brain Research*, 1020(1–2), 196–203.

Tanganelli, S., Perez de la Mora, M., Ferraro, L., *et al.* (1995). Modafinil and cortical gamma-aminobutyric acid outflow. Modulation by 5-hydroxytryptamine neurotoxins. *European Journal of Pharmacology*, 273(1–2), 63–71.

Taylor, M.J., Wilder, H., Bhagwagar, Z. and Geddes, J. (2004). Inositol for depressive disorders. *Cochrane Database of Systematic Reviews*, 2, CD004049.

Terranova, R., Gilotta, S.M. and Luca, S. (1997). Clinical evaluation of the efficacy of pivagabine in the treatment of mood and adjustment disorders. *Arzneimittel-Forschung*, 47(11A), 1325–1328.

Thommessen, B. and Laake, K. (1996). No identifiable effect of ginseng (Gericomplex) as an adjuvant in the treatment of geriatric patients. *Aging (Milano)*, 8(6), 417–420.

Tode, T., Kikuchi, Y., Hirata, J., *et al.* (1999). Effect of Korean red ginseng on psychological functions in patients with severe climacteric syndromes. *International Journal of Gynecology and Obstetrics*, 67(3), 169–174.

Uebelhack, R., Gruenwald, J., Graubaum, H.J. and Busch, R. (2004). Efficacy and tolerability of Hypericum extract STW 3-VI in patients with moderate depression: A double-blind, randomized, placebo-controlled clinical trial. *Advances in Therapy*, 21(4), 265–275.

Ussher, J.M., Dewberry, C., Malson, H. and Noakes, J. (1995). The relationship between health related quality of life and dietary supplementation in British middle managers: A double-blind, placebo controlled study. *Psychology and Health*, 10, 97.

van Gurp, G., Meterissian, G.B., Haiek, L.N., *et al.* (2002). St John's wort or sertraline? Randomized controlled trial in primary care. *Canadian Family Physician*, 48, 905–912.

Verdon, F., Burnand, B., Stubi, C.L., *et al.* (2003). Iron supplementation for unexplained fatigue in non-anaemic women: Double blind randomised placebo controlled trial. *British Medical journal*, 326(7399), 1124.

Vorbach, E.U., Arnoldt, K.H. and Hubner, W.D. (1997). Efficacy and tolerability of St. John's wort extract LI 160 versus imipramine in patients with severe depressive episodes according to ICD-10. *Pharmacopsychiatry*, 30(Suppl 2), 81–85.

Vorbach, E.U., Hubner, W.D. and Arnoldt, K.H. (1994). Effectiveness and tolerance of the hypericum extract LI 160 in comparison with imipramine: Randomized double-blind study with 135 outpatients. *Journal of Geriatric Psychiatry and Neurology*, 7(Suppl 1), S19–23.

Werneke, U., Horn, O. and Taylor, D.M. (2004). How effective is St John's wort? The evidence revisited. *Journal of Clinical Psychiatry*, 65(5), 611–617.

Wesnes, K.A., Ferguson, J. and Petrini, O. (2004). The effects of *Ginkgo biloba* on memory in healthy middle-aged volunteers. Presented at the 44th Annual Meeting of the New Clinical Drug Evaluation Unit of the National Institute of Health. Scottsdale, Arizona.

Wesnes, K.A., Ward, T., McGinty, A. and Petrini, O. (2000). The memory enhancing effects of a *Ginkgo biloba/Panax ginseng* combination in healthy middle-aged volunteers. *Psychopharmacology*, 152(4), 353–361.

Wheatley, D. (1997). LI 160, an extract of St. John's wort, versus amitriptyline in mildly to moderately depressed outpatients — a controlled 6-week clinical trial. *Pharmacopsychiatry*, 30 (Suppl 2), 77–80.

Whiskey, E., Werneke, U. and Taylor, D. (2001). A systematic review and meta-analysis of *Hypericum perforatum* in depression: A comprehensive clinical review. *International Clinical Psychopharmacology*, 16(5), 239–252.

Wiklund, I., Karlberg, J. and Lund, B. (1994). A double-blind comparison of the effect on quality of life of a combination of vital substances including standardized ginseng G115 and placebo. *Current Therapeutic Research*, 55, 32.

Wiklund, I.K., Mattsson, L.A., Lindgren, R. and Limoni, C. (1999). Effects of a standardized ginseng extract on quality of life and physiological parameters in symptomatic postmenopausal women: A double-blind, placebo-controlled trial. Swedish Alternative Medicine Group. *International Journal of Clinical Pharmacology Research*, 19(3), 89–99.

Woelk, H. (2000). Comparison of St John's wort and imipramine for treating depression: Randomised controlled trial. *British Medical Journal*, 321(7260), 536–539.

Zanarini, M.C. and Frankenburg, F.R. (2003). Omega-3 Fatty acid treatment of women with borderline personality disorder: A double-blind, placebo-controlled pilot study. *American Journal of Psychiatry*, 160(1), 167–169.

Zarate, C.A. Jr., Singh, J.B., Carlson, P.J., *et al.* (2007). Efficacy of a protein kinase C inhibitor (tamoxifen) in the treatment of acute mania: A pilot study. *Bipolar Disorders*, 9(6), 561–570.

Zeller, E., Stief, H.J., Pflug, B. and Sastre-y-Hernandez, M. (1984). Results of a phase II study of the antidepressant effect of rolipram. *Pharmacopsychiatry*, 17(6), 188–190.

Zhu, J., Mix, E. and Winblad, B. (2001). The antidepressant and antiinflammatory effects of rolipram in the central nervous system. *CNS Drug Rev*iews, 7(4), 387–398.

Chapter 14

Aberg-Wistedt, A., Jostell, K.G., Ross, S.B. and Westerlund, D. (1981). Effects of zimelidine and desipramine on serotonin and noradrenaline uptake mechanisms in relation to plasma concentrations and to therapeutic effects during treatment of depression. *Psychopharmacology*, 74(4), 297–305.

Adli, M., Hollinde, D.L., Stamm, T., *et al.* (2007). Response to lithium augmentation in depression is associated with the glycogen synthase kinase 3-beta -50T/C single nucleotide polymorphism. *Biological Psychiatry*, 62(11), 1295–1302.

Arias, B., Catalan, R., Gasto, C., *et al.* (2003). 5-HTTLPR polymorphism of the serotonin transporter gene predicts non-remission in major depression patients treated with citalopram in a 12-weeks follow up study. *Journal of Clinical Psychopharmacology*, 23(6), 563–567.

Arias, B., Catalan, R., Gasto, C., *et al.* (2005). Evidence for a combined genetic effect of the 5-HT(1A) receptor and serotonin transporter genes in the clinical outcome of major depressive patients treated with citalopram. *Journal of Psychopharmacology*, 19(2), 166–172.

Arias, B., Serretti, A., Lorenzi, C., *et al.* (2006). Analysis of COMT gene (Val 158 Met polymorphism) in the clinical response to SSRIs in depressive patients of European origin. *Journal of Affective Disorders*, 90(2–3), 251–256.

Arias, B., Serretti, A., Mandelli, L., *et al.* (2009). Dysbindin gene (DTNBP1) in major depression: Association with clinical response to selective serotonin reuptake inhibitors. *Pharmacogenetics and Genomics*, 19(2), 121–128.

Arolt, V., Peters, M., Erfurth, A., *et al.* (2003). S100B and response to treatment in major depression: A pilot study. *European Neuropsychopharmacology*, 13(4), 235–239.

Bares, M., Brunovsky, M., Kopecek, M., *et al.* (2008). Early reduction in prefrontal theta QEEG cordance value predicts response to venlafaxine treatment in patients with resistant depressive disorder. *European Psychiatry*, 23(5), 350–355.

Bares, M., Brunovsky, M., Kopecek, M., *et al.* (2007). Changes in QEEG prefrontal cordance as a predictor of response to antidepressants in patients with treatment resistant depressive disorder: A pilot study. *Journal of Psychiatry Research*, 41(3–4), 319–325.

Bench, C.J., Frackowiak, R.S. and Dolan, R.J. (1995). Changes in regional cerebral blood flow on recovery from depression. *Psychological Medicine*, 25(2), 247–261.

Benedetti, F., Colombo, C., Pirovano, A., *et al.* (2009). The catechol-O-methyltransferase Val(108/158)Met polymorphism affects antidepressant response to paroxetine in a naturalistic setting. *Psychopharmacology (Berl)*, 203(1), 155–160.

Block, W., Träber, F., von Widdern, O., *et al.* (2009). Proton MR spectroscopy of the hippocampus at 3 T in patients with unipolar major depressive disorder: Correlates and predictors of treatment response. *International Journal of Neuropsychopharmacology*, 12(3), 415–422.

Bozina, N., Peles, A.M., Sagud, M., *et al.* (2008). Association study of paroxetine therapeutic response with SERT gene polymorphisms in patients with major depressive disorder. *World Journal of Biological Psychiatry*, 9(3), 190–197.

Brody, A.L., Saxena, S., Silverman, D.H., *et al.* (1999). Brain metabolic changes in major depressive disorder from pre- to post-treatment with paroxetine. *Psychiatry Research*, 91(3), 127–139.

Bruder, G.E., Otto, M.W., McGrath, P.J., *et al.* (1996). Dichotic listening before and after fluoxetine treatment for major depression: Relations of laterality to therapeutic response. *Neuropsychopharmacology*, 15(2), 171–179.

Bruder, G.E., Sedoruk, J.P., Stewart, J.W., *et al.* (2008). Electroencephalographic alpha measures predict therapeutic response to a selective serotonin reuptake inhibitor antidepressant: Pre- and post-treatment findings. *Biological Psychiatry*, 63(12), 1171–1177.

Bruder, G.E., Stewart, J.W., McGrath, *et al.* (2004). Dichotic listening tests of functional brain asymmetry predict response to fluoxetine in depressed women and men. *Neuropsychopharmacology*, 29(9), 1752–1761.

Bruder, G.E., Stewart, J.W., Schaller, J.D. and McGrath, P.J. (2007). Predicting therapeutic response to secondary treatment with bupropion: Dichotic listening tests of functional brain asymmetry. *Psychiatry Research*, 153(2), 137–143.

Bruder, G.E., Stewart, J.W., Tenke, C.E., *et al.* (2001). Electroencephalographic and perceptual asymmetry differences between responders and nonresponders to an SSRI antidepressant. *Biological Psychiatry*, 49(5), 416–425.

Bruder, G.E., Stewart, J.W., Voglmaier, M.M., *et al.* (1990). Cerebral laterality and depression: Relations of perceptual asymmetry to outcome of treatment with tricyclic antidepressants. *Neuropsychopharmacology*, 3(1), 1–10.

Buchsbaum, M.S., Wu, J., Siegel, B.V., *et al.* (1997). Effect of sertraline on regional metabolic rate in patients with affective disorder. *Biological Psychiatry*, 41(1), 15–22.

Castrogiovanni, P., Blardi, P., De Lalla, A., *et al.* (2003). Can serotonin and fluoxetine levels in plasma and platelets predict clinical response in depression? *Psychopharmacology Bulletin*, 37(2), 102–108.

Celada, P., Dolera, M., Alvarez, E. and Artigas, F. (1992a). Effects of acute and chronic treatment with fluvoxamine on extracellular and platelet serotonin in the blood of major depressive patients. Relationship to clinical improvement. *Journal of Affective Disorders*, 25(4), 243–249.

Celada, P., Perez, J., Alvarez, E. and Artigas, F. (1992b). Monoamine oxidase inhibitors phenelzine and brofaromine increase plasma serotonin and decrease 5-hydroxyindoleacetic acid in patients with major depression: Relationship to clinical improvement. *Journal of Clinical Psychopharmacology*, 12(5), 309–315.

Chen, C.H., Ridler, K., Suckling, J., *et al.* (2007) Brain imaging correlates of depressive symptom severity and predictors of symptom improvement after antidepressant treatment. *Biological Psychiatry*, 62(5), 407–414.

Choi, M.J., Kang, R.H., Ham, B.J., *et al.* (2005). Serotonin receptor 2A gene polymorphism (-1438A/G) and short-term treatment response to citalopram. *Neuropsychobiology*, 52(3), 155–162.

Choi, M.J., Kang, R.H., Lim, S.W., *et al.* (2006). Brain-derived neurotrophic factor gene polymorphism (Val66Met) and citalopram response in major depressive disorder. *Brain Research*, 1118(1), 176–182.

Choi, T.K., Koo, M.S., Lee, S.H., *et al.* (2007). Serotonin transporter gene polymorphism associated with venlafaxine treatment response. *European Neuropsychopharmacology*, 17(s4), S228.

Cook, I.A. and Leuchter, A.F. (2001). Prefrontal changes and treatment response prediction in depression. *Seminars in Clinical Neuropsychiatry*, 6(2), 113–120.

Cook, I.A., Leuchter, A.F., Morgan, M.L., *et al.* (2005). Changes in prefrontal activity characterize clinical response in SSRI nonresponders: A pilot study. *Journal of Psychiatry Research*, 39(5), 461–466.

Cook, I.A., Leuchter, A.F., Morgan, M., *et al.* (2002). Early changes in prefrontal activity characterize clinical responders to antidepressants. *Neuropsychopharmacology*, 27(1), 120–131.

Cooper-Kazaz, R., van der Deure, W.M., Medici, M., *et al.* (2009). Preliminary evidence that a functional polymorphism in type 1 deiodinase is associated with enhanced potentiation of the antidepressant effect of sertraline by triiodothyronine. *Journal of Affective Disorders*, 116(1–2), 113–116.

Crowley, J.J., Lipsky, R.H., Lucki, I. and Berrettini, W.H. (2008). Variation in the genes encoding vesicular monoamine transporter 2 and beta-1 adrenergic receptor and antidepressant treatment outcome. *Psychiatric Genetics*, 18(5), 248–251.

Cusin, C., Serretti, A., Zanardi, R., *et al.* (2002). Influence of monoamine oxidase A and serotonin receptor 2A polymorphisms in SSRI antidepressant activity. *International Journal of Neuropsychopharmacology*, 5(1), 27–35.

Davidson, R.J., Irwin, W., Anderle, M.J. and Kalin, N.H. (2003) The neural substrates of affective processing in depressed patients treated with venlafaxine. *American Journal of Psychiatry*, 2003, 160(1), 64–75.

Dmitrzak-Weglarz, M., Rajewska-Rager, A., Gattner, K., *et al.* (2007). Association studies of 5HT2A and 5HTTLPR polymorphisms and drug response in depression patients. *European Neuropsychopharmacology*, 17(s4), S238.

Domschke, K., Lawford, B., Laje, G., *et al.* (in press). Brain-derived neurotrophic factor (BDNF) gene: No major impact on antidepressant treatment response. *International Journal of Neuropsychopharmacology*.

Durham, L.K., Webb, S.M., Milos, P.M., *et al.* (2004). The serotonin transporter polymorphism, 5HTTLPR, is associated with a faster response time to sertraline in an elderly population with major depressive disorder. *Psychopharmacology*, 174(4), 525–529.

Eller, T., Vasar, V., Shlik, J. and Maron, E. (2008). Pro-inflammatory cytokines and treatment response to escitaloprsam in major depressive disorder. *Progress in Neuropsychopharmacology and Biological Psychiatry*, 32(2), 445–450.

Fu, C.H., Williams, S.C., Brammer, M.J., *et al.* (2007). Neural responses to happy facial expressions in major depression following antidepressant treatment. *American Journal of Psychiatry*, 164(4), 599–607.

Fu, C.H., Williams, S.C., Cleare, A.J., *et al.* (2004). Attenuation of the neural response to sad faces in major depression by antidepressant treatment: A prospective, event-related functional magnetic resonance imaging study. *Archives of General Psychiatry*, 61(9), 877–889.

Fu, C.H., Williams, S.C., Cleare, A.J., *et al.* (2008). Neural responses to sad facial expressions in major depression following cognitive behavioral therapy. *Biological Psychiatry*, 64(6), 505–512.

Gallinat, J., Bottlender, R., Juckel, G., *et al.* (2000). The loudness dependency of the auditory evoked N1/P2-component as a predictor of the acute SSRI response in depression. *Psychopharmacology*, 148(4), 404–411.

Gau, Y.T., Liou, Y.J., Yu, Y.W., *et al.* (2008). Evidence for association between genetic variants of p75 neurotrophin receptor (p75(NTR)) gene and antidepressant treatment response in Chinese major depressive disorder. *American Journal of Medical Genetics Part B: Neuropsychiatric Genetics*, 147B(5), 594–599.

Gervasoni, N., Aubry, J.M., Bondolfi, G., *et al.* (2005). Partial normalization of serum brain-derived neurotrophic factor in remitted patients after a major depressive episode. *Neuropsychobiology*, 51(4), 234–238.

Gurguis, G.N., Vo, S.P., Griffith, J.M. and Rush, A.J. (1999a). Neutrophil beta(2)-adrenoceptor function in major depression: G(s) coupling, effects of imipramine and relationship to treatment outcome. *European Journal of Pharmacology*, 386(2–3), 135–144.

Gurguis, G.N., Vo, S.P., Griffith, J.M. and Rush, A.J. (1999b). Platelet alpha2A-adrenoceptor function in major depression: Gi coupling, effects of imipramine and relationship to treatment outcome. *Psychiatry Research*, 89(2), 73–95.

Ham, B.J., Lee, B.C., Paik, J.W., *et al.* (2007). Association between the tryptophan hydroxylase-1 gene A218C polymorphism and citalopram antidepressant response in a Korean population. *Progress in Neuropsychopharmacology and Biological Psychiatry*, 31(1), 104–107.

Hellweg, R., Ziegenhorn, A., Heuser, I. and Deuschle, M. (2008). Serum concentrations of nerve growth factor and brain-derived neurotrophic factor in depressed patients before and after antidepressant treatment. *Pharmacopsychiatry*, 41(2), 66–71.

Hetzel, G., Moeller, O., Evers, S., *et al.* (2005). The astroglial protein S100B and visually evoked event-related potentials before and after antidepressant treatment. *Psychopharmacology (Berl)*, 178(2–3), 161–166.

Hong, C.J., Chen, T.J., Yu, Y.W. and Tsai, S.J. (2006). Response to fluoxetine and serotonin 1A receptor (C-1019G) polymorphism in Taiwan Chinese major depressive disorder. *Pharmacogenomics Journal*, 6(1), 27–33.

Hrdina, P.D., Bakish, D., Ravindran, A., *et al.* (1997). Platelet serotonergic indices in major depression: Up-regulation of 5-HT2A receptors unchanged by antidepressant treatment. *Psychiatry Research*, 66(2–3), 73–85.

Hu, X.Z, Rush, A.J., Charney, D., *et al.* (2007). Association between a functional serotonin transporter promoter polymorphism and citalopram treatment in adult outpatients with major depression. Archives of General Psychiatry, 64(7), 783–792.

Huang, T.L., Lee, C.T. and Liu, Y.L. (2008). Serum brain-derived neurotrophic factor levels in patients with major depression: Effects of antidepressants. *Journal of Psychiatric Research*, 42(7), 521–525.

Hunter, A.M., Cook, I.A. and Leuchter, A.F. (2007). The promise of the quantitative electroencephalogram as a predictor of antidepressant treatment outcomes in major depressive disorder. *Psychiatric Clinics of North America*, 30(1), 105–124.

Hunter, A.M., Leuchter, A.F., Morgan, M.L., *et al.* (2005). Neurophysiologic correlates of side effects in normal subjects randomized to venlafaxine or placebo. *Neuropsychopharmacology*, 30(4), 792–799.

Iga, J., Ueno, S., Yamauchi, K., *et al.* (2007). Altered HDAC5 and CREB mRNA expressions in the peripheral leukocytes of major depression.

Progress in Neuropsychopharmacology and Biological Psychiatry, 31(3), 628–632.

Iosifescu, D.V., Bolo, N.R., Nierenberg, A.A., *et al.* (2008). Brain bioenergetics and response to triiodothyronine augmentation in major depressive disorder. *Biological Psychiatry*, 63(12), 1127–1134.

Iosifescu, D.V., Greenwald, S., Devlin, P., *et al.* (2005). Frontal EEG at 1 week predicts clinical response to SSRIs in MDD. Presented at the 158th Annual meeting of the American Psychiatric Association. Atlanta, Georgia.

Ito, K., Yoshida, K., Sato, K., *et al.* (2002). A variable number of tandem repeats in the serotonin transporter gene does not affect the antidepressant response to fluvoxamine. *Psychiatry Research*, 111(2–3), 235–239.

Joyce, P.R., Mulder, R.T., Luty, S.E., *et al.* (2003). Age-dependent antidepressant pharmacogenomics: Polymorphisms of the serotonin transporter and G protein beta3 subunit as predictors of response to fluoxetine and nortriptyline. *International Journal of Neuropsychopharmacology*, 6(4), 339–346.

Juckel, G., Pogarell, O., Augustin, H., *et al.* (2007). Differential prediction of first clinical response to serotonergic and noradrenergic antidepressants using the loudness dependence of auditory evoked potentials in patients with major depressive disorder. *Journal of Clinical Psychiatry*, 68(8), 1206–1212.

Kang, R.H., Wong, M.L., Choi, M.J., *et al.* (2007a). Association study of the serotonin transporter promoter polymorphism and mirtazapine antidepressant response in major depressive disorder. *Progress in Neuropsychopharmacology and Biological Psychiatry*, 31(6), 1317–1321.

Kang, R.H., Hahn, S.W., Choi, M.J. and Lee, M.S. (2007b). Relationship between G-protein beta-3 subunit C825T polymorphism and mirtazapine responses in Korean patients with major depression. *Neuropsychobiology*, 56(1), 1–5.

Kang, R.H., Choi, M.J., Paik, J.W., *et al.* (2007c). Effect of serotonin receptor 2A gene polymorphism on mirtazapine response in major depression. *International Journal of Psychiatry in Medicine*, 37(3), 315–329.

Karege, F., Widmer, J., Bovier, P. and Gaillard, J.M. (1994). Platelet serotonin and plasma tryptophan in depressed patients: Effect of drug treatment and clinical outcome. *Neuropsychopharmacology*, 10(3), 207–214.

Kato, M., Fukuda, T., Wakeno, M., *et al.* (2006). Effects of the serotonin type 2A, 3A and 3B receptor and the serotonin transporter genes on paroxetine and fluvoxamine efficacy and adverse drug reactions in depressed Japanese patients. *Neuropsychobiology*, 53(4), 186–195.

Kato, M., Wakeno, M., Okugawa, G., *et al.* (2007). No association of TPH1 218A/C polymorphism with treatment response and intolerance to

SSRIs in Japanese patients with major depression. *Neuropsychobiology*, 56(4), 167–171.

Kato, M., Fukuda, T., Serretti, A., *et al.* (2008a). ABCB1 (MDR1) gene polymorphisms are associated with the clinical response to paroxetine in patients with major depressive disorder. *Progress in Neuropsychopharmacology and Biological Psychiatry*, 32(2), 398–404.

Kato, M., Wakeno, M., Okugawa, G., *et al.* (2008b). Antidepressant response and intolerance to SSRI is not influenced by G-protein beta3 subunit gene C825T polymorphism in Japanese major depressive patients. *Progress in Neuropsychopharmacology and Biological Psychiatry*, 32(4), 1041–1044.

Keedwell, P., Drapier, D., Surguladze, S., *et al.* (2009). Neural markers of symptomatic improvement during antidepressant therapy in severe depression: Subgenual cingulate and visual cortical responses to sad, but not happy, facial stimuli are correlated with changes in symptom score. *Journal of Psychopharmacology*, 23(7), 775–788.

Kennedy, S.H., Evans, K.R., Kruger, S., *et al.* (2001). Changes in regional brain glucose metabolism measured with positron emission tomography after paroxetine treatment of major depression. *American Journal of Psychiatry*, 158(6), 899–905.

Kim, D.K., Lim, S.W., Lee, S., *et al.* (2000). Serotonin transporter gene polymorphism and antidepressant response. *Neuroreport*, 11(1), 215–219.

Kim, Y.K., Na, K.S., Shin, K.H., *et al.* (2007). Cytokine imbalance in the pathophysiology of major depressive disorder. *Progress in Neuropsychopharmacology and Biological Psychiatry*, 31(5), 1044–1053.

Knott, V., Mahoney, C., Kennedy, S. and Evans, K. (2000). Pre-treatment EEG and its relationship to depression severity and paroxetine treatment outcome. *Pharmacopsychiatry*, 33(6), 201–205.

Knott, V.J., Telner, J.I., Lapierre, Y.D., *et al.* (1996). Quantitative EEG in the prediction of antidepressant response to imipramine. *Journal of Affective Disorders*, 39(3), 175–184.

Koch, J.M., Kell, S., Hinze-Selch, D. and Aldenhoff, J.B. (2002). Changes in CREB-phosphorylation during recovery from major depression. *Journal of Psychiatric Research*, 36(6), 369–375.

Kraft, J.B., Peters, E.J., Slager, S.L., *et al.* (2007). Analysis of association between the serotonin transporter and antidepressant response in a large clinical sample. *Biological Psychiatry*, 61(6), 734–742.

Kraft, J.B., Slager, S.L., McGrath, P.J. and Hamilton, S.P. (2005). Sequence analysis of the serotonin transporter and associations with antidepressant response. *Biological Psychiatry*, 58(5), 374–381.

Kronenberg, S., Apter, A., Brent, D., *et al.* (2007). Serotonin transporter polymorphism (5-HTTLPR) and citalopram effectiveness and side effects in children with depression and/or anxiety disorders. *Journal of Child and Adolescent Psychopharmacology*. 17(6), 741–750.

Lai, I.C., Hong, C.J. and Tsai, S.J. (2003). Expression of cAMP response element-binding protein in major depression before and after antidepressant treatment. *Neuropsychobiology*, 48(4), 182–185.

Laika, B., Leucht, S. and Steimer, W. (2006). ABCB1 (P-glycoprotein/MDR1) gene G2677T/a sequence variation (polymorphism): Lack of association with side effects and therapeutic response in depressed inpatients treated with amitriptyline. *Clinical Chemistry*, 52(5), 893–895.

Langenecker, S.A., Kennedy, S.E., Guidotti, L.M., *et al.* (2007). Frontal and limbic activation during inhibitory control predicts treatment response in major depressive disorder. *Biological Psychiatry*, 62(11), 1272–1280.

Lanquillon, S., Krieg, J.C., Bening-Abu-Shach, U. and Vedder, H. (2000). Cytokine production and treatment response in major depressive disorder. *Neuropsychopharmacology*, 22(4), 370–379.

Lee, K.M. and Kim, Y.K. (2006). The role of IL-12 and TGF-beta1 in the pathophysiology of major depressive disorder. *International Immunopharmacology*, 6(8), 1298–1304.

Lee, T.W., Yu, Y.W., Chen, T.J. and Tsai, S.J. (2005). Loudness dependence of the auditory evoked potential and response to antidepressants in Chinese patients with major depression. *Journal of Psychiatry and Neuroscience*, 30(3), 202–205.

Lekman, M., Laje, G., Charney, D., *et al.* (2008). The FKBP5-gene in depression and treatment response — an association study in the sequenced treatment alternatives to relieve depression (STAR*D) cohort. *Biological Psychiatry*, 63(12), 1103–1110.

Leuchter, A.F., Cook, I.A., Gilmer, W.S., *et al.* (2009). Effectiveness of a quantitative electroencephalographic biomarker for predicting differential response or remission with escitalopram and bupropion in major depressive disorder. *Psychiatry Research*, 169(2), 124–131.

Leuchter, A.F., Cook, I.A., Lufkin, R.B., *et al.* (1994). Cordance: A new method for assessment of cerebral perfusion and metabolism using quantitative electroencephalography. *NeuroImage*, 1(3), 208–219.

Leuchter, A.F., Cook, I.A., Uijtdehaage, S.H., *et al.* (1997). Brain structure and function and the outcomes of treatment for depression. *Journal of Clinical Psychiatry*, 58(Suppl 16), 22–31.

Leuchter, A.F., Cook, I.A., Witte, E.A., *et al.* (2002). Changes in brain function of depressed subjects during treatment with placebo. *American Journal of Psychiatry*, 159(1), 122–129.

Lingjaerde, O., Bratfos, O., Bratlid, T. and Haug, J.O. (1983). A double-blind comparison of zimelidine and desipramine in endogenous depression. *Acta Psychiatrica Scandinavica*, 68(1), 22–30.

Linka, T., Muller, B.W., Bender, S. and Sartory, G. (2004). The intensity dependence of the auditory evoked N1 component as a predictor of response to Citalopram treatment in patients with major depression. *Neuroscience Letters*, 367(3), 375–378.

Linka, T., Muller, B.W., Bender, S., *et al.* (2005). The intensity dependence of auditory evoked ERP components predicts responsiveness to reboxetine treatment in major depression. *Pharmacopsychiatry*, 38(3), 139–143.

Little, J.T., Ketter, T.A., Kimbrell, T.A., *et al.* (1996). Venlafaxine or bupropion responders but not nonresponders show baseline prefrontal and paralimbic hypometabolism compared with controls. *Psychopharmacology Bulletin*, 32(4), 629–635.

Little, J.T., Ketter, T.A., Kimbrell, T.A., *et al.* (2005). Bupropion and venlafaxine responders differ in pretreatment regional cerebral metabolism in unipolar depression. *Biological Psychiatry*, 57(3), 220–228.

Maes, M., Bosmans, E., De Jongh, R., *et al.* (1997). Increased serum IL-6 and IL-1 receptor antagonist concentrations in major depression and treatment resistant depression. *Cytokine*, 9(11), 853–858.

Maes, M., Meltzer, H.Y., Bosmans, E., *et al.* (1995). Increased plasma concentrations of interleukin-6, soluble interleukin-6, soluble interleukin-2 and transferrin receptor in major depression. *Journal of Affective Disorders*, 34(4), 301–309.

Matrisciano, F., Bonaccorso, S., Ricciardi, A., *et al.* (2009). Changes in BDNF serum levels in patients with major depression disorder (MDD) after 6 months treatment with sertraline, escitalopram, or venlafaxine. *Journal of Psychiatric Research*, 43(3), 247–254.

Mayberg, H.S., Brannan, S.K., Tekell, J.L., *et al.* (2000). Regional metabolic effects of fluoxetine in major depression: Serial changes and relationship to clinical response. *Biological Psychiatry*, 48(8), 830–843.

Mayberg, H.S., Liotti, M., Brannan, S.K., *et al.* (1999). Reciprocal limbic-cortical function and negative mood: Converging PET findings in depression and normal sadness. *American Journal of Psychiatry*, 156(5), 675–682.

Mayberg, H.S., Silva, J.A., Brannan, S.K., *et al.* (2002). The functional neuroanatomy of the placebo effect. *American Journal of Psychiatry*, 159(5), 728–737.

Meltzer, H.Y., Arora, R.C., Baber, R. and Tricou, B.J. (1981). Serotonin uptake in blood platelets of psychiatric patients. *Archives of General Psychiatry*, 38(12), 1322–1326.

McMahon, F.J., Buervenich, S., Charney, D., *et al.* (2006). Variation in the gene encoding the serotonin 2A receptor is associated with outcome of antidepressant treatment. *American Journal of Human Genetics*, 78(5), 804–814.

Michelson, D., Adler, L.A., Amsterdam, J.D., *et al.* (2007). Addition of atomoxetine for depression incompletely responsive to sertraline: A randomized, double-blind, placebo-controlled study. *Journal of Clinical Psychiatry*, 68, 582–587.

Mihaljevic Peles, A., Bozina, N., Sagud, M., *et al.* (2008). MDR1 gene polymorphism: Therapeutic response to paroxetine among patients with major depression. *Progress in Neuropsychopharmacology and Biological Psychiatry*, 32(6), 1439–1444.

Mikova, O., Yakimova, R., Bosmans, E., *et al.* (2001). Increased serum tumor necrosis factor alpha concentrations in major depression and multiple sclerosis. *European Neuropsychopharmacology*, 11(3), 203–208.

Minov, C., Baghai, T.C., Schule, C., *et al.* (2001). Serotonin-2A-receptor and -transporter polymorphisms: Lack of association in patients with major depression. *Neuroscience Letters*, 303(2), 119–122.

Mischoulon, D., Kramer, L., Fava, S., *et al.* (2003). Prevalence of MTHFR C677T and methionine synthase A2756G polymorphisms in major depression, and impact on response to fluoxetine treatment. Presented at the 42nd Annual meeting of the American College of Neuropsychopharmacology. San Juan, Puerto Rico.

Mrazek, D.A., Rush, A.J., Biernacka, J.M., *et al.* (2009). SLC6A4 variation and citalopram response. *American Journal of Medical Genetics Part B: Neuropsychiatric Genetics*, 150B(3), 341–351.

Mulert, C., Juckel, G., Augustin, H. and Hegerl, U. (2002). Comparison between the analysis of the loudness dependency of the auditory N1/P2 component with LORETA and dipole source analysis in the prediction of treatment response to the selective serotonin reuptake inhibitor citalopram in major depression. *Clinical Neurophysiology*, 113(10), 1566–1572.

Mulert, C., Juckel, G., Brunnmeier, M., *et al.* (2007). Prediction of treatment response in major depression: Integration of concepts. *Journal of Affective Disorders*, 98(3), 215–225.

Muller, D.J., Schulze, T.G., Macciardi, F., *et al.* (2002). Moclobemide response in depressed patients: Association study with a functional polymorphism in the monoamine oxidase A promoter. *Pharmacopsychiatry*, 35(4), 157–158.

Murphy, G.M. Jr., Hollander, S.B., Rodrigues, H.E., *et al.* (2004). Effects of the serotonin transporter gene promoter polymorphism on mirtazapine and paroxetine efficacy and adverse events in geriatric major depression. *Archives of General Psychiatry*, 61(11), 1163–1169.

Murphy, G.M., Kremer, C., Rodrigues, H.E. and Schatzberg, A.F. (2003). Pharmacogenetics of antidepressant medication intolerance. *American Journal of Psychiatry*, 160(10), 1830–1835.

Myint, A.M., Leonard, B.E., Steinbusch, H.W. and Kim, Y.K. (2005). Th1, Th2, and Th3 cytokine alterations in major depression. *Journal of Affective Disorders*, 88(2), 167–173.

Ng, C.H., Easteal, S., Tan, S., *et al.* (2006). Serotonin transporter polymorphisms and clinical response to sertraline across ethnicities. *Progress in Neuropsychopharmacology and Biological Psychiatry*, 30(5), 953–957.

Nikisch, G., Eap, C.B. and Baumann, P. (2008). Citalopram enantiomers in plasma and cerebrospinal fluid of ABCB1 genotyped depressive patients and clinical response: A pilot study. *Pharmacologic Research*, 58(5–6), 344–347.

Paddock, S., Laje, G., Charney, D., *et al.* (2007). Association of GRIK4 with outcome of antidepressant treatment in the STAR*D cohort. *American Journal of Psychiatry*, 164(8), 1181–1188.

Paige, S.R., Fitzpatrick, D.F., Kline, J.P., *et al.* (1994). Event-related potential amplitude/intensity slopes predict response to antidepressants. *Neuropsychobiology*, 30(4), 197–201.

Peters, E.J., Slager, S.L., Kraft, J.B., *et al.* (2008). Pharmacokinetic genes do not influence response or tolerance to citalopram in the STAR*D sample. PLoS ONE, 3(4), e1872.

Perez, V., Bel, N., Celada, P., *et al.* (1998). Relationship between blood serotonergic variables, melancholic traits, and response to antidepressant treatments. *Journal of Clinical Psychopharmacology*, 18(3), 222–230.

Perlis, R.H., Moorjani, P., Fagerness, J., *et al.* (2008). Pharmacogenetic analysis of genes implicated in rodent models of antidepressant response: Association of TREK1 and treatment resistance in the STAR(*)D study. *Neuropsychopharmacology*, 33(12), 2810–2819.

Peters, E.J., Slager, S.L., McGrath, P.J., *et al.* (2004). Investigation of serotonin-related genes in antidepressant response. *Molecular Psychiatry*, 9(9), 879–889.

Poland, R., Greenwald, S.D., Devlin, P., *et al.* (2005). Change in frontal EG predictors response to citalopram treatment in MDD. Frontal EEG at 1 week predicts clinical response to SSRIs in MDD. Presented at the 158th Annual meeting of the American Psychiatric Association. Atlanta, Georgia.

Pollock, B.G., Ferrell, R.E., Mulsant, B.H., *et al.* (2000). Allelic variation in the serotonin transporter promoter affects onset of paroxetine treatment response in late-life depression. *Neuropsychopharmacology*, 23(5), 587–590.

Rausch, J.L., Hobby, H.M., Shendarkar, N., *et al.* (2001). Fluvoxamine treatment of mixed anxiety and depression: Evidence for serotonergically mediated anxiolysis. *Clinical Psychopharmacology*, 21(2), 139–142.

Rausch, J.L., Johnson, M.E., Fei, Y.J., *et al.* (2002). Initial conditions of serotonin transporter kinetics and genotype: Influence on SSRI treatment trial outcome. *Biological Psychiatry*, 51(9), 723–732.

Rausch, J.L., Moeller, F.G. and Johnson, M.E. (2003). Initial platelet serotonin (5-HT) transport kinetics predict nortriptyline treatment outcome. *Journal of Clinical Psychopharmacology*, 23(2), 138–144.

Renshaw, P.F., Lafer, B., Babb, S.M., *et al.* (1997). Basal ganglia choline levels in depression and response to fluoxetine treatment: An *in vivo* proton magnetic resonance spectroscopy study. *Biological Psychiatry*, 41(8), 837–843.

Rush, A.J., Erman, M.K., Schlesser, M.A., *et al.* (1985). Alprazolam vs amitriptyline in depressions with reduced REM latencies. *Archives of General Psychiatry*, 42(12), 1154–1159.

Rush, A.J., Giles, D.E., Jarrett, R.B., *et al.* (1989). Reduced REM latency predicts response to tricyclic medication in depressed outpatients. *Biological Psychiatry*, 26(1), 61–72.

Sato, K., Yoshida, K., Takahashi, H., *et al.* (2002). Association between –1438G/A promoter polymorphism in the 5-HT(2A) receptor gene and fluvoxamine response in Japanese patients with major depressive disorder. *Neuropsychobiology*, 46(3), 136–140.

Schroeter, M.L., Abdul-Khaliq, H., Diefenbacher, A. and Blasig, I.E. (2002). S100B is increased in mood disorders and may be reduced by antidepressive treatment. *Neuroreport*, 16;13(13), 1675–1678.

Schroeter, M.L., Abdul-Khaliq, H., Krebs, M., *et al.* (2008). Serum markers support disease-specific glial pathology in major depression. *Journal of Affective Disorders*, 111(2–3), 271–280.

Sen, S., Duman, R. and Sanacora, G. (2008). Serum brain-derived neurotrophic factor, depression, and antidepressant medications: Meta-analyses and implications. *Biological Psychiatry*, 64(6), 527–532.

Serretti, A., Cusin, C., Rausch, J.L., *et al.* (2006). Pooling pharmacogenetic studies on the serotonin transporter: A mega-analysis. *Psychiatry Research*, 145(1), 61–65.

Serretti, A., Kato, M., De Ronchi, D. and Kinoshita, T. (2007). Meta-analysis of serotonin transporter gene promoter polymorphism (5-HTTLPR) association with selective serotonin reuptake inhibitor efficacy in depressed patients. *Molecular Psychiatry*, 12(3), 247–257.

Serretti, A., Lorenzi, C., Cusin, C., *et al.* (2003). SSRIs antidepressant activity is influenced by G beta 3 variants. *European Neuropsychopharmacology*, 13(2), 117–122.

Serretti, A., Zanardi, R., Rossini, D., *et al.* (2001a). Influence of tryptophan hydroxylase and serotonin transporter genes on fluvoxamine antidepressant activity. *Molecular Psychiatry*, 6(5), 586–592.

Serretti, A., Zanardi, R., Cusin, C., *et al.* (2001b). Tryptophan hydroxylase gene associated with paroxetine antidepressant activity. *European Neuropsychopharmacology*, 11(5), 375–380.

Serretti, A., Zanardi, R., Cusin, C., *et al.* (2001c). No association between dopamine D(2) and D(4) receptor gene variants and antidepressant activity of two selective serotonin reuptake inhibitors. *Psychiatry Research*, 104(3), 195–203.

Shelton, R.C., Manier, D.H. and Sanders-Bush, E. (2005). Signal transduction abnormalities in melancholic depression. *International Journal of Neuropsychopharmacology*, 8(1), 5–16.

Smeraldi, E., Zanardi, R., Benedetti, F., *et al.* (1998a). Polymorphism within the promoter of the serotonin transporter gene and antidepressant efficacy of fluvoxamine. *Molecular Psychiatry*, 3, 508–511.

Smits, K.M., Smits, L.J., Peeters, F.P., *et al.* (2008). The influence of 5-HTTLPR and STin2 polymorphisms in the serotonin transporter gene on treatment effect of selective serotonin reuptake inhibitors in depressive patients. *Psychiatric Genetics*, 18(4), 184–190.

Smits, K.M., Smits, L.J., Schouten, J.S., *et al.* (2004). Influence of SERTPR and STin2 in the serotonin transporter gene on the effect of selective serotonin reuptake inhibitors in depression: A systematic review. *Molecular Psychiatry*, 9(5), 433–441.

Spreux-Varoquaux, O., Gailledreau, J., Vanier, B., *et al.* (1996). Initial increase of plasma serotonin: A biological predictor for the antidepressant response to clomipramine? *Biological Psychiatry*, 40(6), 465–473.

Szegedi, A., Rujescu, D., Tadic, A., *et al.* (2005). The catechol-O-methyltransferase Val108/158Met polymorphism affects short-term treatment response to mirtazapine, but not to paroxetine in major depression. *Pharmacogenomics Journal*, 5(1), 49–53.

Szczepankiewicz, A., Rajewska-Rager, A., Dmitrzak-Weglarz, M., *et al.* (2007). Lack of association of 1287A/G NET and Val66Met BDNF polymorphisms with response to antidepressants. *European Neuropsychopharmacology*, 17(s4), S375.

Tadic, A., Muller, M.J., Rujescu, D., *et al.* (2007a). The MAOA T941G polymorphism and short-term treatment response to mirtazapine and paroxetine in major depression. *American Journal of Medical Genetics. Part B, Neuropsychiatric Genetics*, 144(3), 325–331.

Tadic, A., Rujescu, D., Muller, M.J., *et al.* (2007). A monoamine oxidase B gene variant and short-term antidepressant treatment response. *Progress in Neuropsychopharmacology and Biological Psychiatry*, 31(7), 1370–1377.

Tadić, A., Rujescu, D., Müller, M.J., *et al.* (2008). Association analysis between variants of the interleukin-1beta and the interleukin-1 receptor antagonist gene and antidepressant treatment response in major depression. *Neuropsychiatric Disease Treatment*, 4(1), 269–276.

Teranishi, K.S., Slager, S.L., Garriock, H., *et al.* (2007). Variants in PDE11A and PDE1A are not associated with Citalopram response. *Molecular Psychiatry*, 12(12), 1061–1063.

Tsai, S.J., Cheng, C.Y., Yu, Y.W., *et al.* (2003). Association study of a brain-derived neurotrophic-factor genetic polymorphism and major depressive disorders, symptomatology, and antidepressant response. *American Journal of Medical Genetics*, 123B(1), 19–22.

Tsai, S.J., Gau, Y.T., Hong, C.J., *et al.* (2009). Sexually dimorphic effect of catechol-O-methyltransferase val158met polymorphism on clinical response to fluoxetine in major depressive patients. *Journal of Affective Disorders*, 113(1–2), 183–187.

Tsai, S.J., Hong, C.J., Liou, Y.J., *et al.* (2008a). Plasminogen activator inhibitor-1 gene is associated with major depression and antidepressant treatment response. *Pharmacogenetics and Genomics*, 18(10), 869–875.

Tsai, S.J., Liou, Y.J., Hong, C.J., *et al.* (2008b). Glycogen synthase kinase-3beta gene is associated with antidepressant treatment response in Chinese major depressive disorder. *Pharmacogenomics Journal*, 8(6), 384–390.

Tsapakis, E.M., Checkley, S., Kerwin, R.W. and Aitchison, K.J. (2003). Association between the serotonin transporter linked polymorphic region gene (5HTTLPR) and response to tricyclic antidepressants (TCAs). *European Neuropsychopharmacology*, 13(4), S250.

Tzang, R.F., Hong, C.J., Liou, Y.J., *et al.* (2008). Association study of p11 gene with major depressive disorder, suicidal behaviors and treatment response. *Neuroscience Letters*, 447(1), 92–95.

Ulrich, G., Haug, H.J., Stieglitz, R.D. and Fahndrich, E. (1988). EEG characteristics of clinically defined on-drug-responders and non-responders — a comparison clomipramine vs. maprotiline. *Pharmacopsychiatry*, 21(6), 367–368.

Ulrich, G., Renfordt, E., Zeller, G. and Frick, K. (1984). Interrelation between changes in the EEG and psychopathology under pharmacotherapy for endogenous depression. A contribution to the predictor question. *Pharmacopsychiatry*, 17(6), 178–183.

Villafuerte, S.M., Vallabhaneni, K., Sliwerska, E., *et al.* (2009). SSRI response in depression may be influenced by SNPs in HTR1B and HTR1A. *Psychiatric Genetics*, 19(6), 281–291.

Wakeno, M., Kato, M., Okugawa, G., *et al.* (2008). The alpha 2A-adrenergic receptor gene polymorphism modifies antidepressant responses to milnacipran. *Journal of Clinical Psychopharmacology*, 28(5), 518–524.

Walsh, N.D., Williams, S.C., Brammer, M.J., *et al.* (2007). A longitudinal functional magnetic resonance imaging study of verbal working memory in depression after antidepressant therapy. *Biological Psychiatry*, 62(11), 1236–1243.

Wilkie, M.J., Smith, D., Reid, I.C., *et al.* (2007). A splice site polymorphism in the G-protein beta subunit influences antidepressant efficacy in depression. *Pharmacogenetics and Genomics*, 17(3), 207–215.

Wong, M.L., Dong, C., Maestre-Mesa, J. and Licinio, J. (2008). Polymorphisms in inflammation-related genes are associated with susceptibility to major depression and antidepressant response. *Molecular Psychiatry*, 13(8), 800–812.

Yoshida, K., Higuchi, H., Takahashi, H., *et al.* (2008). Influence of the tyrosine hydroxylase val81met polymorphism and catechol-O-methyltransferase val158met polymorphism on the antidepressant effect of milnacipran. *Human Psychopharmacology*, 23(2), 121–128.

Yoshida, K., Ito, K., Sato, K., *et al.* (2002a). Influence of the serotonin transporter gene-linked polymorphic region on the antidepressant response to fluvoxamine in Japanese depressed patients. *Progress in Neuropsychopharmacology and Biological Psychiatry*, 26(2), 383–386.

Yoshida, K., Naito, S., Takahashi, H., *et al.* (2002b). Monoamine oxidase: A gene polymorphism, tryptophan hydroxylase gene polymorphism and antidepressant response to fluvoxamine in Japanese patients with major depressive disorder. *Progress in Neuropsychopharmacology and Biological Psychiatry*, 26(7–8), 1279–1283.

Yoshida, K., Takahashi, H., Higuchi, H., *et al.* (2004). Prediction of antidepressant response to milnacipran by norepinephrine transporter gene polymorphisms. *American Journal of Psychiatry*, 161(9), 1575–1580.

Yoshimura, R., Hori, H., Ikenouchi-Sugita, A., *et al.* (2009). Higher plasma interleukin-6 (IL-6) level is associated with SSRI- or SNRI-refractory depression. *Progress in Neuropsychopharmacology and Biological Psychiatry*, 33(4), 722–726.

Yoshimura, R., Mitoma, M., Sugita, A., *et al.* (2007). Effects of paroxetine or milnacipran on serum brain-derived neurotrophic factor in depressed patients. *Progress in Neuropsychopharmacology and Biological Psychiatry*, 31(5), 1034–1037.

Yu, Y.W., Chen, T.J., Hong, C.J., *et al.* (2003a). Association study of the interleukin-1 beta (C-511T) genetic polymorphism with major depressive disorder, associated symptomatology, and antidepressant response. *Neuropsychopharmacology*, 28(6), 1182–1185.

Yu, Y.W., Chen, T.J., Wang, Y.C., *et al.* (2003b). Association analysis for neuronal nitric oxide synthase gene polymorphism with major depression and fluoxetine response. *Neuropsychobiology*, 47(3), 137–140.

Yu, Y.W., Tsai, S.J., Chen, T.J., *et al.* (2002). Association study of the serotonin transporter promoter polymorphism and symptomatology and antidepressant response in major depressive disorders. *Molecular Psychiatry*, 7(10), 1115–1119.

Yu, Y.W., Tsai, S.J., Hong, C.J., *et al.* (2005). Association study of a monoamine oxidase a gene promoter polymorphism with major depressive disorder and antidepressant response. *Neuropsychopharmacology*, 30(9), 1719–1723.

Yu, Y.W., Tsai, S.J., Liou, Y.J., *et al.* (2006). Association study of two serotonin 1A receptor gene polymorphisms and fluoxetine treatment response in Chinese major depressive disorders. *European Neuropsychopharmacology*, 16(7), 498–503.

Zanardi, R., Benedetti, F., Di Bella, D., *et al.* (2000). Efficacy of paroxetine in depression is influenced by a functional polymorphism within the promoter of the serotonin transporter gene. *Journal of Clinical Psychopharmacology*, 20(1), 105–107.

Zanardi, R., Serretti, A., Rossini, D., *et al.* (2001). Factors affecting fluvoxamine antidepressant activity: Influence of pindolol and 5-HTTLPR in delusional and nondelusional depression. *Biological Psychiatry*, 50(5), 323–330.

Appendix

Alpert, J.E. (2003). Drug–drug interactions in psychopharmacology. In T.A Stern, J.B. Herman, P. Slavin (Eds). *Massachusetts General Hospital Guide to Primary Care Psychiatry*, 2nd edition. New York: McGraw-Hill.

Coulomb, F., Ducret, F., Laneury, J.P., *et al.* (2000). Pharmacokinetics of single-dose reboxetine in volunteers with renal insufficiency. *Journal of Clinical Pharmacology*, 40(5), 482–487.

DeVane, C.L., Donovan, J.L., Liston, H.L., *et al.* (2004). Comparative CYP3A4 inhibitory effects of venlafaxine, fluoxetine, sertraline, and nefazodone in healthy volunteers. *Journal of Clinical Psychopharmacology*, 24(1), 4–10.

DeVane, C.L. and Nemeroff, C.B. (2002). 2002 guide to psychotropic drug interactions. *Primary Psychiatry*, 9, 28–57.

Dodd, S., Boulton, D.W., Burrows, G.D., *et al.* (2001). *In vitro* metabolism of mirtazapine enantiomers by human cytochrome P450 enzymes. *Human Psychopharmacology*, 16(7), 541–544.

Ereshefsky, L. (1996). Drug interactions of antidepressants. *Psychiatr Annals*, 26: 342–350, 1996.

Halas, C.J. (2006). Eszopiclone. *American Journal of Health-System Pharmacy*, 63(1), 41–48.

Greenblatt, D.J., Miller, L.G. and Shader, R.I. (1987). Clonazepam pharmacokinetics, brain uptake, and receptor interactions. *Journal of Clinical Psychiatry*, 48 Suppl, 4–11.

Greenblatt, D.J., von Moltke, L.L., Harmatz, J.S. and Shader, R.I. (1999). Human cytochromes and some newer antidepressants: Kinetics, metabolism, and drug interactions. *Journal of Clinical Psychopharmacology*, 19(5 Suppl 1), 23S–35S.

Kamada, T., Chow, T., Hiroi, T., *et al.* (2002). Metabolism of selegiline hydrochloride, a selective monoamine b-type inhibitor, in human liver microsomes. *Drug Metabolism and Pharmacokinetics*, 17(3), 199–206.

Lantz, R.J., Gillespie, T.A., Rash, T.J., *et al.* (2003). Metabolism, excretion, and pharmacokinetics of duloxetine in healthy human subjects. *Drug Metabolism and Disposition*, 31, 1142–1150.

Nemeroff, C.B., Preskorn, S.H. and Devane, C.L. (2007). Antidepressant drug–drug interactions: Clinical relevance and risk management. *CNS Spectrums*, 12(5 Suppl 7), 1–13.

Nilsen, O.G., Dale, O. and Husebo, B. (1993). Pharmacokinetics of trazodone during multiple dosing to psychiatric patients. *Pharmacology & Toxicology*, 72, 286–289.

Richelson, E. (1997). Pharmacokinetic drug interactions of new antidepressants: A review of the effects on the metabolism of other drugs. *Mayo Clinic Proceedings*, 72(9), 835–847.

Robertson, P. Jr. and Hellriegel, E.T. (2003). Clinical pharmacokinetic profile of modafinil. *Clinical Pharmacokinetics*, 42(2), 123–137.

Sauer, J.M., Ponsler, G.D., Mattiuz, E.L., *et al.* (2003). Disposition and metabolic fate of atomoxetine hydrochloride: The role of CYP2D6 in human disposition and metabolism. *Drug Metabolism Disposition*, 31(1), 98–107.

Schilling, A.D., Yung-Sciame, R. and Leung, L. (2005). Comparison of inhibitory effects of desvenlafaxine succinate, venlafaxine, duloxetine, paroxetine, sertraline, and bupropion in human cytochrome P450 activities. Presented at the Annual Meeting for the International Society for the Study of Xenobiotics. Maui, Hawaii.

Winans, E. (2003). Aripiprazole. *American Journal of Health Systems Pharmacy*, 60(23), 2437–2445.

Index

β-endorphin, 324, 325
β-histine, 282
1-desamo-8-D-arginine vasopressin (DDAVP), 346
17β estradiol, 328, 330
5-hydroxytryptophan (5HTP), 29
5-methoxypsoralen (5-MOP), 344

Acetyl-L-carnitine, 335
Acetylsalicylic acid, 214
Acupuncture, 236
Adinazolam, 201, 294
Agomelatine, 6, 77, 78, 243, 251, 257
Almotriptan, 80
Alprazolam, 163, 277, 278, 292–299, 301
Amantadine, 86, 208, 272, 275, 282, 286, 307–309
Amineptine, 88, 89, 251, 256, 262
Aminoglutethimide, 339
Amisulpride, 90, 189
Amitriptyline, 76, 91, 92, 96–99, 101, 119, 145, 150, 151, 158, 163, 258, 259, 281, 293, 295, 296, 303, 349, 355, 363, 365, 381
Amoxapine, 91, 92, 96
Anetholtrithione, 283
Aripiprazole, 189–192, 279
Ascorbic acid (Vitamin C), 363
Atomoxetine, 85, 187, 277, 374, 381, 382

B vitamin, 362
Baclofen, 298
Bentazepam, 163, 279
Benztropine, 283
Bethanechol, 272, 282
BMS-562086, 340
Bright light therapy, 235
Brofaromine, 134, 140, 202–204, 222
Bromocriptine, 86, 87, 194, 270
Buprenorphine, 325
Bupropion, 6, 18, 23, 24, 46–48, 58, 59, 100, 102, 105, 107, 119, 122–131, 152–154, 157, 176, 185–188, 196, 197, 201, 204, 223, 225, 226, 238, 242, 251, 256, 270, 272–274, 277, 279, 280, 282, 284, 286, 313, 386, 390–392
Buspirone, 74, 78, 79, 157, 184–186, 238, 241, 274, 275, 280, 286, 327

Cabergoline, 86, 87, 194
Captopril, 327
Carbamazepine, 167, 168, 188, 209, 211, 314, 315
Celecoxib, 168, 169
Chlordiazepoxide, 163, 292, 293, 299
Chromium, 214, 362
Cimicoxib, 169
Cisapride, 81, 280

Citalopram, 6, 10, 11, 18, 19, 24, 32, 35, 38–44, 46, 50, 51, 53, 55, 56, 59, 65, 67–70, 93, 95, 147, 156, 185, 186, 213, 224–226, 238, 252, 253, 255, 265, 266, 363, 364, 376–380, 392
Clomipramine, 79, 88, 91–95, 98–100, 102, 145, 152, 161, 163, 184, 279, 296, 304, 349
Clonazepam, 163, 277, 301
Clonidine, 82, 156
Cognitive behavior therapy (CBT)/cognitive therapy (CT), 236
Cognitive behavioral system of psychotherapy — CBASP, 243
Cortisol, 338
CP-101, 606, 209
CP-316, 311, 340
Cyanocobalamin, 353
Cyclazocine, 325
Cyproheptadine, 272

d-cycloserine, 209, 311
Deep brain stimulation (DBS), 235
Dehydroepiandrosterone (DHEA)/Dehydroepiandrosterone Sulfate (DHEAS), 333, 334
Depot-medroxiprogesterone acetate (D-MPA), 333
Desipramine, 41, 89, 92, 98, 99, 101, 124, 130, 145, 147, 149, 150, 152, 153, 161, 163, 175, 184, 196, 204, 216–219, 241, 242, 249, 278, 295, 296, 350, 352, 384
Desvenlafaxine, 6, 102, 110, 111, 242, 251, 257
Dexamethasone, 160
Dexfenfluramine, 76, 77
Dextroamphetamine, 89, 108, 141
DHA, 206, 357–360
Diazepam, 163, 292, 294–299, 301, 303
Diet, 58, 135, 138
Dixyrazine, 150
Donepezil, 172, 173, 282, 283, 322
Dothiepin, 97
Duloxetine, 6, 23, 24, 102, 104, 111–115, 188, 217, 227, 228, 242, 251, 257, 270, 284
Dynamic therapy, 237

EEP, 343
EFP, 343
Electroconvulsive therapy (ECT), 50, 229, 231, 241, 269
Eletriptan, 80
Entacapone, 143
EPA, 169, 170, 205, 206, 357–359
Escitalopram, 6, 18, 24, 32–35, 38–40, 43, 58, 59, 66, 69, 70, 103, 104, 108, 112–114, 123, 153, 154, 164, 165, 253, 254, 277, 279, 378, 382, 383, 390, 391
Estrogen, 62, 118, 159, 160, 199, 328–332, 337, 338
Estrone, 332
Eszopiclone, 163–165, 175, 277, 278, 301
Ethosuximide, 314
Exercise, 239, 240, 281, 282

Famotidine, 282
Felbamate, 311, 314
Fenfluramine, 76, 77, 195
Fengabine, 303, 304
Flesinoxan, 80
Flunitrazepam, 163
Fluoxetine, 5–7, 13, 16–18, 31, 32, 35–40, 42, 44, 45, 48–52, 55–71, 73, 74, 81, 84, 87, 88, 94, 95, 97, 100, 109, 111, 118, 138, 144, 145, 147, 148, 151–156, 159, 160, 163–166, 169, 175, 179–182, 184, 186, 189, 203, 204, 210, 216–219, 224, 225, 243, 252–255, 258, 259, 261, 268, 270, 277–279, 336, 359, 363–366, 378, 380, 383–387, 389, 392, 393
Fluphenazine, 150
Fluvoxamine, 6, 32, 42, 49, 51, 54, 56, 57, 67–70, 115, 159, 252, 258, 259, 280, 393
Folate, 165–167, 176, 212, 242, 348
Folic acid, 166

Folinic acid, 212
Frovatriptan, 80

Gabapentin, 210, 211, 304–306
Galantamine, 172, 173, 213, 283, 321, 322
Ganaxolone, 304
Gepirone, 78, 79, 251, 257
Ginger root, 66
Gingko bilboa, 279, 286
Ginseng, 368
Gonadotropin-releasing hormone (GnRH), 99
Gorei-san (TJ-17), 280
Granisetron, 80, 272, 275, 286
Group therapy, 237
Growth-hormone (GH), 57
GSK 372475, 142
Guanfacine, 82
GW856553, 356

Haloperidol, 316
Hydrocortisone, 338, 339
Hydroxyzine, 327
Hypericin, 364, 365, 367, 368
Hypericum perforatum, 363, 366–369

Igmesine, 326
Imipramine, 27, 28, 30, 76, 88, 91, 92, 94, 95, 97–101, 104, 136, 137, 145, 150–152, 154, 156, 158–161, 163, 166, 169, 196, 200, 220, 221, 230, 249, 258–260, 262, 264, 269, 278, 279, 292–295, 297, 345, 349–352, 363–365, 388, 394
Indalpene, 32
Inositol, 170, 171, 211, 212, 353, 355, 357
Insulin, 60, 61, 66, 346
Interpersonal therapy, 262
Iproniazid, 27, 28
Ipsapirone, 79, 80
Iron/ferrous sulfate, 362
Isocarboxazid, 6, 134, 141, 154

Kava kava, 368, 369
Ketamine, 208, 209, 307–309
Ketoconazole, 339, 340

L-754030, 316
L-acetylcarnitine, 360
L-phenylalanine, 30
L-propionyl-carnitine (LPC), 361
Lamotrigine, 167, 168, 210, 211, 241, 310, 311
Levetiracetam, 304–306
Levodopa, 30, 50
Lithium (Li), 108, 152, 161, 162, 174, 175, 184, 197, 200–202, 204, 205, 216–219, 222, 230, 241, 263–265, 268, 269, 356, 374, 382
Lorazepam, 304
Lormetazepam, 163, 164
Luteinizing-hormone releasing hormone (LHRH), 338
LY354740, 309
LY544344, 309, 310
Lysine vasopressin, 346

M100907, 157
Maca root, 274
Maprotiline, 92, 94, 98, 101, 163, 203, 216, 217, 222, 249, 262, 263, 363, 365
mCPP, 71, 74, 76
Mecamylamine, 213, 242, 322
Medifoxamine, 89
Meditation, 240
Melanocyte-stimulating hormone-release inhibiting factor (MIF), 345
Melatonin, 56, 57, 140, 160, 200, 279, 286, 343, 344
Memantine, 209, 307–309
Meperidine, 141, 325
Mestrolone, 333
Metdroxyyprogesterone, 159
Methylfolate, 212
Methylphenidate, 89, 122, 141, 156, 193, 194, 275, 277, 286
Methyltestosterone, 159
Metyrapone, 159, 160, 175, 200, 339, 340
Mexiletine, 314, 315

Midodrine, 283
Mifepristone, 340–342
Milnacipran, 6, 102, 115, 116, 146, 147, 188, 223, 251, 256, 374, 381, 395
Mirtazapine, 6, 46, 58, 59, 96, 107, 108, 116–121, 149–152, 156, 181–183, 187, 195, 205, 222, 223, 225, 226, 230, 241, 242, 251, 256, 258, 259, 266, 268, 272, 275, 280, 286, 374, 381–384
MK-869, 316
Moclobemide, 32, 72, 95, 97, 134–136, 138–140, 142, 194, 205, 258, 259, 297, 298, 381
Modafinil, 171, 172, 176, 206–208, 241, 242, 275–277, 286, 289, 369, 370
Mosapride, 81, 280

N-acetyl cysteine, 214
Naltrexone, 214, 281, 324
Naratriptan, 80
Nefazodone, 6, 22, 23, 46, 58, 59, 70–76, 97, 107, 119, 159, 187, 228, 238, 251, 256, 258, 259, 266, 272
Nicotine, 319–321
Nimodipine, 171, 175
Nizatadine, 282
Nomifensine, 132
Nortriptyline, 6, 21, 91, 92, 98–101, 163, 202, 203, 222, 223, 230, 231, 242, 249, 281, 295, 381–383, 394

Olanzapine, 35, 37, 155, 175, 176, 189, 275, 282, 286
Omega-3, 170, 205, 206, 289, 356, 358
Ondasetron, 280
ONO-2333Ms, 340
Opipramol, 326
Orlistat, 281
Oxcarbazepine, 314, 315

Papaverine, 214
Paroxetine, 6, 18, 31, 32, 35, 38, 40, 41, 44–46, 48, 49, 51–56, 58–63, 65–70, 77, 94, 95, 97, 100, 109, 111–113, 128, 130, 147, 151, 164, 167, 168, 180, 182, 209, 211, 216, 217, 220, 224, 226, 230, 252, 253, 258, 259, 262, 263, 277, 309, 316–318, 363, 365, 377–380, 382–384, 388, 395
Pemoline, 89
Pergolide, 86, 87, 194
Perphenazine, 150, 263
Phenelzine, 6, 32, 133, 134, 136, 137, 139–141, 145, 154, 195, 220–222, 247, 250, 259, 260, 262, 279
Phenobarbital, 295, 303
Phenytoin, 210, 241, 314–316
Pilocarpine, 282
Pindolol, 80, 145–148, 175, 179, 180, 241
Piperazine sulfate estrone, 332
Piribedil, 86, 87
Pivagabine, 370
Pramipexole, 87, 156, 193, 194, 272
Prazepam, 296
Pregabalin, 210, 272, 304, 305
Progesterone, 62, 159, 328, 332, 333, 340
Propionyl-L-carnitine, 335
Protriptyline, 6, 92, 98, 100
PRX-00023, 80
Psychotherapy, 22, 26, 45, 232, 236–239, 241, 243, 244, 263, 359
Pyridoxine (vitamin B6), 353

Quetiapine, 105, 155, 176, 189–192, 279

R121919, 340
Raloxifene, 199, 338
Ramelteon, 344
Reboxetine, 6, 82–85, 119, 154, 168, 169, 187, 228, 242, 251, 256, 283, 392
Remacemide, 311, 314
Reserpine, 27, 195
Retigabine, 304
Riluzole, 208, 310
Rimostil, 338
Risperidone, 155, 188–190, 265
Ritanserin, 76
Rizatriptan, 80
Rolipram, 354, 355
Ropinirole, 87, 193, 272

S-adenosylmethionine (SAMe), 165, 348, 351
SA4503, 327
Saredutant, 172, 318
Selegiline, 6, 133–135, 138–140, 142, 243, 247, 250
Selenium, 363, 382
Sertraline, 6, 18, 24, 31, 32, 35, 38–40, 42, 44, 46, 48, 49, 51, 52, 56, 58–63, 65, 67–70, 77, 90, 94, 95, 108, 109, 126, 128, 130, 151, 156–159, 181, 182, 187, 196, 197, 204, 215–217, 220, 225, 226, 238, 252–254, 258, 259, 267, 269, 363–365, 381, 382
Sibutramine, 142, 282
Sildenafil, 273, 274, 286
SR58611A, 86, 157
SSR149415, 346
Sumatriptan, 80
Synhexyl, 323

Tamoxifen, 44, 355, 356
Tandospirone, 79, 185
Tegaserod, 81
Testosterone, 57, 99, 140, 159, 198, 242, 333–337, 361
Tetrahydrobiopterin (BH4), 353
Tetrahydrocannabinol (THC), 323
Thioridazine, 149, 150, 194
Thyroid stimulating hormone (TSH), 56, 140
Thyrotropin-releasing hormone (TRH), 158, 198, 342
Thyroxine (T4), 56, 99, 140, 158, 197
Tianeptine, 28, 81, 82, 251, 256
Tibolone, 160
Tolcapone, 143
Topiramate, 210, 281, 282, 311–314
Tramadol, 214, 325
Transcranial magnetic stimulation (TMS), 233
Tranylcypromine, 6, 133, 134, 140, 141, 144, 145, 152, 183, 222
Trazodone, 6, 70–76, 106, 108, 146, 154, 179, 180, 186, 187, 195, 201, 228, 272, 279, 286, 297, 298, 353
Triazolam, 163, 278, 301
Triiodothyronine (T3), 56, 99, 140, 157, 158, 195, 230, 382
Trimipramine, 88, 91, 92, 98, 101, 154, 279
Tropisetron, 80
Tryptophan, 29, 30, 43, 70, 144, 145, 175, 373, 375
Tyrosine, 30, 373

Vagus nerve stimulation, 178, 231, 232, 241
Valerian root, 369
Valproate/Valproic Acid (VPA), 167, 168, 210, 279, 283, 311, 312
Venlafaxine, 6, 18, 23, 24, 46, 48, 49, 54, 55, 58, 59, 74, 77, 78, 83, 97, 102–111, 113, 117–120, 123, 124, 127, 130, 146, 150, 152, 159, 164, 172, 173, 183, 187, 193, 196, 197, 200, 201, 204, 214, 222–227, 231, 234, 238, 242, 251, 257–259, 261, 273, 280, 283, 284, 322, 325, 374, 381, 386, 389, 395
Verdenafil, 273
Viloxazine, 85
Viqualine, 304
Vitamin D, 363
VML-670, 275

Yoga, 240
Yohimbine, 82, 156, 175, 194, 272, 275, 283, 286

Zaleplon, 301
Zalospirone, 79
Zimeldine, 32, 267
Zinc, 169, 304
Ziprasidone, 189
Zolmitriptan, 80
Zolpidem, 164, 165, 175, 277, 278, 301
Zonisamide, 282